BLUEPRINTS
PEDIATRICS

Fifth Edition

BLUEPRINTS
PEDIATRICS

Fifth Edition

Bradley S. Marino, MD, MPP, MSCE
Associate Professor of Pediatrics
Department of Pediatrics
University of Cincinnati College of Medicine

Divisions of Cardiology and Critical Care Medicine
Cincinnati Children's Hospital Medical Center
Cincinnati, Ohio

Katie S. Fine, MD
Private Pediatrician
Charlotte, North Carolina

. Wolters Kluwer | Lippincott Williams & Wilkins
Health

Philadelphia • Baltimore • New York • London
Buenos Aires • Hong Kong • Sydney • Tokyo

Acquisitions Editor: Charley Mitchell
Sr. Managing Editor: Stacey Sebring
Editorial Assistant: Catherine Noonan
Marketing Manager: Jennifer Kuklinski
Production Editor: Kevin Johnson
Art Director: Doug Smock
Compositor: Maryland Composition

Fifth Edition
Copyright © 2009 by Lippincott Williams & Wilkins, a Wolters Kluwer business.

351 West Camden Street   530 Walnut Street
Baltimore, MD 21201   Philadelphia, PA 19106

Printed in China

9 8 7 6 5 4 3 2 1

Library of Congress Cataloging-in-Publication Data

Marino, Bradley S.
Blueprints pediatrics / Bradley S. Marino, Katie S. Fine. —5th ed.
    p. ; cm. — (Blueprints)
Includes bibliographical references and index.
ISBN 978-0-7817-8251-7
1. Pediatrics—Outlines, syllabi, etc. I. Fine, Katie S. (Katie Snead) II. Title. III. Title: Pediatrics. IV. Series.
[DNLM: 1. Pediatrics—Examination Questions. WS 18.2 M339b 2009]
RJ48.3.M37 2009
618.9200076—dc22

2008024249

DISCLAIMER

To purchase additional copies of this book, call our customer service department at **(800) 638-3030** or fax orders to **(301) 223-2320**. International customers should call **(301) 223-2300**.

Visit Lippincott Williams & Wilkins on the Internet: http://www.lww.com. Lippincott Williams & Wilkins customer service representatives are available from 8:30 am to 6:00 pm, EST.

Preface

Blueprints Pediatrics was first published almost 12 years ago as part of a series of books designed to help medical students prepare for USMLE Steps 2 and 3. This examination preparation remains the core mission of the series. To that end, the authors review the subject parameters posted by the testing board before each edition. Our goal is integration of the material into a complete yet concise review guide that is well organized, straightforward, and factually current. However, we have been pleased to hear from our readers that the book is utilized by many students during third year and fourth year medical school rotations. Residents in emergency medicine and family practice as well as nurse practitioners and physicians' assistants have found Blueprints helpful during the pediatric portion of their training. We believe this continued usefulness is because the book covers a broad range of basic yet important topics that must be mastered in order to treat children.

Each chapter in the book contains a single subject for review. Most can be read in under an hour. The topics contained in each chapter are grouped in an orderly fashion, with an end-of-chapter "Key Points" section that allows for review and highlights the concepts most frequently tested. This edition includes 100 questions and answers, as well as access to 50 more posted online. The questions are written in the "clinical vignette" style used on USMLE and Pediatric Board examinations. Thus readers not only can evaluate their grasp of the material but also begin to acclimate themselves to the expected testing environment.

The fifth edition of Blueprints Pediatrics is the strongest to date. It incorporates many of the suggestions we have received from medical students and faculty with regard to content and organization. For the first time, most of the chapters are co-authored by a pediatric expert in the respective content area. This has kept each chapter as up-to-date as possible and created new ways to get the often complex information across in the way most useful to students and practitioners learning pediatrics. In addition, the authors' dual backgrounds in academic medicine and private practice allow us to keep abreast of emerging research and its effect on the understanding of pathology and patient care. For the first time *Blueprints Pediatrics* has included a color section with cardiology figures of the most commonly tested lesions, as well as color photographs to illustrate the appearance of the most commonly tested dermatologic and infectious diseases. We hope you find *Blueprints Pediatrics* to be a beneficial investment, regardless of how you use it.

Bradley S. Marino, MD, MPP, MSCE, and Katie S. Fine, MD

Acknowledgments

This book is a tribute to our patients. Each day we are reminded how truly precious children are and what an honor it is to care for them. We are forever grateful to our colleagues (residents, fellows, and faculty) whose limitless understanding and support allow us to pursue projects such as this. We would specifically like to thank the faculty of Cincinnati Children's Hospital Medical Center, whose editorial comments in the following chapters made sure that the fifth edition of Blueprints Pediatrics represented the latest knowledge in pediatric medicine. In addition, we would like to thank Emily Claybon and Katelyn Mellion for their help in formatting tables and figures, and their overall willingness to always lend a hand. This book has greatly benefited from the remarkable enthusiasm, support, and dedication of Nancy Hoffman, our freelance managing editor.

We would like dedicate this edition of *Blueprints Pediatrics* to our families, without whose support, patience, and encouragement none of this would be possible.

B.M.
K.F.

Contents

Contributors

Shumyle Alam, MD
Assistant Professor of Surgery
Department of Surgery
University of Cincinnati College of Medicine

Division of Pediatric Urology
Cincinnati Children's Hospital Medical Center
Cincinnati, Ohio

Vinod V. Balasa, MD
Assistant Professor of Pediatrics
Department of Pediatrics
University of Cincinnati College of Medicine

Division of Hematology/Oncology
Cincinnati Children's Hospital Medical Center
Cincinnati, Ohio

David I. Bernstein, MD, MA
Professor of Pediatrics
Department of Pediatrics
University of Cincinnati College of Medicine

Director, Division of Infectious Diseases
Cincinnati Children's Hospital Medical Center
Cincinnati, Ohio

Rebecca C. Brady, MD
Assistant Professor of Pediatrics
Department of Pediatrics
University of Cincinnati College of Medicine

Division of Infectious Diseases
Cincinnati Children's Hospital Medical Center
Cincinnati, Ohio

Karen Burns, MD
Assistant Professor
Department of Pediatrics
University of Cincinnati College of Medicine

Division of Hematology/Oncology
Cincinnati Children's Hospital Medical Center
Cincinnati, Ohio

Emily Claybon, MA
Medical Student
Ohio State University College of Medicine
Columbus, Ohio

Mitchell B. Cohen, MD
Professor of Pediatrics
Department of Pediatrics
University of Cincinnati College of Medicine

Director, Division of Gastroenterology, Hepatology and Nutrition
Cincinnati Children's Hospital Medical Center
Cincinnati, Ohio

Robert A. Colbert, MD, PhD
Professor of Pediatrics
Department of Pediatrics
University of Cincinnati College of Medicine

Director, Division of Rheumatology
Cincinnati Children's Hospital Medical Center
Cincinnati, Ohio

Prasad Devarajan, MD
Louise M. Williams Endowed Chair,
Professor of Pediatrics
Department of Pediatrics
University of Cincinnati College of Medicine

Director, Division of Nephrology and Hypertension
Cincinnati Children's Hospital Medical Center
Cincinnati, Ohio

Deborah A. Elder, MD
Assistant Professor of Pediatrics
Department of Pediatrics
University of Cincinnati College of Medicine

Division of Endocrinology
Cincinnati Children's Hospital Medical Center
Cincinnati, Ohio

James M. Greenberg, MD
Professor of Pediatrics
Department of Pediatrics
University of Cincinnati College of Medicine

Director, Division of Neonatology
Cincinnati Children's Hospital Research Foundation
Cincinnati Children's Hospital Medical Center
Cincinnati, Ohio

Stuart Handwerger, MD
Professor of Pediatrics
Department of Pediatrics
University of Cincinnati College of Medicine

Director, Division of Endocrinology
Cincinnati Children's Hospital Medical Center
Cincinnati, Ohio

Claas H. Hinze, MD
Clinical Fellow
Division of Rheumatology
Cincinnati Children's Hospital Medical Center
Cincinnati, Ohio

Carolyn M. Kercsmar, MD
Professor of Pediatrics
Department of Pediatrics
University of Cincinnati College of Medicine

Director, Asthma Center
Division of Pulmonary Medicine
Cincinnati Children's Hospital Medical Center
Cincinnati, Ohio

Catherine Dent Krawczeski, MD
Associate Professor of Pediatrics
Department of Pediatrics
University of Cincinnati College of Medicine

Director, Cardiac Intensive Care
Division of Cardiology
Cincinnati Children's Hospital Medical Center
Cincinnati, Ohio

Angela Lorts MD
Assistant Professor of Pediatrics
Department of Pediatrics
University of Cincinnati College of Medicine

Division of Cardiology
Cincinnati Children's Hospital Medical Center
Cincinnati, Ohio

Anne W. Lucky, MD
Volunteer Professor
Departments of Dermatology and Pediatrics
University of Cincinnati College of Medicine

Acting Director, Division of Dermatology
Cincinnati Children's Hospital Medical Center
Cincinnati, Ohio

Katelyn Mellion, BCE
Research Assistant II
Department of Pediatrics
Division of Cardiology
Cincinnati Children's Hospital Medical Center
Cincinnati, Ohio

Rajaram Nagarajan, MD, MS
Assistant Professor of Pediatrics
Department of Pediatrics
University of Cincinnati College of Medicine

Division of Hematology/Oncology
Cincinnati Children's Hospital Medical Center
Cincinnati, Ohio

Marissa Perman, MD
Resident in Pediatrics
Department of Pediatrics
Cincinnati Children's Hospital Medical Center
Cincinnati, Ohio

Marc Rothenberg, MD, PhD
Professor of Pediatrics
Department of Pediatrics
University of Cincinnati College of Medicine

Director, Division of Allergy and Immunology
Cincinnati Children's Hospital Medical Center
Cincinnati, Ohio

Franklin O. Smith, MD
Marjory J. Johnson Endowed Chair,
Professor of Pediatrics
University of Cincinnati College of Medicine

Director, Division of Hematology/Oncology
Cincinnati Children's Hospital Medical Center
Cincinnati, Ohio

Mary Sutton, MD
Assistant Professor of Pediatrics
Department of Pediatrics
University of Cincinnati College of Medicine

Division of Neurology
Cincinnati Children's Hospital Medical Center
Cincinnati, Ohio

Eric Wall, MD
Associate Professor of Surgery
Department of Surgery
University of Cincinnati College of Medicine

Director, Division of Orthopedic Surgery
Cincinnati Children's Hospital Medical Center
Cincinnati, Ohio

Constance E. West, MD
Associate Professor of Pediatrics
Department of Pediatrics
University of Cincinnati College of Medicine

Director, Division of Pediatric Ophthalmology, and the Abrahamson
Pediatric Eye Institute
Cincinnati Children's Hospital Medical Center
Cincinnati, Ohio

Robert E. Wood, PhD, MD
Professor of Pediatrics and Surgery
Departments of Pediatrics and Surgery
University of Cincinnati College of Medicine

Director, Pediatric Bronchology
Divisions of Pulmonary Medicine and Otolaryngology
Cincinnati Children's Hospital Medical Center
Cincinnati, Ohio

Abbreviations

ABG	arterial blood gas
ACTH	adrenocorticotropic hormone
AIDS	acquired immunodeficiency syndrome
ALL	acute lymphocytic leukemia
ALT	alanine transaminase
AMP	adenosine monophosphate
ANA	antinuclear antibody
AP	anteroposterior
ARDS	adult respiratory distress syndrome
ASD	atrial septal defect
ASO	anti-streptolysin
AST	aspartate transaminase
AZT	zidovudine
BUN	blood urea nitrogen
CAVV	common atrioventricular valve
CBC	complete blood count
CDC	Centers for Disease Control and Prevention
CF	cystic fibrosis
CHF	congestive heart failure
CK	creatine kinase
CNS	central nervous system
CSF	cerebrospinal fluid
CT	computed tomography
DIC	disseminated intravascular coagulation
DMD	Duchenne-type muscular dystrophy
DTP	diphtheria/tetanus/pertussis
DTRs	deep tendon reflexes
DVT	deep venous thrombosis
EBV	Epstein-Barr virus
ECG	electrocardiography
ECMO	extracorporeal membrane oxygenation
EEG	electroencephalography
ELISA	enzyme-linked immunosorbent assay
EMG	electromyography
ESR	erythrocyte sedimentation rate
FEV	forced expiratory volume
FTA-ABS	fluorescent treponemal antibody absorption
FVC	forced vital capacity
G6PD	glucose-6-phosphate dehydrogenase
GI	gastrointestinal
Hgb	hemoglobin
Hib	Haemophilus influenzae type b
HIV	human immunodeficiency virus
HLA	human leukocyte antigen
IFA	immunofluorescent antibody
Ig	immunoglobulin
IM	intramuscular
INH	isoniazid
IV	intravenous
IVC	inferior vena cava
IVIG	intravenous immunoglobulin
JRA	juvenile rheumatoid arthritis
JVP	jugular venous pressure
KUB	kidneys/ureter/bladder
LDH	lactate dehydrogenase
LFTs	liver function tests
LP	lumbar puncture
L/S	lecithin-to-sphingomyelin (ratio)
LV	left ventricle
LVH	left ventricular hypertrophy
MMR	measles-mumps-rubella
MRI	magnetic resonance imaging
NG	nasogastric
NPO	nil per os (nothing by mouth)
NSAID	nonsteroidal anti-inflammatory drug
PCR	polymerase chain reaction
PDA	patent ductus arteriosus
PFTs	pulmonary function tests
PMI	point of maximal intensity
PPD	purified protein derivative
PT	prothrombin time
PTT	partial thromboplastin time
RBC	red blood cell
RF	rheumatoid factor
RPR	rapid plasma reagent (test)
RSV	respiratory syncytial virus

RV	right ventricle	UA	urinalysis
RVH	right ventricular hypertrophy	URI	upper respiratory infection
SIDS	sudden infant death syndrome	US	ultrasound
s/p	status post	VMA	vanillylmandelic acid
T3RU	triiodothyronine resin uptake	VSD	ventricular septal defect
T4	thyroxine	vWF	von Willebrand factor
TSH	thyroid-stimulating hormone	WBC	white blood cell

BLUEPRINTS
PEDIATRICS

Fifth Edition

Emergency Management: Evaluation of the Critically Ill or Injured Child

Bradley S. Marino • *Emily Claybon*

The critically ill or injured child must be evaluated rapidly to minimize morbidity and mortality. Whether presenting to the physician's office, local clinic, community hospital, or tertiary care center, the patient is stabilized by administering basic life-support and pediatric advanced life support measures recommended by the American Heart Association. Once the patient is clinically stable, a problem list can be generated and the cause of the child's symptoms can be determined.

DIFFERENTIAL DIAGNOSIS

Ninety percent of cases of pediatric cardiorespiratory arrest result from respiratory (45%), cardiac (25%), and primary central nervous system (20%) etiologies. Table 1-1 delineates the differential diagnoses of cardiopulmonary arrest in children.

CLINICAL MANIFESTATIONS AND TREATMENT

PRIMARY SURVEY

The **primary assessment** (Fig. 1-1) involves evaluation of Airway, Breathing, Circulation, Disability, and Exposure. The aim of the primary assessment is to identify life-threatening conditions and begin cardiopulmonary resuscitation, if necessary (Fig. 1-2).

The goals of **airway** management are to recognize and relieve obstruction, prevent aspiration of gastric contents, and promote adequate gas exchange. The airway is assessed and, if necessary, secured as follows:

- Immobilize the cervical spine if there is a possibility of spinal cord injury
- Open the airway via the jaw-thrust or chin-lift maneuver and relieve any obstruction caused by the tongue or soft tissues of the neck
- Clear the airway (suction the nose and mouth as indicated)
- Remove any visualized foreign body
- Place an oral or a nasopharyngeal airway, if indicated
- Provide 100% oxygen via nasal cannula, face mask, or nonrebreathing system
- Assist ventilation (e.g., bag mask ventilation), if indicated

Once an airway is established, air exchange (**breathing**) should be evaluated. Examination of chest wall movement will reveal the presence and effectiveness of spontaneous respirations. If spontaneous respiration is present with adequate oxygenation and ventilation, intubation is not indicated. If respiratory effort or chest

TABLE 1-1 The Differential Diagnosis of Cardiopulmonary Arrest in Children

Respiratory	
Upper airway obstruction (e.g., croup, epiglottitis, foreign body, laryngospasm, congenital anomalies, aspiration, bacterial tracheitis, neck trauma, thermal or chemical burns, retropharyngeal abscess, peritonsillar abscess)	Acute hydrocephalus
	Head or spinal cord trauma
	Seizure
	Tumor
	Hypoxic-ischemic injury
Lower airway obstruction (e.g., foreign body, pneumonia, reactive airway disease, bronchiolitis, congenital anomalies)	**Gastrointestinal**
	Abdominal trauma
	Bowel perforation or obstruction
Ventilation-perfusion mismatch (e.g., pneumonia, pulmonary edema, tension pneumothorax, hemothorax, chronic lung disease)	Peritonitis
	Hypovolemic dehydration
	Metabolic
Diffusion abnormality across the alveolus (e.g., ARDS)	Diabetic ketoacidosis
Massive pulmonary embolism	Addison disease
Respiratory muscle failure (e.g., botulism, Guillain-Barré syndrome)	Hyperthyroidism
	Hypoglycemia
Central hypoventilation (e.g., primary apnea, depression of the respiratory center of the brainstem)	Hyperkalemia
	Hypocalcemia
	Hyponatremia
Cardiac	**Multisystem**
Congenital heart disease (e.g., lesions with ductal-dependent systemic blood flow)	Sudden infant death syndrome
	Drug intoxication*
Arrhythmia	Trauma
Myocarditis	Anaphylaxis
Pericarditis	Hypothermia
Cardiac tamponade	Septic shock
Congestive heart failure	**Renal**
Myocardial trauma	Acute and chronic renal failure
Central Nervous System	
Meningitis	
Encephalitis	

*Narcotics, tricyclic antidepressants, barbiturates, benzodiazepines, calcium channel blocker, β-blocker.

wall excursion is not adequate, endotracheal tube placement is indicated. If the child is younger than 8 years, an uncuffed tube should be used to reduce the risk of subglottic edema and stenosis. **The size of the endotracheal tube chosen should equal 4 + (age in years ÷ 4).** Blood oxygenation (via pulse oximetry or arterial blood gas measurement) and blood CO_2 level (by arterial or venous blood gas measurement) should be assessed to help guide respiratory management.

Neonatal intubation is traditionally performed without premedication, but intubation of the infant or child is undertaken with premedication in the following **rapid-sequence** fashion:

1. Preoxygenate with 100% oxygen.
2. Administer a vagolytic drug (e.g., atropine).
3. Administer a sedative, hypnotic, and/or opioid drug (e.g., thiopental, versed, fentanyl).
4. Apply cricoid pressure.
5. Administer a paralyzing dose of a neuromuscular blocking agent (e.g., pancuronium or vecuronium, a nondepolarizing agent; or succinylcholine, a de-

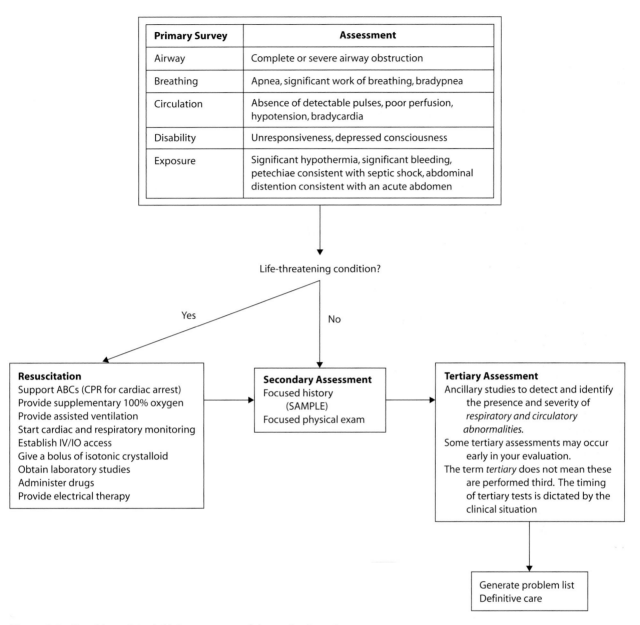

Primary Survey	Assessment
Airway	Complete or severe airway obstruction
Breathing	Apnea, significant work of breathing, bradypnea
Circulation	Absence of detectable pulses, poor perfusion, hypotension, bradycardia
Disability	Unresponsiveness, depressed consciousness
Exposure	Significant hypothermia, significant bleeding, petechiae consistent with septic shock, abdominal distention consistent with an acute abdomen

Life-threatening condition?

Yes   No

Resuscitation
Support ABCs (CPR for cardiac arrest)
Provide supplementary 100% oxygen
Provide assisted ventilation
Start cardiac and respiratory monitoring
Establish IV/IO access
Give a bolus of isotonic crystalloid
Obtain laboratory studies
Administer drugs
Provide electrical therapy

Secondary Assessment
Focused history
    (SAMPLE)
Focused physical exam

Tertiary Assessment
Ancillary studies to detect and identify the presence and severity of *respiratory and circulatory abnormalities.*
Some tertiary assessments may occur early in your evaluation.
The term *tertiary* does not mean these are performed third. The timing of tertiary tests is dictated by the clinical situation

Generate problem list
Definitive care

Figure 1-1 • Algorithm of the initial assessment of the pediatric patient.
(Modified from Nichols DG, Yaster M, Lappe DG, et al. *Golden Hour: The Handbook of Advanced Pediatric Life Support.* St. Louis: Mosby Yearbook, 1991:2,128.)

polarizing agent). If succinylcholine is used, a defasciculating dose of a neuromuscular blocking agent should be given before administration of succinylcholine (e.g., pancuronium or vecuronium).

In the hypotensive, hemodynamically unstable, or unconscious patient, premedication is not indicated. Cricoid pressure should be applied, and the patient should be intubated. Rarely, a patient cannot be intubated or ventilated with a bag and mask, and an emergency needle cricothyrotomy is required to establish an airway.

Circulation is assessed by evaluating pulses (central and peripheral), capillary refill, and blood pressure. A cardiorespiratory arrest is defined as an absence of a pulse in the large arteries of an unconscious patient who is not breathing. *In children, heart rate is the most sensitive measure of intravascular volume status.*

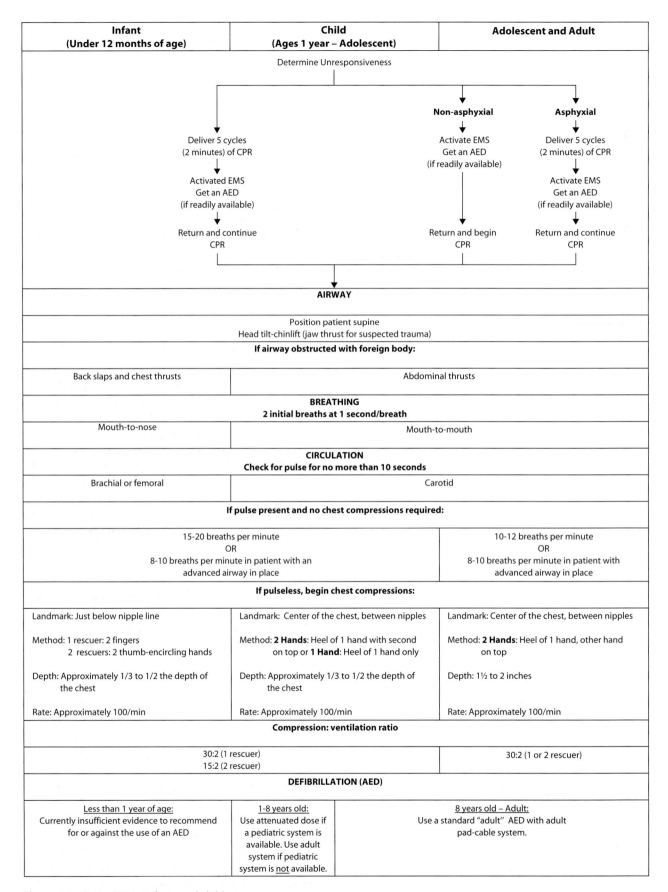

Infant (Under 12 months of age)	Child (Ages 1 year – Adolescent)	Adolescent and Adult
	Determine Unresponsiveness	

		Non-asphyxial	Asphyxial
Deliver 5 cycles (2 minutes) of CPR		Activate EMS Get an AED (if readily available)	Deliver 5 cycles (2 minutes) of CPR
Activated EMS Get an AED (if readily available)			Activate EMS Get an AED (if readily available)
Return and continue CPR		Return and begin CPR	Return and continue CPR

AIRWAY

Position patient supine
Head tilt-chinlift (jaw thrust for suspected trauma)

If airway obstructed with foreign body:

Back slaps and chest thrusts	Abdominal thrusts

BREATHING
2 initial breaths at 1 second/breath

Mouth-to-nose	Mouth-to-mouth

CIRCULATION
Check for pulse for no more than 10 seconds

Brachial or femoral	Carotid

If pulse present and no chest compressions required:

15-20 breaths per minute OR 8-10 breaths per minute in patient with an advanced airway in place	10-12 breaths per minute OR 8-10 breaths per minute in patient with advanced airway in place

If pulseless, begin chest compressions:

Landmark: Just below nipple line Method: 1 rescuer: 2 fingers 2 rescuers: 2 thumb-encircling hands Depth: Approximately 1/3 to 1/2 the depth of the chest Rate: Approximately 100/min	Landmark: Center of the chest, between nipples Method: **2 Hands**: Heel of 1 hand with second on top or **1 Hand**: Heel of 1 hand only Depth: Approximately 1/3 to 1/2 the depth of the chest Rate: Approximately 100/min	Landmark: Center of the chest, between nipples Method: **2 Hands**: Heel of 1 hand, other hand on top Depth: 1½ to 2 inches Rate: Approximately 100/min

Compression: ventilation ratio

30:2 (1 rescuer) 15:2 (2 rescuer)	30:2 (1 or 2 rescuer)

DEFIBRILLATION (AED)

Less than 1 year of age: Currently insufficient evidence to recommend for or against the use of an AED	1-8 years old: Use attenuated dose if a pediatric system is available. Use adult system if pediatric system is <u>not</u> available.	8 years old – Adult: Use a standard "adult" AED with adult pad-cable system.

Figure 1-2 • Basic CPR in infants and children.

Capillary refill is the most sensitive measure of adequate circulation. Blood pressure fluctuations are an insensitive indicator, because hypotension is a late finding in hypovolemia. Cardiorespiratory monitors are helpful to determine the electrical activity of the heart.

If pulselessness is noted on examination of the brachial pulse in the infant or the carotid pulse in the child/adolescent, chest compressions should be started. Vascular access management during cardiopulmonary resuscitation is outlined in Figure 1-3. Vascular access is critical for resuscitative drug administration and fluid resuscitation as indicated. If hypotension due to hemorrhage is suspected, gaining proximal control of the hemorrhage and volume resuscitation with type O-negative blood is vital.

Optimally, a full set of screening tests (including complete blood count, arterial and/or venous blood gas, electrolyte and chemistry panel, and blood glucose) is obtained at the time of vascular access. If ingestion is a possibility, serum and urine toxicology and acetaminophen and salicylate levels may be obtained.

In the patient with tachyarrhythmias (SVT, VT), therapeutic decisions are based on whether the patient is hemodynamically stable or unstable.

Supraventricular Tachycardia (SVT)
- Hemodynamically stable: Vagal maneuvers and adenosine (see Chapter 3).
- Hemodynamically unstable or SVT refractory to medications: Synchronized cardioversion 0.50 to

1.0 J/kg; if initial cardioversion is unsuccessful increase to 2.0 J/kg.

Ventricular Tachycardia (VT) or Ventricular Fibrillation (VF)

- amiodarone procainamide

- Hemodynamically stable VT: Amiodarone or procainamide, and treat hypomagnesemia and/or hypokalemia. Amiodarone and procainamide should not be used together because they both prolong the QT interval and both may cause hypotension. If medication therapy does not convert the VT, synchronized cardioversion 0.5 to 1.0 J/kg may be utilized; if initial cardioversion is unsuccessful increase to 2.0 J/kg (see Chapter 3).
- VF/pulseless VT: Nonsynchronized cardioversion 2.0 J/kg followed by 5 cycles of cardiopulmonary resuscitation (CPR) and new rhythm assessment. Sedate if possible prior to cardioversion, but do not delay cardioversion (see Chapter 3).

Patients with asystole or pulseless electrical activity require 5 cycles of CPR and administration of epinephrine, and an additional 5 cycles of CPR with a new rhythm and pulse check (see Chapter 3).

For a full discussion of drug physiology, indications, dosage, route of administration, effects, and side effects, see the American Academy of Pediatrics and American Heart Association *Pediatric advanced life support provider manual*. Table 1-2 describes the indications and effects of each drug.

For **disability**, a rapid screening neurologic examination is performed to note pupillary response, level of consciousness, and localizing findings. **Exposure** (hypo- or hyperthermia) must be detected and dealt with promptly. Because of children's large surface-to-body mass ratio, they cool rapidly, and passive heat loss can be problematic.

SECONDARY ASSESSMENT

After completion of the primary assessment and appropriate interventions to stabilize the child, the **secondary assessment** should be performed. The components of the secondary assessment are the focused history and focused physical examination. The **SAMPLE** mnemonic may be utilized to identify important aspects of the child's history and presenting complaint (**S**, signs and symptoms; **A**, allergies; **M**, medications; **P**, past medical history; **L**, last meal; **E**, events). The clinician should attempt to gain information that might help explain impaired respiratory, cardiovascular, or neurologic function. A thorough head-to-toe physical examination follows. The severity of the child's illness or injury

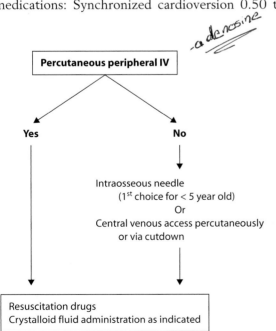

- adenosine

Figure 1-3 • Vascular access management during cardiopulmonary resuscitation.

TABLE 1-2 Drugs Used in Pediatric Cardiorespiratory Resuscitation

Drug	Indication	Action
Adenosine	Supraventricular tachycardia	Adenosine stimulates electrical adenosine receptors in the heart and causes temporary atrioventricular node conduction block and interrupts re-entry circuits that involve the AV node.
Atropine	bradycardia and AV block	Atropine is a parasympatholytic drug that increases heart rate, conduction through the AV node, and cardiac output by blocking vagal stimulation.
Sodium Bicarbonate	Severe refractory metabolic acidosis and/or hyperkalemia, sodium channel blocker overdose (e.g., tricyclic antidepressant)	Sodium bicarbonate increases blood pH.
Elemental calcium (calcium gluconate or calcium chloride)	Hypocalcemia, hyperkalemia, hypermagnesemia, and calcium channel blocker overdose	Calcium increases myocardial contractility, increases ventricular excitability, and increases conduction velocity through the myocardium.
Dextrose (glucose)	Hypoglycemia	Glucose administration increases blood glucose level.
Epinephrine	Asystole, bradycardia, pulseless VT/VF, shock	The α-adrenergic mediated vasoconstriction of epinephrine increases systemic vascular resistance, aortic diastolic pressure, and coronary perfusion. It also increase chronotropy, and inotropy through β_1-adrenergic receptor stimulation. The increased heart rate and stroke volume increase cardiac output. The increased cardiac output and systemic vascular resistance increase blood pressure.
Lidocaine	Pulseless VT/VF, VT with pulse	Lidocaine decreases ventricular automaticity and surresses ventricular arrhythmias. Not as effective as amiodarone to produce return of spontaneous circulation or survival to hospital admission after VF arrest.
Amiodarone	Atrial (refractory SVT) and ventricular arrhythmias (refractory VF, refractory pulseless VT, hemodynamically stable VT)	Amiodarone blocks Na, K, and Ca channels and β-receptors in the myocardium as well as α- and β-receptors in the vascular periphery. Amiodarone slows atrioventricular (AV) conduction, prolongs the AV refractory period and QT interval, and slows ventricular conduction (widens the QRS complex).
Procainamide	SVT, atrial flutter, VT (with pulses)	Procainamide prolongs the refractory period of the atria and ventricles and decreases conduction velocities in the atrium, bundle of His, and ventricle.

Drugs that can be given by endotracheal tube include lidocaine, atropine, naloxone hydrochloride, and epinephrine (high dose).
AV, atrioventricular; SVT, supraventricular tachycardia; VF, ventricular fibrillation; VT, ventricular tachycardia.

should determine the extent of the physical examination.

TERTIARY ASSESSMENT

The **tertiary assessment** consists of ancillary studies to detect and identify the presence and severity of *respiratory* and *circulatory abnormalities*. The term *tertiary* does not mean these are performed third. The timing of tertiary tests is dictated by the clinical situation. Ancillary studies that may assist with the assessment of cardiorespiratory abnormalities include: arterial blood gas, arterial lactate, venous blood gas, central venous oxygen saturation, hemoglobin concentration, oxyhemoglobin saturation via pulse oximetry, invasive arterial pressure monitoring, mixed venous pressure monitoring, exhaled CO_2 monitoring, chest x-ray, echocardiography, and peak expiratory flow rate.

SHOCK

Shock is a syndrome characterized by the inability of the circulatory system to provide adequate delivery of oxygen and nutrients to meet the metabolic demands of the body tissues and vital organs. Children, especially neonates, will initially try to compensate by becoming tachycardic. Hypotension, a late finding, leads to cellular hypoperfusion, metabolic acidosis, and cellular death. Three relationships explain hypotension in shock:

- **Stroke volume** is determined by preload (ventricular end diastolic volume), afterload (systemic vascular resistance), and myocardial contractility
- **Cardiac output** = stroke volume × heart rate
- **Blood pressure** = cardiac output × systemic vascular resistance

Shock may be compensated, uncompensated, or irreversible. In **compensated shock**, homeostatic mechanisms maintain essential organ perfusion. Blood pressure, urine output, and cardiac function all seem to be normal. In **uncompensated shock**, homeostatic mechanisms fail because of ischemia, endothelial injury, and the elaboration of toxic materials. Eventually, cellular function deteriorates and multiorgan system dysfunction results. When this process has caused irreparable functional loss in essential organs, a terminal or **irreversible** shock state is reached.

Shock can be categorized into hypovolemic, cardiogenic, distributive, and obstructive types (Table 1-3). **Hypovolemic shock** results from decreased intravascular volume, which results in decreased venous return and myocardial preload. Because of the reduction in myocardial preload, there is a resultant decrease in stroke volume, cardiac output, and blood pressure. This is the most common etiology of shock in children. **Cardiogenic shock** is the result of "pump failure." Inadequate stroke volume results in diminished cardiac output and hypotension. **Distributive shock** results from an abnormality in vasomotor tone that leads to maldistribution of a normal circulatory volume and a state of relative hypovolemia. Because of peripheral pooling, preload is reduced, causing a decrease in stroke volume, cardiac output, and blood pressure. Systemic vascular resistance is also decreased due to vasomotor dysfunction. Because both systemic vascular resistance and cardiac output are reduced, severe hypotension results. **Septic shock**, a cause of distributive shock, results when certain pathogens infect the blood. The early compensated stage of septic shock is characterized by decreased systemic vascular resistance (distributive shock), whereas in the late uncompensated phase, hypovolemia from third spacing and pump failure due to myocardial depression becomes more apparent. **Obstructive shock** is a condition of impaired cardiac output caused by physical obstruction of blood flow into or out of the heart. Cardiac tamponade and tension pnemothorax cause obstruction of blood flow into the heart, while pulmonary embolism and congenital heart disease lesions with ductal-dependent systemic blood flow produce obstruction of blood flow out of the heart. Lesions that obstruct blood flow into the heart decrease preload stroke volume and cardiac output. Lesions that obstruct blood flow out of the heart may cause

■ **TABLE 1-3** The Etiologies of Shock
Hypovolemic
Water and electrolyte losses (diarrhea, emesis)
Inadequate fluid intake
Osmotic diuresis (e.g., diabetic ketoacidosis)
Hemorrhage (internal and external)
Plasma losses ("third spacing" or capillary leak)
Burns
Cardiogenic
Congenital heart disease
Myocarditis
Ischemic heart disease
Cardiomyopathies (inherited or acquired abnormality of ventricular function)
Arrhythmia
Myocardial traumatic injury
Poisoning or drug toxicity (e.g., β-blocker, calcium channel blocker ingestion, chemotherapy)
Distributive
Anaphylaxis
Neurologic injury (head or spinal cord)
Septic shock
Obstructive
Cardiac tamponade
Tension pneumothorax
Massive pulmonary embolism
Congenital heart lesions with ductal-dependent systemic blood flow

myocardial pump failure, secondary cardiogenic shock, and decreased stroke volume and cardiac output.

CLINICAL MANIFESTATIONS

History and Physical Examination

The history should focus on potential causes. Hypovolemic shock is likely if there is a history of vomiting, diarrhea, polyuria, burns, trauma, surgery, gastrointestinal bleeding, intestinal obstruction, long periods in the sun, or pancreatitis. A history of congenital heart disease, arrhythmias, or chemotherapy (doxorubicin) administration may indicate cardiogenic shock. Distributive shock should be contemplated when there is a history of toxic ingestion, anaphylaxis, or head or spinal cord injury. In addition, any immunocompromised patient who presents with a history of fever and is ill-appearing may be in septic shock.

Serial vital signs are critical in the diagnosis and management of children with shock. In early "warm" compensated septic shock, vasodilation, warm extremities, tachycardia, a widened pulse pressure, and adequate urine output are seen. In contrast, symptoms of hypovolemic, cardiogenic, and late "cold" uncompensated septic shock include vasoconstriction, tachycardia, cold extremities, poor peripheral pulses, altered consciousness, pallor, sweating, ileus, and oliguria.

DIAGNOSTIC EVALUATION

During the stabilization period, the clinician must determine into which category of shock the patient's illness falls. Any patient with shock should be placed on a cardiac monitor. The level of tachycardia is the best determinant of the level of intravascular depletion or vasomotor abnormality. Hypotension is a late finding and occurs only after 40% of the intravascular volume has been depleted. Diagnostic tests are determined on the basis of the specific causes suspected.

TREATMENT

The treatment of shock is aimed at ensuring perfusion of critical vascular beds (coronary, cerebral, hepatic, renal) and preventing or correcting metabolic abnormalities arising from cellular hypoperfusion. Management of hypoxia reduces the level of metabolic acidosis. Correcting metabolic acidosis results in better cellular function, better myocardial performance, and decreased systemic and pulmonary vascular resistance.

Hypovolemic shock is treated with normal saline or lactated Ringer's solution (see Chapter 7 for details). If hemorrhage is the cause of the hypovolemia, type O-negative, cross-matched whole blood or packed red cells may be given. In cardiogenic shock resulting from a congenital heart defect, surgery, a catheter-based interventional procedure (e.g., balloon angioplasty or valvuloplasty, balloon atrial septostomy), or inotropic support may be indicated. Children with severe ischemic injury to the heart, dilated cardiomyopathy, or myocarditis may ultimately need a heart transplant. In distributive shock due to anaphylaxis, intravenous steroids, diphenhydramine, subcutaneous epinephrine, and albuterol nebulizers are employed. Sometimes intubation for laryngospasm and vasopressors for intractable hypotension are needed. Septic shock is treated with vasopressors, fluids, and broad-spectrum antibiotics. Antibiotics are considered a resuscitation medication for septic shock. Pneumothorax is treated by needle or chest tube removal of the air from the pleural space. Pericardial tamponade is treated by pericardiocentesis. Neonates with lesions with ductal-dependent systemic blood flow should be started on PGE_1 therapy as soon as possible to maintain ductal patency and systemic blood flow.

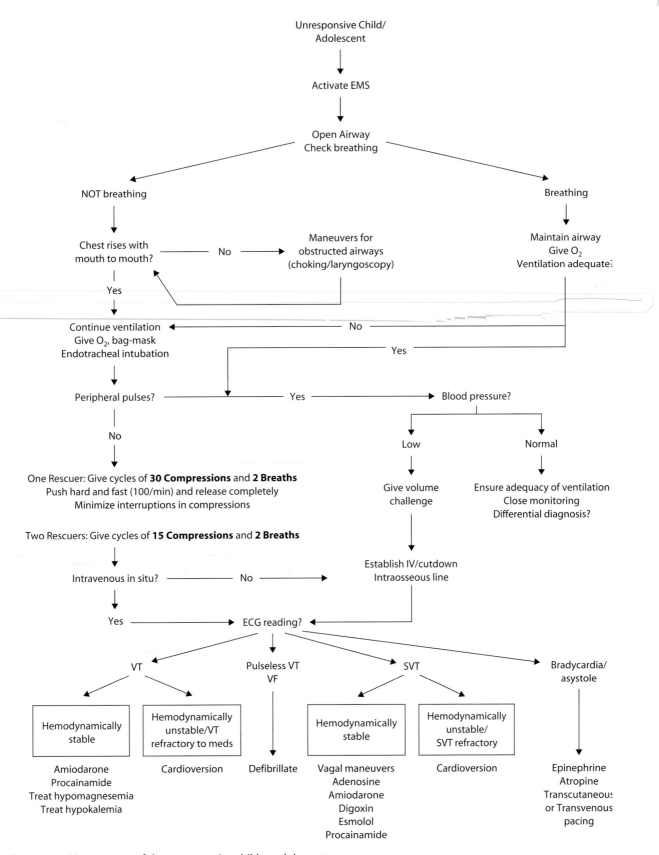

Figure 1-4 • Management of the unresponsive child or adolescent.

KEY POINTS

- No matter what the cause of cardiorespiratory arrest, the algorithms outlined for pediatric basic and advanced cardiac life support should be followed. A primary assessment (**A**irway, **B**reathing, **C**irculation, **D**isability, **E**xposure) should be performed, followed by resuscitative measures, if necessary.

- Approximately half of the causes of pediatric arrest are due to respiratory arrest, which can be brought about by upper airway obstruction, lower airway obstruction, restrictive lung disease, or any etiology that results in inadequate gas exchange.

- Management of the unresponsive child or adolescent is shown in Figure 1-4.

- If resuscitation does not establish cardiac output, the following mechanical or metabolic causes should be investigated: hypothermia, tension pneumothorax, hemothorax, cardiac tamponade, profound hypovolemia, profound metabolic imbalance, toxin ingestion, and closed head injury.

- Determine the category of shock and whether the patient has early or late manifestations.

- Hypovolemic shock accounts for most cases of shock.

- In hypovolemic shock, blood pressure depression is a late finding, and the level of tachycardia is the most sensitive measure of intravascular fluid status.

- In septic shock, antibiotics are a resuscitation medication and their administration should not be delayed.

Chapter 2

Poisoning, Burns, and Injury Prevention

Katie S. Fine

Nowhere does the old adage "an ounce of prevention is worth a pound of cure" resonate more true than in pediatrics. As a group, injuries are the most significant cause of morbidity and mortality in children and adolescents. When an untoward event occurs, timely evaluation and treatment may limit disability and preserve quality of life.

ACUTE POISONING

Poisoning is one of the more common pediatric medical emergencies, resulting in over a million emergency department visits per year. Children **younger than 5 years** of age account for over half of all cases of poisonous ingestion. These are more likely to involve only one substance and usually denote **accidental** ingestion, although abuse by caretakers must be considered. **Adolescents** account for a much smaller percentage; such ingestions are often **intentional**, represent a suicide attempt or gesture, and may involve multiple substances. Recreational drug use in this population may also lead to unintentional but fatal overdoses. Intentional ingestions are more likely to require medical intervention and result in death.

CLINICAL MANIFESTATIONS

History and Physical Examination

The history should include the substance and amount ingested, time elapsed since ingestion, early symptoms, subsequent behavior, and any attempts at treatment. The physical examination begins with the primary survey to evaluate the need for emergency cardiopulmonary support (Chapter 1). Other findings which aid in diagnosis include temperature and other vital signs; odors on the breath/skin/clothing; pupil size and reactivity; and skin color and feel. The characteristic clinical manifestations and treatment of the most common poisonings in children are listed in Table 2-1.

DIFFERENTIAL DIAGNOSIS

The possibility of toxicologic ingestion should be considered in any patient presenting with acute-onset illness involving multiple organ systems, including altered mental status, acute behavior changes, respiratory compromise, seizures, arrhythmias, and/or coma.

DIAGNOSTIC EVALUATION

Initial screening studies include assessment of oxygen saturation, a pulse oxygenation check, dextrose-stick, electrocardiogram, serum electrolytes and osmolarity, and a venous blood gas to determine pH, PCO_2, bicarbonate level, and base deficit/excess. Blood and urine toxicology screens are often helpful, but specific substances may not be detected on routine laboratory screens (e.g., iron, organophosphates).

TREATMENT

Parents should be instructed to immediately call 911 or their local poison control center. Although the data regarding relative benefits and risks of ipecac use in the home is still evolving, the American Academy of Pediatrics has recently reaffirmed its

■ TABLE 2-1 Signs, Symptoms, and Treatment of Specific Pediatric Poisonings

Substance[1]	Clinical Manifestations	Suggested Labs[2]	Antidote/Treatment
Acetaminophen	Nausea/vomiting, anorexia; may progress over days to jaundice, abdominal pain, liver failure	Serum acetaminophen level 4 to 24 hrs after ingestion[3]; (late) serum hepatic transaminases ($\uparrow$), prothrombin time ($\uparrow$)	A: Oral N-acetylcysteine (most effective within 8 to 10 hrs of ingestion) 140 mg/kg PO × 1, then 70 mg/kg PO q 4 hrs × 17 dosages T: Gastric emptying (w/in 1 hr) Activated charcoal (w/in 4 hrs)
Anticholinergic agents (atropine, scopolamine, first-generation antihistamines)	"Mad as a hatter, red as a beet, blind as a bat, hot as a hare, dry as a bone"; drowsiness, delirium, hallucinations, seizure; skin flushing; fixed dilated pupils; fever, cardiac dysrhythmias; dry mouth, speech and swallowing difficulties, nausea, vomiting	Drug screen	A: Physostigmine in select cases of severe anticholinergic signs and symptoms T: Gastric emptying (early), activated charcoal/cathartic; whole bowel irrigation for sustained-release preparations; cardiorespiratory support, seizure control; benzodiazepines/haloperidol for agitation
Carbon monoxide	Lethargy, irritability, confusion, dizziness, headache; nausea; irregular breathing, cyanosis; palpitations; progression to coma, death	Blood carboxyhemoglobin levels; blood gas (metabolic acidosis with normal PaO_2); urine dipstick (myoglobinuria); EKG	A: Oxygen T: Normobaric oxygen 100% until asymptomatic and carboxyhemoglobin level ≤5%; hyperbaric oxygen if available for severe poisoning
Ethanol[4] (wine/beer/liquor; also found in cold preparations and mouthwash)	Lethargy, CNS depression, nausea/vomiting, ataxia, respiratory depression, coma, hypotension, hypothermia (in young children)	Serum ethanol level, blood glucose ($\downarrow$), electrolytes ($\downarrow$ potassium), blood pH ($\downarrow$), $\uparrow$ osmolal gap	A: None T: Supportive care, glucose if needed, correction of electrolytes, parenteral fluids
Ethylene glycol (radiator fluid, de-icing solution)	Anorexia, vomiting, lethargy, respiratory/cardiovascular collapse	Serum ethylene glycol level; serum ammonia ($\uparrow$); arterial blood gas monitoring (metabolic acidosis); serum electrolytes ($\uparrow$ anion gap); $\uparrow$ osmolal gap; serum calcium ($\downarrow$); urinalysis (calcium oxalate crystals)	A: None T: Fomepizole (preferred) or ethanol to prevent metabolism; sodium bicarbonate to correct metabolic acidosis; hemodialysis; respiratory and cardiovascular support
Hydrocarbons (in fuels, household cleaners, polishes, and other solvents)	Tachypnea, coughing, respiratory distress, cyanosis, fever (aspiration); nausea/vomiting, gastrointestinal discomfort (oral ingestion); mental status changes	Arterial blood gas monitoring, chest x-ray (initial and 4 to 6 hrs after exposure)	A: None T: Avoid gastric emptying.[5] Prevent aspiration, which results in chemical pneumonitis and possibly proliferative alveolar thickening and chronic lung function abnormalities. Supportive respiratory care.
Ibuprofen	Nausea/vomiting, anorexia, stomach pain; gastrointestinal bleeding (obvious or occult) Massive ingestion: mental status changes/stupor/coma; seizures	Serum ibuprofen level 4 hrs after ingestion[6]; serum transaminase levels ($\uparrow$), alkaline phosphatase ($\uparrow$); metabolic acidosis with $\uparrow$ anion gap	A: None T: Gastric lavage (early); activated charcoal/cathartic; respiratory support/seizure control

◼ TABLE 2-1 Signs, Symptoms, and Treatment of Specific Pediatric Poisonings *(continued)*

Substance[1]	Clinical Manifestations	Suggested Labs[2]	Antidote/Treatment
Iron	Nausea/vomiting, diarrhea, gastrointestinal blood loss, acute liver failure, seizures, shock, coma	Serum iron level (3 to 5 hrs postingestion), serum pH ($\downarrow$), glucose ($\uparrow$), bilirubin and liver function tests ($\uparrow$), PT (prolonged), WBC ($\uparrow$); abdominal radiograph (radiopaque material)	A: Deferoxamine chelation T: Gastric lavage (early); whole bowel irrigation; dialysis (late, severe)
Methanol (in windshield washer fluid; toxic in very small amounts; toxicity related to formation of formic acid)	Nausea/vomiting, inebriation; $\uparrow$ minute ventilation to offset metabolic acidosis as methanol is metabolized; ocular findings 18 to 24 hrs after ingestion (blurred vision, optic disc hyperemia/edema)	Serum methanol level; arterial blood gases; severe metabolic acidosis; osmolal gap	A:None. T: Ethanol to block metabolism; sodium bicarbonate for metabolic acidosis; folate to hasten formic acid elimination; hemodialysis in severe cases
Organophosphates (insecticides)	SLUDGE (salivation, lacrimation, urination, defecation, gastric cramping, emesis); small but reactive pupils; sweating; muscle fasciculations; confusion; coma	Plasma or red blood cell cholinesterase activity ($\downarrow$)	A: Atropine sulfate followed by pralidoxime chloride T: Gastric lavage (early), activated charcoal (if ingested)
Opiates	Bradycardia, hypotension, decreased respiratory rate, pinpoint pupils, somnolence, coma	Toxicologic screen (urine and serum)	A: Naloxone[7] T: Gastrointestinal decontamination if appropriate; respiratory support
Salicylates (aspirin, antidiarrheal medications)	Hyperpnea/tachypnea (respiratory alkalosis/ metabolic acidosis), fever, nausea, vomiting, dehydration, tinnitus, agitation, seizures	Blood gas ($\uparrow$pH, $\downarrow$PCO$_2$, $\downarrow$bicarbonate), glucose ($\uparrow$), electrolytes ($\downarrow$potassium), PT and PTT (prolonged), serum salicylate level	A: None T: Gastric emptying/activated charcoal,[8] alkalinization of the serum to increase renal excretion and prevent entry into CNS; correct hypokalemia, which inhibits salicylate excretion; fluid/electrolyte management; hemodialysis in severe cases
Sympathomimetic agents (**decongestants**; also amphetamines, cocaine)	Tachycardia, hypertension, fever, large but reactive pupils, sweating, agitation, delirium/psychosis, seizures	Electrolytes ($\downarrow$potassium), blood glucose ($\uparrow$), EKG	A: None T: Gastric lavage/activated charcoal/cathartics; sedatives for severe agitation; cardiorespiratory support
Theophylline	Tachycardia, hypotension, tachypnea, vomiting, agitation, seizures	Serum theophylline level (every 2 to 4 hrs), blood glucose ($\uparrow$), potassium ($\downarrow$), pH ($\downarrow$), calcium ($\uparrow$), phosphate ($\downarrow$), EKG	A: None T: Activated charcoal/whole bowel decontamination; hemodialysis in severe ingestions

continues

■ **TABLE 2-1** Signs, Symptoms, and Treatment of Specific Pediatric Poisonings *(continued)*

Substance[1]	Clinical Manifestations	Suggested Labs[2]	Antidote/Treatment
Tricyclic antidepressants	Anticholinergic effects as above; tachycardia, hypertension progressing to hypotension, confusion, drowsiness, dry mucous membranes, dilated but responsive pupils, agitation, seizures, coma, dysrhythmias[9]	ECG (prolonged PR interval, widened QRS complex, prolongation of the QT interval, AV block, ventricular arrhythmias); these effects may be delayed	A: None[10] T: Gastric lavage/activated charcoal[11]; sodium bicarbonate (blood alkalinization) for conduction abnormalities; all patients with tricyclic antidepressant ingestions should be admitted and monitored in an intensive care unit

[1]Substances in bold represent the most common pediatric toxicologic emergencies.
[2]All patients with suspected ingestions should receive serum and urine toxicology screens, because ingestion of multiple substances is common, especially in intentional poisonings.
[3]An accepted nomogram exists for predicting the severity of the toxicity based on a blood acetaminophen measurement taken at least 4 hrs after ingestion.
[4]Physicians should have a high suspicion of co-ingestions in adolescents with ethanol intoxication. The clinical manifestations of co-ingestion of a central nervous system stimulant may be attenuated, whereas ingestion with a depressant may potentiate the effects of the alcohol.
[5]Some specific exceptions.
[6]An accepted nomogram exists for predicting the severity of the toxicity based on a blood ibuprofen measurement taken 4 hrs after ingestion.
[7]Naloxone administration may result in withdrawal symptoms (tachypnea, tachycardia, sweating, agitation, seizures) in chronic users.
[8]Aspirin ingestion causes delayed gastric emptying, so gastrointestinal decontamination plays a significant role.
[9]Although extremely rare, fatal dysrhythmias have occurred up to several days after ingestion.
[10]Despite the anticholinergic effects of tricyclic antidepressants, physostigmine is *contraindicated* in these ingestions.
[11]Tricyclic antidepressant ingestion causes delayed gastric emptying, so gastrointestinal decontamination plays a significant role.

recommendation that syrup of ipecac no longer routinely be kept in the home or given by parents following accidental ingestions.

Patients who present in unstable condition must be evaluated and treated according to the ABCDEs discussed in Chapter 1. With regard to ingestions, the "D" in the mnemonic may stand for: dextrose (as several commonly ingested agents precipitate hypoglycemia); empiric drug treatment (relating to possible antidotes or cardiac stabilizers, etc.); and appropriate decontamination. Treatment decisions should be based on the estimated maximal potential dose ingested.

Gastric lavage both removes and dilutes stomach contents. It is generally only effective if performed in the first hour after ingestion or when the compound ingested slows gastric emptying (aspirin, tricyclic antidepressants). Pill fragments recovered may aid in diagnosis. Gastric lavage is contraindicated in patients who are vomiting and those thought to have ingested corrosive/caustic substances, hydrocarbons, or agents known to cause neurologic depression (increasing the risk of an unprotected airway). **Activated charcoal** by mouth or nasogastric tube minimizes absorption by binding the substance and hastening its elimination; however, activated charcoal is ineffective in ingestions with alcohol, hydrocarbons, iron, and lithium. **Whole bowel irrigation** is an option for ingestions involving iron; the procedure is usually undertaken following activated charcoal administration as well. Hemodialysis is beneficial for selected ingestions to prevent life-threatening complications.

PREVENTION

The pediatric medical community has played a major role in decreasing the number and severity of poisonings, including lobbying for child-resistant medicine bottle and household cleaner caps and incorporating anticipatory guidance into health maintenance visits. Specific topics include "child-proofing" the home, keeping medicines in a lockbox, and securing cleaning products out of the child's reach.

LEAD POISONING

Lead poisoning is one of the most important preventable health problems in primary care pediatrics. The elimination of lead in house paint (in 1977) and gasoline (in 1988) has decreased the average blood lead level by 75%. The primary source of lead today is lead-containing paint present in buildings constructed before 1950. Children breathe in lead dust, ingest paint chips, and play in lead-contaminated soil. Other sources of exposure include ingredients used in some cultural customs and folk remedies (e.g., kohl, greta, pay-loo-ah) and industrial materials/emissions. Lead poisoning disproportionately effects lower socioeconomic populations.

Lead is not a naturally occurring substance in the body; any amount detected is abnormal. Although there is no direct correlation between blood levels and morbidity, levels of 10 to 19 μg/dL are considered "borderline" elevated, and the term "**lead poisoning**" is reserved for levels of **20 μg/dL** or greater. However, blood levels <10 μg/dL may also adversely affect neurodevelopment.

CLINICAL MANIFESTATIONS

The great majority of affected children are asymptomatic. Early symptoms of lead poisoning include irritability, hyperactivity, apathy, decreased play, anorexia, intermittent abdominal pain, and constipation. Children with chronically elevated lead levels may manifest developmental delay, behavioral problems, attention disorders, and poor school performance. **Acute encephalopathy**, characterized by increased intracranial pressure, vomiting, ataxia, confusion, and seizures, is the most serious complication of severe lead poisoning.

TREATMENT

The most effective therapy involves **removing the poison** from the child's environment. Lead paint should be stripped and surfaces cleaned with high-phosphate detergent and a special high-efficiency particle accu-mulator vacuum. These removal techniques invariably increase the amount of lead dust in the air, so the inhabitants must be temporarily housed elsewhere. Many treatment centers recommend optimizing the patient's iron and calcium intake through diet and/or a multivitamin, although specific benefits are unproven. All children with elevated blood lead levels should receive developmental screening.

All elevated screening (capillary) blood tests should be confirmed with a venous sample before treatment is initiated unless the child is acutely symptomatic. Management of elevated blood lead levels in the asymptomatic child is detailed in Table 2-2. The **symptomatic** child should be immediately removed from the home, placed in a lead-free environment, and provided chelation therapy. Children with levels between 45 and 69 mg/dL may be treated with inpatient intravenous **edetate calcium-disodium** (EDTA) or outpatient **oral succimer** (DMSA). Intramuscular **dimercaprol** (BAL) is added to EDTA for the inpatient (required) treatment of the child with levels over 70 mg/dL. **Chelation must be administered in a lead-free environment.** A rebound increase in blood lead levels occurs even in the absence of lead exposure, due to the release of lead from bone stores.

PREVENTION

Targeted screening is based on risk assessment information gathered during well-child visits. The Centers for Disease Control and Prevention recommends lead screening at 12 and 24 months for patients living in areas with many pre-1950 homes and unusually high percentages of elevated blood lead levels. Siblings of affected children should also be screened. New

■ **TABLE 2-2** Management of Elevated Blood Lead Levels in Asymptomatic Children	
Venous Lead Level	**Recommendations**
10 to 14 μg/dL	risk reduction and nutritional education
15 to 19 μg/dL	above, plus repeat test in 1 to 3 months; coordinate home inspection and other services with local lead poisoning prevention programs
	if still elevated at 3 months, consider abdominal radiograph and bowel decontamination
20 to 44 μg/dL	above, plus consider abdominal radiograph/decontamination at initial elevation
45 to 69 μg/dL	above, plus chelation therapy within 48 hours; consider obtaining free erythrocyte protoporphyrin or zinc protoporphyrin level to help assess response to treatment
≥70 μg/dL	above, with immediate in-patient chelation therapy

screening recommendations from the Centers for Disease Control are expected in early 2008.

TRAFFIC AND MOTOR VEHICLE ACCIDENTS

Motor vehicle injuries remain the leading cause of accidental death in pediatric patients. In adolescents, alcohol ingestion is a significant risk factor for vehicular injury and death.

The routine use of **seat belts** and **child car seats** has been shown to be highly effective in reducing the incidence of severe injury and death. All states require car seat restraint of passengers under 40 pounds. Children 20 pounds or heavier *and* 1 year of age or older may ride facing forward, whereas lighter/younger infants must face the rear. When a child passenger has reached the height/weight limit for his or her car seat (usually up to 40 lbs), a booster seat should be employed. The child should be restrained in a booster seat until the standard lap belt fits correctly (across the chest and thighs) and the child is tall enough for the legs to bend at the knees with the feet hanging down. This usually does not occur until the child is 8 to 12 years old or approximately 57 inches in height. Older children should remain belted with lap and shoulder straps at all times. Because front seat air bags are designed for the adult passenger, children should always ride belted in the back seat to avoid injury from air bag deployment. Despite being required in many states to obtain a learner's permit, **driver education programs do not decrease the rate of accidents involving teenage drivers**.

Head trauma is the accidental injury most associated with death in children. **Bike helmets** decrease the risk of significant closed head trauma due to traffic accidents involving bicycles. In many jurisdictions, laws mandate their use by children. Children younger than 10 years should be supervised while walking or playing near streets to avoid accidental injury.

DROWNING

Drowning is a frequent cause of morbidity and mortality in the pediatric population. Incidence peaks in the older infant/toddler age group and again in adolescence. Rates are twice as high in blacks and three times higher in boys. **Bathtubs** are the most common site of drowning in the first year of life. Large buckets and residential pools are particularly dangerous for

toddlers, whereas natural water sources account for most adolescent injuries.

Reliable predictors of outcome include water temperature, time of submersion, presence of aspiration (and pulmonary parenchymal injury), and effectiveness of early resuscitation efforts. Submersion for more than 5 minutes in warm water associated with significant aspiration and minimal response to initial cardiopulmonary resuscitation (CPR) virtually always results in major disability or death.

All patients with a history of near drowning should be evaluated with serial chest x-rays and blood gas measurements for 24 hours. Those with hypoxemia and mental status changes require aggressive respiratory and circulatory support.

Toddlers and young children must be supervised at all times while in the bathtub or around pools or other bodies of water. Residential and commercial swimming pools should be fenced in (with unscalable fences) and have locked gates. Isolation fencing (fencing limited to the immediate pool area) is more effective at preventing accidental drowning than perimeter property fencing. CPR training is available to parents through the American Heart Association and many area hospitals. Learning to swim is an important preventive measure but does not take the place of close supervision.

FOREIGN BODY ASPIRATION

The natural curiosity of children coupled with the toddler's tendency to put everything in the mouth make **foreign body aspiration** a frequent occurrence in the pediatric population. Aspiration is the accidental inspiration of foreign material into the respiratory tract. Most objects and foodstuffs are immediately expelled from the trachea by coughing. Unfortunately, foreign bodies that lodge in the upper or lower respiratory tract are more problematic.

EPIDEMIOLOGY

The highest incidence of foreign body aspiration is noted in children 6 to 30 months old. Aspiration into the lower airways is much more common than tracheal obstruction. While the angle of the right main stem bronchus in adults favors right-sided aspiration, no such propensity exists in children given the symmetric bronchial angles in this age group. Many children do not have fully erupted second molars until age 30 months; inappropriate food choices include nuts, popcorn, hot dogs, hard vegetables, meat with bones, and seeds. Food, coins, and small toys constitute the most commonly aspirated objects. Inadequate supervision and pediatric anatomy result in increased risk.

DIFFERENTIAL DIAGNOSIS

Patients who do not acutely obstruct their airways may present up to a week after the initial event with no witnessed episode of choking. Wheezing and respiratory distress may be mistaken for asthma; pneumonia is a consideration when breath sounds are decreased. Of note, findings on auscultation in cases of foreign body aspiration are localized to one side of the chest only. Chronic foreign body aspiration should be considered in patients with recurrent focal pneumonias and/or lung abscesses.

CLINICAL MANIFESTATIONS

Following an initial episode of choking and coughing, many children may be asymptomatic for a period of time. When symptoms occur, presentation varies depending on where the foreign body lodges in the respiratory tree (Table 2-3). If the obstruction is **complete**, the chest radiograph demonstrates significant one-sided atelectasis, and the heart is drawn toward the affected lung throughout the entire respiratory cycle. However, a **partial** obstruction allows air to enter during inspiration, where it becomes trapped (ball-valve obstruction). In these cases, the inspiratory film may appear normal, but the expiration radiograph will show a hyperinflated obstructed lung with mediastinal shift away from the blockage (Fig. 2-1). Decubitus films may be helpful in infants and young children. Radiographs should include the neck area as well.

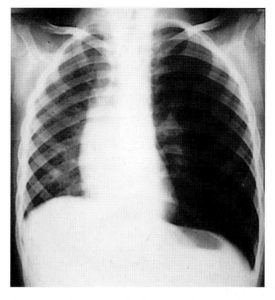

Figure 2-1 • Expiratory film in foreign body aspiration with partial obstruction; the obstructed left lung is hyperinflated, whereas the heart and mediastinum are shifted to the right.

TREATMENT

Airway intervention is contraindicated in the child in the field who is actively coughing, crying, or speaking. If the airway is compromised, the choking response protocol (abdominal thrusts) is the same for children as for adults, with the exception that the blind oropharyngeal sweep is omitted in children. For infants, back thumps and chest thrusts are alternated, with the infant's body angled slightly head-down.

Foreign bodies must be removed from the airway to alleviate symptoms. **Rigid bronchoscopy** is the treatment of choice. Thereafter, prognosis depends

TABLE 2-3 Signs and Symptoms of Foreign Body Aspiration	
Location of Obstruction	**Associated Signs and Symptoms**
Trachea	
Total obstruction	Acute asphyxia, severe retractions with poor chest wall movement
Extrathoracic, partial	Inspiratory and expiratory stridor, retractions
Intrathoracic, partial	Expiratory wheeze; there is frequently inspiratory stridor as well
Main stem bronchus	Cough and expiratory wheeze; there may be blood-tinged sputum
Lobar/segmental bronchus	Decreased breath sounds over affected lobe; wheezing, rhonchi

on the degree of lung damage, which is directly related to time interval to diagnosis. Most patients recover quickly with minimal sequelae.

PREVENTION

Infants are not developmentally prepared to protect their airways from small morsels of food, including hard candy, nuts, and popcorn. Small toys, coins, buttons, and balloons should be kept out of the toddler's reach. Federal legislation requires toys with small parts to be labeled as inappropriate for children younger than 3 years of age.

BURNS

Burns are the third leading cause of injury in children, behind motor vehicle accidents and drowning, and are the second most frequent cause of accidental death. An estimated 15% to 25% of burns are the result of **abuse**. Fortunately, the great majority of burns are not life-threatening. Patients who survive severe burns are often left with significant scarring and disability.

EPIDEMIOLOGY

The great majority of burns are **scald** injuries, resulting from contact with hot liquids. These may occur in association with spillage of hot food or drinks or be due to bathing injuries. Scald burns that end in straight lines without associated splash marks suggest abuse. **Contact** burns are the next most common and result from direct contact with a hot surface (iron, stove). Contact burns due to cigarettes are the most common burn injury in abused children. **Flame** burns are less frequent but result in a high mortality rate due to associated smoke inhalation injury. Typical scenarios for an **electrical** burn involve a young child putting conductive material into a wall socket or an infant sucking on the connected end of an extension cord. **Chemical burns** result from exposure to strong acidic or alkaline material.

RISK FACTORS

Boys and children younger than 4 years old, particularly those with disabilities, are at the greatest risk for burn injury.

CLINICAL MANIFESTATIONS

Clinical severity is based on affected body surface area and depth. Partial-thickness burns are divided into first-degree and second-degree burns. **First-degree** burns involve only the epidermis; the skin is red, dry, and tender but does not blister. First-degree burns usually heal within a week with no residual scarring. **Second-degree** burns may be superficial (less than half the depth of the dermis) or deep (involving most of the dermis but leaving appendages such as sweat glands and hair follicles intact). Superficial partial-thickness burns are often caused by scald injuries. They are painful and exhibit blisters and/or weeping but generally resolve in a few weeks with little scarring. Deep second-degree injuries may or may not be painful. They result in significant scarring and may require skin grafting. **Third degree burns** extend into the subcutaneous tissue and are nontender due to sensory nervous tissue loss.

Specific injury sites and patterns are characteristic of abuse (Fig. 2-2).

TREATMENT

Burned areas should be placed immediately in luke-warm water or covered with wet gauze or cloth. Minor burns (superficial burns involving 10% of the total body surface area or less) respond to gentle cleansing, **silver sulfadiazine** (an antimicrobial agent), and daily dressing changes until re-epithelialization occurs. Burns that are severe, circumferential, extensive (more than 10% to 15% of the body), or that involve the face, hands, perineum, or

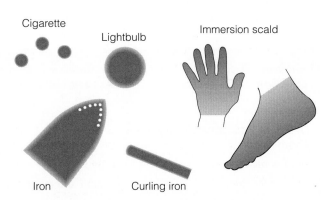

Cigarette
Lightbulb
Immersion scald
Iron
Curling iron

Figure 2-2 • Burn injury patterns consistent with abuse.

feet require more specialized care. Treatment includes appropriate management of airway, breathing, and circulation issues; effective electrolyte and fluid therapy to account for increased fluid loss; specialized nutritional support; prevention of infection; pain management; excision and skin grafting; optimization of cosmetic recovery; and early mobility and rehabilitation.

PREVENTION

Installing and maintaining **smoke detectors** and decreasing **water heater thermostat** settings are the two most successful preventive measures for avoiding burn injury. All sleepwear for children should be constructed of flame-retardant material. Smoking cessation decreases the likelihood that matches or lighters will be left where children can experiment with them. Parents should be counseled to practice escape routes and reinforce the "stop, drop, and roll" technique for extinguishing fire with their children.

CHILD ABUSE AND NEGLECT

Injuries intentionally perpetrated by a caretaker that result in morbidity or mortality constitute **physical abuse**. **Sexual abuse** is defined as the involvement of a child in any activity meant to provide sexual gratification to an adult. Failure to provide a child with appropriate food, clothing, medical care, schooling, and a safe environment constitutes **neglect**.

EPIDEMIOLOGY

Almost half the children who are brought for medical attention as a result of physical abuse are under 1 year of age; the great majority are preschool-aged. It is estimated that 10% of emergency room visits involving children younger than 5 years result from abuse. Parents, the mother's boyfriend, and stepparents are the most frequent perpetrators. Reports of abuse that increase in number and severity of injury over time are highly correlated with increased mortality.

Reports of sexual abuse have skyrocketed over the past few decades. The abuse may occur at any age. Relatives and family acquaintances account for most cases; molestation by strangers is uncommon. In 80% of reports, the victims are girls; most are abused by stepfathers, fathers, or other male family members. Male sexual abuse is probably under-recognized.

Neglect results in more deaths than physical and sexual abuse combined. It is the most common cause of failure to thrive in developed nations.

RISK FACTORS

Abuse and neglect occur at all socioeconomic levels but are more prevalent among the poor. Children with special needs (mental retardation, cerebral palsy, prematurity, chronic illness) and those younger than 3 years of age are at particular risk. Caretakers who have themselves suffered abuse, who are alcohol or substance abusers, or who are under extreme stress are more likely to abuse or neglect.

DIFFERENTIAL DIAGNOSIS

Most cases of suspected abuse are subsequently substantiated by child protective services. Care should be taken to differentiate bruises from Mongolian spots, which commonly occur in the buttocks area. Occasionally, osteogenesis imperfecta has been mistaken for abuse. Skin conditions such as bullous impetigo may mimic cigarette burns or other forms of abuse. Children with extensive bruising should undergo coagulation studies to rule out hematologic abnormalities (von Willebrand, etc.).

CLINICAL MANIFESTATIONS

History

An injury that is **inconsistent with the stated history**, or **a history that changes over time**, coupled with **delay in obtaining appropriate medical care** strongly suggests abuse. Age-inappropriate sexual behavior and knowledge are consistent with sexual abuse. Victims of physical or sexual abuse may act out by abusing others, attempting suicide, running away, or engaging in high-risk behaviors. Abuse places children at an increased risk for poor school performance, low self-esteem, and depression.

Physical Examination

Growth parameters are often stunted in abused children. As with burns, the location and pattern of injury may strongly suggest abuse (Fig. 2-3). Bruises,

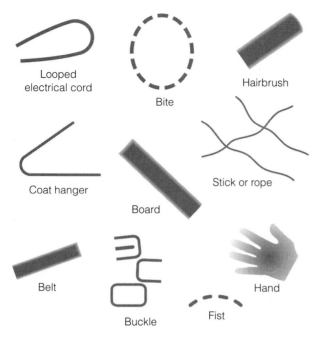

Figure 2-3 • Body marks consistent with abuse.

burns, or lacerations in different stages of healing occur in chronic or repeated abuse. Bruises associated with normal play are generally limited to the shins and elbows. Bruises on the chest, head, neck, or abdomen and bruises on a nonambulatory child are extremely suspicious. Vigorous shaking may lead to **shaken baby syndrome** (SBS), which results from acceleration/deceleration forces to the head. Virtually pathognomoic injuries include intracranial (subdural) hemorrhage, diffuse axonal injury, and widespread retinal hemorrhages, which may result in permanent vision loss. SBS has the highest mortality rate of any reported form of child abuse. Falls from beds, changing tables, cribs, counters, or toilet seats do not cause the injuries seen in SBS.

DIAGNOSTIC EVALUATION

A skeletal survey and bone scan reveal areas of past injury that may not be evident on physical examination. Fractures which are highly specific for abuse include bilateral fractures, bucket handle fractures, metaphyseal chip fractures, and fractures of the (especially posterior) ribs, scapula, sternum, or spinous processes. Fractures that occur before ambulation are usually inflicted. CT scans will reveal intracranial injuries, which in infants are highly suggestive of abuse; 95% of intracranial injuries and two-thirds of all head injuries in infants are due to abuse. When sexual abuse is suspected, rectal, oral, vaginal, and urethral specimens should be examined for *Neisseria gonorrhoeae*, *Chlamydia trachomatis*, and other sexually transmitted diseases. Other studies include blood tests for syphilis and human immunodeficiency virus.

TREATMENT/PREVENTION

Healthcare workers are **required by law** to report any suspicion of child abuse or neglect to state protection agencies. Victims should be immediately removed from their homes and placed in protective custody at a hospital or a state facility. Many family intervention programs that focus on social support, nursing staff visits, and parenting skills are being evaluated across the country in an attempt to provide children with safer home environments. Pediatricians can aid in preventing child abuse by providing parents with realistic expectations for their child's behavior at each health maintenance appointment. It is also important to recognize when the family and/or caregiver experiences an acute crisis or social isolation; referral for supportive services may make a significant difference in the home environment of the child.

SUDDEN INFANT DEATH SYNDROME

By definition, sudden infant death syndrome (**SIDS**) is the unexpected death of an infant less than 1 year of age for which the etiology remains unclear despite a thorough history and postmortem evaluation. The cause of SIDS remains unproven but is thought to be related to delayed maturation of brainstem respiratory or cardiovascular control and arousal mechanisms.

RISK FACTORS

Although multiple factors have been associated with an increased risk for SIDS, none has proven prognostic value (Table 2-4). Incidence peaks between 3 and 5 months of age. More cases are reported during the winter months.

■ TABLE 2-4 SIDS: Risk Factors
Prone sleeping position*
Child/Birth Factors
Male gender
Low birthweight/intrauterine growth restriction*
Prematurity*
Multiple gestation
African-American or American Indian race
Maternal Factors
Maternal smoking during pregnancy*
Young maternal age
Lower socioeconomic status
Higher parity
Single parenthood
Fewer years of maternal education
Environmental Factors
Soft bedding
Potentially obstructive materials in the bed
*Factors with highest risk.

■ TABLE 2-5 Differential Diagnosis of ALTEs
Idiopathic (apnea of infancy)
Infection
Respiratory
Respiratory syncytial virus
Pertussis
Systemic
Sepsis
Meningitis
Metabolic disease
Gastroesophageal reflux
Aspiration
Seizures
Cardiac arrhythmias
Abuse

DIFFERENTIAL DIAGNOSIS

Cases that initially appear to be SIDS may in fact result from infection, congenital heart disease, metabolic disorders, seizures, accidental trauma, or abuse.

Apparent life-threatening events (ALTEs) are characterized by choking, gagging, or apnea in combination with changes in color (cyanosis) and muscle tone. They understandably are extremely frightening to the caregiver. A differential diagnosis list is found in Table 2-5.

PREVENTION

Infants should be placed on their backs while sleeping. Contrary to popular belief, 24-hour home apnea monitoring does not decrease the risk of SIDS. Use of monitors should be reserved for infants with documented episodes of apnea, bradycardia, or desaturation.

 KEY POINTS

- Along with a careful history, information gathered from vital signs, physical examination, and early laboratory data may suggest the substance ingested by conforming to a specific toxidrome (Table 2-1).
- The great majority of children with lead poisoning are asymptomatic.
- After an initial episode of coughing and/or choking, the patient with foreign body aspiration may be asymptomatic for up to several days. Physical examination findings in a patient with foreign body aspiration are generally localized to one side of the chest.
- Child neglect is the most common cause of failure to thrive in developed countries.

- An injury that is inconsistent with the history, a history that changes over time, and a delay in seeking appropriate medical care all strongly suggest abuse.
- Shaken baby syndrome includes intracranial bleeding, diffuse axonal injury, and retinal hemorrhages. Intracranial injuries in absence of substantiated major trauma are virtually pathognomonic of abuse in infants.
- Babies should be put to sleep on their backs (supine).
- The use of a home apnea monitor does not decrease an infant's risk of SIDS.

Chapter 3

Cardiology

Angela Lorts • *Catherine D. Krawczeski* • *Bradley S. Marino*

The field of pediatric cardiology has experienced a remarkable evolution over the past half century due to advances in diagnostic techniques, interventional cardiac catheterization and cardiac surgical procedures, pediatric anesthesia, neonatal medicine, and intensive care. **Functional heart murmurs** are very common in childhood and do not signify disease. The incidence of structural heart disease is approximately 8 in 1,000 live births. Critical **congenital heart disease** (CHD), requiring surgery or an interventional cardiac catheterization procedure in the neonatal period, occurs in approximately 1 in 400 live births. Children may acquire **structural heart disease** later in life, or they may suffer from **functional heart disease** (i.e., myocarditis or cardiomyopathy) or **arrhythmias**.

HEART MURMURS

Heart murmurs are very common in children; they are heard on routine physical examinations in approximately a third of patients. **Functional ("innocent") heart murmurs** are the result of normal physiologic flow turbulence. Each of these murmurs has specific characteristics that usually allow it to be confidently diagnosed by physical examination alone (Table 3-1). It is equally important to recognize the signs and symptoms of potentially pathologic murmurs to facilitate rapid diagnosis and intervention, if necessary (Table 3-2).

CLINICAL MANIFESTATIONS

History

Infants with heart disease may have a history of difficulty feeding, tachypnea, irritability, diaphoresis, cyanosis, and/or failure to thrive. Significant symptoms in older patients include shortness of breath, dyspnea on exertion, exercise intolerance, palpitations, paroxysmal nocturnal dyspnea, orthopnea, and syncope. Chest pain is a frequent complaint in older children and adolescents; however, it is rarely cardiac in origin. Children who have syndromes often associated with heart disease (e.g., Turner, Down, William, Noonan, DiGeorge/velocardiofacial) are at a higher risk for a pathologic murmur. The family history should include questions regarding syncope, sudden death, heart attacks, or stroke before 50 years of age; connective tissue disorders (Marfan syndrome); hyperlipidemia; hypercholesterolemia; arrhythmia; valvular disease; cardiomyopathy; and CHD.

PHYSICAL EXAMINATION

The physical examination includes a comparison of the child's weight and height to normal values for age and gender and to previous measurements on a growth curve. Careful attention should be paid to vital signs, including heart rate (Table 3-3), respiratory rate, and blood pressure. The examiner should assess for cyanosis and digital clubbing (indicating a right-to-left shunt), as well as signs of congestive heart failure (extremity edema and hepatomegaly). Pulses should be palpated in both upper and lower extremities and compared. The examiner should inspect and palpate the chest for placement of the apical impulse and any heaves or thrills. Auscultation allows detection and characterization of heart sounds (normal and extra) and murmurs. Murmurs may be systolic, diastolic, or continuous and should be graded according to their intensity.

■ TABLE 3-1 Functional Heart Murmurs

Murmur	Typical Age at Presentation	Characteristics	Source
Peripheral pulmonary stenosis (PPS)	Neonate (birth to 2 mo)	Medium-pitched systolic ejection murmur best heard at the left upper sternal border, radiating through to the back	Turbulence of flow where the main pulmonary artery branches into left and right arteries
Vibratory (Still murmur)	2 to 8 yr	Grade II to III midsystolic musical or vibratory murmur heard best near the left lower sternal border and apex	Vibrations in ventricular or mitral structures caused by flow in the left ventricle
Venous hum	3 to 7 yr	Continuous, soft humming murmur heard at the neck or right upper chest that disappears in the supine position	Turbulent flow in the jugular venous/superior vena cava systems
Carotid bruit	3 to 8 yr	Systolic ejection murmur heard best at the neck	Turbulence of flow where the brachiocephalic vessels attach to the aorta
Pulmonary flow murmur	6 yr to adolescence	Systolic ejection murmur best heard at the left upper sternal border	Turbulence of flow where the main pulmonary artery connects to the right ventricle (across the pulmonary valve)

■ TABLE 3-2 Concerning Signs on Cardiac Examination

Heaves, thrills, or other abnormal or increased precordial activity
Brachiofemoral delay and/or decreased femoral pulses
Abnormal first or second heart sound (abnormal splitting)
Extra heart sounds
Gallop rhythms (S_3, S_4, or summation gallop)
Ejection click
Opening snap
Pericardial rub

Murmurs
  Very loud, harsh, or blowing
  Does not change in intensity relative to patient positioning

DIAGNOSTIC EVALUATION

Pulse oximetry assesses for decreased oxygen saturation in the blood. The chest radiograph evaluates heart size and pulmonary vascularity. The heart size should be less than 50% of the chest diameter in children over age 1 year. Pulmonary vascularity is usually increased in lesions with large left to right shunts, for example, ventricular septal defects, and may be diminished in

■ TABLE 3-3 Resting Heart Rates

Age	Low	High
<1 mo	80	160
1 to 3 mo	80	200
2 to 24 mo	70	120
2 to 10 yr	60	90
11 to 18 yr	40	90

lesions such as tetralogy of Fallot. All patients with suspected pathologic murmurs should receive an electrocardiogram (ECG) and echocardiogram (ECHO).

TREATMENT

The treatment of heart disease may be medical, surgical, interventional (cardiac catheterization), or a combination of these, depending on the specific abnormality.

EVALUATION OF THE CYANOTIC NEONATE

Cyanosis is a physical sign characterized by a bluish tinge of the mucous membranes, skin, and nail beds. Cyanosis results from hypoxemia (decreased arterial oxygen saturation). Cyanosis does not become clinically evident until the absolute concentration of deoxygenated hemoglobin is at least 3.5 g per dL. Factors that influence the degree of cyanosis include the total hemoglobin concentration (related to the hematocrit) and factors that affect the O_2 dissociation curve (pH, PCO_2, temperature, and ratio of adult to fetal hemoglobin). Cyanosis will be evident sooner (and more pronounced) under the following conditions: (a) high hemoglobin concentration (polycythemia), (b) decreased pH (acidosis), (c) increased PCO_2, (d) increased temperature, and (e) increased ratio of adult to fetal hemoglobin. Cyanosis should not be confused with acrocyanosis (blueness of the distal extremities only). Acrocyanosis is caused by peripheral vasoconstriction and is a normal finding during the first 24 to 48 hours of life.

DIFFERENTIAL DIAGNOSIS

Cyanosis in the newborn may be cardiac, pulmonary, neurologic, or hematologic in origin (Table 3-4). Cyanosis is one of the most common presentations of CHD in the newborn (Table 3-5). Pulmonary disorders may lead to cyanosis as a result of primary lung disease, airway obstruction, or extrinsic compression of the lung. Neurologic causes of cyanosis include central nervous system dysfunction and respiratory neuromuscular dysfunction.

CLINICAL MANIFESTATIONS

History and Physical Examination

A complete birth history that includes maternal history; prenatal, perinatal, and postnatal complications;

history of labor and delivery; and neonatal course should be obtained. Exactly when the child developed cyanosis is critical because certain congenital heart defects present at birth, whereas others may take as long as 1 month to become evident.

The initial physical examination should focus on the vital signs and the cardiac and respiratory examinations, assessing for evidence of right, left, or biventricular congestive heart failure and respiratory distress. Blue or dusky mucous membranes are consistent with cyanosis. Rales, stridor, grunting, flaring, retractions, and evidence of consolidation or effusion should be evaluated on pulmonary examination. On cardiovascular examination, the precordial impulse is palpated, and the clinician should evaluate for systolic or diastolic murmurs, the intensity of S1, S2 splitting abnormalities, and the presence of an S3 or S4 gallop, ejection click, opening snap, or rub. Examination of the extremities should focus on the strength and symmetry of the pulses in the upper and lower extremities, evidence of edema, and cynaosis of the nail beds. Hepatosplenomegaly may be consistent with right ventricular or biventricular heart failure.

DIAGNOSTIC EVALUATION

The goal of the initial evaluation of the cyanotic neonate is to determine whether the cyanosis is cardiac or noncardiac in origin. Preductal and postductal oxygen saturation and four extremity blood pressures should be documented. An ECG, chest radiograph, and hyperoxia test should be performed.

Preductal (right upper extremity) **and postductal** (lower extremity) **oxygen saturation measurements** permit evaluation for *differential* cyanosis and reverse *differential* cyanosis. **When the preductal saturation is higher than the postductal measurement, differential cyanosis exists.** Possible diagnoses associated with differential cyanosis include persistent pulmonary hypertension of the newborn (PPHN; see Chapter 13) and left ventricular outflow tract obstructive lesions such as interrupted aortic arch, critical coarctation of the aorta, and critical aortic stenosis. Deoxygenated blood from the pulmonary circulation enters the descending aorta through a patent ductus arteriosus (PDA), decreasing the postductal oxygen saturation. **When the preductal saturation is lower than the postductal saturation, reverse differential cyanosis exists.** Possible diagnoses associated with reverse differential cyanosis include transposition of the great arteries with either PPHN or coarctation of the aorta. Oxygenated

TABLE 3-4 Differential Diagnosis of Cyanosis in the Neonate

Cardiac	Pneumonia
Ductal-independent mixing lesions	Persistent pulmonary hypertension of the newborn
Truncus arteriosus	**Airway obstruction**
Total anomalous pulmonary venous return	Choanal atresia
D-transposition of the great arteries[a]	Vocal cord paralysis
Lesions with ductal-dependent PBF	Laryngotracheomalacia
Tetralogy of Fallot with pulmonary atresia[b]	**Extrinsic compression of the lungs**
Critical pulmonic stenosis	Pneumothorax
Tricuspid valve atresia[b] with normally related great arteries[b]	Chylothorax
	Hemothorax
Pulmonic valve atresia with intact ventricular septum	**Neurologic**
Lesions with ductal-dependent SBF	*CNS dysfunction*
Hypoplastic left heart syndrome	Drug-induced depression of respiratory drive
Interrupted aortic arch	Postasphyxial cerebral dysfunction
Critical coarctation of the aorta	Central apnea
Critical aortic stenosis	*Respiratory neuromuscular dysfunction*
Tricuspid valve atresia with transposition of the great arteries[b]	Spinal muscular atrophy
	Infant botulism
Pulmonary	Neonatal myasthenia gravis
Primary lung disease	**Hematologic**
Respiratory distress syndrome	Methemoglobinemia
Meconium aspiration	Polycythemia

[a]A patent ductus arteriosus may improve mixing, especially with an intact ventricular septum.
[b]Most forms.
PBF, pulmonary blood flow; SBF, systemic blood flow.

blood from the pulmonary circulation enters the descending aorta through a PDA, increasing the postductal oxygen saturation.

Four extremity blood pressure measurements that show a systolic blood pressure in the upper extremities greater than 10 mm Hg higher than that in the

TABLE 3-5 Most Common Congenital Heart Disease Leading to Cyanosis in the Newborn

Tetralogy of Fallot
Transposition of the great vessels
Tricuspid atresia
Pulmonary atresia with intact ventricular septum
Truncus arteriosus
Total anomalous pulmonary venous connection
Critical pulmonary stenosis

lower extremities are consistent with coarctation of the aorta, or other lesions with ductal-dependent systemic blood flow with a restrictive ductus arteriosus. The **chest radiograph** is obtained to determine the size of the heart and whether the pulmonary vascularity is increased or decreased. The **ECG** evaluates the heart rate, rhythm, axis, intervals, forces (atrial dilatation, ventricular hypertrophy), and repolarization (abnormal Q-wave pattern, ST/T waves, and corrected QT interval).

A **hyperoxia test** should be carried out in all neonates with a resting pulse oximetry reading less than 85%, visible cyanosis, or circulatory collapse. The hyperoxia test consists of obtaining a baseline right radial (preductal) arterial blood gas measurement with the child breathing room air ($FIO_2 = 0.21$), and then repeating the measurement with the child inspiring 100% oxygen ($FIO_2 = 1.00$). PaO_2 should be measured directly via arterial puncture.

Pulse oximetry measurements are not appropriate for interpretation of the hyperoxia test. A PaO_2 greater than 250 mm Hg on 100% oxygen essentially rules out cardiac disease. These patients are more likely to have a pulmonary cause for their cyanosis. A PaO_2 less than 50 mm Hg on 100% oxygen is very suggestive of a cardiac lesion.

The combined results of the tests just described will point the clinician in the right direction as to the source of the cyanosis and may also suggest a likely diagnosis. If a cardiac cause is deemed likely, an echocardiogram **(ECHO)** and cardiology consultation should be obtained.

TREATMENT

Cyanotic infants require immediate assessment of the ABCs (Chapter 1) and stabilization. **Prostaglandin E1** (PGE1) administration, via continuous intravenous infusion, should be started in any unstable infant with a strong suspicion of CHD. In newborns with mixing lesions or defects that have ductal-dependent pulmonary or systemic blood flow, PGE1 acts to maintain patency of the ductus arteriosus until definitive surgical treatment can be accomplished. Rarely, the patient with CHD may become progressively more unstable after the institution of PGE1 therapy, indicating a defect that has obstructed pulmonary venous flow, for example, total anomalous venous return with obstruction.

CYANOTIC CONGENITAL HEART DISEASE: DUCTAL-INDEPENDENT MIXING LESIONS

TRUNCUS ARTERIOSUS

Truncus arteriosus (Color Plate 1) is a rare form of cyanotic CHD that consists of a single arterial vessel arising from the base of the heart, which gives rise to the coronary, systemic, and pulmonary arteries. The number of valve leaflets varies from two to six, and the valve may be insufficient or stenotic. A ventricular septal defect (VSD) is always present. There is complete mixing of systemic and pulmonary venous blood in the truncal vessel. This lesion, along with other conotruncal anomalies (tetralogy of Fallot, interrupted aortic arch, VSD, isolated arch anomalies, and vascular rings), is associated with 22q11 microdeletion (i.e., **DiGeorge syndrome**).

Clinical Manifestations

The clinical picture varies depending on the amount of pulmonary blood flow. On physical examination a nonspecific murmur and minimal cyanosis may be present at birth. Congestive heart failure develops in a matter of weeks as the pulmonary vascular resistance falls and pulmonary blood flow increases at the expense of systemic blood flow. On cardiac examination, a systolic ejection murmur is heard at the left sternal border, there is usually a loud ejection click, and a single second heart sound (S2). Pulse pressure is widened and bounding arterial pulses are palpated. A chest radiograph reveals mild cardiomegaly, increased pulmonary vascularity, and occasionally a right aortic arch (30% of the time). Seventy percent of children with truncus arteriosus have biventricular hypertrophy on ECG. Hypocalcemia and absence of the thymic shadow (on chest radiograph) may occur if the patient has DiGeorge syndrome in addition to truncus arteriosus.

Treatment

At most centers, surgical repair is performed in the neonatal period. This involves closing the VSD, separation of the pulmonary arteries from the truncal vessel, and placing a conduit between the right ventricle and the pulmonary arteries.

D-TRANSPOSITION OF GREAT ARTERIES

D-transposition of great arteries (D-TGA) (Color Plate 2) accounts for 5% of congenital heart defects and is the most common form of cyanotic CHD presenting in the first 24 hours of life. There is a 3:1 male predominance. In this defect, the aorta arises anteriorly from the morphologic right ventricle, and the pulmonary artery arises posteriorly from the left ventricle. The pulmonary and systemic circuits thus are in parallel rather than in series; the systemic circuit (deoxygenated blood) is recirculated through the body, whereas the pulmonary circuit (oxygenated blood) recirculates through the lungs. An adequate sized patent foramen ovale (PFO) is required to allow mixing of the systemic and pulmonary circulations and is necessary for survival. The three basic variants are D-TGA with intact ventricular septum (60%), D-TGA with VSD (30%), and D-TGA with VSD and pulmonic stenosis (10%).

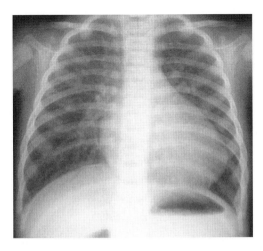

Figure 3-1 • Chest x-ray of transposition of the great arteries. (Image courtesy of Dr. Bradley Marino.)

Clinical Manifestations

Cyanosis is present from birth; the degree varies according to how much mixing across the patent foramen ovale is taking place. The infant may also be tachypneic. On cardiac examination, a loud, single S2 is appreciated. A systolic murmur indicates the presence of a VSD and/or pulmonic stenosis. The chest radiograph usually reveals mild cardiomegaly and increased pulmonary vascular markings. An "egg-shaped silhouette" is characteristic and results from the anterior aorta being superimposed on the posterior pulmonary artery, thereby narrowing the mediastinum (Fig. 3-1). The ECG generally reveals right axis deviation and right ventricular hypertrophy.

Treatment

PGE1 administration is often necessary to keep the ductus arteriosus open and increase aorta (deoxygenated) to pulmonary artery (oxygenated) shunting. A balloon atrial septostomy (Rashkind procedure) may need to be performed to increase atrial level mixing. The arterial switch procedure, which restores the left ventricle as the systemic ventricle, is generally performed during the first week of life.

TOTAL ANOMALOUS PULMONARY VENOUS CONNECTION

Total anomalous pulmonary venous connection (TAPVC) (Color Plate 3) is a rare lesion (1% to 2% of CHDs) in which the pulmonary veins are not connected to the left atrium. The pulmonary veins come to a confluence behind the left atrium, which then drains anomalously into the right atrium either directly or indirectly through other systemic venous pathways.

There are four variants:

- **Supracardiac** (50% of cases): Blood drains via a vertical vein into the innominate vein or directly into the superior vena cava.
- **Cardiac** (20% of cases): Blood drains into the coronary sinus or directly into the right atrium.
- **Infradiaphragmatic** (20% of cases): Blood drains via a vertical vein into the portal or hepatic veins.
- **Mixed** (10% of cases): Blood returns to the heart via a combination of the routes just described.

TAPVC can occur *with* or *without obstruction*. Pulmonary venous flow is obstructed when the anomalous vein enters a vessel at an acute angle or courses between or through other mediastinal structures. The presence or absence of obstruction determines whether there is pulmonary venous hypertension and severe cyanosis (obstruction) or increased pulmonary blood flow and mild cyanosis (no obstruction). Because there is no pulmonary venous return to the left side of the heart, shunting of blood from right to left (through an ASD or PFO) is necessary for blood flow to the systemic vascular bed.

Clinical Manifestations

The clinical presentation varies greatly depending on mode of venous return and whether it is obstructed. The infant without obstruction may present with mild cyanosis at birth and progressive congestive heart failure. There is an active precordium with a right ventricular heave, a wide and fixed split S2 with a loud pulmonary component, and a systolic ejection murmur at the left upper sternal border. On chest radiograph, cardiomegaly is noted with increased pulmonary vascularity. There is often a characteristic contour of the heart called a "snowman" which is seen when the pulmonary veins drain via a vertical vein into the innominate vein and ultimately the right superior vena cava. On ECG, right-axis deviation and right ventricular hypertrophy are seen.

Infants with pulmonary venous obstruction display marked cyanosis and respiratory distress. A loud, single (or narrowly split) S2 is heard on cardiac examination, and tachypnea with respiratory distress may be present. The chest radiograph generally shows normal heart size with markedly increased pulmonary vascular markings and diffuse pulmonary edema. Right ventricular hypertrophy is seen on ECG.

Treatment

Corrective surgery is performed emergently in the newborn period if pulmonary venous obstruction is present. If the anomalous pulmonary veins are unobstructed (typically cardiac subtype), repair is elective and takes place prior to the child exhibiting symptoms of congestive heart failure during infancy.

CYANOTIC CONGENITAL HEART DISEASE: LESIONS WITH DUCTAL-DEPENDENT PULMONARY BLOOD FLOW

TRICUSPID ATRESIA

Tricuspid atresia (Color Plate 4) is a rare defect (<1% of CHD) that is characterized by complete atresia of the tricuspid valve. This lesion leads to severe hypoplasia or absence of the right ventricle. Tricuspid atresia can be divided into two types: tricuspid atresia with normally related great arteries (NRGA) or tricuspid atresia with transposition of the great arteries (TGA). Ninety percent of cases of tricuspid atresia have an associated VSD. The systemic venous return is shunted from the right atrium to the left atrium through the PFO or an ASD, and the left atrium and left ventricle handle both systemic and pulmonary venous return. Oxygenated and deoxygenated blood is mixed in the left atrium. The VSD allows blood to pass from the left ventricle to the right ventricular outflow chamber and pulmonary arteries. The vast majority of patients with tricuspid atresia with NRGA also have pulmonary stenosis. Depending on the degree of pulmonary stenosis, cyanosis may be severe in the neonatal period.

In 30% of cases, transposition of the great vessels is also present, which results in blood passing from the left ventricle through the VSD to the right ventricular outflow and the ascending aorta. Tricuspid atresia with TGA is often associated with coarctation of the aorta and/or aortic arch hypoplasia. Unlike tricuspid atresia with NRGA, which often has ductal-dependent pulmonary blood flow, tricuspid atresia with TGA is a cyanotic lesion with ductal-dependent systemic blood flow.

Clinical Manifestations

The clinical features of tricuspid atresia are dependent of the degree of pulmonary stenosis present. Most commonly, neonates will have significant pulmonary stenosis or even pulmonary atresia. These infants present with progressive cyanosis, poor feeding, and tachypnea during the first 2 weeks of life. If pulmonary atresia is present, severe cyanosis is noted when the ductus arteriosus becomes restrictive or closes. Less commonly, infants may have minimal or no pulmonary stenosis. These infants may have normal to increased pulmonary blood flow and may have no symptoms or symptoms of congestive heart failure. On cardiac examination, abnormalities include the holosystolic murmur of a ventricular septal defect at the left lower sternal border and (possibly) the continuous murmur of a PDA. On ECG, there is left axis deviation, right atrial enlargement, and left ventricular hypertrophy. Findings on chest radiograph include normal heart size and decreased pulmonary vascular markings.

Neonates with tricuspid atresia and TGA also present with cyanosis, poor feeding, and tachypnea. If severe arch hypoplasia or coarctation of the aorta is present, the patient may present with shock after closure of the ductus arteriosus. Clinical severity depends on the degree of arch obstruction. The chest radiograph may reveal cardiomegaly and increased pulmonary vascular markings as the pulmonary vascular resistance falls and the child's pulmonary blood flow increases, resulting in congestive heart failure.

Treatment

Treatment of tricuspid atresia is variable depending on the amount of pulmonary blood flow and the presence or absence of an aortic arch abnormality. A child with tricuspid atresia with NRGA and restriction to pulmonary blood flow should have PGE1 started to maintain ductal patency. Surgical management for tricuspid atresia with decreased pulmonary blood flow may involve placing a modified Blalock-Taussig shunt to maintain pulmonary blood flow. The modified Blalock-Taussig shunt is a Gore-Tex tube placed between the subclavian artery and the pulmonary artery. If the pulmonary blood flow is adequate, surgery will not be required during the neonatal period. Rarely, infants with increased pulmonary blood flow may require banding of the pulmonary artery to restrict flow. Regardless of the neonatal course, all infants with tricuspid atresia will undergo further surgeries to separate the pulmonary and systemic circulations. In infancy, a cavopulmonary anastomosis (anastamosis of the superior vena cava to the pulmonary artery, called a hemi-Fontan or bidirectional Glenn) is performed to provide stable pulmonary blood flow. A final surgery is performed at 2 to 4 years of age. This procedure, the Fontan procedure, redirects the inferior vena cava and hepatic vein flow into the pulmonary circulation.

A child with tricuspid atresia with TGA should have PGE1 started to maintain ductal patency and systemic blood flow. Surgical management for tricuspid atresia with TGA depends on the degree of arch obstruction. Patients with hemodynamically significant arch obstruction will require a more extensive surgery with reconstruction of the aortic arch and placement of a reliable source of pulmonary blood flow.

TETRALOGY OF FALLOT

Tetralogy of Fallot (TOF) (Color Plate 5) is the most common CHD (10%) presenting in childhood. Fifteen percent of all patients with TOF have 22q11 microdeletion; 50% of patients with 22q11 microdeletion have TOF. The four defects include an anterior malalignment VSD, which results in valvar and subvalvar pulmonary valve stenosis, right ventricular hypertrophy, and an "overriding" large ascending aorta (Fig. 3-2). Infants with TOF are cyanotic because of right-to-left shunting across the VSD. The degree of right ventricular outflow obstruction determines the timing and severity of the cyanosis. In neonates, blood shunted from the aorta to the pulmonary artery through the PDA provides additional pulmonary blood flow. Infants with severe obstruction and ductus-dependent blood flow present within hours of birth. Cyanosis may not develop in children with mild obstruction until later in the infant period. Associated lesions include other VSDs, right aortic arch, left anterior descending (LAD) coronary artery from the right coronary artery coursing across the right ventricular outflow tract, and aortopulmonary collateral arteries.

Clinical Manifestations

Infants present with cyanosis and tachypnea of varying severity. They may have characteristic periodic episodes of cyanosis, rapid and deep breathing, and agitation known as "**tet spells**," caused by an increase in right ventricular outflow tract resistance, which leads to increased right-to-left shunting across the VSD. Such spells may last minutes to hours and may resolve spontaneously or lead to progressive hypoxia, metabolic acidosis, and death.

On cardiac examination, a right ventricular heave may be palpable, and a loud systolic ejection murmur is heard in the left upper sternal border. The heart size is generally normal on chest radiograph, with decreased pulmonary vascular markings. The right ventricular hypertrophy will lead to upturning of the apex on chest x-ray ("boot shaped" heart). Twenty-five percent of children with TOF have a right-sided aortic arch. The ECG reveals right axis deviation and right ventricular hypertrophy.

Treatment

The treatment of "tet spells" is aimed at diminishing right-to-left shunting by increasing systemic vascular resistance, decreasing pulmonary vascular resistance, and/or increasing preload. The older child who has "tet spells" may squat to increase their

A. Right ventricular hypertrophy   **B.** VSD   **D.** Right ventricular outflow obstruction   **C.** Overriding aorta

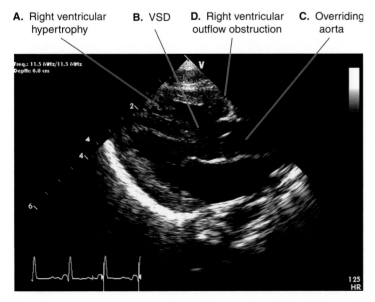

Figure 3-2 • Echocardiogram of tetralogy of Fallot. Characteristic features include: (**A**) right ventricular hypertrophy; (**B**) ventricular septal defect; (**C**) overriding aorta; (**D**) right ventricular outflow tract obstruction (not visualized in this image).
(Image courtesy of Dr. Bradley Marino.)

venous return and improve their systemic perfusion. In the infant, initial measures include calming the patient and vagal maneuvers (holding the child in a knee-chest position), and the administration of supplemental oxygen and morphine sulfate to diminish the agitation and hyperpnea and minimize oxygen consumption. If these measures are not successful, volume expansion and vasoconstrictors may be given to increase systemic blood pressure and systemic vascular resistance. In addition, β-blockers may be given to decrease infundibular spasm, and sodium bicarbonate may be given to reduce acidosis and decrease pulmonary vascular resistance. In most institutions, surgical repair is performed during the first 3 to 6 months of life or after the first hypercyanotic episode ("tet spell"). Neonates with TOF with critical pulmonary valve stenosis are generally repaired at presentation. In some cases of TOF with multiple VSDs, left anterior descending coronary artery from the right coronary artery coursing across the right ventricular outflow tract, or pulmonary atresia, a modified Blalock-Taussig shunt may be placed during the neonatal period prior to definitive repair later.

EBSTEIN ANOMALY

Ebstein anomaly (Color Plate 6) is an extremely rare anomaly in which the septal leaflet of the tricuspid valve is displaced inferiorly into the right ventricular cavity and the anterior leaflet of the tricuspid valve is sail-like and redundant. This results in a portion of the right ventricle being incorporated into the right atrium. Functional hypoplasia of the right ventricle results, as well as tricuspid regurgitation. In severe cases of Ebstein anomaly, the majority of the pulmonary blood flow comes from the PDA and not the right ventricle. A PFO is present in 80% of neonates with the anomaly, and there is a right-to-left shunt at the atrial level. The right atrium is massively dilated, which may result in supraventricular tachycardia (SVT). Wolff-Parkinson-White (WPW) syndrome is associated with Ebstein anomaly. Ebstein anomaly is associated with maternal lithium use.

Clinical Manifestations

Neonates with severe disease present with cyanosis and congestive heart failure in the first few days of life. The cardiac examination reveals a widely fixed split S_2 and a gallop rhythm. A tricuspid regurgitant

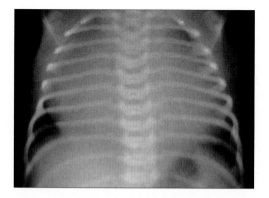

Figure 3-3 • Chest x-ray of Ebstein anomaly. (Image courtesy of Dr. Bradley Marino.)

blowing holosystolic murmur is heard at the left lower sternal border. Chest radiograph shows extreme cardiomegaly with notable right atrial enlargement and decreased pulmonary vascular markings (Fig. 3-3). Characteristic ECG findings include right bundle branch block with right atrial enlargement. WPW syndrome is indicated by a delta wave and a short PR interval.

Children with milder forms of the disease may present later in childhood with fatigue, exercise intolerance, palpitations, and/or mild cyanosis with clubbing.

Treatment

Severely cyanotic newborns require PGE1 infusion to maintain pulmonary blood flow through the PDA.

In general, all attempts are made to avoid surgical intervention. Surgery on the abnormal tricuspid valve has yielded poor results. Patients with the most severe forms of Ebstein anomaly may require heart transplantation.

CYANOTIC CONGENITAL HEART DISEASE: LESIONS WITH DUCTAL-DEPENDENT SYSTEMIC BLOOD FLOW

HYPOPLASTIC LEFT HEART SYNDROME

Hypoplastic left heart syndrome (HLHS) (Color Plate 7) is the second most common congenital cardiac lesion presenting in the first week of life and the most common cause of death from CHD in the 1st month of life. In this syndrome, there is hypoplasia of the left ventricle, aortic valve stenosis or atresia, mitral valve stenosis or atresia, and hypoplasia of the ascending aorta. These lesions reduce or eliminate blood flow through the left side of the heart. Oxygenated blood from the pulmonary veins is shunted left to right through an atrial defect. Right ventricular cardiac output goes to both the pulmonary arteries and through the ductus arteriosus to the descending aorta. Systemic blood flow is completely ductal-dependent, and coronary perfusion is retrograde when aortic atresia or critical aortic stenosis is present.

Clinical Manifestations

As the ductus arteriosus closes, neonates with HLHS will have severely diminished systemic blood flow and rapidly present in shock. They manifest signs of poor systemic perfusion with poor pulses, tachycardia, and tachypnea. A right ventricular heave may be present. A single S_2 will be present and possibly a continuous murmur consistent with flow through the PDA. The chest radiograph reveals pulmonary edema and progressive cardiac enlargement. The ECG is consistent with right ventricular hypertrophy, and there is poor R wave progression across the precordial leads.

Treatment

PGE1 should be started to maintain ductal-dependent systemic blood flow. Only a palliative procedure is available; there is no corrective surgery for this lesion. The stage I (or Norwood) palliation, which is performed in the first week of life, allows the majority of neonates to survive infancy. The stage I procedure involves amalgamation of the pulmonary artery and aorta to provide unobstructed systemic blood flow, atrial septectomy, and modified Blalock-Taussig shunt or right ventricular to pulmonary artery conduit to provide a stable source of pulmonary blood flow. After the stage I procedure, a cavopulmonary anastomosis (bidirectional Glenn procedure or Hemi-Fontan) is performed at 3 to 6 months of age, and a modified Fontan completion procedure is generally performed between 2 to 5 years of age. Some centers do not perform the stage I palliation and proceed directly to heart transplantation.

INTERRUPTED AORTIC ARCH

Interrupted aortic arch is essentially an extreme form of coarctation of the aorta (Fig. 3-4). There are three types of interrupted aortic arch: Type A is interruption beyond the left subclavian artery, type B is interrup-

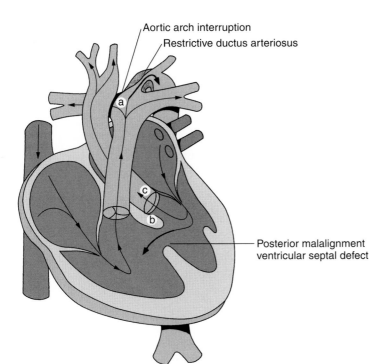

Aortic arch interruption
Restrictive ductus arteriosus

Posterior malalignment ventricular septal defect

Figure 3-4 • Interrupted aortic arch with restrictive PDA. Typical anatomic findings include: **(A)** atresia of a segment of the aortic arch between the left subclavian artery and the left common carotid (the most common type of interrupted aortic arch–"type B"); **(B)** posterior malalignment of the infundibular septum resulting in a large VSD and a narrow subaortic area; **(C)** a bicuspid aortic valve, which occurs in 60% of patients.

tion between the left subclavian and left common carotid arteries, and type C is interruption between the left common carotid and the brachiocephalic artery. Systemic blood flow depends on patency of the ductus arteriosus, which shunts blood from the pulmonary artery to the aorta. Interrupted aortic arch is often associated with a 22q11 microdeletion.

Clinical Manifestations

Neonates with interrupted aortic arch have ductal-dependent systemic blood flow and present with circulatory collapse as the ductus closes. The clinical presentation is similar to that of HLHS after the ductus arteriosus closes.

Treatment

PGE1 therapy should begin immediately to maintain systemic blood flow via right-to-left shunting at the PDA. Surgical treatment involves an extended end-to-end anastomosis of the interrupted aortic segments.

ACYANOTIC CONGENITAL HEART DISEASE

Acyanotic cardiac defects that result in *increased pulmonary blood flow* (left-to-right shunts) include ASD, VSD, PDA, and common atrioventricular canal. Acyanotic lesions that result in *pulmonary venous hypertension* include coarctation of the aorta and aortic valve stenosis. The acyanotic structural anomaly that results in *normal or decreased pulmonary blood flow* is pulmonary valve stenosis.

ATRIAL SEPTAL DEFECTS

Atrial septal defects account for 8% of CHD and have a 2:1 female-to-male predominance. There are three types of atrial septal defects:

- Ostium secundum defect, seen in the midportion of the atrial septum.
- Ostium primum defect, located in the lower portion of the atrial septum.
- Sinus venosus defect, found at the junction of the right atrium and the superior or inferior vena cava.

The degree of atrial shunting depends on the size of the ASD and the relative compliance of the ventricles in diastole. Because right ventricular diastolic compliance is usually greater than left ventricular diastolic compliance, left-to-right shunting occurs at the atrial level and results in right atrial and right ventricular enlargement and increased pulmonary blood flow.

Clinical Manifestations

Atrial septal defects are usually asymptomatic, although exercise intolerance may be noted in older children. Paradoxical embolism may occur. Supraventricular tachycardia from atrial enlargement may also occur. On examination, a right ventricular heave is often present. A systolic ejection murmur in the pulmonic (left upper sternal border) area and a mid-diastolic rumble in the lower right sternal border reflect the increased flow across the pulmonary and tricuspid valves. S_1 is loud, and S_2 is widely split on both inspiration and expiration ("fixed" splitting). The chest radiograph reveals enlargement of the heart and main pulmonary artery with increased pulmonary vascularity. The ECG often shows right ventricular enlargement. Right-axis deviation is seen in secundum defects, whereas primum defects have characteristic extreme left-axis deviation.

Treatment

Spontaneous closure of small secundum ASDs (the most common type) often occurs in the first year of life. In both symptomatic and asymptomatic children with suitable secundum ASDs, transcatheter device closure may be undertaken after 2 years of age. Moderate- to large-size secundum ASDs that have not spontaneously closed and are not candidates for device closure must be addressed surgically. Ostium primum and sinus venosus ASDs will not close spontaneously and must be addressed surgically. Surgical closure involves pericardial patch or suture closure. Subacute bacterial endocarditis prophylaxis is indicated in primum and sinus venosus ASDs; patients with secundum defects do not require such precautions.

VENTRICULAR SEPTAL DEFECTS

The VSD is the most common congenital heart defect, accounting for 25% of all congenital heart defects. The five types of VSDs are as follows (as seen in Fig. 3-5):

- Muscular
- Inlet
- Conoseptal hypoplasia
- Conoventricular
- Malalignment

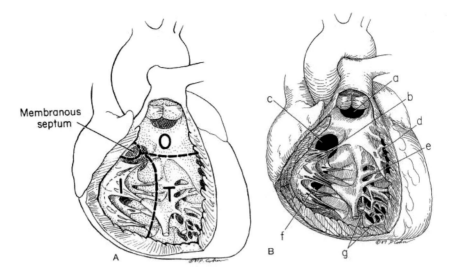

Figure 3-5 • **(A)** Ventricular septum viewed from right ventricular side is made of four components; I, inlet component extends from tricuspid annulus to attachments of tricuspid valve; T, trabecular septum extends from inlet out to apex and up to smooth-walled outlet; O, outlet septum or infundibular septum, which extends up to pulmonary valve, and membranous septum. **(B)** Anatomic position of defects: a, outlet defect; b, papillary muscle of the conus; c, perimembranous defect; d, marginal muscular defects; e, central muscular defects; f, inlet defect; g, apical muscular defects. (From Allen HD, Gutgesell HP, et al. *Moss and Adams Heart Disease in Infants, Children, and Adolescents*, 6th ed. Philadelphia: Lippincott Williams & Wilkins, 2001.)

Muscular and conoventricular VSDs are the most common types. Muscular ventricular septal defects occur in the muscular portion of the septum and may be single or multiple and located in the posterior, apical, or anterior portion of the septum. The inlet VSD is an endocardial cushion defect and occurs in the inlet portion of the septum beneath the septal leaflet of the tricuspid valve. Conoseptal hypoplasia VSDs are positioned in the outflow tract of the right ventricle (RV) beneath the pulmonary valve. The conoventricular VSD occurs in the membranous portion of the ventricular septum. Malalignment VSDs result from malalignment of the infundibular septum. Anterior malalignment results in TOF, and posterior malalignment results in aortic stenosis or subaortic stenosis with arch hypoplasia or interruption.

When the VSD is small (restrictive), shunt flow is left to right from the high pressure LV to the lower pressure RV. Small shunts result in relatively normal pulmonary blood flow and pulmonary vascular resistance (PVR). When the VSD is large (nonrestrictive), LV and RV pressure are equal and PVR and systemic vascular resistance (SVR) determine shunt flow. When the PVR is less than the SVR, the shunt flow is left to right. The amount of LV and left atrial dilatation is directly proportional to the size of the left-to-right shunt. Right ventricular hypertrophy occurs when PVR increases. If left untreated, the large VSD may result in elevated pulmonary arterial pressures and may lead to pulmonary vascular obstructive disease, pulmonary hypertension, and **Eisenmenger syndrome**. In severe cases of Eisenmenger syndrome, the VSD shunt reverses right to left when the PVR exceeds the SVR.

Clinical Manifestations

Clinical symptoms are related to the size of the shunt. A small shunt produces no symptoms, whereas a large shunt gives rise to signs of congestive heart failure and growth failure. The smaller the defect, the louder the harsh systolic murmur, heard best at the mid- to lower left sternal border. As the PVR increases in patients with nonrestrictive VSDs, shunting from left-to-right decreases, the murmur shortens, and the pulmonary (late) component of S_2 increases in intensity. Eisenmenger syndrome results in a right ventricular heave, pulmonary valve ejection click, short systolic ejection murmur, diastolic murmur of pulmonary valve insufficiency, and a loud, single S_2.

Small VSDs have a normal chest radiograph and electrocardiogram. Moderate-size VSDs may show mild cardiomegaly and slightly increased pulmonary vascularity on chest radiograph. Large left-to-right shunts result in cardiomegaly, increased pulmonary vascularity, and enlargement of the left atrium and left ventricle. The ECG is consistent with left atrial, left ventricular, or biventricular hypertrophy. Right ventricular hypertrophy predominates when pulmonary vascular resistance is high.

Treatment

Most small VSDs close without intervention (40% by 3 years, 75% by 10 years); in cases which do not, surgery is unnecessary. Muscular VSDs are the most likely to close spontaneously. The treatment for large VSDs, with significant left-to-right shunting and variable levels of congestive heart failure, is surgical closure before pulmonary vascular changes become irreversible. Surgical closure usually involves Dacron patch closure. In some cases, transcatheter device placement in the interventricular septum may be used for VSD closure. Congestive heart failure is treated with digoxin, diuretics, and systemic afterload reduction with an angiotensin-converting enzyme (ACE) inhibitor. Patients with unrepaired VSDs require bacterial endocarditis prophylaxis.

COMMON ATRIOVENTRICULAR CANAL DEFECT

The common atrioventricular canal defect (Fig. 3-6) is most commonly seen in children with Down syndrome. The lesion results from deficiency of the endocardial cushions and results in an ostium primum ASD and inlet VSD with lack of septation of the mitral and tricuspid valves (common atrioventricular valve [CAVV]). The various forms of atrioventricular canal defects account for 5% of all CHD. In an **incomplete atrioventricular canal defect**, the CAVV leaflets attach directly to the top of the muscular portion of the ventricular septum. As a result, there is no communication beneath the atrioventricular valves between the right and left ventricles. The communication at the atrial level is an ostium primum ASD. The mitral valve is cleft, and there may be some degree of mitral regurgitation. In **complete common atrioventricular canal**, there is a CAVV that is not attached to the muscular ventricular septum. As a result, there is a large inlet VSD located between the CAVV and the top of the muscular ventricular septum. In this defect, there is a left-to-right shunting at the ostium primum ASD and inlet VSD. Because of the increase in pulmonary blood flow, pulmonary hypertension and pulmonary vascular disease may develop over time. In untreated cases, Eisenmenger syndrome may develop.

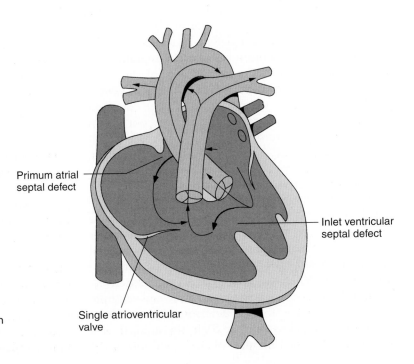

Primum atrial septal defect

Inlet ventricular septal defect

Single atrioventricular valve

Figure 3-6 • Complete common atrioventricular canal. Typical anatomic findings include: large atrial and ventricular septal defects of the endocardial cushion type; single atrioventricular valve; left-to-right shunting, which is noted at the atrial and ventricular level when pulmonary vascular resistance falls during the neonatal period.

Clinical Manifestations

The clinical manifestations and treatment of incomplete common atrioventricular canal are the same as those described for an ASD. There may be a blowing systolic murmur heard best at the left lower sternal border and apex, consistent with mitral regurgitation through the mitral valve cleft.

In complete common atrioventricular canal, the degree of congestive heart failure depends on the magnitude of the left-to-right shunting and the amount of CAVV regurgitation. If shunting or valve regurgitation is significant, congestive heart failure is seen early in infancy, with tachypnea, dyspnea, and failure to thrive. On examination, a blowing holosystolic murmur is heard at the left lower sternal border, and S_2 is widely split and fixed. Cardiac enlargement and increased pulmonary vascularity are visible on the chest radiograph. The ECG reveals a superior axis, which is characteristic of a canal defect and dilatation of both right and left atria.

Treatment

Prior to surgical repair, congestive heart failure may be treated with digoxin, diuretics, and an ACE inhibitor. The symptomatic patient with complete common atrioventricular valve (CAVV) is generally repaired during infancy. The asymptomatic child with incomplete canal without pulmonary hypertension may undergo elective repair within the first few years of life. Infants with a large VSD component should be repaired by 6 months to decrease the risk of pulmonary artery hypertension and pulmonary vascular obstructive disease. The ASD and VSD portions are closed, and the CAVV is divided into left and right sides. Suture closure of the cleft leaflets of the septated left-sided atrioventricular inflow is performed to make the LV inflow as competent as possible. Complete heart block occurs in 5% of patients undergoing repair, and residual mitral insufficiency is not uncommon.

PATENT DUCTUS ARTERIOSUS

Persistent patency of the ductus arteriosus accounts for 10% of CHD. The incidence of PDA is higher in premature neonates. The ductus arteriosus connects the underside of the aorta and the left pulmonary artery just distal to the takeoff of the left subclavian artery from the aorta (Fig. 3-7). The direction of

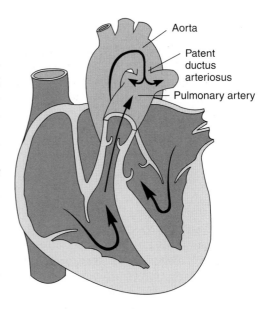

Figure 3-7 • Patent ductus arteriosus. The ductal arteriosus connects the underside of the aorta to the takeoff of the left pulmonary artery. When pulmonary vascular resistance falls, blood flows from left-to-right from aorta to pulmonary artery. (From Pillitteri A. *Maternal and Child Nursing*, 4th ed. Philadelphia: Lippincott Williams & Wilkins, 2003.)

blood flow through a PDA depends on the relative resistances in the pulmonary and systemic circuits. In the nonrestrictive (large) PDA, a left-to-right shunt is present as long as the systemic vascular resistance is greater than the pulmonary vascular resistance. If pulmonary vascular resistance rises above systemic vascular resistance, a right-to-left shunt develops.

Clinical Manifestations

Symptoms are related to the *size* of the defect and the *direction* of flow. A small PDA causes no symptoms or abnormalities on chest radiograph or ECG. A large PDA with left-to-right shunting may result in congestive heart failure and failure to thrive. Bounding pulses are palpable. A continuous murmur begins after S_1, peaks at S_2, and trails off during diastole. The chest radiograph of a large patent ductus arteriosus shows cardiomegaly, increased pulmonary vascularity, and left atrial and ventricular enlargement. The ECG shows left or biventricular hypertrophy. If pulmonary vascular resistance rises above systemic resistance (pulmonary hypertension), flow at the PDA reverses, and cyanosis is noted.

Treatment

Indomethacin decreases PGE1 levels and is often effective in closing the ductus in the premature neonate. A PDA usually closes in term infants in the first month of life. If the ductus remains patent, coil embolization or device closure in the cardiac catheterization laboratory or surgical ligation may be performed.

COARCTATION OF THE AORTA

Coarctation of the aorta (Color Plate 8) accounts for 8% of congenital heart defects and has a male-to-female predominance of 2:1. When coarctation of the aorta occurs in a female, **Turner syndrome** must be considered. The obstruction (narrowing) is usually located in the descending aorta at the insertion site of the ductus arteriosus. The coarctation results in obstruction to blood flow (between the proximal and distal aorta) and increased left ventricular afterload.

Clinical Manifestations

The degree of narrowing determines clinical severity. Infants may be asymptomatic or present with irritability, difficulty feeding, and failure to thrive. More than half of infants with coarctation will have no symptoms in infancy. Neonates with critical coarctation have ductal-dependent systemic blood flow and may present with circulatory collapse as the ductus closes, similar to HLHS and interrupted aortic arch. On examination, the femoral pulses are often weak and delayed or even absent, and there is upper extremity hypertension. On cardiac examination, there is a nonspecific ejection murmur at the heart apex. If the coarctation is associated with a bicuspid aortic valve, an apical ejection click will be heard. The chest radiograph and ECG are normal in mild lesions. In patients with more severe obstruction, the chest radiograph may reveal an enlarged aortic knob and cardiomegaly. Right ventricular hypertrophy is seen in the neonatal ECG; left ventricular hypertrophy is more common in the older patient.

Treatment

In neonates with critical coarctation of the aorta, the child's systemic blood flow is ductal-dependent, and PGE1 should be started prior to surgical intervention. Treatment may be surgical, with end-to-end anastomosis or patch aortoplasty, or interventional, with balloon dilation angioplasty with or without stent placement. Timing and type of therapy depend on age at diagnosis, severity of illness, and related defects. Restenosis at the surgical repair site is not uncommon, especially in neonates. Persistent hypertension after intervention in the older child may require β-blocker therapy.

AORTIC STENOSIS

In aortic stenosis, the valvular tissue is thickened, rigid, and domed in systole. Most commonly, the valve is bicuspid. The increased pressure generated in the left ventricle, as it attempts to direct blood flow across a stenotic valve, results in left ventricular hypertrophy and, over time, decreased compliance and ventricular performance.

Clinical Manifestations

The level of symptomatology is related to the severity of the stenosis and the level of ventricular function. Infants with minimal stenosis are asymptomatic (although with a murmur). The neonate with critical aortic stenosis has ductal-dependent systemic blood flow and may present with circulatory collapse if the ductus closes. The cardiac examination is characterized by a harsh systolic ejection murmur heard at the right upper sternal border that is preceded by an ejection click. In severe aortic stenosis, a thrill may be palpable. The more pronounced the stenosis, the louder the murmur. However, if ventricular function is highly compromised, only a soft murmur may be appreciated. The chest radiograph shows cardiomegaly. Pulmonary edema may be noted in cases with ventricular dysfunction. Left ventricular hypertrophy is seen on the ECG. In some cases, a strain pattern of ST depression and inverted T waves consistent with ischemia may be noted.

Treatment

In neonates with critical aortic stenosis, the child's systemic blood flow is ductal-dependent, and PGE1 should be started prior to surgical or catheter-based intervention. If intervention is required, relief of the aortic valve gradient may be accomplished by balloon valvuloplasty. Balloon valvuloplasty may result in progressive aortic regurgitation that may require aortic valvuloplasty or aortic valve replacement with a mechanical, homograft, or autograft valve (Ross procedure).

PULMONIC STENOSIS

Pulmonic valve stenosis accounts for 5% to 8% of CHDs. The valve is domed with only a small central opening, and there is poststenotic dilatation of the main pulmonary artery. Right ventricular hypertrophy occurs over time as the ventricle attempts to maintain cardiac output. In *critical pulmonic stenosis*, a decrease in the compliance of the right ventricle increases right atrial pressure and may open the foramen ovale, producing a right-to-left shunt.

Clinical Manifestations

Most patients are asymptomatic. Severe or critical pulmonary stenosis may cause dyspnea on exertion and angina. Right-sided congestive heart failure is rare, except in infants with critical pulmonic stenosis who may have ductal-dependent pulmonary blood flow. Characteristically, the ejection click of pulmonic stenosis varies with inspiration, and a harsh systolic ejection murmur is heard at the left upper sternal border. In severe stenosis, a thrill and right ventricular heave are palpable. On chest radiograph, heart size and pulmonary vascularity are normal, but the pulmonary artery segment is enlarged. The degree of right ventricular hypertrophy and right-axis deviation present on ECG correlates with the degree of stenosis.

Treatment

In neonates with critical pulmonary stenosis, the child's pulmonary blood flow is ductal-dependent, and PGE1 should be started prior to surgical or catheter-based intervention.

Table 3-6 lists the findings for the ten most common congenital heart lesions.

ACQUIRED STRUCTURAL HEART DISEASE

RHEUMATIC HEART DISEASE

Acute rheumatic fever causes carditis in 50% to 80% of patients. Rheumatic heart disease results from single or multiple episodes of acute rheumatic fever. **Mitral regurgitation** is the most common valvular residual lesion of acute rheumatic carditis. Aortic insufficiency may also occur, with or without mitral regurgitation. Late-stage disease may progress to mitral and/or aortic stenosis. Patients with severe valvular involvement manifest signs and symptoms of chronic congestive heart failure. Chapter 12 discusses acute rheumatic fever.

■ **TABLE 3-6** Findings for the Ten Most Common Congenital Heart Lesions				
Lesion	**Presentation**	**Physical Examination**	**ECG**	**Radiograph**
Atrial septal defect	Murmur	Fixed split S_2	Mild RVH	±CE, ↑ PBF
Ventricular septal defect	Murmur, CHF	Holosystolic murmur	LVH, RVH	±CE, ↑ PBF
Patent ductus arteriosus	Murmur, ±CHF	Continuous murmur	LVH, ± RVH	±CE, ↑ PBF
AV canal defect	Murmur, ±CHF	Holosystolic murmur	"Superior" axis	±CE, ↑ PBF
Pulmonic stenosis	Murmur, ±cyanosis	Click, SEM	RVH	±CE, NL, or ↓ PBF
Tetralogy of Fallot	Murmur, ±cyanosis	SEM	RVH	±CE, ↓ PBF
Aortic stenosis	Murmur, ±CHF	Click, SEM	LVH	±CE, NL, PBF
Coarctation of the aorta	Hypertension	↓ Femoral pulses	LVH	±CE, NL, PBF
Transposition of the great arteries	Cyanosis	Marked cyanosis Loud S_2	RVH	±CE, NL, or ↑ PBF
Single ventricle	(Variable)	(Variable)	(Variable)	(Variable)

CE, cardiac enlargement; CHF, congestive heart failure; LVH, left ventricular hypertrophy; NL, normal; PBF, pulmonary blood flow; RVH, right ventricular hypertrophy; SEM, systolic ejection murmur.

KAWASAKI DISEASE

Cardiac effects may include pericarditis, myocarditis, and coronary arteritis. It is the development of **coronary artery aneurysms**, with their potential for occlusion, however, that makes the disease life-threatening. Coronary artery aneurysms develop during the subacute phase (11th to 25th day) in approximately 25% of cases but regress in most patients. Early therapy with intravenous immunoglobulin decreases the incidence of coronary artery aneurysms to less than 10%. High-dose aspirin therapy given during the acute inflammatory period lessens the likelihood of aneurysm development. Low-dose aspirin is continued for 6 to 8 weeks (or indefinitely if the aneurysms do not resolve). An ECHO is used to assess ventricular function and detect and follow coronary artery aneurysms. Evidence of myocardial ischemia warrants a cardiac catheterization and in some cases may require bypass surgery if obstruction exists. Chapter 11 offers a thorough discussion of Kawasaki disease.

ENDOCARDITIS

Pathogenesis

Bacterial endocarditis (BE) is a microbial infection of the endocardium. Although it may occur on normal valves, BE is more likely to occur where there is turbulent flow on congenitally abnormal valves, valves damaged by rheumatic fever, acquired valvular lesions (mitral valve prolapse), and prosthetic replacement valves. Factors that may precipitate BE include intravenous drug abuse, an indwelling central venous catheter, and/or prior cardiac surgery. In 2007 the American Heart Association's Endocarditis Committee, together with national and international experts on BE, extensively reviewed published studies in order to determine whether dental, gastrointestinal, or genitourinary tract procedures are possible causes of BE. These experts determined that there is no conclusive evidence that links dental, gastrointestinal, or genitourinary tract procedures with the development of BE. The prior practice of giving patients antibiotics prior to a dental procedure is no longer recommended **except** for patients with the highest risk of adverse outcomes resulting from BE:

- Prosthetic cardiac valve
- Previous endocarditis

- Congenital heart disease only in the following categories:
  - Unrepaired cyanotic congenital heart disease, including those with palliative shunts and conduits
  - Completely repaired congenital heart disease with prosthetic material or device, whether placed by surgery or catheter intervention, during the first 6 months of after the procedure (Prophylaxis is recommended because endothelialization of prosthetic material occurs within 6 months after the procedure.)
  - Repaired congenital heart disease with residual defects at the site or adjacent to the site of a prosthetic patch or prosthetic device (which inhibits endothelialization)
- Cardiac transplantation recipients with cardiac valvular disease

In children, α-hemolytic streptococci (*Streptococcus viridans*) and *Staphylococcus aureus* are the most common etiologic agents. *S. viridans* accounts for approximately 67% of cases, whereas *S. aureus* is present in an estimated 20% of cases. When the infection is a complication of cardiac surgery, *Staphylococcus epidermidis* and fungi should be considered. Gram-negative organisms cause approximately 5% of cases of endocarditis in children and are more likely in neonates, immunocompromised patients, and intravenous drug abusers.

Clinical Manifestations

Fever is the most common finding in children with bacterial endocarditis. Often, a new or changing murmur is auscultated. Children with endocarditis usually display nonspecific symptoms, including chest pain, dyspnea, arthralgia, myalgia, headache, and malaise. Embolic phenomena such as hematuria and strokes may occur. Other embolic phenomena (Roth spots, splinter hemorrhages, petechiae, Osler nodes, and Janeway lesions) are relatively rare in children with bacterial endocarditis.

Diagnostic Evaluation

Typical laboratory findings include elevated white blood count, erythrocyte sedimentation rate (ESR), and C-reactive protein (CRP). Anemia is common. Hematuria may be seen on urinalysis. Multiple blood cultures increase the probability of discovering the pathogen. An ECHO is used to define vegetations and/or thrombi in the heart.

Treatment

Medical management consists of 6 weeks of intravenous antibiotics directed against the isolated pathogen. Surgery is indicated for endocarditis when medical treatment is unsuccessful, refractory congestive heart failure exists, serious embolic complications occur, myocardial abscesses develop, or when there is refractory infection of a prosthetic valve.

FUNCTIONAL HEART DISEASE

MYOCARDITIS

Most cases of myocarditis in the developed world result from viral infection of the myocardium, predominantly adenovirus, coxsackie A and B, and echovirus. It is unclear whether the myocardial damage results from direct viral invasion or an autoimmune antibody response.

Clinical Manifestations

If myocardial damage is mild, patients are asymptomatic; the diagnosis may be made by finding ST- and T-wave changes on an ECG done for an unrelated reason. Severe myocardial damage presents with fulminant congestive heart failure and arrhythmia. Common symptoms include fever, dyspnea, fatigue, and chest pain (usually caused by a secondary pericarditis). Tachycardia, evidence of congestive heart failure, and S3 ventricular gallop may be appreciated on examination. The ECG often reveals ST-segment depression, T-wave inversion, and low voltage. Arrhythmias and conduction defects may also be present. Heart size on chest radiograph varies from mild to markedly enlarged. The ECHO reveals ventricles that are dilated and/or poorly functioning. Pericardial effusion is common. Viral etiology should be investigated by viral culture and polymerase chain reaction (PCR) from the throat, stool, blood, and pericardial fluid, if present. In select cases, endomyocardial biopsy is indicated to confirm diagnosis.

Treatment

Therapy for patients with viral myocarditis is supportive to maintain perfusion and oxygen delivery. Ventricular arrhythmias, conduction abnormalities, and congestive heart failure are treated as indicated. Intravenous immunoglobulin is often given despite limited data, to minimize further damage to the myocardium. The prognosis for patients with myocarditis is directly related to the extent of myocardial damage.

CORONARY ARTERY DISEASE

Coronary artery disease is rare in childhood. The atherosclerotic process appears to begin early in life. Evidence indicates that progression of atherosclerotic lesions is influenced by genetic factors (familial hypercholesteremia) and lifestyle (cigarette smoking; high cholesterol diet, high saturated-fat diet). Certain diseases place children at increased risk for hypercholesteremia (e.g., some storage and metabolic diseases, renal failure, diabetes, hepatitis, systemic lupus erythematosus). Because many lifetime habits are formed during childhood, the opportunity exists for prevention of coronary artery disease.

DILATED CARDIOMYOPATHY

Dilated or congestive cardiomyopathy is characterized by myocardial dysfunction and ventricular dilation. In idiopathic cases (most common), the cause is theorized to be a recent undiagnosed episode of myocarditis. Dilated cardiomyopathy can also be caused by neuromuscular disease (Duchenne muscular dystrophy) or drug toxicity (anthracyclines). It may also be familial with associated gene/protein abnormalities.

Clinical Manifestations

Signs and symptoms are related to the resultant congestive heart failure and pulmonary edema. Symptoms include dyspnea, orthopnea, and paroxysmal nocturnal dyspnea. The cardiac examination reveals an S_3 gallop rhythm and often a murmur consistent with mitral regurgitation. As right heart failure worsens, dependent edema, a right ventricular heave, and pulsus alternans (beat-to-beat variability in pulse magnitude) may be noted. The heart is enlarged on chest radiograph, often accompanied by pulmonary edema. The ECG is notable for broadening of the QRS complexes and nonspecific ST- and T-wave ischemic changes. Ventricular function is evaluated by ECHO.

Treatment

Initial treatment includes fluid restriction and diuretics (to reduce preload), inotropic agents and vasodilators (to improve myocardial contractility and decrease afterload), and anticoagulants (to prevent thrombus formation). Antiarrhythmic medications are reserved for treatment of potentially fatal ventricular arrhythmias. If medical therapy fails, heart transplantation may be necessary.

HYPERTROPHIC OBSTRUCTIVE CARDIOMYOPATHY

Also known as idiopathic hypertrophic subaortic stenosis, hypertrophic cardiomyopathy is a disorder in which the ventricular septum is significantly thickened, resulting in left ventricular outflow tract obstruction. The thickened stiff left ventricle has compromised diastolic function and preserved systolic function. Abnormal motion of the mitral valve results in mitral insufficiency. Inheritance is autosomal dominant with incomplete penetrance.

Clinical Manifestations

Most cases are asymptomatic and discovered as a result of evaluation of a heart murmur. When present (generally in adolescence), symptoms include dyspnea on exertion, chest pain, and syncope. A systolic ejection murmur at the left lower sternal border and/or apex may be accompanied by the soft, holosystolic murmur of mitral regurgitation and an S_3 gallop. There may be a left ventricular heave and thrill. The chest radiograph shows normal vascularity and mild left ventricular enlargement. The ECG illustrates left-axis deviation, left ventricular hypertrophy, and possible ST- and T-wave changes consistent with ischemia or strain. The ECHO is diagnostic.

Unfortunately, hypertrophic cardiomyopathy may also present as sudden death during physical activity in an otherwise healthy, asymptomatic person with undiagnosed disease.

Treatment

Therapy is centered on preventing fatal ventricular arrhythmias and improving left ventricular filling by slowing the intrinsic heart rate and decreasing the stiffness of the left ventricle. Medications that reduce the risk of arrhythmia and decrease chronotrophy and inotrophy include calcium channel blockers and β-adrenergic blocking agents. The avoidance of competitive sports is essential because sudden death during exertion is a significant risk (4% to 6% of affected patients a year).

ARRHYTHMIAS

Arrhythmias in children are much less common than in adults but can be just as life-threatening. Arrhythmias result from disorders of impulse formation, impulse conduction, or both, and they are generally classified as follows.

Bradyarrhythmias
- Sinus node dysfunction
- Conduction block

Tachyarrhythmias
- Narrow QRS
- Wide QRS

Premature Beats
- Atrial
- Ventricular

Arrhythmias may result from congenital, functional, or acquired structural heart disease; electrolyte disturbances (potassium, calcium, and magnesium); drug toxicity; poisoning; or an acquired systemic disorder. Table 3-7 lists the etiologies predisposing children to arrhythmias.

BRADYARRHYTHMIAS

Bradyarrhythmias result from either depressed automaticity at the sinus node (sinus node dysfunction) or conduction block at the atrioventricular node or bundle of His (AV block). Bradyarrhythmias that may result from sinus node dysfunction include sinus bradycardia, junctional bradycardia, ectopic atrial bradycardia, and sinus pauses. Bradyarrhythmias that may result from AV block include first-degree heart block, second-degree heart block, and third-degree (complete) heart block.

Differential Diagnosis

Figure 3-8 shows the rhythm strips of various bradycardias. **Sinus bradycardia** is caused by a decreased rate of impulse generation at the sinus node. It may be associated with increased vagal tone, hypoxia, central nervous system disorders with increased intracranial pressure, hypothyroidism, hyperkalemia, hypothermia, drug intoxication (digoxin, β-blockers, calcium channel blockers), and prior atrial surgery. It is also a normal finding in healthy athletic teenagers. The ECG reveals a normal P wave with normal AV

■ TABLE 3-7 Factors Predisposing to Arrhythmias

Congenital heart disease:	Friedreich ataxia (atrial tachycardia or fibrillation)
Supraventricular arrhythmias:	Muscular dystrophies (Duchenne, periodic paralysis)
Ebstein anomaly, atrial septal defects, atrial surgery, L-transposition of the great arteries, after Fontan operation	Glycogen storage diseases (Pompe disease)
Ventricular arrhythmias:	Collagen vascular diseases (rheumatic carditis, systemic lupus erythematosus, periarteritis nodosa, dermatomyositis)
Aortic valve disease, pulmonary valve disease, after tetralogy of Fallot repair, anomalous left coronary artery, RV dysplasia	Endocrine disorders (hyperthyroidism, adrenal dysfunction)
Heart block (varying degrees):	Metabolic and electrolyte disturbances (hypomagnesemia, hyperkalemia, hypocalcemia, hypoxia)
After open-heart surgery (ventricular septal defect, Ebstein anomaly, L-transposition of the great arteries)	Lyme disease
Isolated conduction system disorders	Drug toxicity
Maternal lupus erythematosus	Chemotherapeutic agents
Prolonged QT-interval	Tricyclic antidepressants
Inherited syndromes (Romano-Ward, Jervell and Lange-Nielson)	Cocaine
Associated with systemic illness	Antiarrhythmia drugs (Digitalis, β-adrenergic blockers, calcium blockers)
Infectious myocarditis	Asthma medications (sympathomimetics)
Kawasaki disease	Blunt chest trauma (myocardial contusion)
Idiopathic dilated or hypertrophic cardiomyopathy	Increased intracranial pressure

RV, right ventricle.

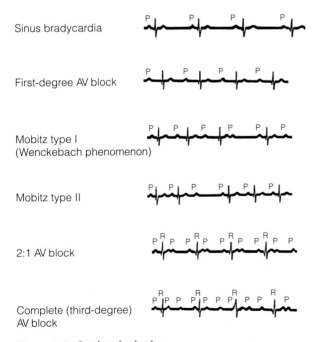

Sinus bradycardia

First-degree AV block

Mobitz type I (Wenckebach phenomenon)

Mobitz type II

2:1 AV block

Complete (third-degree) AV block

Figure 3-8 • Bradyarrhythmias.

conduction at rates less than 100 beats per minute (bpm) in the neonate and 60 bpm in the older child. When sinus bradycardia becomes too slow, sinus pauses or escape rhythms (ectopic atrial bradycardia or ectopic atrial rhythm, junctional bradycardia or junctional rhythm, or a slow idioventricular ventricular rhythm) may occur. Patients with sinus bradycardia can increase their heart rate appropriately when stimulated.

First-degree heart block usually results from slowing of atrioventricular conduction at the level of the AV node. First-degree heart block is associated with increased vagal tone; medication administration (digoxin and β-blocker); infectious etiologies (viral myocarditis, Lyme disease); hypothermia; electrolyte abnormalities (hypo/hyperkalemia, hypo/hypercalcemia, and hypomagnesemia); CHD (ASD, atrioventricular canal defect, Ebstein anomaly, TAPVC, and L-transposition of the great arteries or "corrected transposition"); rheumatic fever; and cardiomyopathy. First-degree AV block is characterized on ECG by PR interval prolongation for age and rate. Otherwise, the rhythm is regular, originates in the sinus node, and has a normal QRS morphology.

Second-degree heart block refers to episodic interruption of AV nodal conduction ("dropped beats"). Some P waves are followed by QRS complexes; others are not.

- **Mobitz type I** (Wenckebach) denotes progressive prolongation of the PR interval over several beats until a QRS is dropped. This cycle repeats itself often, although the number of beats in a cycle may not be constant. The QRS configuration is normal. Etiologies for this rhythm are the same as those for first-degree heart block.
- **Mobitz type II** is caused by abrupt failure of atrioventricular conduction below the AV node in the bundle of His-Purkinje fiber system. It is a more serious bradycardia than first-degree heart block or Wenckebach because it can progress to complete heart block. On ECG, there is sudden AV conduction failure with a dropped QRS after a normal P wave. No preceding PR interval prolongation is seen in normal conducted impulses.
- **Fixed-ratio AV block** is an arrhythmia in which the QRS complex follows only after every second (third or fourth) P wave, causing 2:1 (3:1 or 4:1) AV block. There is a normal PR interval in conducted beats. There is usually a normal or slightly prolonged QRS. Fixed-ratio block results from either AV node or His bundle injury, and intracardiac recordings are required to distinguish the site of injury. Patients may progress to complete heart block.

Third-degree heart block exists when no atrial impulses are conducted to the ventricles. The atrial rhythm and rate are normal for the patient's age, and the ventricular rate is slowed markedly (40 to 55 bpm). If an escape rhythm arises from the AV node (*junctional rhythm*), the QRS interval is of normal duration, but if an escape rhythm arises from the distal His bundle or Purkinje fibers, the QRS interval is prolonged (*idioventricular rhythm*). Congenital complete AV block can be an isolated abnormality or can be associated with L-transposition of the great arteries, atrioventricular canal defect, or maternal lupus erythematosus. Other causes include open-heart surgery (especially after large ventricular septal defect closure), cardiomyopathy, or Lyme disease. Newborns with congenital complete heart block may present with hydrops fetalis.

Treatment

No intervention is necessary for bradycardia if cardiac output is maintained. Figure 3-9 shows a management algorithm for bradycardia.

No treatment is necessary for first- or second-degree heart block (Mobitz type I). Mobitz type II, fixed-ratio AV block, and third-degree heart block all require pacemaker placement. In Mobitz type II and fixed-ratio AV block, prophylactic pacemaker insertion is essential to protect the patient should he or she progress to complete heart block with inadequate cardiac output away from medical care.

If the child with complete heart block is hemodynamically unstable, transcutaneous or transvenous pacing can be performed acutely, and permanent transvenous or epicardial pacemaker placement can be performed later. Third-degree heart block is managed with either ventricular demand pacing or AV sequential pacing.

TACHYARRHYTHMIAS

Tachyarrhythmias arise from abnormal impulse formation caused by enhanced automaticity or a reentrant circuit. Narrow-complex tachycardias have a QRS morphology identical to that of normal sinus rhythm. Most SVTs are narrow-complex in appearance. Narrow-complex tachycardias may be caused by increased automaticity (e.g., sinus tachycardia, ectopic atrial tachycardia, junctional ectopic tachycardia, atrial fibrillation) or a reentrant circuit. Reentrant circuits are categorized into orthodromic reentrant tachycardia (ORT) or antidromic reentrant tachycardia (ART). In ORT, the SVT propagates down the AV node and up the bypass tract. Because the ventricles are depolarized in the normal fashion (down the AV node), the QRS *complex is narrow*. In ART, the SVT propagates down the bypass tract and up the AV node. Because the ventricles are depolarized down the bypass tract and the ventricles depolarize at different times, the QRS *complex is widened*. Narrow-complex AV reciprocating tachycardias include AV node reentrant tachycardia; WPW syndrome orthodromic tachycardia (accessory pathway not concealed on ECG-short PR interval with delta wave); orthodromic atrioventricular reciprocating tachycardia (accessory pathway concealed on ECG; normal PR interval and no delta wave); sinoatrial reentrant tachycardia; and atrial flutter. Narrow-complex tachycardias are relatively well tolerated acutely. Patients with WPW syndrome have antegrade impulse propagation through

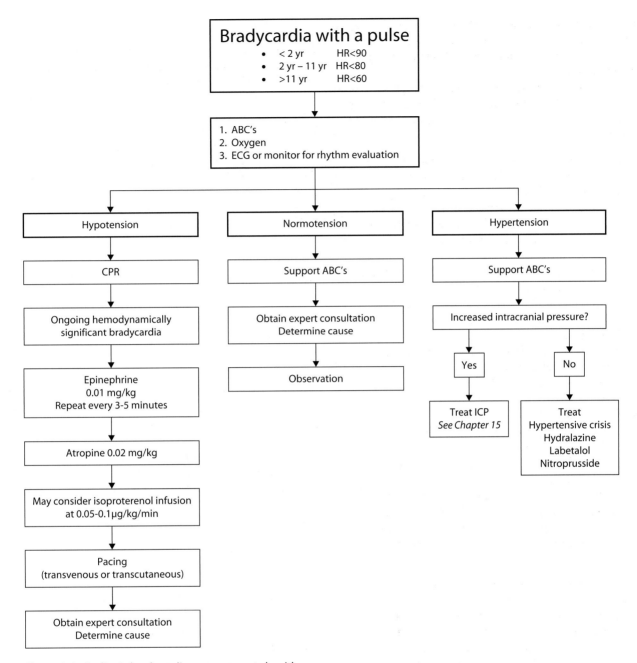

Figure 3-9 • Pediatric bradycardia management algorithm.

both the AV node and the accessory pathway. Characteristic findings on ECG include a short PR interval and delta wave (Fig. 3-10).

Conversely, wide-complex tachycardias, defined as tachycardias with a QRS more than 0.12 s, are a medical emergency. Wide-complex tachycardias include ventricular tachycardia, ventricular fibrillation, WPW syndrome antidromic reentrant tachycardia, and orthodromic SVT with aberrancy.

Differential Diagnosis

The causes of tachyarrhythmia are as follows:

Narrow-Complex Tachycardias

- *Sinus tachycardia*: Fever, stress, dehydration, and anemia.
- *ORT (most common nonsinus tachycardia SVT)*: Most cases result from a concealed bypass tract

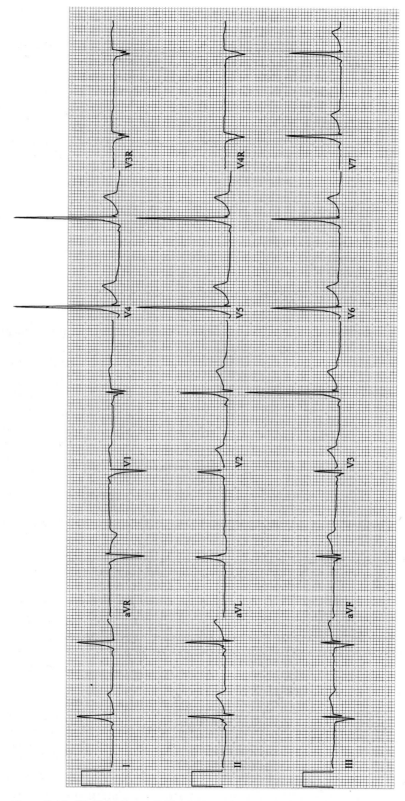

Figure 3-10 • Wolff-Parkinson-White ECG. Upslurring of QRS represents delta wave. Note short PR interval.

AV node reentrant tachycardia, WPW syndrome, Ebstein anomaly (associated with WPW syndrome), or L-transposition of the great arteries.

- *Atrial flutter*: Atrial surgery (D-TGA status post Mustard/Senning procedure, ASD status post repair Hemi-Fontan, Fontan), myocarditis, structural heart disease with dilated atria (Ebstein anomaly, tricuspid atresia, rheumatic heart disease of the mitral valve), severe tricuspid regurgitation.
- *Atrial fibrillation*: Most often seen with left atrial enlargement (rheumatic heart disease of the mitral valve, VSD, systemic to pulmonary artery palliative shunt placement); other causes that result in right atrial or biatrial enlargement include Ebstein anomaly, WPW syndrome, and myocarditis (Fig. 3-11).

Wide-Complex Tachycardia

- *Ventricular tachycardia*: Congenital or acquired heart disease resulting in ventricular dilatation or hypertrophy or ventricular suture line, drug ingestion, or WPW syndrome with ART.
- *Ventricular fibrillation*: Terminal rhythm that develops after hypoxia, ischemia, or high-voltage electrical injury; predisposing factors include WPW syndrome and long QT syndrome (Fig. 3-12).

Treatment

Narrow-Complex Tachycardia

Treatment of sinus tachycardia involves correcting the underlying cause of the tachycardia. Treatment for stable narrow-complex tachycardia progresses from vagal maneuvers to pharmacotherapy to cardioversion. Figure 3-13 outlines the management of pediatric supraventricular tachycardia. Vagal maneuvers (ice to face and carotid massage) enhance vagal tone to slow conduction in the AV node and often result in termination of the arrhythmia.

If vagal maneuvers are ineffective, adenosine may be given to block the AV node and break the reentrant SVT. The reentrant SVT, whose circuit involves the AV node (AV node reentrant tachycardia, WPW syndrome—type ORT, concealed bypass tract—type ORT), is likely to break with the administration of adenosine. Adenosine is ineffective on a narrow-complex tachycardia that results from increased automaticity or a reentrant mechanism that does not involve the AV node (sinus tachycardia, ectopic atrial tachycardia, junctional ectopic tachycardia, atrial flutter, or sinoatrial reentrant tachycardia). If adenosine returns the child to normal sinus rhythm and WPW is not suspected (no delta wave seen after conversion of tachycardia), the child may be started on digoxin to reduce the risk of future events. A β-blocker should be used if adenosine therapy reveals WPW syndrome (short PR interval and delta wave noted after conversion of tachycardia). The use of digoxin in patients with WPW may slow the conduction across the AV node, leading to preferential depolarization down the accessory pathway in an antidromic fashion. This antidromic conduction may result in ventricular fibrillation if atrial fibrillation or some other fast atrial arrhythmia is present.

Treatment for hemodynamically stable atrial flutter may include digoxin, β-blockers, procainamide, amiodarone, flecainide, or sotalol.

If atrial fibrillation has been present for more than a few days, anticoagulation is needed before converting the rhythm to decrease the risk of embolization of possible intra-atrial clots. An alternative to anticoagulation is transesophageal echocardiography to assess for clots. If no clots are seen, cardioversion may proceed, although with a slightly increased risk of thromboembolism relative to anticoagulation.

When narrow-complex tachycardia is present and the patient is hemodynamically unstable, cardioversion is indicated. Synchronized cardioversion is required to avoid the inadvertent development of ventricular fibrillation.

Most chronic cases of SVT with the exception of atrial fibrillation are amenable to radiofrequency ablation.

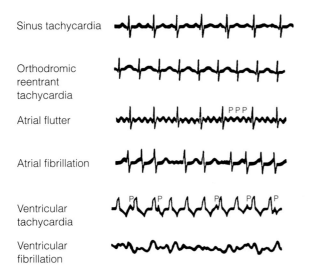

Sinus tachycardia

Orthodromic reentrant tachycardia

Atrial flutter

Atrial fibrillation

Ventricular tachycardia

Ventricular fibrillation

Figure 3-11 • Tachyarrhythmia.

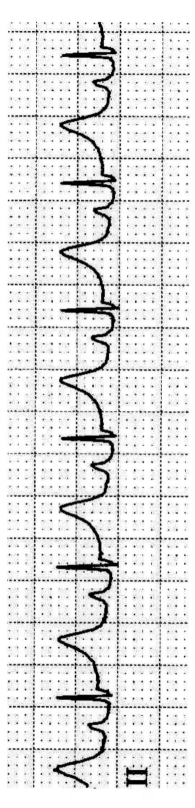

Figure 3-12 • Long QT syndrome ECG.
(Image courtesy of Dr. Bradley Marino.)

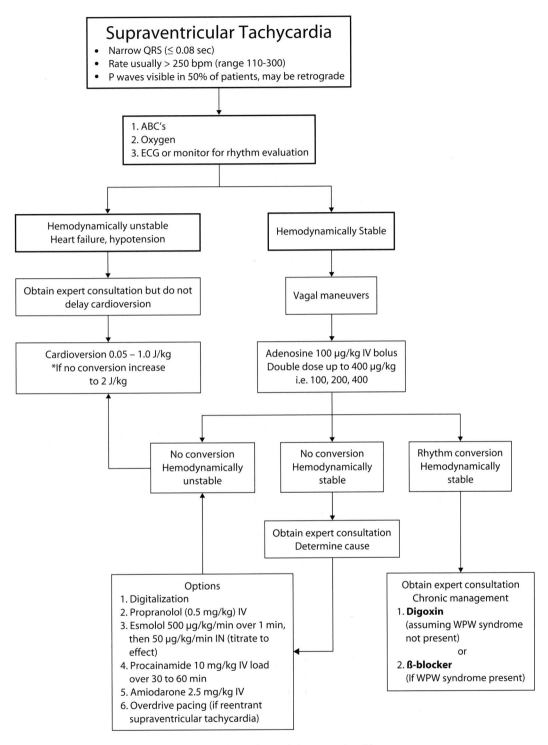

Figure 3-13 • Pediatric supraventricular tachycardia management algorithm.

Wide-Complex Tachycardia

Wide-complex tachycardia caused by WPW syndrome with antidromic conduction or orthodromic SVT with aberrancy should be treated as if the patient has ventricular tachycardia. Hypotensive or unresponsive patients should be treated immediately with cardiopulmonary resuscitation and synchronized cardioversion. After cardioversion, sinus rhythm can be maintained with intravenous amiodarone. Normotensive patients with acute-onset ventricular tachycardia can be treated with intravenous amiodarone in an attempt to break the arrhythmia without cardioversion. Many

chronic cases of ventricular tachycardia are amenable to radiofrequency ablation. Figure 3-14 outlines management for ventricular tachycardia.

Children with ventricular fibrillation or pulseless ventricular tachycardia should receive CPR and must be defibrillated with nonsynchronized cardioversion. Giving epinephrine may turn fine fibrillation into coarse fibrillation and allow successful defibrillation. Figure 3-15 outlines the management algorithm for a pulseless arrest, which may result from ventricular fibrillation, pulseless ventricular tachycardia, pulseless electrical activity or asystole.

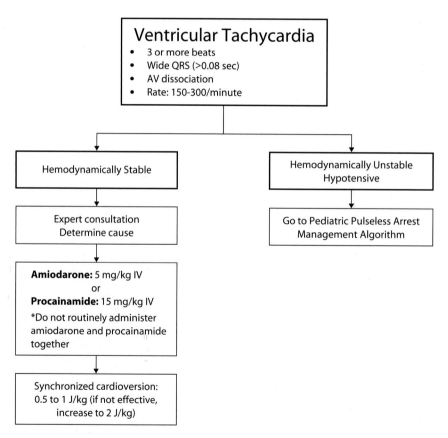

Figure 3-14 • Pediatric ventricular tachycardia management algorithm.

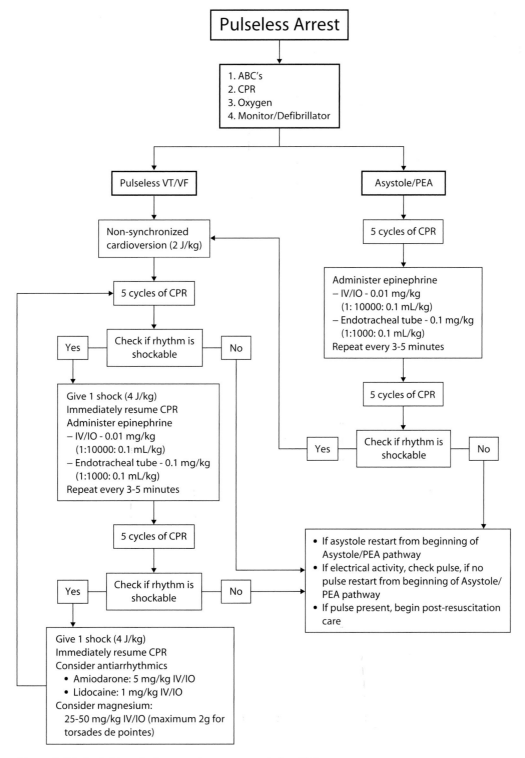

Figure 3-15 • Pediatric pulseless arrest management algorithm.

KEY POINTS

- The absolute concentration of deoxygenated hemoglobin determines the presence of cyanosis.

- Cyanosis in the newborn may be cardiac, pulmonary, neurologic, or hematologic in origin. Following stabilization of a cyanotic infant, the goal of the preliminary workup (chest radiograph, electrocardiogram, and hyperoxia test) is to determine whether the lesion is cardiac or noncardiac in origin.

- Comparison of preductal to postductal measurements of oxygen saturation allows the clinician to evaluate for differential cyanosis.

- Prostaglandin E1 (PGE1) therapy should be started in all unstable infants with suspected congenital heart disease (CHD).

- Patients with the highest risk of adverse outcomes resulting from bacterial endocarditis include those with: prosthetic cardiac valves; previous endocarditis; unrepaired cyanotic congenital heart disease including those with palliative shunts and conduits; completely repaired congenital heart disease with prosthetic material or a device within 6 months of the procedure; repaired congenital heart disease with residual defects at the site or adjacent to the site of a prosthetic patch or prosthetic device; and car-

diac transplantation recipients with cardiac valvular disease. According to the new 2007 bacterial endocarditis prophylaxis guidelines, these patients warrant dental prophylaxis.

- Most cases of myocarditis in North America result from viral infection of the myocardium.

- Dilated or congestive cardiomyopathy is characterized by myocardial dysfunction and ventricular dilation; it is usually idiopathic.

- Hypertrophic cardiomyopathy may present as sudden death during physical exertion in an asymptomatic, otherwise healthy individual.

- Therapy for hypertrophic cardiomyopathy is centered on preventing fatal ventricular arrhythmias and improving left ventricular filling by slowing the intrinsic heart rate and decreasing the stiffness of the left ventricle. Medications that reduce the risk of arrhythmia and decrease chronotrophy and inotrophy include calcium channel blockers and β-adrenergic blocking agents.

- Narrow-complex tachycardias tend to be well tolerated acutely, whereas wide-complex tachycardias often result in hemodynamic instability and are considered a medical emergency.

Chapter 4

Development

Katie S. Fine

DEVELOPMENTAL MILESTONES

Both intellectual and physical development in infants and children occur in predictable, sequential manners. Table 4-1 presents the typical progression of developmental milestones. Notable skills are subdivided into **gross motor**, **visual motor** (or fine motor–adaptive), **language**, and **social** milestones.

The two developmental screens most commonly employed by pediatricians are the **Denver II** developmental screening test and the Clinical Adaptive Test/Clinical Linguistic and Auditory Milestone Scale (**CAT/CLAMS**). The Denver II evaluates children birth-6 years of age and divides streams of development into gross motor, fine motor–adaptive, language, and personal-social. The CAT rates problem-solving/visual motor ability and the CLAMS assesses language development between birth and 36 months of age.

Sometimes development does not progress as expected. **Developmental delay** is diagnosed when performance lags significantly compared with average attainment in a given skill area. The **developmental quotient** (DQ) reflects a child's present developmental achievement: DQ = (developmental age/chronological age) × 100. A DQ below 70 constitutes developmental delay. **Developmental dissociation** refers to a substantial difference in the rates of development between two skill areas. An example of a developmental discrepancy between gross motor and language development is a child with speech delay due to isolated mental retardation whose gross motor development is normal.

Language is the best indicator of future intellectual potential. Language development is divided into two streams, receptive and expressive; each form is assigned a separate DQ. Overall, language delay is the most commonly diagnosed form of developmental delay in preschool children.

Age-adjusted parameters are used when evaluating the developmental achievement of former preterm infants. Until 2 years of age, a child's chronological age should take into account the gestational age at birth. For example, at his or her 9-month checkup, an infant born at 28 weeks' gestation should be able to perform skills typical for a 6-month-old.

DEVELOPMENTAL DELAY

MENTAL RETARDATION

Mental retardation, as defined in the DSM-IV-TR, involves: (a) IQ (intellectual quotient) ≤70; (b) onset prior to 18 years of age; and (c) impaired adaptive functioning (in at least two of the following areas: communication, self-care, home living, social/interpersonal skills, use of community resources, self-direction, academic skills, work, leisure, health, and safety). The most commonly used IQ tests in the pediatric population are the **Wechsler** scales (preschool and school age) and the **Stanford-Binet** (school age). An IQ of 50 to 70 denotes **mild** retardation (the great majority of affected individuals), 35 to 55 defines **moderate** retardation, 20 to 40 correlates with **severe** retardation, and below 20 to 25 signifies **profound** retardation.

The cause of mental retardation is identified in only about half of cases. Mental retardation may come to the attention of the pediatrician when the

■ TABLE 4-1 Commonly Quizzed Developmental Milestones

Age	Gross Motor	Fine (Visual) Motor	Language	Social/Adaptive
Birth–1 month	Raises head slightly in prone position	Follows with eyes to midline only; hands tightly fisted	Alerts/startles to sound	Fixes on face (at birth)
2 months	Raises chest and head off bed in prone position	Regards object and follows through 180-degree arc; briefly retains rattle	Coos and vocalizes reciprocally	Social smile; recognizes parent
4 months	Lifts onto extended elbows in prone position; steady head control with no head lag; rolls over front to back	Reaches for objects with both hands together; bats at objects; grabs and retains objects	Orients to voice; laughs and squeals	Initiates social interaction
6 months	Sits, but may need support; rolls in both directions	Reaches with one hand; transfers objects hand-to-hand	Babbles	Recognizes object or person as unfamiliar
9 months	Sits without support; crawls; pulls to stand	Uses pincer grasp; finger-feeds	Imitates speech sounds (nonspecific "mama," "dada"); understands "no"	Plays gesture games ("pat-a-cake"); understands own name; object permanence; stranger anxiety
12 months	Cruises; stands alone; takes a few independent steps	Can voluntarily release items	Discriminative use of "mama," "dada," plus 1 to 4 other words; follows command with gesture	Imitates; comes when called; cooperates with dressing
15 months	Walks well independently	Builds a two-block tower; throws ball underhand	4 to 6 words in addition to above; uses jargon; responds to one-step verbal command	Begins to use cup; indicates wants or needs
18 months	Runs; walks up stairs with hand held; stoops and recovers	Builds a three-block tower; uses spoon; spontaneous scribbling	Uses 10 to 25 words; points to body parts when asked; uses words to communicate needs or wants	Uses words to communicate wants or needs; plays near (but not with) other children
24 months	Walks unassisted up and down stairs; kicks ball; throws ball overhand; jumps with two feet off the floor	Builds four- to six-block tower; uses fork and spoon; copies a straight line	Uses 50+ words, two- and three-word phrases; uses "I" and "me"; 50% of speech intelligible to stranger	Removes simple clothing; parallel play
36 months	Pedals tricycle; broad jumps	Copies a circle	Uses 5 to 8 word sentences; 75% of speech intelligible to stranger	Knows age and gender; engages in group play; shares
4 years	Balances on one foot	Copies a cross; catches ball	Tells a story; 100% of speech intelligible to stranger	Dresses self; puts on shoes; washes and dries hands; imaginative play
5 years	Skips with alternating feet	Draws a person with six body parts	Asks what words mean	Names four colors; plays cooperative games; understands "rules" and abides by them
6 years	Rides a bike	Writes name	Identifies written letters and numbers	Knows right from left; knows all color names

52

child exhibits developmental delay in one or more areas. Obvious dysmorphisms occasionally suggest a specific disorder (e.g., Down, fragile X, or fetal alcohol syndrome). Laboratory testing may be beneficial when a genetic cause is suggested and the parents desire more children or when the potential diagnosis may affect prognosis or life span. Co-morbid conditions (cerebral palsy, behavioral disorders, seizures) are not uncommon, depending on the underlying etiology. Treatment is interdisciplinary, supportive, and symptom-specific, with the goal of maximizing adaptive functioning and quality of life.

SPEECH AND LANGUAGE DELAY

An individual's ability to speak impacts his or her capacity to communicate with others and develop social relationships. Speech delay is the most common developmental concern raised by parents. As many as 15% of children have some sort of speech/language delay at one time or another during the preschool years. Persistent speech delay which significantly interferes with communication suggests a speech disorder. In most cases, there is no underlying biologic abnormality (genetic syndrome, neuromuscular disease) associated with the disorder.

Language disorders result in the inability to understand or acquire the vocabulary, grammatical rules, or conversation patterns of language. **Speech disorders** involve difficulty producing the sounds and rhythms of speech. **Phonetic disorders** are problems with articulation. Speech and phonetic disorders are expressive disorders, whereas language disorders often affect both expressive and receptive language skills.

Dysfluency produces interruptions in the flow of speech. Developmental dysfluency is observed in many preschoolers, resolves by age 4 years, and is not pathologic. True dysfluency (**stuttering**), characterized by signs of tension and struggle when speaking, sound repetition, or complete speech blockage, significantly impedes the ability to communicate.

Parental concern is a good predictor of the need for further workup. Since many young children are uncomfortable speaking freely in front of strangers, a detailed history is often necessary to characterize the quantity and quality of the patient's speech. **Any child with suspected language delay should receive a full audiologic (hearing) assessment**, followed by referral to a speech pathologist for further workup and treatment (if indicated). The most common cause of mild-to-moderate hearing loss in young children is otitis media with effusion. Early and intensive speech therapy often results in significant and sustained improvement in communication skills over time.

VARIATIONS IN DEVELOPMENTAL PATTERNS

ATTENTION-DEFICIT/HYPERACTIVITY DISORDER

Attention-deficit/hyperactivity disorder (ADHD) is a syndrome characterized by **inattention**, **hyperactivity**, and **impulsivity** which are inconsistent with the developmental stage of the child and manifested through maladaptive behaviors. Classic ADHD is more common in boys and is usually diagnosed in elementary school. School performance and peer relationships often suffer, placing the child at risk for low self-esteem. A variant of ADHD in which inattentiveness is the sole distinguishing feature is more common in girls, who are often diagnosed later than their hyperactive peers. Symptoms persist into adulthood in the majority of patients.

Clinical Manifestation

To be diagnosed with ADHD, a patient must meet specific criteria detailed in the DSM-IV-TR and summarized in Table 4-2. Moreover, the inattention, hyperactivity, and impulsiveness must be present by age 7 years, persist for at least 6 months, and be observed consistently in multiple environments (e.g., school and home). Signs of ADHD may be minimized in settings which are novel, highly supervised, or narrowly focused on the patient. Thus, an affected child may not display any behaviors typical of ADHD in the pediatrician's office.

Assessment

ADHD is a clinical diagnosis. The initial assessment of a child with possible ADHD relies firmly on history obtained from parents and teachers. Age-appropriate rating scales (e.g., Conner's Parent and Teacher Rating Scales) are available and standardized. A complete physical examination should be performed, but is noncontributory in the majority of cases.

■ **TABLE 4-2** Characteristic Features of Attention-Deficit/Hyperactivity Disorder

Inattention
Has a short attention span, is easily distractible
Fails to attend to details
Demonstrates difficulty organizing activities, completing tasks
Avoids activities that require sustained mental effort
Is forgetful in daily activities
Has difficulty following directions
Hyperactivity
Excessively active for age
Fidgets and squirms; restless
Unable to remain seated
Unable to play quietly or entertain oneself
Talks excessively
Impulsivity
Has difficulty waiting one's turn
Often interrupts others

Management

The goal of therapy is to provide sustained symptom reduction throughout the day with an acceptable minimum of adverse effects. Patients with ADHD benefit from a multidisciplinary approach. Emotional supports should be made available for the patient and parents. A behavior management program must be developed to assist both the parents and teachers with positive reinforcement and discipline. Educational assessment should be considered for children with school underperformance; up to 25% of students with ADHD also have a learning disability. Oppositional defiant disorder is the most common comorbid psychiatric diagnosis; others may include mood, anxiety, and conduct disorders.

Pharmacologic intervention is proven to be superior to behavior modification alone. Psycho-stimulants, including **methylphenidate**, **dextroamphetamine**, and **mixed amphetamine salts**, have a long history of use and are available in immediate- and extended-release formulations. All are designated as controlled substances. These drugs work by increasing the availability of dopamine and norepinephrine in the CNS. Side effects include insomnia and anorexia; rarely tics and dyskinesias may develop. An inactive prodrug form of dextroamphetamine called **lisdexamfetamine** which is metabolized to an active formula by the body has recently been approved for treatment of ADHD in the United States. The nonstimulant **atomoxetine** is a highly-specific norepinephrine reuptake inhibitor with a low incidence of side effects and low abuse potential. The Federal Drug Administration requires "black box" warning labels on both the stimulants and atomoxetine (risk of sudden cardiac death for the former; suicidal ideation for the latter). The recommendation that patients stop taking their medications for ADHD on the weekends and during vacations has been discarded; symptom control during nonschool hours is of great benefit to the patient in terms of family and social relationships and performance in extracurricular activities.

AUTISM SPECTRUM DISORDER

Autism spectrum disorder encompasses a collection of chronic, nonprogressive disabilities characterized by impairments in **social interaction**, **communication**, and **behavior** (Table 4-3). Both autism and **Asperger syndrome** are classified as autism spectrum disorders. The reported prevalence of these conditions has been rising over the past 20 years, although it is unclear whether this is due to improved reporting, more inclusive criteria, or a higher rate of disease. Autism is

■ **TABLE 4-3** Characteristics of Autism Spectrum Disorders

Social Interaction
• limited eye contact and facial expression
• difficulty developing peer relationships
• indifference to social overtures
• lack of social reciprocity
• inflexibility
• no engagement in pretend play
Communication
• impaired reciprocal communication
• language development deviant, rather than simply delayed
• echolalia, perseverative speech
Behaviors
• restrictive, stereotyped patterns of behavior
• repetitive, self-stimulatory behaviors (e.g., rocking, spinning)
• preoccupation or fascination with a single object or subject

more common in males. It is usually diagnosed between 18 months and 3 years of age, although symptoms such as impaired attachment are often present from infancy. Autism is currently thought to be a multifactorial disorder; ongoing research may eventually identify genetic abnormalities and/or environmental triggers. *Long-term epidemiologic studies have not found any association between the MMR vaccine or thimerosal (a former vaccine preservative) and the development of autism.*

Clinical Manifestations

Children with classic **autism** have significant language and communication abnormalities and do not engage in meaningful social interactions. They avoid eye contact, exhibit little or no reciprocal communication, and do not engage in pretend play. Affected children usually display stereotypic and/or repetitive behavior patterns and may have an attachment to or fascination with unusual objects.

Asperger syndrome is characterized by difficulty forming relationships/relating to others *and* development of intense interest in very specific topics (e.g., dinosaurs, ancient Egyptian mummies, electronics). While people with Asperger syndrome may not have disordered language production, they do not understand abstract forms of language such as metaphors and sarcasm, and they are unable to interpret nonverbal behavior. Children with Asperger syndrome usually want to form friendships, but their inability to pick up on subtle social cues makes this difficult.

Management

Treatment of autism spectrum disorders consists of intensive behavioral and sensory integration therapy, speech and language training, social modeling, family support, and pharmacologic intervention which targets specific symptoms such as anxiety, hyperactivity, and perseverative behaviors. Special restrictive diets, supplements, immunotherapy, secretin administration, heavy metal detoxification, and craniosacral therapy are all forms of alternative treatments which

remain unproven by scientific study. What is clear is that early recognition and intervention lead to better clinical outcomes. The American Academy of Pediatrics recommends routine screening of all children prior to age 2 years. The best prognostic indicator of future success is the extent of language development present during the preschool years.

KEY POINTS

- Until 2 years of age, a child's chronological age should be adjusted for gestational age at birth when assessing developmental achievement.
- The Wechsler preschool scale is used to assess IQ in preschoolers.
- Language is the best indicator of intellectual potential.
- Any child with a suspected speech or language disorder should be referred for a full hearing evaluation.
- Dysfluency may be developmental between 3 to 4 years of age. Dysfluency which is accompanied by tension, struggle, and/or total word blockage OR severely limits communication should be considered true dysfluency (stuttering) necessitating referral to a speech therapist.
- The predominant elements of attention-deficit-/hyperactivity disorder are inattentiveness, hyperactivity, and impulsivity.
- Pharmacologic interventions for ADHD include stimulant medications, the new prodrug lisdexamfetamine, and the nonstimulant atomoxetine.
- Autism spectrum disorder represents a continuum of chronic, nonprogressive developmental disabilities involving impairments in social interaction, communication, and behavior. Autism and Asperger syndrome are categorized as autism spectrum disorders.
- Administration of the MMR vaccine and thimerosal has not been associated with the development of autism.

5 Dermatology

Marissa Perman • *Anne Lucky* • *Bradley S. Marino*

SKIN MANIFESTATIONS OF VIRAL INFECTIONS

Hand-foot-and-mouth disease is a common acute disease of young children during the spring and summer caused by Coxsackie A viruses. There is usually a prodrome of fever, anorexia, and oral pain, followed by crops of ulcers on the tongue and oral mucosa and a vesicular rash on the hands, feet, and occasionally the buttocks. The individual vesicles often have a "football" shape with surrounding erythema. Diagnosis is made by the history and the constellation of symptoms. Treatment is supportive.

Giannoti-Crosti Syndrome or papular acrodermatitis of childhood is a typically asymptomatic erythematous papular eruption occurring commonly from one to six years of age following an upper respiratory illness. It is symmetrically distributed on the face, extensor surfaces of the arms, legs, and buttocks, and strikingly spares the trunk (Color Plate 9). Papules may coalesce into larger edematous plaques or become purpuric. Several viruses have been associated with this syndrome including hepatitis B (rare in the United States), Epstein-Barr virus (EBV), and varicella. Treatment is supportive, and the rash typically resolves without treatment, but resolution may take up to 8 weeks. A thorough history and physical examination to assess for signs and symptoms associated with hepatitis B should be obtained, and if suggestive, hepatitis B serologies should be ordered.

Varicella (chickenpox) is a highly contagious disease caused by primary infection with varicella-zoster virus (VZV). It is usually a mild, self-limited disease in immunocompetent children. Its severity can range from a few lesions and a low-grade fever to hundreds of lesions and a temperature up to 105°F

(40.6°C). Fatal disseminated disease may occur in immunocompromised children or in neonates whose mothers develop the infection within 1 week of delivery. Adolescents and adults often have a more severe clinical course. After an incubation period of 10 to 21 days, there is a prodrome consisting of mild fever, malaise, anorexia, and occasionally a scarlatiniform or morbilliform rash. The characteristic pruritic rash occurs the following day, appearing first on the trunk and then spreading peripherally. The rash begins as red papules which develop rapidly into clear vesicles that are approximately 1 to 2 mm in diameter (the so-called "dewdrop on a rose petal"). The vesicles then become cloudy, rupture, and form crusts (Fig. 5-1). The lesions occur in widely scattered "crops," so several stages are usually present at the same time. Vesicles often are present on mucous membranes as well. Patients are infectious from 24 hours before the appearance of the rash until all the lesions are crusted, which usually occurs 1 week after the onset of the rash.

Chickenpox is a clinical diagnosis. In unclear cases, a Tzanck test, looking for multinucleated giant cells, can be performed on a vesicle, or a pharyngeal swab or swab of vesicular fluid can be sent for viral culture. Most centers now perform direct fluorescent antibody (DFA) testing, which can rapidly identify the presence of infected cells. Other confirmatory techniques include viral culture for varicella (which may take as long as a week) and polymerase chain reaction (PCR) testing. Progressive varicella with meningoencephalitis, hepatitis, and pneumonitis may occur in immunocompromised children and is associated with a 20% mortality rate. Immunization with varicella vaccine has significantly reduced the frequency of this infection in the United States.

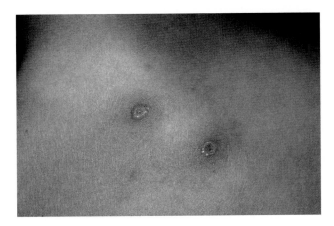

Figure 5-1 • Ruptured, crusted vesicles from varicella.
(Image courtesy of Dr. Anne W. Lucky.)

Treatment of varicella is supportive and includes antipyretics and daily bathing to reduce the risk of secondary bacterial infection. In some patients, ibuprofen has been associated with an increased risk of streptococcal cellulitis when given in the setting of primary varicella. Pruritus can be treated with oral antihistamines. Immunocompromised children who are exposed to VZV are given varicella-zoster immune globulin within 96 hours of the exposure and observed closely. Administration of the varicella vaccine within 72 hours of exposure may prevent or lessen disease severity.

Herpes zoster (shingles) represents a reactivation of VZV infection and occurs predominantly in adults who previously have had varicella and have circulating antibodies. However, if varicella occurs early in life, the risk for shingles in childhood is higher. After primary infection, VZV retreats to the dorsal root ganglia; as a result, it follows a dermatomal distribution when reactivated. Although herpes zoster occurs in children, it is uncommon in healthy children less than 10 years of age. An attack of zoster begins with pain and/or pruritus along the affected sensory nerve and is accompanied by fever and malaise. A vesicular eruption then appears in crops confined to the dermatomal distribution and clears in 7 to 14 days. Typical of all herpes virus infections, the lesions are grouped vesicles on an erythematous base (Color Plate 10). The rash may last as long as 4 weeks, with pain persisting for weeks or months. Other complications from herpes virus include encephalopathy, aseptic meningitis, Guillain-Barré syndrome, pneumonitis, thrombocytopenic purpura, cellulitis, and arthritis.

Herpes zoster can be quite painful, and narcotics are sometimes needed. Systemic administration of antivirals, such as acyclovir, may be considered for use in immunocompromised patients, patients older than 12 years, children with chronic disease, and those who have received systemic steroids for any reason.

Molluscum contagiosum is a cutaneous viral infection caused by a poxvirus and is very common in childhood. It is manifested by small, flesh-colored, pearly, umbilicated, dome-shaped papules in moist areas such as the axillae, buttocks, and groin region, but can appear anywhere (Fig. 5-2). The papules spread via touching, auto-inoculation, and scratching. They are often seen in wrestlers and sauna bathers. Lesions may resolve spontaneously over one to two years, but families typically request treatment sooner. Treatment depends on the experience of the practitioner and includes curettage, crythotherapy, cantharidin (an extract from the blister beetle that causes blistering of the epidermis), oral cimetidine, and imiquimod cream.

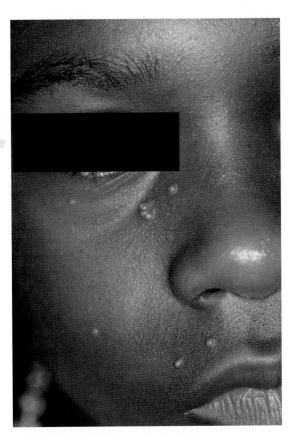

Figure 5-2 • Molluscum on the face. Note how the lesions have central umbilication.
(Image courtesy of Dr. Anne W. Lucky.)

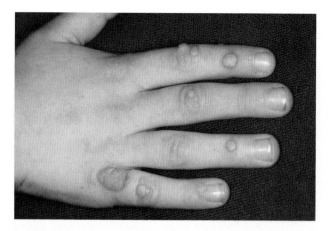

Figure 5-3 • Verruca vulgaris on the dorsal surface of the digits. (Image courtesy of Dr. Anne W. Lucky.)

Verrucae, commonly known as warts, are caused by the human papillomavirus (HPV). Warts are typically benign in otherwise healthy individuals and are spread by skin-to-skin contact or fomites. They may also develop at sites of trauma. There are four common types including verruca vulgaris (common wart) (Fig. 5-3), verruca plantaris (plantar wart), verruca plana (flat wart), and condyloma accuminata (genital warts). Treatment of warts in the pediatric population is based on the type and location of the wart and includes topical salicylic acid, liquid nitrogen, imiquimod cream, oral cimetidine, intralesional *Candida* antigen, and squaric acid dibutylester. Patients may require multiple treatments, especially in the case of recalcitrant warts.

PROBABLE VIRAL EXANTHEMS

Pityriasis Rosea is an exanthem of unknown etiology, but a viral prodrome, often upper respiratory in nature, is sometimes found in the history. The rash has a distinct morphology that typically begins with a herald patch, a 2 to 10 cm oval salmon-pink plaque on the trunk, neck, upper extremities, or thigh (Color Plate 11). This is followed by several smaller lesions distributed in a "Christmas tree pattern" over the trunk and upper extremities that develop over days to weeks. The lesions often have a "collarette" of scale which may cause the lesions to be confused with tinea corporis. Some patients develop lesions with a more papular appearance, especially younger children and African-Americans. The rash fades over four to twelve weeks and is typically asymptomatic in most patients but can be pruritic in some. Usually, pityriasis rosea is self-limited, and no treatment is needed. Topical and oral antihistamines as well as mild topical steroids can be used for pruritus. Sunlight has been shown to hasten resolution of the lesions.

Unilateral thoracic exanthem (asymmetric periflexural exanthem of childhood) is a rash with varying morphologies that occurs in children ages 1 to 5 years and begins as an exanthem on one side of the trunk that spreads centripetally. The rash is seen more commonly in the winter and spring months and may follow symptoms of low-grade fever, lymphadenopathy, respiratory, or gastrointestinal complaints. A viral etiology has been presumed, although no specific virus has been implicated. Often confused with contact dermatitis, the lesions vary from erythematous macules or papules with a surrounding halo to morbilliform, eczematous, scarlatiniform or reticulate configurations that may spread to the opposite side from initial involvement (Fig. 5-4). Pruritus is common and can

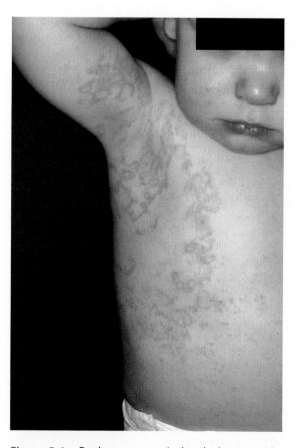

Figure 5-4 • Erythematous reticulated plaques with central clearing and scattered erythematous papules involving the right trunk and periflexural region following a viral URI. The lesions subsequently desquamated before resolving completely over several weeks.
(Image courtesy of Dr. Anne W. Lucky.)

be treated in the same manner as pityriasis rosea-associated pruritus. Lesions resolve over 6 to 8 weeks without treatment and may desquamate or leave post-inflammatory pigment changes.

SKIN MANIFESTATIONS OF BACTERIAL INFECTIONS

Bacterial infections of the skin are common, and in most cases they are the result of group A β-hemolytic streptococcal or *Staphylococcus aureus* (*S. aureus*) infection.

Bullous impetigo, which is caused by a toxin-producing strain of *S. aureus*, begins as red macules that progress to bullous (fluid-filled) eruptions on an erythematous base (as seen on Color Plate 12). These lesions range from a few millimeters to a few centimeters in diameter. After the bullae rupture, a clear, thin, varnish-like coating forms over the denuded area. *S. aureus* can be cultured from the vesicular fluid. Bullous impetigo lesions can be mistaken for cigarette burns, raising the suspicion of abuse.

Nonbullous impetigo, which is caused by both group A β-hemolytic streptococci and *S. aureus*, begins as papules that progress to vesicles and then to pustules measuring approximately 5 mm in diameter with a thin erythematous rim. The pustules rupture, leaving a honey-colored thin exudate that then forms a crust over a shallow ulcerated base (Color Plate 13). Local lymphadenopathy is common with streptococcal impetigo. Fever is uncommon. The causative organism can usually be isolated from the lesions.

Limited nonbullous impetigo can be treated topically with topical antibiotics such as mupirocin ointment. If the lesions of bullous and nonbullous impetigo are numerous, they can be treated with a first-generation cephalosporin such as cephalexin, an oral drug that is effective against both *Staphylococci* and group A *Streptococcus*. In settings where methicillin-resistant *S. aureus* (MRSA) is suspected, agents such as clindamycin or trimethoprim-sulfamethoxazole may be more appropriate. The caretaker can remove any honey-colored crusts with twice-daily cool compresses.

Staphylococcal scalded skin syndrome (SSSS), which is caused by exfoliative toxin-producing isolates of *S. aureus*, is most common in infancy and rarely occurs beyond 5 years of age. Onset is abrupt, with diffuse erythema, marked skin tenderness, irritability, and fever. Within 12 to 24 hours of onset, superficial flaccid bullae develop and then rupture almost immediately, leaving a beefy red, weeping surface (Color Plate 14). Although widespread areas may be affected, accentuation is seen on periorificial areas of the face, as well as flexural areas around the neck, axillae, and inguinal creases. Exfoliation is caused by a toxin and may affect most of the body. There is usually a positive Nikolsky sign (separation of the epidermis after light rubbing). The initial focus of staphylococcal infection may be minor such as conjunctivitis or rhinitis or inapparent. Unruptured bullae contain sterile fluid.

Mild to moderate cases of SSSS are treated with an oral antistaphylococcal medication. Children with severe cases should be treated as though they have a second-degree burn, with meticulous fluid management and intravenous oxacillin or clindamycin.

Folliculitis is an infection of the shaft of the hair follicle, usually with *S. aureus*. Superficial folliculitis is common and easily treated. The buttocks and the lower legs in girls who shave are frequent sites of infection. Deep forms of this infection include furuncles (boils) and carbuncles. Furuncles begin as superficial folliculitis and are most frequently found in areas of hair-bearing skin that are subject to friction and maceration, especially the scalp, buttocks, and axillae. Carbuncles are larger accumulations of furuncles.

Superficial folliculitis responds to aggressive hygiene with antiseptic cleansers and topical mupirocin. Folliculitis of the male beard is unusually recalcitrant and requires an oral anti-staphylococcal drug. Simple furunculosis is treated with moist heat. Larger and deeper furuncles, which are becoming increasingly more common in the community (particularly with the spread of MRSA), may need to be incised and drained. Antibiotic therapy following incision and drainage is under debate. Rarely, folliculitis can be caused by *Pseudomonas aeuroginosa* in the specific setting of bathing in contaminated hot tubs. These lesions are self-limited when the exposure is discontinued.

SUPERFICIAL FUNGAL INFECTIONS

Essentially, two fungal species cause the most common superficial infections: *Trichophyton* and *Microsporum*, although *Trichophyton tonsurans* is the most common cause of **tinea capitis** in the United States. *Microsporum canis* is also common and is spread from animals. On the scalp, tinea capitis manifests as patches of scaling and hair loss, broken off hairs known as "black dots,"

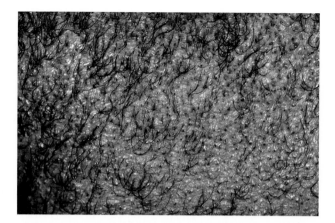

Figure 5-5 • Tinea capitis causing characteristic "black dot" alopecia.
(Image courtesy of Dr. Anne W. Lucky.)

(Fig. 5-5) and boggy, pustular masses known as kerions. The latter can be associated with pain, itching, a diffuse morbilliform eruption, and lymphadenopathy. On the skin, **tinea corporis** frequently manifests as annular plaques with peripheral scaling, giving the appearance of rings (hence the name "ring-worm"). **Tinea pedis**, usually an infection with *Microsporum rubrum* classically presents as scaling in a "moccasin" distribution, and frequently also involves the interdigital spaces of the toes. **Tinea cruris**, also caused by *Microsporum rubrum*, presents with erythema, scaling, and maceration in inguinal creases. Most superficial skin infections can be treated with topical antifungal agents. However, systemic antifungal drugs are necessary to eradicate dermatophyte infections of the nails or hair. Table 5-1 presents tinea infections and their treatments.

Tinea (pityriasis) versicolor is caused by infection with a yeast, *Malassezia furfur*, and is characterized by superficial tan or hypopigmented oval scaly patches on the neck, upper part of the back, chest, and upper arms. Dark-skinned individuals tend to have hypopigmented lesions during the summer when uninfected skin tans from sunlight exposure. However, individual patients may demonstrate both dark- and light-colored lesions at the same time (hence the name versicolor). Treatment includes selenium sulfide shampoo or other topical or systemic antifungal agents. Recurrence in the summertime is common.

Diaper rash may result from atopic dermatitis, primary irritant dermatitis, or primary or secondary *Candida albicans* infection. Eighty percent of diaper rashes lasting more than 4 days are colonized with *Candida*. Fiery red papular lesions with peripheral papules, pustules, and scales in the skin folds and satellite lesions are typical for candidal diaper rash. Barrier creams along with topical antifungal or nystatin creams are the first-line treatments of choice.

ACNE VULGARIS

Acne vulgaris is a very common, self-limited, multifactorial disorder of the sebaceous follicles noted during the teenage years. Lesions may begin as early as 8 to 10 years of age. Prevalence increases steadily throughout adolescence and then decreases in adulthood. Although girls often develop acne at a younger age than boys, severe disease affects boys ten times more frequently because of higher androgen levels. In fact, 15% of all teenage boys have severe acne (Fig. 5-6).

The **pathogenesis** of acne includes multiple factors such as androgen stimulation of the sebaceous glands, follicular plugging, proliferation of *Propionibacterium acnes* (*P. acnes*), and inflammatory changes. There is a predilection for the sebaceous follicle-rich areas of the face, chest, and back. Closed comedones (whiteheads), and open comedones (blackheads) are noninflammatory and nonscarring. Pustules, papules, and nodules (formerly called cysts) are inflammatory and

TABLE 5-1 Common Tinea Infections and Their Treatments	
Infection	**Treatment**
Tinea capitis (scalp)	Oral griseofulvin, 4 to 6 wks
	Selenium sulfide shampoo to kill spores; does not eradicate infection
Tinea corporis (body)	Topical antifungals (e.g., clotrimazole) for at least 4 wks; oral griseofulvin if refractory
Tinea cruris (genitocrural) "jock itch"	Same as tinea corporis
Tinea pedis ("athlete's foot")	Same as tinea corporis, plus proper foot hygiene

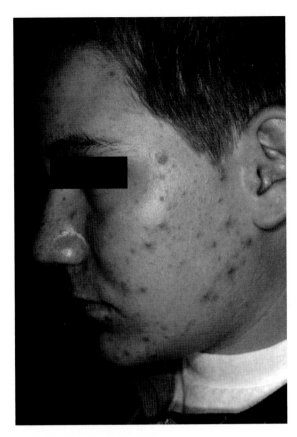

Figure 5-6 • Typical inflammatory acne lesions.
(Image courtesy of Dr. Anne W. Lucky.)

A thorough **physical examination** including distribution, morphology, and severity of lesions should be recorded. The back and chest should be examined and treated as well as the face. Severe inflammatory and especially nodular acne may result in hypertrophic or pitted scarring.

Treatment should be individualized depending on the patient's gender and the severity, type, and distribution of lesions. Mild acne generally responds to topical therapy without scarring. Benzoyl peroxide works by decreasing the colonization of *P. acnes*. Topical retinoids (e.g., tretinoin, adapalene, and tazarotene) have strong anticomedogenic activity; however, side effects may limit use and include dryness, burning, and, most important, photosensitivity by reducing the thickness of the stratum corneum layer. The use of sunscreen with a sun protective factor (SPF) of at least 15 is necessary. Topical antibiotics (clindamycin and erythromycin) are used to prevent and decrease colonization of *P. acnes*, but their sole use for acne treatment promotes bacterial resistance. Topical antibiotics are also available in combination with benzoyl peroxide, which prevents bacterial resistance. There is growing resistance to antibiotic therapy for acne, and oral antibiotics should be used in severely affected patients or those who do not respond to conventional topical therapy. The systemic antibiotics used include tetracycline, doxycycline, minocycline, and erythromycin. In females, oral contraceptives may also be helpful by suppressing androgen production and are now approved for acne therapy. Oral isotretinoin is very effective for acne, but because of its teratogenicity and high adverse effect profile, strict monitoring is needed. Isotretinoin is usually prescribed by a dermatologist. See Figure 5-7 for a guide to acne therapy.

PSORIASIS

Psoriasis is a common but often undiagnosed childhood disease with 10% of cases beginning before 10 years of age, and 35% before 20 years of age. There is often a positive family history, and HLA inheritance is part of the mode of transmission.

This non-pruritic, papulosquamous eruption consists of erythematous papules that coalesce to form dry plaques with sharply demarcated borders and silvery scales. The scales tend to build up into layers, and their removal may result in pinpoint bleeding (**Auspitz sign**). Psoriasis often appears at sites of physical, thermal, or mechanical trauma. This is known as the **Koebner phenomenon**, a diagnostic feature of the dis-

carry the potential for scarring. Atrophic and hypertrophic scars or keloids may occur. At puberty, there is androgen-dependent sebaceous follicle stimulation leading to increased sebum production. Female patients with severe acne often have high levels of circulating androgens.

Risk factors include family history and puberty. In girls, **polycystic ovary syndrome** (PCOS) is a common underlying factor. Rarely, Cushing disease or any other condition that results in androgen excess can predispose to acne. Poor hygiene and food intake are NOT risk factors for acne.

It is important to obtain a good **medical history** including when the acne started and whether there is a family history of acne. A full menstrual history should be taken to determine whether there is a hormonal pattern to flares associated with the menstrual cycle. It is also important to discuss the patient's skin care, including how the patient's acne has been treated in the past, and any medications the patient is currently taking because some drugs can cause or exacerbate acne.

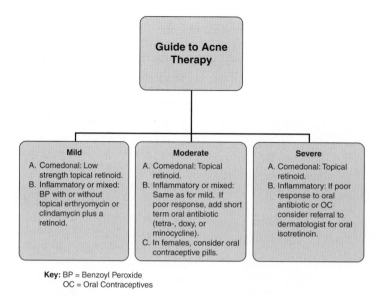

Guide to Acne Therapy

Mild
A. Comedonal: Low strength topical retinoid.
B. Inflammatory or mixed: BP with or without topical erthryomycin or clindamycin plus a retinoid.

Moderate
A. Comedonal: Topical retinoid.
B. Inflammatory or mixed: Same as for mild. If poor response, add short term oral antibiotic (tetra-, doxy, or minocycline).
C. In females, consider oral contraceptive pills.

Severe
A. Comedonal: Topical retinoid.
B. Inflammatory: If poor response to oral antibiotic or OC consider referral to dermatologist for oral isotretinoin.

Key: BP = Benzoyl Peroxide
OC = Oral Contraceptives

Figure 5-7 • Therapy for mild, moderate, and severe acne.
BP = Benzoyl Peroxide
OC = Oral Contraceptive

ease. It is usually symmetric, with plaques appearing over the knees, elbows, and in childhood, the scalp, periocular, and genital areas. The nails often demonstrate punctate stippling or pitting, distal detachment of the nail plate (onycholysis), and accumulation of subungual debris. Examination of the palms and soles reveals scaling and fissuring.

Psoriatic arthritis may also be present in a subset of patients. Occasionally, atopic dermatitis may be confused with psoriasis; however, eczema is often pruritic and concentrated in flexural creases, whereas psoriasis is not usually pruritic and favors extensor surfaces. Scalp lesions may be confused with seborrheic dermatitis or tinea capitis.

Psoriasis is characterized by remissions and exacerbations. Group A β-hemolytic streptococcal infections are a common exacerbating cause of psoriasis in a genetically-susceptible individual. The most important aspect of treating psoriasis is to educate the patient and family that the disease is chronic and recurrent. It cannot be cured but can be controlled with conscientious therapy. No matter the location or severity of the rash, the goal of psoriasis therapy is to keep the skin well-hydrated. Topical steroids are the mainstay of therapy; the least potent but effective dose should be used because adrenal suppression can occur. Topical vitamin D cream and tar can also be helpful. For more severe cases, natural sunlight or ultraviolet B (UVB) light is useful. In severe cases, methotrexate and biological immunosuppressants such as etanercept can be tried under supervision of a dermatologist.

ERUPTIONS SECONDARY TO ALLERGIC REACTIONS

Atopic dermatitis, urticaria, and angioedema are discussed in Chapter 11.

ERYTHEMA MULTIFORME

Erythema multiforme is an acute, self-limited, hypersensitivity reaction that is uncommon in children. The most frequent etiologic agents include viral infections such as herpesvirus, adenovirus, and Epstein-Barr virus.

Clinical Manifestations

In erythema multiforme (EM), a symmetric distribution of lesions evolves through multiple morphologic stages: erythematous macules, papules, plaques, vesicles, and target lesions. The lesions evolve over days, not hours and often have a target-like appearance. Erythema multiforme is often confused with polycyclic urticaria which also can appear targetoid, but urticarial lesions are not fixed and do not have necrotic centers. Urticarial lesions tend to have edematous, erythematous borders with central clearing, and individual lesions resolve within 12 to 24 hours. In contrast, lesions in EM are typically fixed and develop dusky, necrotic centers. EM lesions also tend to occur over the dorsum of the hands and feet, palms and soles, and extensor surfaces of extremities, but may spread to the trunk. Burning and itching are common. Systemic manifestations include fever, malaise, and myalgias. The most common cause of recurrent erythema multiforme in children is herpes simplex virus type I.

Stevens-Johnson syndrome (SJS) is a distinct hypersensitivity reaction and a variant of toxic epidermal necrolysis. There is a prodrome for 1 to 14 days of fever, malaise, myalgias, arthralgias, arthritis, headache, emesis, and diarrhea. This is followed by the sudden onset of high fever, erythematous and purpuric macules with dusky centers, and inflammatory bullae of two or more mucous membranes (oral mucosa, lips, bulbar conjunctiva, and anogenital area; Color Plate 15). In the most severe cases, involvement of most of the gastrointestinal, respiratory, or genitourinary tracts may be seen. Untreated, this syndrome has a mortality rate of approximately 10%. The most common causes of SJS include drugs such as nonsteroidal anti-inflammatory drugs, penicillins, sulfonamides, and many anti-epileptic medications, mycoplasma infections, and (less likely) immunizations.

Toxic epidermal necrolysis (TEN) is the most severe form of cutaneous hypersensitivity, and likely a more severe variant of SJS. Although its occurrence in children is rare, it is associated with a 30% mortality rate. The pathogenesis appears to be related to upregulated expression of Fas ligand, a mediator of apoptosis. The etiology is similar to SJS. Onset is acute, with high fever, a burning sensation of the skin and mucous membranes, and/or oral and conjunctival erythema and erosions. The presentation of the skin resembles that of staphylococcal scalded skin, with widespread erythema, tenderness, blister formation, and full detachment of the epidermis causing denudation (positive Nikolsky sign). Mucous membrane involvement is severe, and the nails may be shed. Systemic complications include elevated liver enzymes, renal failure, and fluid and electrolyte imbalance. Sepsis and shock are frequent causes of death.

Treatment

For uncomplicated erythema multiforme, symptomatic treatment and reassurance are all that are necessary. Oral antihistamines, moist compresses, and oatmeal baths are helpful. The lesions resolve over a 1- to 3-week period, with some hyperpigmentation. The use of corticosteroids is controversial. Treatment of the patient with SJS includes hospitalization with barrier isolation, fluid and electrolyte support, treatment of common secondary infections of the skin, moist compresses on bullae, and colloidal baths. For oral mucosal lesions, mouthwashes with viscous lidocaine, diphenhydramine, and Maalox (aluminum hydroxide, magnesium hydroxide) are comforting. Because corneal ulceration, keratitis, uveitis, and panophthalmitis are possible, an ophthalmology consultation is recommended. Children with toxic epidermal necrolysis are treated as though they had a full-body second-degree burn. Fluid therapy and reverse barrier isolation are critical to survival; many patients are treated in an intensive care or burn center unit. Intravenous immunoglobulin has been used with some success in several series of patients with TEN, presumably because of its effects of binding or modulating the effect of Fas ligand.

ALLERGIC DRUG REACTIONS

Allergic reactions to drugs typically present as urticarial or morbilliform exanthems which can develop within 1 to 2 weeks of starting a new medication. The risk of an allergic drug reaction may be increased if the patient has a concurrent viral illness similar to patients with mononucleosis treated with ampicillin. The eruption may clear after the inciting agent is removed, but it may take several days to weeks. Following the acute eruption, many patients tend to desquamate. Treatment is based on symptoms. The decision to discontinue the medication is based on the risks and benefits of the need for treatment in the primary illness, and possible alternative medications.

HYPERPIGMENTED LESIONS

With the incidence of melanoma increasing, it is very important to identify suspicious lesions and understand risk factors. Children with fair skin, excessive sun exposure, and multiple nevi are at increased risk for both melanoma and nonmelanoma skin cancer such as basal cell and squamous cell carcinomas.

Congenital nevi are usually larger than acquired nevi and can vary considerably in color and shape. They tend to get darker, thicker, and hairier with time, although giant nevi often will become lighter. Congenital nevi are classified based on their size. Large or giant nevi are greater than 20 cm^2 (see Fig. 5-8), small nevi are less than 2 cm^2, and intermediate nevi are in between in size. Although there is controversy about the magnitude, large and medium-sized congenital nevi appear to have an increased risk of developing melanoma. Congenital nevi must be followed annually for changes and may require complete excision. The increased lifetime risk of melanoma in giant nevi is estimated to be between 5% and 15%. There is also an association with neurocutaneous melanosis; thus patients with large lesions over the head and spine, or with multiple associated satellite nevi, require an MRI of the brain and spinal cord to evaluate for central nervous system (CNS) involvement. Any nevi over the sacral spine may indicate underlying spinal abnormalities, especially tethered cord.

Many children develop **acquired nevi** during infancy and childhood, reaching a maximum number in early adulthood. Patients with more than 15 common acquired moles may have an increased risk for melanoma in the future. Nevi need to be assessed by using the ABCD rules: watching for Asymmetry, irregular Borders, variations in Color, and Diameter larger than 6 mm. Nevi that change rapidly or exhibit atypical features may need to be excised.

A **Spitz** (spindle and epithelial cell) nevus is a smooth pink to brown to jet black dome-shaped papule which usually enlarges rapidly after its appearance. These nevi are usually benign but may need to be removed if they grow rapidly as malignant forms have been reported rarely.

Halo nevi are moles which develop up to 1 cm depigmented surrounding rings. These represent an immune reaction against the pigment cells. Halo nevi may completely regress, leaving a white macule that eventually fills in. They are generally benign in children but may be associated with the presence of vitiligo or melanoma at another site.

Prevention

A large amount of childhood sun exposure and frequent sunburns are associated with increased risk for the development of moles and skin cancer. Sun protection with a sunblock having an SPF of 15 or more against UVB and ultraviolet A (UVA) light is recommended. Re-applying sunscreen during exposure, avoiding long periods of sun exposure in mid-day, and sun-protective clothing are equally important for adequate protection.

INFANTILE HEMANGIOMAS

Infantile hemangiomas are vascular tumors which are common in infancy, noted in 1% to 2% of neonates. They are more common in females, Caucasians, and premature infants. They are classified as superficial, deep, or mixed, and are generally not present at birth. Superficial hemangiomas are bright red and noncompressible, whereas deep hemangiomas are subcutaneous, compressible, and often have a bluish hue and superficial telangiectasias. Mixed lesions have characteristics of both superficial and deep hemangiomas (Color Plate 16). Infantile hemangiomas can be found in any location but are commonly seen on the head and neck. Hemangiomas must be distinguished from more aggressive vascular tumors, such as hemangioendotheliomas, and from vascular malformations which may involve capillaries, veins, arteries, lymphatics, or combinations of these. Vascular malformations tend not to resolve and become more troublesome with time.

The evolution of infantile hemangiomas is generally predictable. They present during the first month of life, maintain a period of growth over the next several months to a year, and then begin to slowly involute. Involution is marked by decreasing size and change in color from a bright to duller red or purple to grey. Involution may take many years; however most lesions typically resolve by 10 years of age. There may be residual textural change in the skin or superficial telangiectasias.

Treatment is based on individual findings including: size, location, overlying changes, and rate of growth. The most common management is to provide anticipatory guidance and support to the family while following the lesion on a regular basis.

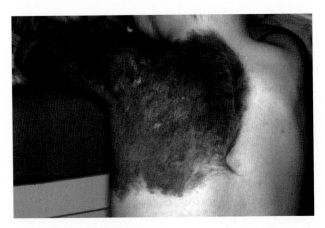

Figure 5-8 • Giant congenital (hairy) nevus on the back. (Image courtesy of Dr. Anne W. Lucky.)

Lesions requiring active intervention are those that pose life-threatening or functional risks. Large hemangiomas may cause heart failure; lesions involving the airway may cause obstruction; periocular lesions are mandatory to treat to prevent astigmatism or blindness; facial lesions may produce severe disfigurement or interfere with eating; genital and perianal lesions may ulcerate and cause significant pain; lumbosacral lesions may indicate underlying spinal abnormalities; and multiple (greater than 5) lesions may be associated with liver and other internal hemangiomas.

Treatment varies with each situation, but may include local or systemic corticosteroids, antibiotics and dressings, or excision where indicated. Laser treatment has a limited role, often helping with ulcerations. In severe cases, vincristine or alpha interferon may be necessary.

KEY POINTS

- Children with chickenpox are contagious from 24 hours before the onset of rash until all lesions have crusted over.
- *Staphylococcus aureus* and Group A β-hemolytic *Streptococcus* cause most bacterial skin infections.
- *Trichophyton tonsurans* is the most common cause of tinea capitis.
- Severe inflammatory and nodular acne are associated with scarring.
- Acne is best treated with combination therapy, and choice of therapy depends on the type of acne.
- Psoriasis can be treated but not be cured, and is characterized by remissions and exacerbations, often following streptococcal infections. Psoriasis occurs at skin points of repeated trauma, and the rash is nonpruritic.
- Erythema multiforme is most commonly caused by herpes simplex virus type I.
- Nevi need to be assessed for change as well as asymmetry, irregular borders, color, and size.
- Sun protection against ultraviolet B and A (UVB and UVA) light is recommended to decrease the risk of melanoma as well as nonmelanoma skin cancer.
- Infantile hemangiomas are vascular tumors that appear in the first month of life and often regress without treatment over several years of life.

Endocrinology

Deborah Elder • Stuart Handwerger • Bradley S. Marino

DIABETES MELLITUS

Diabetes mellitus (DM) is a chronic metabolic disorder characterized by hyperglycemia and abnormal energy metabolism due to diminished or absent insulin secretion or action at the cellular level.

TYPE 1 DIABETES MELLITUS

Pathogenesis

Type 1 diabetes mellitus (T1DM) is a chronic metabolic disorder characterized by autoimmune **destruction** of pancreatic beta-cells resulting in hyperglycemia and abnormal energy metabolism caused by absent or diminished insulin secretion. Although the precise trigger of T1DM is unknown, genetic, autoimmune, and environmental factors have all been implicated.

After 90% of beta-cell function has been destroyed, loss of insulin secretion becomes clinically significant, resulting in hyperglycemia. With the loss of insulin (the major anabolic hormone), a catabolic state develops which decreases peripheral glucose utilization and increases hepatic glucose production through gluconeogenesis and glycogenolysis. The lack of insulin prevents glucose from entering the cell, and hyperglycemia results. The production of ketoacids is brought about by an increase in the catabolic mediators glucagon, epinephrine, growth hormone (GH), and cortisol. These messengers trigger lipolysis, fatty acid release, and ketoacid synthesis. When the blood glucose concentration exceeds 180 mg/dL, the resultant glycosuria causes an osmotic diuresis with increased urine output (polyuria). If insulin deficiency is

severe, ketones are produced in significant quantities, the blood's native buffering capacity is overwhelmed, and **diabetic ketoacidosis** (DKA) results.

DKA is characterized by hyperglycemia, metabolic acidosis (ketoacidosis), dehydration, and lethargy. It is a medical emergency that, in severe cases, may progress to coma and death. The most common cause of DKA in the known diabetic is inadequate insulin dosing. The condition may also be triggered by insulin resistance, which is exacerbated by an intercurrent illness or extreme physiologic stress. Frequently, new-onset diabetics present in DKA. The most severe complication of DKA management is cerebral edema.

In addition to DKA, the other major complication seen in T1DM is hypoglycemia from insulin overdose, decreased caloric intake, or increased exercise without a concomitant increase in calories.

Epidemiology and Risk Factors

T1DM is the most common endocrine disease in childhood. The overall prevalence of T1DM is 0.25% to 0.5% of the population or 1/400 children and 1/200 adults in the United States. Peak age of onset is 10 to 12 years, but the disease may be diagnosed in children less than 1 year of age. Males and females are equally affected. T1DM accounts for 10% of all diabetes cases diagnosed. The main risk factor for T1DM is a positive family history. The presence of DR3 and DR4 major histocompatibility antigens increases the lifetime risk for an individual developing T1DM, as does having a first-degree relative with T1DM. There is a 50% concordance rate among identical twins. The presence of **anti-islet cell antibodies in 85%** of individuals with recent-onset DM and the increased incidence of other autoimmune diseases in children with T1DM suggest an autoimmune etiology. The environmental role in disease pathogenesis remains unclear. No particular virus has been determined to be directly responsible.

Clinical Manifestations

History and Physical Examination

A history of new-onset weight loss, polydipsia, polyphagia, and polyuria is consistent with T1DM. The physical examination is generally normal in T1DM unless DKA is present.

When DKA is suspected in a child with known T1DM, important historical information includes the usual insulin dose, the last insulin dose, the child's diet over the previous day, and whether the child has been ill and emotionally or physically stressed. The child with DKA appears acutely ill and suffers from moderate to profound dehydration. Symptoms include polyuria, polydipsia, fatigue, headache, nausea, emesis, and abdominal pain. The child's mental status may vary from confused to comatose. On physical examination, tachycardia and hyperpnea (Kussmaul respirations) are generally noted. There may be a fruity odor to the breath because of the ketosis. Intravascular volume depletion may be so marked that hypotension is present. Although cerebral edema is uncommon, it frequently is fatal. Changing mental status, unequal pupils, decorticate or decerebrate posturing, and/or seizures indicate cerebral edema. Early identification and aggressive management of increased intracranial pressure are pivotal to improve outcome.

Symptoms of hypoglycemia are caused by catecholamine release (trembling, diaphoresis, flushing, and tachycardia) and to cerebral glucopenia (sleepiness, confusion, mood changes, seizures, and coma).

Differential Diagnosis

Secondary diabetes may occur when there is insulin antagonism from excess glucocorticoids (Cushing syndrome or iatrogenic), hyperthyroidism, pheochromocytoma, GH excess, or with medications such as thiazide diuretics.

Other forms of diabetes include: (i) **cystic fibrosis-related diabetes** (CFRD) resulting from beta-cell destruction from auto-digestion of the pancreas and chronic inflammation, and (ii) **maturity-onset diabetes of the young** (MODY), a clinically heterogeneous group of disorders characterized by nonketotic diabetes inherited in autosomal dominant fashion with onset before the age of 25. The primary abnormality in MODY results from a defect in one of six genes that are involved in insulin secretion (one encodes glucokinase [MODY2] and the other 5 are transcription factors).

Diagnostic Evaluation

Glucosuria, ketonuria, and a random plasma glucose level greater than 200 mg/dL are consistent with a diagnosis of diabetes mellitus. If early diabetes is suspected, a 2-hour postprandial blood glucose concentration is the first value to become abnormal. A fasting blood glucose concentration greater than 126 mg/dL and a 2-hour postprandial blood glucose concentration greater than 200 mg/dL are suggestive of diabetes. Islet cell antibodies in the serum may be found in 85% of new-onset insulin-dependent diabetics. Poorly controlled diabetics have high levels of glycosylated hemoglobin (HbA1c%).

In children with suspected DKA, the serum glucose concentration is grossly elevated, and the venous pH and serum PCO_2 are low. Metabolic acidosis from ketosis results in a diminished serum pH. The response to metabolic acidosis is a compensatory respiratory alkalosis and a drop in serum PCO_2. Because of the osmotic diuresis, blood urea nitrogen is elevated, and there is loss of phosphate, calcium, and potassium. Although there is a total body loss of potassium, serum potassium may be low, normal, or even high depending on the level of acidosis. When acidosis is present, protons move from the extracellular space to the intracellular space and potassium moves from the intracellular space to the extracellular space to maintain electroneutrality. Until the catabolic state is reversed with insulin, the urine is positive for ketones; until the serum concentration of glucose falls below 180 mg/dL, the urine is positive for glucose.

Treatment

The immediate goals of treatment of new-onset DM and DKA are reversal of the catabolic state through exogenous **insulin therapy** and restoration of **fluid** and electrolyte balances.

The child with T1DM is treated through insulin replacement, diet, exercise, psychological support, and regular medical follow-up. Patient education has a vital role. Current therapy requires frequent blood glucose monitoring and carbohydrate counting. The patient learns how to tailor insulin dosing based on the glucose level and the current meal. The newly diagnosed diabetic requires 0.5 to 1.0 units per kg of insulin per day. Most diabetics take insulin two to three times a day. Conventional therapy utilizes doses where two thirds of the total daily dose is given before breakfast and one third before dinner and bedtime. The human insulin is divided between short-acting Humalog insulin and intermediate-acting neutral protamine Hagedorn (NPH) insulin. Families are now attracted to "Basal-Bolus" methods of insulin administration where a basal insulin is administered (glargine) once each day and short acting insulin is given prior to carbohydrate consumption. This allows for a more flexible meal plan and schedule. Insulin pump therapy has now become available to deliver a basal amount of insulin throughout the day, with bolus doses of short-acting insulin given at mealtimes. At times of medical, surgical, or emotional stress, additional insulin may be needed. Glycosylated hemoglobin levels should be monitored every 3 months to assess average glycemic control.

If hypoglycemia occurs, a child may ingest a carbohydrate snack to increase the serum glucose concentration. If the child is vomiting, instant glucose or cake icing may be applied to the buccal mucosa to provide glucose. If the child is stuporous or having a seizure, intravenous glucose or intramuscular glucagon may be given.

DKA is a medical emergency. Initial fluid resuscitation consists of administering normal saline or a lactated Ringer solution of 10 mL per kg intravenous bolus. While the fluid bolus is running in, the total fluid deficit is calculated based on the amount of dehydration.

The fluid deficit should be replaced over a 48-hour period. The level of hyperglycemia is assessed, and an insulin drip is started at 0.1 U/kg/hour. The goal is to decrease the serum glucose 50 to 100 mg/dL/hour. A glucose level that falls too quickly could precipitate cerebral edema. When serum glucose approaches 250 to 300 mg per dL, dextrose should be added to normal saline and the electrolyte solution to avoid hypoglycemia. Hyperglycemia, acidosis, and ketone production correct with insulin therapy. Until there is adequate insulin, the body will continue to produce ketoacids. Frequent monitoring of blood glucose level, electrolytes, and acid-base status is crucial.

Prognosis

The Diabetes Control and Complications Trial demonstrated that intensive management and tight glycemic control reduce the risk of diabetes complications by 50% to 75%. Complications from diabetes include microvascular disease of the eye (retinopathy), kidney (nephropathy), and nerves (neuropathy). Microvascular disease is generally not observed until the child has been insulin dependent for a minimum of 10 years. Accelerated large vessel atherosclerotic disease may lead to myocardial infarction or stroke. Diabetic children should have annual urine collections to screen for microalbuminuria, annual ophthalmologic examinations, and annual screening for hyperlipidemia.

TYPE 2 DIABETES MELLITUS

Pathogenesis

Type 2 diabetes mellitus (T2DM) is a polygenic condition that results from relative insulin resistance and beta-cell dysfunction. This insulin resistance initially causes a compensatory increase in insulin secretion; however, with time there is a progressive decline in glucose-stimulated insulin secretion.

Epidemiology

T2DM now accounts for 10% to 40% of newly diagnosed diabetes in adolescents. The increasing incidence parallels the high prevalence of obesity. Most cases occur during early adolescence around the onset of puberty. Prevalence is highest in Native Americans (PIMA Indians), African Americans, and Hispanics but is seen in all ethnic groups. Genetic susceptibility is important; however, environmental factors, including obesity, physical inactivity, and diet, play a major role.

History and Physical Examination

Many patients are asymptomatic at presentation. Others may have symptoms similar to those of T1DM. There is usually a positive family history. On physical examination, obesity is noted, with a body mass index (BMI) usually greater than 30 kg/m^2. Often associated with T2DM is **acanthosis nigricans**, a skin condition involving hyperpigmentation and thickening of the skin folds, found primarily on the back of the neck and flexor areas.

Treatment

Currently, the mainstay of treatment is insulin therapy. In addition to medical therapy, lifestyle changes in diet and exercise are particularly important. Metformin is the only oral hypoglycemic agent used for the treatment of T2DM in children older than 10 years; other oral agents are primarily anecdotal. More research is needed in this area.

HYPOGLYCEMIA

The definition of hypoglycemia is a plasma glucose value of less than 50 mg/dL or a whole blood glucose level less than 60 mg/dL.

Etiology

Hypoglycemia may result from: (i) hyperinsulinism (congenital, insulinoma, exogenous administration of insulin or insulin secreting agents); (ii) ketotic hypoglycemia (childhood, age 18 months to 5 years, intolerance of fasting states, ketonuria usually present); (iii) hormone deficiency (ACTH with or without growth hormone deficiency); (iv) glycogen storage disease (glucose 6-phosphatase deficiency); (v) disorders of gluconeogenesis (hereditary fructose intolerance, fructose 1,6-diphosphatase deficiency); and/or (vi) defects in fatty acid oxidation.

Clinical Manifestation

Features of hypoglycemia can be classified into two categories. The first is activation of the autonomic nervous system causing a release of epinephrine, which manifests symptoms of sweating, shakiness, tachycardia, and anxiety. The second is of neuroglucopenic origin, resulting in headaches, visual disturbances, lethargy, irritability, mental confusion, loss of consciousness, and/or coma.

Evaluation

During a hypoglycemia event the circulating levels of certain hormones and other biomarkers of fuels can assess the integrity of the metabolic and hormonal systems. It is essential to obtain a "**critical sample**" when the plasma glucose level is less than 50 mg/dL. The critical sample should assess: a chemistry panel with bicarbonate, insulin, c-peptide, cortisol, growth hormone, free fatty acids, beta-hydroxybutyrate, acetoacetate, lactate, and ammonia.

A comparison of expected normal values to the critical sample is necessary to determine the etiology of hypoglycemia. In the fasting state of a normal individual, it would be expected for glycogen stores to be depleted and levels of gluconeogenic substrates, free fatty acids, and beta-hydroxybutyrate (the major ketone body) to rise significantly. GH and cortisol will be up-regulated during a fast and certainly elevated during a hypoglycemic event. Insulin levels should then decline to undetectable levels (<2 μU/mL).

Total and free carnitine, acyl carnitine profile, and serum amino acids should be collected in a nonfasting state.

DISORDERS OF WATER REGULATION

DIABETES INSIPIDUS

In **central** diabetes insipidus, there is loss of arginine vasopressin secretion (antidiuretic hormone) from the posterior pituitary gland which results in an inability to concentrate the urine. Diabetes insipidus may occur after head trauma or with a brain tumor or central nervous system (CNS) infection. Surgical interruption of the pituitary stalk during craniopharyngioma removal often results in diabetes insipidus. Only rarely is diabetes insipidus an isolated idiopathic disorder.

Clinical Manifestations

The child with diabetes insipidus has abrupt-onset polydipsia and polyuria. If water intake is inadequate, severe dehydration and hypernatremia occur. If the cause of the diabetes insipidus is a brain tumor impinging on the pituitary gland, focal neurologic signs and visual abnormalities may be noted.

The increased urine output may reach 5 to 10 L/day, with a urine specific gravity and urine osmolality that are quite low. Over time, serum sodium and serum osmolality increase as hemoconcentration occurs from free water loss. In unclear cases, the water deprivation test is used to document diabetes insipidus. To establish a diagnosis of diabetes insipidus, one must have dilute urine (specific gravity <1.010) and urine osmolality <300 mOsm/kg in the setting of hyper tonicity (hypernatremia and plasma osmolality >295 mOsm/kg). Demonstration of antidiuretic hormone (ADH) secretion is critical in differentiating

ADH-deficient (central) diabetes insipidus from nephrogenic diabetes insipidus, a rare X-linked recessive disease in which the collecting ducts do not respond to ADH (Chapter 14).

Treatment

Desmopressin acetate (DDAVP), an ADH analogue, is given intranasally, subcutaneously, or orally to stimulate the kidneys to retain water and reverse the polyuria, polydipsia, and hypernatremia.

SYNDROME OF HYPONATREMIA WITH INAPPROPRIATE INCREASED SECRETION OF VASOPRESSIN

Syndrome of hyponatremia with inappropriate increased secretion of vasopressin (SIADH) may be identified in children with encephalitis, brain tumors, head trauma, or psychiatric disease. Many drugs are capable of interfering with free water clearance (lisinopril, cabamazepine, tricyclic antidepressants, and others). Children with tuberculous meningitis and SIADH have a particualrly poor prognosis, as do those with liver failure and SIADH.

Clinical Manifestations

Patients present with normovolemic hyponatremia, relatively concentrated urine, and normal renal, thyroid, and adrenal function. Symptoms are related to the degree of hyponatremia and how rapid the hyponatremia progressed. A patient is unlikely to have symptoms with a sodium of >125 mEq/L. Headache, nausea, lethargy, and other CNS findings may occur when sodium falls ≤125 mEq/L.

Management

SIADH is a diagnosis of exclusion. Other causes of hyponatremia must be ruled out (hyperglycemia, increased serum lipids or protein). A serum osmolality <280 mOsm/kg combined with urine osmolality >200 mOsm and urine sodium concentration >20 mEq/L are consistent with SIADH. The patient should appear euvolemic.

Most cases of SIADH are self-limited, and the mode of management is **fluid restriction**. In a child, this involves limiting oral fluid intake to 1,000 mL/m^2/day. In a young child this may not provide sufficient calories for growth. Demeclocycline, which

produces a reversible nephrogenic diabetes insipidus, may also be utilized to treat SIADH, but only in chronic cases. Treatment for the acute symptomatic hyponatremia may be managed by the administration of hypertonic fluids. The goal is to raise the serum sodium level by 0.5 mEq/hour to a maximum of 12 mEq/L in the first 24 hours. Serum sodium should be monitored every 3 to 4 hours.

SHORT STATURE

Short stature is a common concern of parents. Normal causes include **familial (genetic) short stature** and **constitutional delay**. Eighty percent of cases of short stature are attributable to these two causes. Pathologic causes may result in either disproportionate or proportionate short stature. Etiologies that result in proportionate short stature are much more prevalent. Disorders that result in disproportionate short stature affect the long bones predominantly and include rickets, which is caused by activated vitamin D deficiency, and achondroplasia, an autosomal dominant disorder.

Diseases that cause proportionate short stature may result from either a prenatal or postnatal insult to the growth process. Prenatal etiologies include intrauterine growth retardation, placental dysfunction, intrauterine infections, teratogens, and chromosomal abnormalities. The most common chromosomal abnormalities that result in short stature are trisomy 21 and Turner syndrome. Postnatal causes include malnutrition, chronic systemic diseases, psychosocial deprivation, drugs, and endocrine disorders. Common endocrine defects that result in short stature include hypothyroidism, GH deficiency, and glucocorticoid excess and precocious puberty. Of note, with precocious puberty there is initial acceleration of growth; however, final adult height is compromised, leaving the individual with subsequent short stature compared to the genetic potential.

DIFFERENTIAL DIAGNOSIS

Children with familial short stature establish growth curves at or below the fifth percentile by 2 years of age. They are otherwise completely healthy, with normal physical examinations. These children have normal bone age values, and puberty occurs at the expected time. Short stature is usually found in at least one parent, but height inheritance is complex, and the diminutive ancestor may be more distant.

Children with constitutional delay of growth develop at or below the 5th percentile at normal growth velocities. This results in a curve parallel to the 5th percentile. Puberty is significantly delayed, which results in a delay in the bone age. Because these children fail to enter puberty at the usual age, their short stature and sexual immaturity are accentuated when their peers enter puberty. Family members are usually of average height, but there is often a history of short stature in childhood and delayed puberty. The parents of children with constitutional delay should be counseled that their child's growth is a normal variant and the child will likely mature to the height expected for their family.

GH deficiency accounts for approximately 5% of cases of short stature referred to endocrinologists. Children with classic GH deficiency grow at a diminished growth velocity (less than 5 cm per year) and have delayed skeletal maturation. A history of birth asphyxia, neonatal hypoglycemia, or physical findings of microphallus, cleft palate, or other midline defects are suggestive of idiopathic GH deficiency. GH deficiency secondary to hypothalamic or pituitary tumor usually is associated with other neurologic or visual impairments. In an older child with more recent onset of subnormal growth, the index of suspicion for a tumor should be high. Insulin-like growth factor-I (IGF-I) and its binding protein-3 (IGF-BP3) are used to screen for growth hormone deficiency. Formal GH testing with timed sampling for GH is indicated if these screening tests are low for age and pubertal status, or if clinical suspicion is high for GH deficiency.

Primary hypothyroidism causes marked growth failure through diminished growth velocity and skeletal maturation. Thyroxine (T4), free T4, triiodothyronine resin uptake (T3RU), thyroid-stimulating hormone (TSH), and thyroid antibodies should be measured (even in the absence of symptoms) to rule out any degree of hypothyroidism when evaluating short stature. Primary hypothyroidism is treated with levothyroxine (Synthroid).

Cushing disease is a rare cause of short stature. Hypercortisolism, from either exogenous steroid therapy or endogenous over-secretion, may have a profound growth-suppression effect. Usually, other stigmata of Cushing syndrome are present if growth suppression has occurred.

Chronic systemic diseases may result in short stature from lack of caloric absorption or increased metabolic demands. Cyanotic heart disease, cystic fibrosis, poorly controlled DM, chronic renal failure, human immunodeficiency (HIV) infection, and severe rheumatic illness are disorders that increase metabolic demands and diminish growth. Alternatively, inflammatory bowel disease, celiac sprue, and cystic fibrosis may reduce caloric absorption and produce short stature.

Some children who live in emotionally or physically abusive or neglectful environments develop functional GH deficiency. Children with psychosocial deprivation may have bizarre behaviors that include food hoarding, pica, and encopresis, as well as immature speech, disturbed sleep-wake cycles, and an increased pain tolerance. Clinically, they resemble children with primary GH deficiency, with marked retardation of bone age and pubertal delay. If GH testing is done while the child remains in the hostile environment, there is a blunted GH response; when the child is removed from the deprived environment, GH testing reverts to normal and catch-up growth is noted.

One of the manifestations of Turner syndrome (discussed in detail in Chapter 9) is short stature. The clinical manifestations of Turner syndrome may sometimes be subtle. Given that the incidence of Turner syndrome is 1 in 2,500 females, gonadotropins and karyotype testing are indicated in the female adolescent with short stature and delayed puberty. Elevated gonadotropins (indicating primary ovarian failure) and a 45,XO karyotype are diagnostic.

Chronic administration of certain medications may result in poor growth. Such drugs include steroids, dextroamphetamine (Dexedrine), and methylphenidate (Ritalin).

CLINICAL MANIFESTATIONS

History

Important historical information includes the child's prenatal and birth history, the pattern of growth, presence of chronic disease, long-term medication use, achievement of developmental milestones, and growth and pubertal patterns of the patient's parents and siblings. Evaluating the child's growth charts is vitally important. A thorough feeding history, including what, how, and by whom the child is fed, is also required.

Physical Examination

The majority of physical examinations performed on children with short stature are normal. It is critical to plot the child's height and weight on the appropriate growth curve for age. In addition to height, arm span and upper-to-lower-body segment ratio are measured to check for pathologic disproportionate causes of short stature and suggestive midline defects. In young children, the head circumference should also be evaluated to check for failure to thrive. In children with failure to thrive, weight and height are diminished, and the head circumference is often spared. When examining the child with short stature, the physician may find dysmorphic features in a pattern suggestive of a particular syndrome. The integument should be examined for cyanosis indicating potential congenital heart disease, abnormal pigmentation noted in Cushing syndrome, the stigmata of hypothyroidism, and bruises and poor hygiene indicative of psychosocial deprivation. The thyroid is palpated to determine its size, its consistency, and the presence of thyroid nodules. The lungs and heart are examined to identify chronic cardiopulmonary disease. Abdominal tenderness or bloating may indicate inflammatory bowel disease or celiac sprue. Tanner staging for both boys and girls must be documented to help differentiate among familial short stature, constitutional delay, and precocious puberty. A thorough neurologic and funduscopic examination may reveal underlying CNS disease resulting in GH deficiency.

DIAGNOSTIC EVALUATION

Because most cases of short stature result from either familial short stature or constitutional delay, diagnostic studies are generally not necessary unless abnormalities are found on examination. A bone age (anteroposterior radiograph of the left wrist) assessment helps delineate familial short stature from constitutional delay. An advanced bone age likely indicates precocious puberty; a normal bone age, familial short stature, and a delayed bone age, constitutional delay.

Thyroid function tests must be completed to evaluate for hypothyroidism. Urinalysis and renal function tests are needed to rule out chronic renal disease. A complete blood count with differential and an erythrocyte sedimentation rate may reveal evidence of chronic systemic infection. The child's nutritional status may be examined through the serum albumin and total protein counts. A screen for insulin-like growth factor-1 (IGF-1) and insulin-like growth factor binding protein-3 (IGF-BP3) may be ordered to look for GH deficiency. If a chromosomal anomaly is considered, obtaining a karyotype may be helpful. An MRI of the head may identify a hypothalamic or pituitary process that results in decreased GH secretion from the pituitary. Other laboratory testing to consider: tissue transglutaminase antibodies (celiac sprue), chemistry profile with Ca, Mg, Phos (renal function), luteinizing hormone (LH), follicle-stimulating hormone (FSH), estrogen or testosterone (to assess puberty status), and prolactin (mild elevation could suggest a disruption of the pituitary stalk).

TREATMENT

The child with familial short stature has few therapeutic options. For most children with constitutional delay, reassurance that the child's short stature is a normal variant suffices. In some select patients with no signs of puberty by 14 years of age, a 4 to 6 month treatment with the appropriate sex hormone may help to modestly increase stature and pubertal development for psychological support until true pubertal development begins.

Children with GH deficiency are managed with biosynthetic human GH by subcutaneous injection every day, or by a depot form of growth hormone that is given one to two times per month. Accelerated growth velocity on GH treatment results in catch-up growth in most children. An MRI of the brain should be ordered prior to initiating GH therapy. GH therapy is needed into adulthood because of its effects on bone mass and lipid metabolism. If puberty is delayed beyond 14 years of age, the addition of sex steroids may be considered, both to augment the growth response to GH and to stimulate secondary sexual development.

There is now FDA indication to treat children who carry the diagnosis of idiopathic short stature (final adult height prediction below the 3rd percentile) with growth hormone and children small for gestation age and failure to have catch-up growth by 2 years of age.

Primary hypothyroidism is treated with levothyroxine (Synthroid). After several weeks of therapy, the growth velocity generally returns to normal. Unlike GH therapy, levothyroxine therapy does not promote catch-up growth.

To manage the short stature associated with Cushing disease, the physician must identify and treat the etiology. Girls with short stature caused by Turner syndrome may receive GH to increase their final adult height. Short stature caused by psychosocial deprivation is treated by removing the child from the environment. Short stature caused by medications is reversed by discontinuing the offending medication.

THYROID DYSFUNCTION

HYPERTHYROIDISM

Most cases of hyperthyroidism in children are caused by Graves disease. Other causes include a hyperfunctioning "hot" thyroid nodule or acute suppurative thyroiditis. **Graves disease**, an autoimmune disorder, is caused by circulating thyroid-stimulating immunoglobulins binding to thyrotropin receptors on thyroid cells, which results in diffuse hyperplasia and increased levels of free T_4. Neonatal Graves disease follows transplacental passage of maternal thyroid-stimulating immunoglobulins. In hyperthyroidism, T4 levels are elevated, T3RU is elevated, and TSH is suppressed.

Clinical Manifestations

Symptoms include a voracious appetite (without weight gain or with weight loss), heat intolerance, emotional lability, restlessness, excessive sweating, frequent loose stools, and poor sleep. Exophthalmos is uncommon in children. Older children may complain of palpitations. There is often a change in behavior and school performance. On physical examination, the child may be flushed, fidgety, and warm, with proptosis, a hyperactive precordium, resting tachycardia, and a widened pulse pressure. The thyroid gland is generally enlarged, smooth, firm (but not hard), and nontender, with a bruit on auscultation of the gland. Often a fine tremor is noted, and proximal muscle weakness is present. Acute-onset tachycardia, hyperthermia, diaphoresis, fever, nausea, and vomiting indicate thyroid storm (**malignant hyperthyroidism**), which may be life-threatening but is rare in children.

Infants with neonatal Graves disease tend to stare, are jittery and hyperactive, and have an increased appetite and poor weight gain. Tachycardia is usually present, and thyromegaly may be palpable. The cardiovascular system is the most sensitive to elevated thyroxine levels, and these infants may have evidence of congestive heart failure.

Treatment

Neonatal Graves disease generally resolves over the first several months of life as maternal antibodies are cleared. In the infant hemodynamically compromised by hyperthyroidism, parenteral fluids, digoxin, propranolol and antithyroid medications may be necessary.

Medical Management

The use of antithyroid drugs (propylthiouracil [PTU] or methimazole) to treat Graves disease requires a prolonged period (usually 2 to 5 years) and close supervision by a physician. Less than 60% of these patients will achieve permanent remission with drug therapy alone. The antithyroid medication may cause a hypothyroid state necessitating the addition of thyroxin to normalize circulating T_4 levels. It may take greater than one year for the TSH to recover from suppression and normalize. A small percentage of patients are sensitive to these medications and will experience hives. PTU has been associated with idiopathic hepatic toxicity and agranulocytosis.

Most physicians will delay the use of radioiodine (I^{131}) for the treatment of thyrotoxicosis until adolescence so as not to expose a child to radiation. It is preferred in children to ablate the gland and induce a hypothyroid state rather than underdose and create a situation that would require a second dose of I^{131}.

HYPOTHYROIDISM

Congenital hypothyroidism is discussed in Chapter 13. The most common cause of juvenile or acquired hypothyroidism is **Hashimoto thyroiditis**, a chronic lymphocytic thyroiditis that results in autoimmune destruction of the thyroid gland. Other causes of hypothyroidism include panhypopituitarism, ectopic thyroid dysgenesis, administration of antithyroid medications, and surgical or radioactive iodine ablation for treatment of hyperthyroidism. The incidence of hypothyroidism in girls is four times greater than in boys. There is often a family history of Graves disease or Hashimoto thyroiditis. Most children present during adolescence; it is unusual to develop thyroiditis before 5 years of age.

Clinical Manifestations

Symptoms include cold intolerance, diminished appetite, lethargy, and constipation. Physical findings include slow linear growth, delayed puberty, immature body proportions, coarse puffy facies, dry thin hair, dry skin, and deep tendon reflexes with delayed relaxation.

Diagnostic Evaluation

Thyroid function tests reveal a depressed total T_4 serum concentration and a depressed T_3RU level. If primary hypothyroidism is present, an elevated serum TSH concentration is noted. If secondary hypothyroidism is present, the TSH level may be depressed, normal, or mildly elevated. The detection of thyroid autoantibodies indicates an autoimmune basis for disease, whereas palpation of a thyroid nodule should prompt evaluation with a thyroid scan.

Treatment

Patients with hypothyroidism require thyroid hormone replacement with levothyroxine. Both Free T4 and TSH should be monitored frequently at the outset of therapy and yearly once normal values are achieved. Hypothyroidism which persists untreated for longer than 6 to 9 months results in linear growth attenuation and may have a deleterious effect on final adult height.

ADRENAL DYSFUNCTION

CONGENITAL ADRENAL HYPERPLASIA

The clinical characteristics of congenital adrenal hyperplasia depend on which enzyme in the pathway of steroidogenesis is deficient. Figure 6-1 is a schematic of steroidogenesis in the adrenal cortex.

21-Hydroxylase deficiency accounts for 90% of the cases of congenital adrenal hyperplasia. The disease is inherited as an autosomal recessive trait and tends to occur as either classic salt-wasting 21-hydroxylase deficiency or as virilizing 21-hydroxylase deficiency. 21-Hydroxylase is needed to produce aldosterone and cortisol. 21-Hydroxylase deficiency results in a buildup of the precursors of aldosterone and cortisol. Specifically, 17-hydroxyprogesterone increases, which is then metabolized to dehydroepiandrosterone and androstenedione, which are weak androgens. Androstenedione is then converted to testosterone. Both forms of 21-hydroxylase deficiency result in decreased cortisol and aldosterone secretion, increased adrenocorticotropin hormone

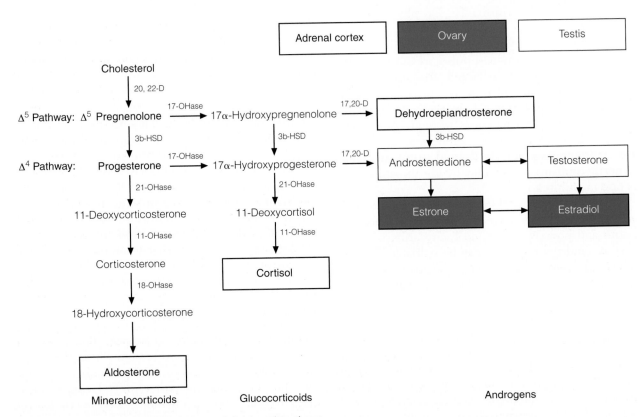

Figure 6-1 • A schematic of steroidogenesis in the adrenal cortex.

(ACTH), and increased 17-hydroxyprogesterone and 17-hydroxypregnenolone.

11-Hydroxylase deficiency accounts for 5% of the cases of congenital adrenal hyperplasia and is also inherited as an autosomal recessive trait. Similar to 21-hydroxylase deficiency, 11-hydroxylase deficiency impairs the production of aldosterone and cortisol. 11-Hydroxylase converts 11-deoxycortisol to cortisol and deoxycorticosterone to corticosterone in the aldosterone pathway. With reduction or absence of 11-hydroxylase, cortisol and aldosterone precursors build up and are shunted to androgen synthesis.

Clinical Manifestations

In congenital 21-hydroxylase deficiency, female infants are born with ambiguous genitalia. Clitoromegaly and labioscrotal fusion may result in erroneous male sex assignment. There is normal ovarian development, and internal genital structures are female. Male infants born with the defect have no genital abnormalities. Unless identified by newborn screen, male infants may present with poor feeding, failure to thrive, lethargy, dehydration, hypotension, hyponatremia, and hyperkalemia. Symptoms of emesis, salt wasting, dehydration, and shock develop in the first 2 to 4 weeks of life. Hyponatremia and hyperkalemia result from lack of aldosterone, and hypoglycemia results from decreased levels of cortisol.

The diagnosis of 21-hydroxylase deficiency is made by documenting elevated serum levels of 17-hydroxyprogesterone greater than 5,000 ng/dL (usually much higher).

In 11-hydroxylase deficiency, there is overproduction of deoxycorticosterone, which has mineralocorticoid activity and results in hypernatremia, hypokalemia, and hypertension. Diagnosis is based on the measurement of increased levels of 11-deoxycortisol and deoxycorticosterone in the serum, or their metabolites in the urine. Serum androstenedione and testosterone are also elevated, and renin and aldosterone levels are depressed.

Treatment

Cortisol therapy reduces ACTH secretion and overproduction of androgens, and mineralocorticoid administration is adjusted to normalize serum renin levels. Cortisol doses may range from 10 to 20 mg/m^2/day divided 2 to 3 times each day. If salt loss occurs, oral fludrocortisone (florinef) is used for mineralocorticoid replacement (0.05 to 0.1 mg each day).

Neonates and infants may require higher florinef dosing and even sodium supplements. Families require education of steroid "**stress dosing**" of the cortisol. They are asked to give larger doses of the cortisol in times of physiologic stress (fever >101°F, vomiting illness, trauma, surgical procedures). In general 50 mg/m^2/day as a bolus and then divided every 8 hours for 24 hours until clinically stable is an appropriate stress dose. IM or IV hydrocortisone may be administered in the vomiting child or child with mental status changes.

Surgical correction of female genital abnormalities is accomplished early. The linear growth and sexual development of children with 21-hydroxylase deficiency must be monitored closely. Undertreatment, as indicated by elevated 17-hydroxyprogesterone, androstenedione, and renin levels and by accelerated advancement of skeletal maturity, leads to excessive growth, premature sexual pubarche, and virilization of the child. Ultimately, undertreatment may lead to premature epiphyseal fusion and adult short stature. Over treatment with cortisol suppresses growth and may cause symptoms of hypercortisolism.

ADDISON DISEASE

Addison disease, or primary adrenal insufficiency, may be congenital or acquired and results in decreased cortisol secretion. Depending on the disease process, there may be a concomitant decrease in aldosterone release. In the newborn, primary adrenal insufficiency may be caused by adrenal hypoplasia, ACTH unresponsiveness, adrenal hemorrhage, or ischemic infarction with sepsis (Waterhouse-Friderichsen syndrome). In older children and adolescents, autoimmune adrenal insufficiency is most common. It may occur alone or in association with another autoimmune endocrinopathy such as thyroiditis or type 1 DM. Tuberculosis, hemorrhage, fungal infection, neoplastic infiltration, and HIV infection may also cause destruction of the adrenal gland. Adrenoleukodystrophy is an X-linked recessive disorder of long-chain fatty acid metabolism that results in adrenal insufficiency and progressive neurologic dysfunction.

In contrast to primary adrenal insufficiency, **secondary adrenal insufficiency** is caused by an ACTH deficiency. The most common cause of ACTH deficiency is chronic steroid therapy that results in suppression of pituitary ACTH. Congenital hypopituitarism or pituitary tumors (craniopharyngioma) also result in depressed pituitary ACTH secretion.

Clinical Manifestations

Symptoms of adrenal insufficiency include weakness, nausea, vomiting, weight loss, headache, emotional lability, and salt craving. Postural hypotension is common. Increased pigmentation over joints and on scar tissue, lips, nipples, and the buccal mucosa is observed in primary adrenal insufficiency because of increased ACTH secretion. Melanocyte-stimulating hormone is a byproduct of the ACTH biosynthetic pathway. The postural hypotension and salt craving are caused by a lack of aldosterone. **Adrenal crisis** is a medical emergency characterized by fever, vomiting, dehydration, and shock. It may be precipitated by intercurrent illness, trauma, or surgery.

Electrolyte abnormalities include hyponatremia, hyperkalemia, hypoglycemia, and mild metabolic acidosis from dehydration. An elevated baseline ACTH with a concurrent low cortisol level is consistent with primary adrenal insufficiency. If the corticotropin stimulation test is abnormal (cortisol of less than 20 micrograms/dL), adrenal insufficiency should be suspected.

Treatment

Adrenal crisis, also known as Addisonian crisis, is a life-threatening condition that should be treated without delay. Correction of electrolyte abnormalities and dehydration is required immediately with 5% dextrose in normal saline and **stress dose** intravenous glucocorticoids.

Long-term management of adrenal insufficiency consists of maintenance doses of oral glucocorticoids and mineralocorticoids. The glucocorticoid dose is increased during times of acute metabolic stress to avoid adrenal insufficiency.

CUSHING SYNDROME

Cushing syndrome is a constellation of symptoms and signs that result from any form of cortisol excess. It is caused by either endogenous overproduction of cortisol or excessive exogenous treatment with pharmacologic doses of cortisol. Endogenous causes include Cushing disease (pituitary overproduction of ACTH) and adrenal tumors. Cushing disease, also known as **bilateral adrenal hyperplasia**, is the most common etiology of Cushing syndrome in children older than 7 years. In most instances, it is caused by a microadenoma of the pituitary gland resulting in ACTH oversecretion. In infants and children younger than 7 years of age, adrenal tumors predominate. Most adrenal tumors that cause Cushing syndrome are adenomas. Ectopic ACTH secretion may occur with some tumors; however, this is exceedingly rare in children.

Clinical Manifestations

The classic signs and symptoms of Cushing syndrome include slow growth with pubertal arrest, "moon" facies, central obesity, abdominal striae, acne, hirsutism, facial flushing, hyperpigmentation, hypertension, fatigue, muscle weakness, acne, buffalo hump, and emotional and mental changes. Most adrenal tumors are virilizing.

Initial laboratory studies include documentation of an elevated serum cortisol level and an increased 24-hour urine free cortisol test. If hypercortisolism is demonstrated, the dexamethasone suppression test is performed to document the presence of Cushing syndrome. Dexamethasone is given in the late evening, and a cortisol level is measured the next morning. Failure of the dexamethasone to suppress the morning cortisol level is consistent with Cushing syndrome. A prolonged dexamethasone suppression test is used to differentiate Cushing disease from an adrenal tumor. When evaluating a child with Cushing syndrome, obtaining an MRI scan of the pituitary and CT scan of the adrenal glands is helpful in determining if additional pathology exists.

Treatment

Adrenal tumors require surgical removal. Similarly, bilateral adrenal hyperplasia is treated with surgical excision of the pituitary adenoma. Transsphenoidal microsurgery is the most effective method of microadenoma removal. Perioperative stress dosing of glucocorticoids is needed to avoid adrenal insufficiency. Postoperatively, the patient may develop a mineralocorticoid deficiency in addition to the glucocorticoid deficiency.

DISORDERS OF PUBERTY

PRECOCIOUS PUBERTY

True precocious puberty is defined as secondary sex characteristics presenting in girls before 7 years of age and in boys before 9 years of age, and may be either gonadotropin-dependent or gonadotropin-independent. True central (gonadotropin-dependent) precocious puberty is more common in girls than in boys. Precocious puberty in girls is usually idiopathic, whereas in boys there is a greater incidence of CNS pathology. Tumors causing gonadotropin-dependent precocious puberty (GDPP) include gliomas, embryonic germ cell tumors, and hamartomas. Other causes of GDPP include hydrocephalus, head injury, and CNS infection or congenital malformation.

Gonadotropin-independent precocious puberty (GIPP) is extremely rare but does occur due to McCune-Albright syndrome (polyostotic fibrous dysplasia of bone and café au lait spots), familial precocious puberty in boys (familial testitoxicosis), Leydig cell tumors, and ectopic human chorionic gonadotropin (HCG) production by neoplasms such as hepatic and pineal tumors.

Precocious thelarche refers to isolated early breast development. The usual age of onset for precocious thelarche is 12 to 24 months. Premature thelarche is likely caused by small transient bursts of estrogen from the prepubertal ovary or from increased sensitivity to low levels of estrogen in the prepubertal female. This is an isolated finding in a girl with a normal growth rate and bone age.

Premature adrenarche refers to the early appearance of sexual hair before 8 years of age in girls and 9 years of age in boys. This benign condition is caused by early maturation of adrenal androgen secretion. This is an isolated finding in children with a normal growth rate and bone age.

Clinical Manifestations

In precocious thelarche, gonadotropin and serum estrogen levels are in the prepubertal range, and linear growth acceleration and advancing skeletal maturation are not present. This nonprogressive, benign condition is distinguished from true precocious puberty by the normal growth rate and bone age noted with premature thelarche.

In premature adrenarche, the levels of adrenal androgens are normal for pubertal stage but elevated for chronologic age. The child's bone age is usually slightly advanced. Children with premature adrenarche must be evaluated for other causes of increased androgen production, such as congenital adrenal hyperplasia, polycystic ovarian syndrome, or adrenal tumor. In children with evidence of significant androgen effect (advanced bone age, growth acceleration, and acne), measurement of adrenal steroids and androgens before and after ACTH administration is used to identify those with congenital adrenal hyperplasia.

Clinical Manifestations

The clinical manifestations of GDPP include premature development of secondary sexual characteristics and an accompanying growth spurt. If the GDPP is secondary to pathology of the CNS, focal neurologic signs are often present. Diagnosis is based on advanced bone age and pubertal levels of gonadotropins (LH and FSH) and estrogen or testosterone. A pubertal pattern of elevated gonadotropins after infusion of gonadotropin-releasing hormone (GnRH) is indicative of GDPP. In GIPP, gonadotropins are low, and GnRH has no effect on gonadotropin levels.

Treatment

Premature thelarche is a benign condition that does not require any treatment. Premature adrenarche that is not caused by congenital adrenal hyperplasia, tumor, or polycystic ovarian syndrome is also a benign condition.

GDPP is treated with injections of long-acting preparations of GnRH (leuprolide). GnRH analogues suppress gonadotropin release and thereby decrease secondary sex characteristics, slow skeletal growth, and prevent the fusion of long bone epiphyseal plates. GIPP is managed by treating the underlying disease process.

PUBERTAL DELAY

Pubertal delay is characterized by a delay in the onset of puberty or in the rate of progression through normal sexual development. In females, this refers to the absence of secondary sex characteristics at 13 years of age or the absence of menarche 3 years from the onset of sexual development. In males, pubertal delay denotes the absence of secondary sex characteristics at 14 years of age or the failure to complete genital growth 5 years from the onset of puberty. Constitutional delay is the cause in 90% to 95% of cases. In these children the bone age is delayed, growth is slow, and puberty simply appears late. There is usually a positive family history.

Differential Diagnosis

Systemic disease may delay puberty in both sexes. Pubertal delay may be caused by primary gonadal failure (hypergonadotropic hypogonadism). Examples of this include Turner syndrome (45X) or autoimmune ovarian failure (in girls) and Klinefelter syndrome

(47XXY) in boys. Hypogonadotropic hypogonadism is caused by hypothalamic/pituitary axis dysfunction. Examples include Kallmann syndrome (mutation in *KAL* gene), isolated gonadotropic deficiency, hypothalamic and pituitary tumors, hypopituitarism, and anorexia nervosa. Other endocrine disorders (e.g., hypothyroidism) may also delay or advance puberty.

Clinical Manifestations

The history and physical examination should include an examination of growth trends, the timing of puberty in other family members, and an assessment of the patient's current Tanner staging. Laboratory evaluation is helpful, including bone age, testosterone and estradiol levels, gonadotropins, FSH, LH, prolactin, and thyroid function testing. Screening to look for systemic disease is also indicated.

Treatment

In the case of constitutional delay, a short course of sex steroids may be needed to initiate pubertal development. Psychosocial support is also important. If permanent hypogonadism is determined to be the etiology, sex steroid replacement is initiated at the normal time of puberty and continued for a lifetime.

DISORDERS OF CALCIUM

Disorders of calcium and phosphorus metabolism result from abnormalities in the two major regulators of calcium homeostasis: parathyroid hormone (PTH) and vitamin D. Total serum calcium is tightly regulated within a narrow range normally between 9 and 10.5 mg/dL. Calcium is bound to albumin. As a result, the total calcium may be low while the ionized calcium is normal (1.1 to 1.4 mmol/L). PTH is secreted by the parathyroid glands in response to low levels of calcium. PTH increases serum calcium by releasing stored calcium from bone, increases renal retention of calcium, and increases the production of the active vitamin D metabolite (1-25(OH)$_2$D).

HYPOCALCEMIA

Etiology

Hypocalcemia may be the result of: (i) inadequate PTH secretion (hypoparathyroidism) or action (pseudohypoparathyroidism), (ii) vitamin D deficiency or resistance, or (iii) other disorders such as hypomagnesemia, hyperphosphatemia, hypoproteinemia, and/or drug toxicity.

There are congenital and familial forms of **hypoparathyroidism**. Pseudohypoparathyroidism is due to a PTH receptor mutation and creates a PTH-resistant state. Other causes of hypoparathyroidism include autoimmune disease, surgical removal of the parathyroid glands, and hypomagnesemia (magnesium is required for PTH secretion). Hypoparathyroidism is also seen with DiGeorge syndrome and Kenny-Caffey syndrome. Of note, many cases of hypoparathyroidism are idiopathic in nature.

Vitamin D deficiency may be due to nutritional deprivation. Higher risk individuals include infants who are exclusively breastfed and people who are highly pigmented, take medications that rapidly metabolize vitamin D, and live in areas with limited sunlight exposure. Vitamin D requires enzymes in the liver and kidney to convert the fat soluble form of vitamin D to its most active form (calcitriol 1,25 OH$_2$ vitamin D). In addition, there are vitamin D resistance syndromes.

Hypocalcemia may also be seen in Bartter syndrome, renal tubular acidosis, and as a side effect of the administration of particular drugs (furosemide, calcitonin, and antineoplastic agents).

Clinical Manifestations

A patient with hypocalcemia may present with carpo-pedal spasm facial twitching, jitteriness, tetany, or seizures. Laryngospasm may cause shortness of breath or apnea. The electrocardiogram may reveal a prolonged corrected QT interval.

Vitamin D deficiency often presents with rachitic bone disease and poor growth parameters in children.

The electrolyte pattern may identify and diagnose the defect of hypocalcemia. In hypoparathyroidism, the serum calcium is low and serum phosphorus is elevated due to a lack of renal stimuli by PTH to excrete phosphorus. This pattern is also seen in pseudohypoparathyroidism (ineffective PTH effect). Low serum calcium and low serum phosphorus is consistent with vitamin D deficiency. In vitamin D deficiency PTH levels are extremely elevated in an attempt to normalize the serum calcium at the expense of bone resorption, resulting in excessive renal phosphorus wasting.

Treatment

The treatment of functional hypoparathyroidism is replacement with oral calcium supplements and an active metabolite of vitamin D (calcitriol 1,25 OH_2 vitamin D). Hypocalcemia as a result of vitamin D deficiency may be treated with 25(OH)D. Resistance to vitamin D must be treated with calcitriol 1,25 OH_2 vitamin D.

HYPERCALCEMIA

Hypercalcemia may be due to: (i) hyperparathyroidism; (ii) hypervitaminosis D; (iii) immobilization; (iv) neoplasia; or (v) familial hypocalciuric hypercalcemia. Hypercalcemia can also be associated with William syndrome or multiple endocrine neoplasia syndrome (hyperparathyroidism).

Clinical Manifestations

Hypercalcemia may be asymptomatic or present with vomiting, lethargy, seizures, polyuria, and hypertension. Patients may also present with renal calculi on abdominal ultrasonography, pathological fractures, or a short QT interval on electrocardiograph.

Treatment

Medical management of symptomatic hypercalcemia is hydration with intravenous saline. Furosemide may be given (1 mg/kg) in 6 to 8 hour intervals. Bisphosphonate infusions (pamidronate) have also been found to be useful to inhibit osteoclast function. A sestamibi parathyroid scan may be indicated to identify a surgically removable adenoma of the parathyroid gland. Hypercalcemia caused by vitamin D excess may be treated by glucocorticoids or ketoconazole to suppress the renal activation of 1-25$(OH)_2$D.

It is equally important to identify the individual with familial hypocalciuric hypercalcemia, a benign condition, so that unnecessary aggressive management is avoided.

KEY POINTS

- DM is a chronic metabolic disorder characterized by hyperglycemia and abnormal energy metabolism due to absent or diminished insulin secretion or action at the cellular level.

- T1DM results from a lack of insulin production by the β-cells of the pancreas. Long-term complications from T1DM include microvascular disease (retinopathy, nephropathy, and neuropathy) and accelerated large vessel atherosclerotic disease.

- The percentage of T2DM cases in children is rising.

- The definition of hypoglycemia is a plasma glucose value of less than 50 mg/dL. Hypoglycemia may be the result of hyperinsulinemia, pituitary disease (ACTH deficiency with or without GH deficiency), glycogen storage disease, disorders of gluconeogenesis, or defects in fatty acid oxidation.

- In central diabetes insipidus, there is loss of ADH secretion and an inability to concentrate the urine. This may occur after head trauma, with a brain tumor, or CNS infection.

- A low serum osmolality with inappropriately elevated urine osmolality and urine sodium are consistent with SIADH. SIADH is treated with fluid restriction. Hypertonic fluids may be administered in acute symptomatic hyponatremia as long as the serum sodium is not corrected too rapidly.

- Eighty percent of cases of short stature result from normal growth and development and are caused by either familial (genetic) short stature or constitutional delay of growth and puberty.

- Most cases of hyperthyroidism in children are caused by Graves disease, which is an autoimmune-induced thyroid hyperplasia. Medical therapy for Graves disease consists of antithyroid medication administration. Neonatal Graves disease results from transplacental passage of maternal thyroid-stimulating immunoglobulins.

- The most common cause of juvenile or acquired hypothyroidism is Hashimoto thyroiditis, which is a chronic lymphocytic thyroiditis that results in autoimmune destruction of the thyroid gland. Hypothyroidism is treated with synthetic levothyroxine.

- 21-Hydroxylase deficiency accounts for 90% of the cases of congenital adrenal hyperplasia. In congenital 21-hydroxylase deficiency, female infants are born with ambiguous genitalia, whereas male infants born with the defect have no genital abnormalities. The

KEY POINTS *(continued)*

diagnosis of congenital adrenal hyperplasia is made by documenting elevated levels of 17-hydroxyprogesterone in the serum.

- Primary adrenal insufficiency may be congenital or acquired and results in decreased cortisol and aldosterone secretion, whereas secondary adrenal insufficiency is caused by adrenocorticotropin hormone (ACTH) deficiency.

- Cushing syndrome is a constellation of symptoms and signs that result from high cortisol levels and is caused by either endogenous overproduction of cortisol or excessive exogenous treatment with pharmacologic doses of cortisol.

- True precocious puberty is defined as secondary sex characteristics presenting in girls before 7 years of age and in boys before 9 years of age, and may be either gonadotropin-dependent or independent. The most common cause of pubertal delay is constitutional delay.

- Inadequate PTH secretion (hypoparathyroidism) or action (pseudohypoparathyroidism) and vitamin D deficiency are likely causes of hypocalcemia in the pediatric patient. The treatment of functional hypoparathyroidism is replacement with oral calcium supplements and an active metabolite of vitamin D (calcitriol 1,25 OH_2 vitamin D).

Fluid, Electrolyte, and pH Management

Katie S. Fine

At birth, free water accounts for 90% of body weight. Body composition changes dramatically over the first year of life as muscle mass increases. By 1 year of age, a child's total body water approaches the adult level of 60% body weight. **Electrolyte homeostasis**, **fluid distribution**, and **pH balance** are critical to the maintenance of normal physiology. The younger the patient, the more intolerant he or she is to challenges to these systems.

MAINTENANCE FLUIDS

The amount of fluid needed to maintain normal body function is directly related to caloric expenditure, which in turn is related to a child's weight. The **Holliday-Segar method** is useful for calculating daily maintenance fluids: 100 mL/kg/day for the first 10 kg, plus 50 mL/kg/day for the next 10 kg, plus 25 mL/kg/day for each additional kg thereafter. For practical purposes, it is often more useful to calculate an hourly rate using 4 mL/kg/hr (first 10 kg body weight), 2 mL/kg/hr (second 10 kg body weight), 1 mL/kg/hr (each additional kilogram).

An example of calculating maintenance fluid requirements for a 22-kg child follows.

Daily rate: (100 mL/kg/day × 10 kg) + (50 mL/kg/day × 10 kg) + (25 mL/kg/day × 2 kg) = 1,550 mL/day

Hourly rate: 1,550 mL/day divided by 24 hr/day = 65 mL/hr

Short-cut method: (4 mL/hr × 10 kg) + (2 mL/hr × 10 kg) + (1 mL/hr × 2 kg) = 62 mL/hr

For each 100 cc of maintenance fluids, a child needs 3 mEq of sodium and 2 mEq of potassium, as well as a carbohydrate source (dextrose). In general, one-fourth normal saline with 5% dextrose (10% in infants) and 20 mEq/L KCl meets maintenance glucose and electrolyte needs. One-half normal saline with KCl is often used in adolescents and adults.

DEHYDRATION

Dehydration in the pediatric patient is usually secondary to **vomiting** and/or **diarrhea**. Infants and toddlers are particularly susceptible because of the limited ability of the immature kidney to conserve water and electrolytes and because of the child's dependence on caretakers to meet his or her needs. When addressing dehydration, it is important to consider **maintenance fluid** needs as well as **replacement** of the initial deficit and **ongoing losses**.

Clinical Manifestations

History

A careful history limits the differential diagnosis list and provides information concerning the acuity, source, and quantity of fluid lost, all of which influence treatment. Recent **weight loss** and **decreased urine output** are important benchmarks of the degree of deficiency. The color, consistency, frequency, and volume of stool and/or emesis may influence initial diagnostic and therapeutic measures.

Many chronic medical illnesses may present acutely with dehydration, including diabetes, metabolic disorders, cystic fibrosis, and congenital adrenal hyperplasia. Polyuria in the presence of physical signs of dehydration may indicate diabetes mellitus,

■ TABLE 7-1 Clinical Estimation of Degree of Dehydration*

	Mild	Moderate	Severe
Weight loss	<5%	5% to 10%	>10%
Vital signs			
Heart rate	increased	increased	greatly increased
Respiratory rate	normal	normal	increased
Blood pressure	normal	normal (orthostasis)	decreased
Skin			
Capillary refill	<2 seconds	2 to 3 seconds	>3 seconds
Mucous membranes	normal/dry	dry	dry
Anterior fontanelle	normal	depressed	depressed
Eyes			
Tearing	normal/absent	absent	absent
Appearance	normal	sunken	sunken
Mental status	normal	altered	depressed
Lab values			
Urine osmolarity	600 mOsm/L	800 mOsm/L	maximal
Urine specific gravity	1.020	1.025	maximal
Blood urea nitrogen	<20	elevated	high
Blood pH	normal	mildly acidotic	moderate/profound acidosis
Stage of shock	not in shock	compensated shock	uncompensated shock

*Infants will exhibit greater weight loss per degree of dehydration (5% mild, 10% moderate, 15% severe), whereas adolescents will exhibit less weight loss per degree of dehydration (3% mild, 5% to 6% moderate, 7% to 9% severe).

diabetes insipidus, or renal tubular acidosis. Children who are neglected or refuse to drink because of severe oropharyngeal pain may also become significantly dehydrated.

Physical Examination

There is no single physical or laboratory finding that will accurately assess a patient's degree of dehydration (Table 7-1). It is important to remember that a child's primary initial mechanism of compensation for decreased plasma volume is **tachycardia**. **Hypotension**, a sensitive early indicator in adults, is a very late and ominous finding in children.

Diagnostic Evaluation

Serum electrolyte levels help guide the *choice* of fluid composition and *rate* of replacement. Dehydration may be isotonic, hypotonic (hyponatremic), or hypertonic (hypernatremic), depending on the nature of the fluid lost and the replacement fluids provided by the caretaker.

Isotonic dehydration is the most common form and suggests that either compensation has occurred or that water losses roughly parallel sodium losses. **Hypotonic (hyponatremic) dehydration** is defined by a serum sodium less than 130 mEq/L. Children who lose electrolytes in their stool and are supplemented with free water or very dilute juices may present in this manner. **Hypertonic (hypernatremic) dehydration** (Na ≥150 mEq/L) is uncommon in children, but implies an excessive loss of free water compared with electrolyte loss (e.g., diabetes insipidus). Of note, patients with hyponatremic dehydration tend to appear more dehydrated than they truly are, while those with hypernatremic dehydration may not appear as clinically compromised because intravascular volume is preserved.

Usually, the serum bicarbonate concentration is decreased secondary to metabolic acidosis. However, protracted vomiting may result in alkalosis and a high bicarbonate level due to acid lost from gastric secretions (see Metabolic Alkalosis below). With significant dehydration, perfusion of the kidneys may be impaired. This will be reflected in elevations of the serum blood urea nitrogen (BUN) and creatinine (Cr) levels as glomerular filtration rate falls. A BUN/Cr ratio greater than 20 is consistent with intravascular depletion and prerenal failure.

Treatment

Oral rehydration therapy (ORT) is the preferred treatment for mild-to-moderate dehydration. The World Health Organization recommends that solutions contain 90 mEq/L sodium, 20 mEq/L potassium, and 20 g/L glucose. Commercial preparations that approximate these concentrations are available. Free water may precipitate hyponatremia and is contraindicated. ORT is particularly labor intensive, requiring small volumes of fluid given very frequently. Administered correctly, it is extremely effective.

Severe dehydration leads to life-threatening **hypovolemic shock**. Children in hypovolemic shock should receive 20 mL/kg intravenous boluses of isotonic fluid (normal saline or Ringer's lactate) until their blood pressure normalizes (see Chapter 1). Both fluids are isotonic, resulting in improved intravascular volume without fluid shifts. Clinical estimation of degree of dehydration and serum electrolyte studies tailor subsequent management.

Most **deficits** are replaced over 24 hours, with half given in the first 8 hours and the rest over the next 16 hours. One notable exception is the child with hypernatremic dehydration, in whom the deficit should be replaced over 48 to 72 hours to prevent excessive fluid shifts and cerebral edema. **Ongoing losses** (usually in stool) are replaced milliliter for milliliter with intravenous fluid comparable in electrolyte content to that being lost.

For example, an 18-kg infant with a normal serum sodium who is judged to be 10% dehydrated has lost an estimated 2,000 mL of fluid (1,000 mL = 1 kg). Half the deficit is replaced over the first 8 hours, with the balance given over the next 16 hours. Maintenance therapy must also be included. The child received a 20-mL/kg bolus initially.

1. 2,000 mL ÷ 2 = 1,000 mL (one-half the total deficit); 360 mL (20 mL/kg) has already been replaced. Therefore, 640 mL is given over the first 8 hours at 80 mL/hr. This should be added to the 56 mL/hr the child requires to meet maintenance needs. Rate = 80 mL/hr + 56 mL/hr = 136 mL/hr.
2. The second half (1,000 mL) is replaced over the next 16 hours (63 mL/hr) along with the maintenance rate (56 mL/hr). Rate = 63 mL/hr + 56 mL/hr = 119 mL/hr.

The composition of the **replacement fluid** varies depending on the initial laboratory values. Replacement (and maintenance) fluid should not contain potassium until the patient urinates. Sodium bicarbonate therapy may be indicated if the pH and serum bicarbonate levels remain dangerously low after initial isotonic boluses. In general, ongoing gastrointestinal losses are replaced with one-half normal saline. Urine electrolyte and osmolality studies should be obtained if ongoing losses result from an abnormal renal process.

Patients with profound hyperglycemia or electrolyte disturbances due to an ongoing underlying pathologic process (e.g., diabetic ketoacidosis) may require more specialized management discussed elsewhere in this review.

HYPONATREMIA

Hyponatremia (serum sodium level <130 mEq/L) may occur in the face of decreased, normal, or increased total body sodium content. In children, the most common setting is **dehydration**. Other causes include syndrome of inappropriate secretion of antidiuretic hormone (SIADH), water intoxication, renal or congestive heart failure, and adrenal insufficiency.

Clinical Manifestations

History and Physical Examination

The severity of clinical manifestations depends on both the **level of sodium** in the extracellular space and the **rate of change** from normal. Falling levels that occur over several days are better tolerated than rapid losses. Anorexia and nausea are early, nonspecific complaints. Neurologic findings include confusion, lethargy, and decreased deep tendon reflexes. **Seizures** and **respiratory arrest** are late, life-threatening complications.

Diagnostic Evaluation

The laboratory workup of hyponatremia includes serum electrolytes, glucose, blood urea nitrogen and creatinine, serum osmolality, liver function tests, protein, and lipid levels as well as urine sodium (U_{Na}) concentration and specific gravity (USG). These laboratory values quantitate the severity of the deficit and may suggest an underlying cause. The measured serum sodium needs to be "corrected" in the setting of hyperglycemia. For every 100 mg/dL rise in glucose (above "normal" 100 mg/dL), add 1.6 mEq Na to the *measured* value to get the *true* value.

Treatment

Dehydration is treated with fluid resuscitation as discussed previously. Hyponatremia due to SIADH, water intoxication, or renal failure requires fluid restriction and treatment of the underlying disorder. Adrenal insufficiency is treated with fluid resuscitation and stress-dose hydrocortisone. The cautious use of 3% hypertonic saline is limited to life-threatening situations (i.e., intractable seizures). Serum sodium correction should not exceed 1 to 2 mEq/L per hour because of the risk of central-pontine myelinolysis.

HYPERNATREMIA

Hypernatremia is uncommon in children in the absence of dehydration (discussed earlier). Signs and symptoms include muscle weakness, irritability, and lethargy. Seizures and coma are the major complications. Hypernatremic dehydration is treated with infusion of isotonic saline. Serum sodium correction should not exceed 1 to 2 mEq/L per hour due to the risk of cerebral edema.

HYPERKALEMIA

Normal serum potassium values range from 3.5 to 5.7 mEq/L; a measurement of 5.8 mEq/L or greater is considered **hyperkalemia**. In children, the most common cause of an abnormally high potassium level is artifactual hyperkalemia, due to the hemolysis of red cells during sample collection. Transcellular shifts in hydrogen ions increase serum potassium without changing total body content; for every unit reduction in arterial pH, plasma potassium increases 0.2 to 0.4 mEq/L. Disorders and medications that interfere with renal excretion of the electrolyte precipitate true hyperkalemia.

Differential Diagnosis

Common causes of hyperkalemia include the following:

- Acidosis
- Severe dehydration
- Potassium-sparing diuretics (spironolactone)
- Excessive parenteral infusion
- Renal failure

Other less common but important conditions to consider include the following:

- Adrenal corticoid deficiency (i.e., Addison disease)
- Renal tubular acidosis
- Massive crush injury with rhabdomyolysis
- Beta-blocker or digitalis ingestions
- Excessive supplementation

Clinical Manifestations

Paresthesias and weakness are the earliest symptoms; flaccid paralysis and tetany occur late. Cardiac involvement produces specific progressive **ECG changes**; T-wave elevation ("peaking") is followed by loss of P waves, widening QRS complexes, and ST segment depression (see Fig. 7-1). Ventricular fibrillation and cardiac arrest occur at serum levels greater than 9 mEq/L.

Treatment

Calcium gluconate infusion protects the heart by stabilizing the myocyte cell membrane. Infusion of sodium bicarbonate or insulin (and glucose) drives potassium into the cells. Hyperventilation prompts the transfer of hydrogen ions out of the cell in exchange

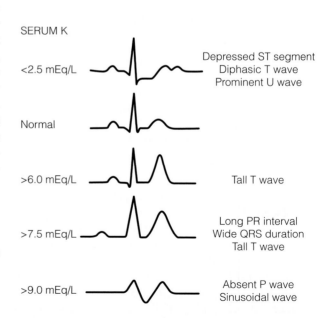

SERUM K

<2.5 mEq/L		Depressed ST segment Diphasic T wave Prominent U wave
Normal		
>6.0 mEq/L		Tall T wave
>7.5 mEq/L		Long PR interval Wide QRS duration Tall T wave
>9.0 mEq/L		Absent P wave Sinusoidal wave

Figure 7-1 • ECG findings consistent with hyperkalemia (Lead II).

for potassium ions, effectively lowering the serum potassium. Cation exchange resins (e.g., Kayexylate) and hemodialysis are the only measures that actually remove potassium from the body.

HYPOKALEMIA

Hypokalemia in the pediatric population is usually encountered in the setting of alkalosis secondary to vomiting, administration of loop diuretics (furosemide), or diabetic ketoacidosis. Signs and symptoms include weakness, tetany, constipation, polyuria, and polydipsia. Muscle breakdown leading to myoglobinuria may compromise renal function. ECG changes (prolonged Q-T interval, T wave flattening) are noted at levels less than or equal to 2.5 mEq/L; cardiac arrhythmias (ventricular tachycardia/fibrillation) can occur and are more likely if the patient is being treated with digoxin. Blood pressure changes and urine electrolyte content assist in diagnosis (Fig. 7-2). Treatment consists of correcting pH (when increased) and replenishing potassium stores orally or intravenously.

METABOLIC ACIDOSIS

The extracellular fluid **pH** (the negative logarithm of the hydrogen ion concentration) is maintained in a very narrow range (normal 7.4), largely as a result of the **bicarbonate buffer system**. Hydrogen ions (H^+) combine with HCO_3^- to form H_2CO_3, which is transformed into water and CO_2. The kidneys control excretion of HCO_3 (bicarbonate), whereas CO_2 is expired by the lungs. The addition of excessive H^+, the loss of HCO_3^-, or abnormal renal or pulmonary function can all affect this buffering system and lead to acid–base disturbances.

Metabolic acidosis (pH ≤ 7.35) results from the loss of HCO_3^- or the addition of H^+ in the extracellular fluid. It is the most common acid–base disorder encountered in the pediatric population. Causes include increased acid intake or production, decreased renal excretion, or increased renal or gastrointestinal bicarbonate loss. $PaCO_2$ begins to drop almost immediately due to increased ventilation; the compensation is complete within 24 hours. In the presence of a metabolic acidosis, the expected $PaCO_2 = 1.5 \times HCO_3^- + 8 (\pm 2)$. If the measured $PaCO_2$ is higher than expected, then there is a concurrent primary respiratory acidosis. If it is lower than expected, there is a concurrent primary respiratory alkalosis (see "Respiratory Acidosis and Alkalosis").

Clinical Manifestations

Hyperpnea is the most consistent clinical finding in metabolic acidosis. Severe acidemia affects multiple organ systems: cardiac contractility is impaired, cardiac output is reduced, and the heart becomes vulnerable to arrhythmias. Protein breakdown is accelerated, and mental status changes occur. Other signs and symptoms are specific to the underlying disorder. Important laboratory studies include serum electrolytes, blood urea nitrogen, creatinine, glucose, venous or arterial blood gas, and urine dipstick for pH and glucose. These studies help quantify the acidosis

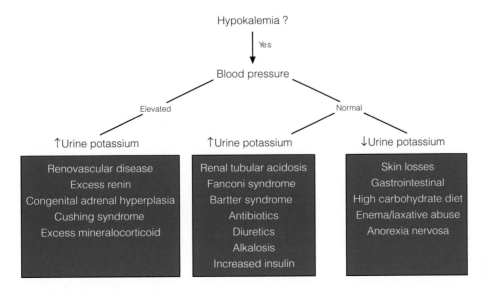

Figure 7-2 • Evaluation of hypokalemia.

■ **TABLE 7-2** Changes in the Anion Gap

Increased Anion Gap*	Normal Anion Gap	Decreased Anion Gap
Hypokalemia	Diarrhea	Hyperkalemia
Hypocalcemia	Renal tubular acidosis	Hypercalcemia
Hypomagnesemia	Hyperalimentation	Hypermagnesemia
Hyperphosphatemia	Hypoaldosteronism	Hypoalbuminemia
Lactic acidosis	Lithium ingestion	
Diabetic ketoacidosis		
Renal failure/Uremia		
Salicylate ingestion		
Ethylene glycol, ethanol, methanol ingestion		

*The mnemonic **MUDPILES** is helpful for recalling several clinical conditions that result in metabolic acidosis with a high anion gap: **m**ethanol ingestion; **u**remia; **d**iabetic ketoacidosis; **p**araldehyde ingestion; **i**soniazid ingestion, iron ingestion, and inborn errors of metabolism; **l**actic acidosis; **e**thanol ingestion; and **s**alicylate ingestion.

and may suggest the causative condition. The difference between the sums of the measured cations ($Na^+ + K^+$) and anions ($Cl^- + HCO_3^-$), termed the **anion gap**, is normally 12 ± 4; Table 7-2 lists conditions associated with changes in the anion gap.

Treatment

The intravenous administration of sodium bicarbonate should be reserved for cases in which the serum pH is less than 7.0 and the cause is unknown or slow to reverse (i.e., most normal anion gap acidosis). Boluses are reserved for extreme situations; in general, the infusion should be slow and relatively isotonic. Patients receiving alkali therapy require frequent monitoring of blood pH, sodium, potassium, and calcium. Complications include alkalosis (overcorrection), hypokalemia, hypernatremia/hyperosmolarity, and hypocalcemia.

METABOLIC ALKALOSIS

Metabolic alkalosis (pH ≥ 7.45) is much less common than acidosis in children. "Contraction" alkalosis results from the loss of fluid high in H^+ or Cl^-, as may occur with protracted gastric vomiting (pyloric stenosis, bulimia) or chronic thiazide or loop diuretic administration. Patients with cystic fibrosis may develop metabolic alkalosis due to excessive electrolyte losses in the sweat. Other causes include laxative abuse and other chloride-wasting diarrheas. Volume expansion and chloride replacement correct the alkalosis unless

it results from disorders of mineralocorticoid excess (e.g., renal artery stenosis, adrenal disorders, steroid use); potassium supplements are also necessary in these cases.

Diagnosis and resolution of the underlying disorder guide management decisions. Complications of severe alkalosis include reduction in coronary blood flow and arrhythmias, hypoventilation, seizures, and decreased potassium, magnesium, and phosphate levels.

RESPIRATORY ACIDOSIS AND ALKALOSIS

Normal $PaCO_2$ levels range from 35 to 45 mm Hg. Any process that causes respiratory insufficiency (CNS depression, chest wall muscle weakness, pulmonary or cardiopulmonary diseases) results in a primary elevation in the $PaCO_2$, termed respiratory acidosis. This is followed by renal bicarbonate reabsorption and a compensatory rise in the serum bicarbonate measurement (secondary metabolic alkalosis). Conversely, respiratory alkalosis results from a primary reduction in the $PaCO_2$. The kidney responds by increasing the urine bicarbonate concentration (secondary metabolic acidosis). Causes of respiratory alkalosis include lung disease, mechanical ventilation, or any process (metabolic or neurological) which results in a sustained increase in the respiratory rate.

Of note, both respiratory acidosis and alkalosis may occur as compensation for other primary metabolic pH disturbances.

KEY POINTS

- Tachycardia is an early sign of dehydration in children. Hypotension occurs very late in children, and its absence does not rule out significant dehydration requiring intervention.

- If IV fluids are required, initial 20 mL/kg boluses of normal saline or Ringer's lactate should be given until the patient's condition stabilizes.

- Potassium should not be added to replacement or maintenance fluids until urine output is assured.

- Hyponatremia in the pediatric patient is most frequently due to dehydration; other causes include SIADH, water intoxication, renal or heart failure, and adrenal insufficiency.

- Serum sodium levels need to be "corrected" in the setting of hyperglycemia.

- Neither hyponatremia nor hypernatremia should be corrected too quickly due to the risk of severe central nervous system complications.

- Progressive ECG changes associated with hyperkalemia include peaked T waves, loss of P waves, and widening of the QRS complex.

- Emergent treatment for life-threatening hyperkalemia includes hyperventilation and calcium gluconate, sodium bicarbonate, and/or insulin/glucose infusion.

- The equation $P_aCO_2 = 1.5 \times HCO_3^- + 8\,(\pm 2)$ can help distinguish between primary and secondary metabolic acidosis.

- An increased respiratory rate is the most consistent physical finding in metabolic acidosis.

- $NaHCO_3$ (sodium bicarbonate) should be used only when acidosis is severe or difficult to correct.

Gastroenterology

Mitchell Cohen • *Bradley S. Marino*

ABDOMINAL PAIN

Abdominal pain is a common pediatric problem encountered by primary care physicians, medical subspecialists and surgical specialists. Chronic abdominal pain is defined as at least three bouts of pain severe enough to affect activities over a period of at least 3 months. The exact prevalence of chronic abdominal pain in children is not known. It appears to account for 2% to 4% of all pediatric office visits; approximately 15% of middle school and high school students experience weekly abdominal pain. In children without objective evidence of an underlying organic disorder, chronic abdominal pain is most frequently functional.

DIFFERENTIAL DIAGNOSIS

Infectious conditions (including bacterial and viral gastroenteritis) are a common cause of acute abdominal pain. Mesenteric lymphadenitis may cause persistent pain following an infection. Extraintestinal infections may also cause abdominal pain. These include group A streptococcal infections, urinary tract infections, and lower lobe pneumonias. Pelvic inflammatory disease (PID) is an important consideration in adolescent females. Infectious mononucleosis is one of several systemic infections that can cause abdominal pain.

Gall bladder diseases, including cholecystitis, choledocolithiasis and biliary cholic, pancreatitis, gastritis, and peptic ulcer disease, are less common in children but warrant consideration especially when the pain is localized to the right upper quadrant or epigastrium and is worsened by meals. *Helicobacter pylori* is a cause of gastritis and ulcer disease. Abdominal pain is a primary feature in Henoch-Schonlein purpura (HSP), but also may be seen in other vasculitides, including Kawasaki disease, polyarteritis nodosa, and lupus erythematosus, and can also be a manifestation of sickle cell crisis.

If the pain is recurrent, the differential diagnosis must be expanded. Constipation and functional abdominal pain including functional dyspepsia, irritable bowel syndrome (IBS), and abdominal migraine are among the most frequent causes of recurrent abdominal pain in children. Lactase deficiency may cause recurrent pain with exposure to milk sugar in dairy food. Inflammatory bowel disease (ulcerative colitis and Crohn disease) are chronic conditions often associated with diarrhea, anemia and poor growth in which pain is a major symptom. Celiac disease may present with abdominal pain, although anemia and poor growth without pain are also common manifestations. A less frequent cause of intestinal inflammation is an eosinophilic gastrointestinal disorder of the small intestine or colon.

Appendicitis is the most common surgical cause of abdominal pain. Intussusception is an important pediatric disease that presents with intermittent but severe pain and may also manifest with striking lethargy. Incarcerated hernia, volvulus, bowel obstruction, and testicular torsion represent surgical emergencies. Trauma can lead to significant intra-abdominal injury and pain.

Urologic obstruction at any level is an important consideration. Ureteropelvic junction obstruction, hydronephrosis, and renal stones can cause significant pain.

Gynecologic causes are an important part of the differential diagnosis in adolescent girls. Pregnancy should always be considered, especially if symptoms are consistent with an ectopic pregnancy. Dysmenorrhea, ovarian cysts, mittelschmerz, PID, cervicitis, endometriosis, and ovarian or adnexal torsion are all potential problems in this population.

Psychiatric causes of abdominal pain are uncommon in children. True malingering is unusual, as are conversion disorders. However, many children do experience abdominal pain in the setting of stress, especially in the context of school, and mild intermittent pain also can be seen in children with depression. Although children with chronic abdominal pain and their parents are more often anxious or depressed, the presence of anxiety, depression, behavior problems, or recent negative life events does not appear to be useful in distinguishing between functional and organic abdominal pain. Nonetheless, inquiry into recent social changes in the family unit or at school may provide great insight into the etiology of the pain.

CLINICAL MANIFESTATIONS

History

The history should localize the pain and determine its quality, temporal characteristics, and exacerbating and alleviating factors. With "inflammatory" pain, the child tends to lie still, whereas with "colicky" pain, the child cannot remain still. Colicky pain usually results from obstruction of a hollow viscus. It is important to ascertain whether the child has had previous abdominal surgery; with a history of previous laparotomy, small bowel obstruction becomes more likely. Pain may be accompanied by anorexia, nausea, emesis, diarrhea, or constipation. If the pain wakes the child at night, an organic cause is more likely, but night time pain does not exclude functional disorders. Both bilious emesis and nonbilious emesis may be seen in small bowel obstruction although bilious emesis raises the level of suspicion considerably. Bloody emesis may result from an upper gastrointestinal (GI) bleeding source (Mallory-Weiss tear, esophagitis, gastritis, or duodenitis). Bloody diarrhea with mucopus suggests bacterial enterocolitis. Stooling characteristics are also important because constipation is a common etiology of chronic abdominal pain.

In the setting of chronic abdominal pain, the growth curve should be examined for any alterations in weight gain or linear growth, which may be a sign of a chronic illness such as inflammatory bowel disease (IBD) or celiac disease.

The presence of alarm symptoms or signs including, but not limited to, involuntary weight loss, deceleration of linear growth, gastrointestinal blood loss, significant vomiting, chronic severe diarrhea, persistent right upper or right lower quadrant pain, unexplained fever, and/or family history of IBD is generally an indication to pursue further diagnostic testing.

Physical Examination

One goal of the abdominal examination is to ascertain whether the child has an abdominal process that requires surgical intervention. Watching the child walk, climb onto the examination table, and interact with both parents and staff before formally examining the child's abdomen, helps one to gain an appreciation for the degree of incapacitation or emotional overlay that may be present. The abdomen should be inspected, auscultated, and palpated. Peritoneal signs include rebound tenderness, guarding, psoas or obturator signs, and rigidity of the abdominal wall. Right lower quadrant tenderness requires the consideration of appendicitis. Rectal skin tags or fistulae may suggest the diagnosis of Crohn disease. Unless the diagnosis is thought to be uncomplicated viral gastroenteritis, a rectal examination is most often indicated to detect tenderness or hard stool and to obtain stool for occult blood testing. If the patient is an adolescent female, a pelvic examination is often indicated as part of the appropriate evaluation. Cervical motion tenderness is consistent with PID.

The examination of children with functional abdominal pain is often devoid of positive physical findings. Alarm signs on abdominal examination include localized tenderness in the right upper or right lower quadrants, a localized fullness or mass effect, hepatomegaly, splenomegaly, costovertebral angle tenderness, tenderness over the spine, and perianal abnormalities.

DIAGNOSTIC EVALUATION

The diagnostic test strategy is dictated by the history and findings on the physical examination. Surgical consultation should be sought if there is concern for appendicitis, volvulus, testicular torsion, or other conditions requiring urgent surgery. A complete blood count with differential, serum electrolytes and chemistries, amylase, lipase, stool hemoccult examination, urinalysis, and radiographic studies should be performed if there has been abdominal trauma or an acute surgical condition is suspected. Blood should also be typed for possible transfusion. A computed tomography (CT) scan may be useful when appendicitis is being considered. When uncomplicated viral gastroenteritis is the most likely cause and the child is well hydrated, no studies need be performed, but if bacterial enterocolitis is being considered, stool should be obtained for culture. Group A streptococcal pharyngitis and PID require appropriate cultures. To diagnose a urinary tract infection, a urinalysis and urine culture should be performed. Celiac disease is best diagnosed with serologic screening studies, e.g., tissue transglutaminase (IgA) or anti-endomysial antibodies (IgA). Screening for IBD is best performed by history and physical examination, but a CBC and ESR or CRP may be helpful screening tools. In many cases, especially when functional pain is thought to be the cause of the pain, less diagnostic testing may be more helpful than more testing. This will enable the focus to remain on appropriate treatment strategies.

TREATMENT

Treatment is directed at the underlying cause of the pain. Infections may require antimicrobial therapy. Lactase deficiency and celiac disease improve with dietary intervention. Constipation is well treated with polyethylene glycol and a bowel rehabilitation plan. Diagnostic trials of histamine-2 receptor antagonists or proton pump inhibitor therapy may be very helpful when esophagitis, gastritis, duodenitis, or non-ulcer dyspepsia is suggested. Functional abdominal pain is best treated with a biopsychosocial model. Medical treatment might include acid reduction therapy for pain associated with dyspepsia, antispasmodic agents, smooth muscle relaxants or low dosages of tricyclic psychotropic agents for pain, or nonstimulating laxatives or antidiarrheals for pain associated with altered bowel pattern.

APPENDICITIS

Appendicitis is the most common indication for abdominal surgery in childhood. Appendicitis results from bacterial invasion of the appendix, which is more likely when the lumen is obstructed by a fecalith, parasite, or lymph node. Appendicitis occurs most frequently in children between 10 and 15 years of age. Less than 10% of patients are younger than 5 years.

CLINICAL MANIFESTATIONS

Classically, fever, emesis, anorexia, and diffuse periumbilical pain develop. Subsequently, pain and abdominal tenderness localize to the right lower quadrant as the parietal peritoneum becomes inflamed. Guarding, rebound tenderness, and obturator and psoas signs are commonly found. The appendix tends to perforate approximately 36 hours after pain begins. The incidence of perforation and diffuse peritonitis is higher in children younger than 2 years, when diagnosis may be delayed. Atypical presentations are common in childhood, especially with retrocecal appendicitis, which may present with periumbilical pain and diarrhea. Retrocecal appendicitis usually does not induce right lower quadrant pain until after perforation. Bacterial enterocolitis caused by *Campylobacter* and *Yersinia* species may mimic appendicitis because both can result in right lower quadrant abdominal pain and tenderness. Diagnosis of appendicitis is established clinically by history and by physical examination, which should include a rectal examination to detect tenderness or a mass. A moderately elevated white blood cell count with a left shift is often seen in appendicitis. A plain film of the abdomen may demonstrate a fecalith. An inflamed appendix may be noted on ultrasound, but CT scans have a higher yield.

TREATMENT

Laparotomy and appendectomy should be performed before perforation. When appendicitis results in perforation, the patient should be given broad spectrum antibiotics, e.g., ampicillin, gentamicin, and metronidazole, to treat peritonitis from intestinal flora. The mortality rate rises significantly with perforation.

INTUSSUSCEPTION

Intussusception results from telescoping of one part of the intestine into another. Intussusception causes impaired venous return, bowel edema and ischemia, necrosis, and perforation. It is one of the most common causes of intestinal obstruction in infancy. Most intussusceptions are ileocolic; the ileum invaginates into the colon at the ileocecal valve. Previous viral or bacterial enteritis may cause hypertrophy of the Peyer patches or mesenteric nodes, which are hypothesized to act as the lead point in intussusception. A specific lead point is identified in only approximately 5% of cases but should be sought in neonates or in children older than 5 years. Recognizable lead points in intussusception include Meckel diverticulum, an intestinal polyp, lymphoma, or a foreign body. Intussusception has also been associated with HSP, but in this setting is usually ileo-ileal. It can be very difficult to distinguish HSP complicated by intussusception from the inflammatory abdominal pain seen in simple HSP.

CLINICAL MANIFESTATIONS

Violent episodes of irritability, colicky pain, and emesis are interspersed with relatively normal periods. Rectal bleeding occurs in 80% of patients but less commonly in the form of the classic "currant jelly" stools (stools containing bright red blood and mucus). The degree of lethargy shown by the child may be striking. A tubular mass is palpable in approximately 80% of patients. A plain abdominal film may show a paucity of gas in the right lower quadrant or evidence of obstruction with air fluid levels. An ultrasound examination may be very helpful as a screening tool. A contrast enema or air enema, which often proves therapeutic as well as diagnostic, demonstrates a characteristic coiled spring appearance to the bowel.

TREATMENT

Fluid resuscitation with normal saline or lactated Ringer solution is usually necessary. Hydrostatic reduction with barium enema or pneumatic reduction with air enema is successful in 75% of cases if performed in the first 48 hours. Peritoneal signs are an absolute contraindication to this procedure. Laparotomy and direct reduction is indicated when reduction by enema is either unsuccessful or contraindicated. The immediate recurrence rate is approximately 15%. When a specific lead point is identified, the recurrence rate is higher.

EMESIS

Vomiting is one of the most common presenting symptoms in pediatrics and can be caused by both gastrointestinal (GI) and non-GI pathologies. Complications of severe, persistent emesis include dehydration and hypochloremic, hypokalemic metabolic alkalosis. Forceful emesis can result in a Mallory-Weiss tear of the esophagus at the gastroesophageal junction or erosion of the gastric cardia; chronic emesis can result in distal esophagitis.

DIFFERENTIAL DIAGNOSIS

Table 8-1 lists the most common causes of vomiting in infants and children.

CLINICAL MANIFESTATIONS

History

In infants, the history should differentiate between true vomiting (forceful expulsion of gastric contents) and effortless regurgitation ("spitting up"). The latter is often due to gastroesophageal reflux. Frequency, appearance (bloody or bilious), amount, and timing of the emesis are important. Emesis shortly after feeding in the infant is probably gastroesophageal reflux. If the emesis is projectile and the child is 1 to 3 months of age, pyloric stenosis must be considered. Poor weight gain and emesis may indicate pyloric stenosis or a metabolic disorder. Macrolide antibiotics are known to cause emesis and diarrhea; chemotherapeutic agents and some toxic ingestions cause emesis. If the child has a ventriculo-peritoneal shunt, vomiting may be a sign of shunt obstruction and increased intracranial pressure. Emesis with seizure or headache or both may indicate an intracranial process. Diarrhea, emesis, and fever are seen with gastroenteritis. Fever, abdominal pain, and emesis are typical for appendicitis, whereas bilious emesis and abdominal pain are seen with intestinal obstruction. Emesis and syncope may result from pregnancy.

Physical Examination

On physical examination, the initial assessment should focus on the child's vital signs and hydration status. Chapter 7 discusses signs and symptoms of dehydration. A bulging fontanelle or papilledema implicates increased intracranial pressure as the cause of the emesis. Emesis is common in infectious pharyngitis. The lung fields should be auscultated for crackles or an asymmetric examination to rule out pneumonia. Emesis and vaginal discharge in the female adolescent warrant a pelvic examination to evaluate for PID. The abdominal examination should focus on bowel sounds and the presence of distention, tenderness, or masses. Hypoactive bowel sounds may indicate ileus or obstruction, whereas hyperactive bowel sounds suggest

■ TABLE 8-1 Differential Diagnosis of Vomiting in Children

Infectious	Gastrointestinal: Infant
Viral gastroenteritis, e.g., Rotavirus and Norovirus	Gastroesophageal reflux
Bacterial enterocolitis/sepsis	Cow or soy milk protein intolerance
Hepatitis	Bowel obstruction[a]
Food poisoning	Duodenal atresia
Pelvic inflammatory disease	Pyloric stenosis
Peritonitis	Malrotation with or without volvulus
Pharyngitis/tonsillitis	Incarcerated hernia
Pneumonia	Intussusception
Otitis media	Meckel diverticulum with torsion
Urinary tract infection	Hirschsprung disease
Metabolic	**Gastrointestinal: Child**
Diabetic ketoacidosis	Appendicitis
Inborn errors of metabolism	Eosinophilic gastroenteritis
Addisonian crisis/adrenal insufficiency	Pancreatitis
Reye syndrome	Hepatitis
Other	Cholecystitis
Renal failure	Bowel obstruction
Hepatic failure	Malrotation
Congestive heart failure or pericarditis	Incarcerated hernia
Lead poisoning	Intussusception
Munchausen syndrome and Munchausen syndrome by proxy	Meckel diverticulum with torsion
	Adhesions
Central Nervous System	Superior Mesenteric Artery Syndrome
Increased intracranial pressure	Posttraumatic obstruction[b]
Ventricular-peritoneal shunt malfunction	**Respiratory**
Meningitis	Post-tussive emesis
Encephalitis	Reactive airway disease
Labyrinthitis	**Medications**
Migraine	Chemotherapeutic agents
Seizure	Cancer chemotherapy
Tumor	Digoxin and other cardiac drugs
Gynecologic	Antibiotics, e.g.,erythromycin
Pregnancy	Theophylline
	Caustic agents
	Ipecac
	Emotional/Behavioral
	Psychogenic
	Bulimia
	Rumination

[a]Malrotation with or without volvulus is much more likely in an infant than in a child.
[b]From duodenal hematoma, ruptured viscus.

gastroenteritis. Abdominal mass with emesis may indicate intussusception or malignancy. Tenderness on examination is suggestive of appendicitis, pancreatitis, cholecystitis, peritonitis, or PID.

DIAGNOSTIC EVALUATION

Specific laboratory studies depend on the suspected cause. Appropriate cultures, a complete blood count, and serum electrolytes may help determine the cause of vomiting and the metabolic complications secondary to vomiting. A chest radiograph will help rule out pneumonia. If a surgical process within the abdomen is considered, upright and supine abdominal films should be obtained, along with a complete blood count and electrolyte and chemistry panels. Amylase and lipase should be sent to detect pancreatitis. If vomiting is prolonged or the patient is significantly dehydrated, electrolytes will help guide replacement therapy. An ammonia level, serum amino acids, and urine organic acids should be sent if metabolic disease is suspected. Urinalysis and urine culture should be obtained to assess the degree of dehydration and rule out urinary tract infection.

TREATMENT

If the cause appears to be a self-limited nonsurgical infectious process (viral gastroenteritis or bacterial enterocolitis) and the patient is not significantly dehydrated, outpatient therapy is indicated. Oral rehydration therapy (ORT), discussed in Chapter 7, is recommended for dehydrated infants. For older children, fluids should be encouraged, with advancement to a regular diet as tolerated. Children who are severely dehydrated or unable to effectively hydrate themselves orally should be admitted to the hospital.

A surgical consultation should be obtained if indicated. If ventriculo-peritoneal shunt malfunction is a possibility, the standard of care dictates that a CT of the head and a shunt series be obtained in tandem with a neurosurgical consultation.

PYLORIC STENOSIS

Pyloric stenosis is an important cause of gastric outlet obstruction and vomiting in the first 2 to 3 months of life. Peak incidence occurs at 2 to 4 weeks of life, with an incidence of 1 in 500 infants. Male infants are affected 4:1 over female infants, and pyloric stenosis occurs more frequently in infants with a family history of the condition. Current evidence suggests that erythromycin therapy may precipitate pyloric stenosis.

Clinical Manifestations

Projectile nonbilious vomiting is the cardinal feature of the disorder. Physical findings vary with the severity of the obstruction. Dehydration and poor weight gain are common when the diagnosis is delayed. Hypokalemic, hypochloremic metabolic alkalosis with dehydration is seen secondary to persistent emesis in the most severe cases. The classic finding of an olive-sized, muscular, mobile, nontender mass in the epigastric area occurs in most cases but may be difficult to palpate. Visible gastric peristaltic waves may be seen. Ultrasonography reveals the hypertrophic pylorus. Upper GI study may show the classic "string sign."

Treatment

Initial treatment involves nasogastric tube placement and correction of dehydration, alkalosis, and electrolyte abnormalities. Pyloromyotomy should take place as soon as the metabolic anomalies are corrected.

MALROTATION AND VOLVULUS

Malrotation occurs when the small intestines rotate abnormally in utero, resulting in malposition in the abdomen and abnormal posterior fixation of the mesentery. When the intestine attaches improperly to the mesentery, it is at risk for twisting on its vascular supply; the twisting phenomenon is called **volvulus**. The most common age of presentation is less than 1 month of age.

Clinical Manifestations

The history almost always includes bilious emesis. In older children, a history of past attacks is occasionally elicited. Physical examination may reveal abdominal distention or shock. Blood-stained emesis or stool may be noted. Abdominal radiographs typically show gas in the stomach with a paucity of air in the intestine. An upper GI series with small bowel follow-through confirms the diagnosis by illustrating the abnormal position of the ligament of Treitz and the cecum. A positive stool test for blood may indicate significant bowel ischemia. Unexplained lactic acidosis may be an important sign of intestinal ischemia.

Treatment

Operative correction of the malrotation and the volvulus should be undertaken as soon as possible because bowel ischemia, metabolic acidosis, and sepsis can progress quickly to death.

GASTROESOPHAGEAL REFLUX

Gastroesophageal reflux (GER), defined as the passage of gastric contents into the esophagus, and GER disease (GERD), defined as symptoms or complications of GER, are common pediatric problems. Clinical manifestations of GERD in children include vomiting, poor weight gain, dysphagia, abdominal or substernal pain, esophagitis and respiratory disorders.

DIFFERENTIAL DIAGNOSIS

If the infant is having forceful emesis or projectile vomiting, reflux is *not* the most likely cause, and the differential diagnosis for emesis should be broadened (see Table 8-1). In the infant with recurrent vomiting, a thorough history and physical examination, with attention to warning signals, is generally sufficient to allow the clinician to establish a diagnosis of uncomplicated GER (the "happy spitter").

CLINICAL MANIFESTATIONS

History

It is important to determine if the infant is "spitting up" or having projectile emesis, and if the emesis is bloody or bilious.

Physical Examination

In most cases, the physical examination of the child with GER is normal. In severe cases, infants present with poor weight gain or failure to thrive.

DIAGNOSTIC EVALUATION

In most infants with vomiting, and in most older children with regurgitation and heartburn, a history and physical examination are sufficient to reliably diagnose GER, recognize complications, and initiate management.

The upper gastrointestinal (GI) series is neither sensitive nor specific for the diagnosis of GER, but is useful for the evaluation of the presence of anatomic abnormalities, such as pyloric stenosis, malrotation, and annular pancreas in the vomiting infant, as well as hiatal hernia and esophageal stricture in the older child.

Esophageal pH monitoring is a valid and reliable measure of acid reflux. Esophageal pH monitoring or impedance manometry with esophageal pH monitoring is useful to establish the presence of abnormal acid reflux, determine if there is a temporal association between acid reflux and frequently occurring symptoms, and assess the adequacy of therapy in patients who do not respond to treatment with acid suppression.

Endoscopy with biopsy can assess the presence and severity of esophagitis, strictures, and Barrett esophagus, as well as exclude other disorders such as Crohn disease and eosinophilic or infectious esophagitis in older children. Eosinophilic esophagitis (EE) does not respond to antacid therapy and may be a cause of chronic poorly responsive reflux symptoms. A characteristic endoscopic appearance and biopsy is diagnostic for EE. A normal appearance of the esophagus during endoscopy does not exclude GER.

A trial of time-limited medical therapy for GER is useful for determining if GER is causing a specific symptom.

TREATMENT

Diet and Lifestyle Changes

Esophageal pH monitoring has demonstrated that infants have significantly less GER when placed in the prone position than in the supine position. However, prone positioning is associated with a higher rate of the sudden infant death syndrome (SIDS). In infants from birth to 12 months of age with GERD, the risk of SIDS generally outweighs the potential benefits of prone sleeping. In children older than 1 year it is likely that there is a benefit to left side positioning during sleep and elevation of the head of the bed.

There is evidence to support a 1 to 2 week trial of a hypoallergenic formula in formula fed infants with vomiting. Milk-thickening agents do not improve reflux index scores but do decrease the number of episodes of vomiting. Children and adolescents with GERD should avoid food triggers. While these may be individualized based on history, caffeine, spicy foods, and high fat foods that delay gastric emptying may provoke symptoms. Obesity, exposure to tobacco smoke, and alcohol are also associated with GER.

Medications

Histamine2-receptor antagonists (H 2 RAs) produce relief of symptoms and mucosal healing. Proton pump inhibitors (PPIs), the most effective acid suppressant medications, are superior to H 2 RAs in relieving symptoms and healing esophagitis. Chronic antacid therapy is generally not recommended since more convenient and safe alternatives (H 2 RAs and PPIs) are available.

Surgical Therapy

Case series indicate that surgical therapy generally results in favorable outcomes. The potential risks, benefits, and costs of successful prolonged medical therapy versus fundoplication have not been well studied in infants or children in various symptom presentations.

DIARRHEA

Diarrhea is defined as an increase in the frequency and the water content of stools. Viral gastroenteritis is the most common cause of acute diarrheal illness throughout the world. The complications of acute diarrhea include dehydration, electrolyte and acid-base disturbances, bacteremia and sepsis, and malnutrition in chronic cases. **Enteritis** refers to small bowel inflammation, whereas **colitis** refers to large bowel inflammation.

DIFFERENTIAL DIAGNOSIS

Table 8-2 lists the most common causes of diarrhea in the pediatric population in developed countries.

■ TABLE 8-2 Differential Diagnosis of Diarrhea in Children	
Acute Diarrhea	**Chronic Recurrent Diarrhea**
Intestinal infections	*Immunodeficiency*
Viral, e.g., Rotavirus, Norovirus, Adenovirus, Astrovirus	Acquired immunodeficiency
	Congenital immunodeficiency
Bacterial, e.g., *Shigella, Salmonella, Campylobacter, Escherichia coli* (enterohemorrhagic, i.e., *E. coli* O157:H7, enteroaggregative and others), Yersinia, *Clostridium difficile*, Vibrio spp, e.g., *V. cholerae*, possibly Aeromonas spp, Plesiomonas spp	*Infectious*
	Clostridium difficile
	Parasites, e.g., *Giardia*, Cryptosporidium
	Gastrointestinal
Parasitic, e.g., *Giardia*, Cryptosporidium, *Entamoeba histolytica*	Cow/soy milk intolerance
Extraintestinal infections	Ulcerative colitis
Otitis media	Crohn disease
Urinary tract infection	Lactase deficiency
Gastrointestinal	Irritable bowel syndrome
Intussusception	Encopresis with overflow incontinence
Appendicitis	Excessive fructose or sorbitol intake
Osmotic diarrhea, i.e., hyperconcentrated infant formula, medications	Pancreatic insufficiency, e.g., cystic fibrosis
	Celiac disease
Toxic ingestion	Neuroendocrine tumor
Iron, mercury, lead, fluoride ingestion	*Allergy*
Medication induced	Food allergies
Antibiotics, chemotherapeutic agents	Eosinophilic gastrointestinal disorders
	Vasculitis
	Henoch-Schönlein purpura

CLINICAL MANIFESTATIONS

History

The history should ascertain whether the diarrhea is acute or chronic/recurrent and establish the frequency and appearance of the stools (bloody with mucopus, or watery). Dietary indiscretions and manipulations may result in diarrhea. Small infants have diarrhea when they are fed concentrated formula. Weight loss or lack of weight gain in association with diarrhea indicates more severe disease. Certain medications, especially antibiotics and chemotherapeutic agents, may cause diarrhea. Viral and bacterial gastroenteritis are both highly contagious, so sick contacts are likely.

Physical Examination

Chapter 7 discusses signs and symptoms of dehydration, which are critical in the evaluation of a patient with diarrhea. An attempt should be made to determine the degree of dehydration to guide therapy. The abdominal examination focuses on bowel sounds and the presence of distention, tenderness, or masses. Hypoactive bowel sounds point to intestinal obstruction. Hyperactive sounds are consistent with gastroenteritis. Abdominal mass with diarrhea could indicate intussusception or malignancy.

DIAGNOSTIC EVALUATION

When evaluating a child with diarrhea, inspecting the stool is critical to evaluation and formulation of a treatment plan. If there is a history of blood and/or mucous in the stool, if the child needs hospitalization, or the child is younger than 3 months of age, bacterial cultures should be obtained. Rapid tests for rotavirus are available; however, laboratory tests need not be routinely performed in children with signs and symptoms of acute gastroenteritis. Serum electrolytes are sometimes useful in assessing children with moderate to severe dehydration who require intravenous (IV) or nasogastric (NG) fluids. A normal bicarbonate concentration may be useful in ruling out or characterizing dehydration. For persistent diarrhea, the diagnostic evaluation should proceed in a stepwise fashion, including a complete blood count and stool tests for bacterial pathogens (including C. *difficile*, and parasitic pathogens, i.e., giardia and cryptosporidium). Subsequent evaluation may include tests for immunodeficiency, pancreatic insufficiency and celiac disease, etc., as appropriate.

TREATMENT

Acute gastroenteritis (AGE) is often self-limited and most often results in inconvenience and expense to the family in terms of work lost. However, the goals of treatment are primarily prevention and/or management of dehydration and secondarily improvement of symptoms, the latter being an appropriate concern of the family. Immunization with rotavirus vaccine is an important approach to limit severe diarrhea, prevent dehydration, and reduce the likelihood of hospitalization when rotaviral illness occurs.

When a child has mild to moderate diarrhea, continued use of the child's preferred, usual, and age-appropriate diet should be encouraged to prevent or limit dehydration. Regular diets are generally more effective than restricted and progressive diets, and in numerous trials have consistently produced a reduction in the duration of diarrhea. The historical BRAT diet (consisting of bananas, rice, applesauce, and toast) is unnecessarily restrictive, but may be offered as part of the child's usual diet. Clear liquids are not recommended as a substitute for oral rehydration solutions (ORS) or regular diets in the prevention or therapy of dehydration. The vast majority of patients with mild to moderate AGE do not develop clinically important lactose intolerance and do not need to be milk-restricted. In selected patients with documented, persistent clinical lactose intolerance, lactose-free formulas are recommended. The vomiting child should be offered frequent small feedings (every 10 to 60 minutes) of any tolerated foods or ORS.

Dehydration should be treated with ORS, for a period of 4 to 6 hours or until an adequate degree of rehydration is achieved. When the care provider is unable to replace the estimated fluid deficit and keep up with ongoing losses using oral feedings alone, or the child is severely dehydrated with an obtunded mental status, IV fluids or NG ORS should be given for a period of 4 to 6 hours or until adequate rehydration is achieved. It is appropriate to involve the family in the decision regarding the method of fluid replacement. Refeeding of the usual diet should be started at the earliest opportunity after an adequate degree of rehydration is achieved. Following rehydration therapy in the child with mild to moderate dehydration, regular diets may be supplemented with ORS containing at least 45 mEq Na^+/L, and targeted to deliver 10 mL/kg for each stool or emesis. It is important to reassess hydration status by phone or in the office when a child refuses ORS. This can be a sign of severe illness or refusal may indicate an absence of salt craving, and, as such, resolution of dehydration.

Antidiarrheal agents and antiemetics are not recommended for the routine management of children with AGE. However, ondansetron may decrease vomiting and hospitalization rates in those patients who require IV or NG fluids. It is recommended that antimicrobial therapies be used only for selected children with AGE who present with special risks or evidence of a serious bacterial infection. The infant with salmonellosis represents just such a special case.

If the stool culture is positive for salmonella and the infant is afebrile and does not appear toxic, the infant can be reexamined and observed at home. If the stool culture is positive and the infant is febrile, the infant's age determines therapy:

- The infant younger than 3 months is admitted to the hospital; a blood culture is obtained, and intravenous antibiotics are started. A lumbar puncture and urinalysis should also be considered in this age group.
- The infant older than 3 months is admitted to the hospital; a blood culture should be sent, but antibiotics may be withheld pending the results of the blood culture.
- Any infant with a positive stool culture who looks toxic or has a positive blood culture is admitted for intravenous antibiotics and evaluation for pyelonephritis, meningitis, pneumonia, and osteomyelitis.

Treatment for *C. difficile* involves discontinuation of concurrent antimicrobial therapy and enteral therapy with metronidazole or vancomycin. *Giardia lamblia* and *Cryptosporidium* are also common causes of persistent diarrhea and, if found, treatment is available with metronidazole or nitazoxanide.

It is recommended that probiotics be considered as adjunctive therapy, as they have been shown to reduce the duration of diarrhea. The family preference may be central to the decision to use probiotics. Parameters influencing the family's decision may include cost, degree of potential benefit, availability, and unverified effectiveness of commercial products.

CONSTIPATION

Constipation is defined as the infrequent passage of hard, dry stools. Constipated infants fail to empty the colon completely with bowel movements and over time stretch the smooth muscle of the colon, resulting

in a functional ileus. In contrast to constipation, **obstipation** is the absence of bowel movements. Beyond the neonatal period, the most common cause (90% to 95%) of constipation is voluntary withholding or "functional" constipation. Intentional withholding is often noted from the very beginning of toilet training. A family history of similar problems is often obtained. Stool retention may be caused by conflicts in toilet training but is usually caused by pain on defecation, which creates a fear of defecation and further retention. Voluntary withholding of stool increases distention of the rectum, which decreases rectal sensation, necessitating an even greater fecal mass to initiate the urge to defecate. Complications of stool retention include impaction, abdominal pain, overflow diarrhea resulting from leakage around the fecal mass, anal fissure, rectal bleeding, and urinary tract infection caused by extrinsic pressure on the urethra.

Encopresis, which is daytime or nighttime soiling by formed stools in children beyond the age of expected toilet training (3 to 5 years), is another complication of constipation. In older children, it is important to ask specifically about soiling, because such information may not be expressed because of embarrassment. These children are unable to sense the need to defecate because of stretching of the internal sphincter by the retained fecal mass.

Organic causes of failure to defecate include decreased peristalsis, decreased expulsion, and anatomic malformation. Organic etiologies are delineated in the following section.

DIFFERENTIAL DIAGNOSIS

Nonorganic
- Functional constipation (intentional withholding)
- Dysfunctional toilet training

Organic
- Dietary: Low-fiber diet, inadequate fluid intake
- GI: Functional ileus, Hirschsprung disease, anal stenosis, rectal abscess or fissure, stricture following necrotizing enterocolitis (NEC), collagen vascular disease
- Drugs or toxins: Lead, narcotics, phenothiazines, vincristine, anticholinergics
- Neuromuscular: Meningomyelocele, tethered spinal cord, infant botulism, absent abdominal muscles (prune belly syndrome)
- Metabolic: Cystic fibrosis, hypokalemia, hypercalcemia
- Endocrine: Hypothyroidism

CLINICAL MANIFESTATIONS

History and Physical Examination

Abdominal pain caused by constipation is often diffuse and constant. The pain may be accompanied by nausea, but vomiting is unusual. Stools are hard, difficult to pass, and infrequent. Discussion of withholding behavior (potty dance) can be helpful in identifying functional etiologies of constipation. An organic cause of constipation (cystic fibrosis, Hirschsprung disease) is more likely in a patient who did not pass meconium in the first 24 to 48 hours of life. Findings that suggest concern for a non-organic etiology of constipation include: failure to grow, pilonidal dimple covered with a tuft of hair, absent anal wink, tight empty rectum in the presence of a palpable fecal mass, anteriorly displaced anus, and decreased lower extremity tone or strength.

DIAGNOSTIC EVALUATION

Most often no diagnostic studies are needed. If the diagnosis is unclear, a plain abdominal film can be helpful because a colon full of feces makes the diagnosis of constipation. Thyroid studies, including free T4 and TSH levels are indicated if hypothyroidism is suspected. If hypokalemia or hypocalcemia is a potential cause, an electrolyte and chemistry panel may be obtained. A rectal mucosal biopsy is required to make the diagnosis of Hirschsprung disease. A lead level assists in diagnosing plumbism as the cause of constipation.

TREATMENT

The general approach to the child with functional constipation includes the following steps: determine whether fecal impaction is present, treat the impaction if present, initiate treatment with oral medication, provide parental education and follow-up, and adjust medications as necessary.

Polyethylene glycol (PEG) 3350 is efficacious for disimpaction in children. When daily medication is necessary in the treatment of constipation, PEG 3350 also appears to be superior to other osmotic agents in palatability and acceptance by children. The goal is to achieve a soft (mashed potato or pudding consistency stool) on a daily or more frequent basis. Data in children under a year of age indicate that PEG 3350 is safe and effective in this age group as well. There is extensive experience with other therapies including mineral oil, magnesium hydroxide, and lactulose or sorbitol. Long-term studies show that these therapies are effective and safe. Because mineral oil, magnesium hydroxide, lactulose, and sorbitol seem to be equally efficacious, the choice among these is based on safety, cost, the child's preference, ease of administration, and the practitioner's experience. A behavioral program of daily sit downs and positive reinforcement is often helpful in structuring the approach for the family. While dietary changes are anticipated by families as part of the treatment plan, no randomized controlled studies have demonstrated an effect on stools of increasing intake of fluids, nonabsorbable carbohydrates, or dietary fiber in children. Forceful implementation of diet is undesirable. The education of the family and the demystification of constipation, including an explanation of the pathogenesis of constipation, are important steps in treatment. Providing hope to a frustrated family is key. If fecal soiling is present, an important goal for both the child and the parent is to remove negative attributions. It is especially important for parents to understand that soiling from overflow incontinence is not a willful and defiant maneuver.

HIRSCHSPRUNG DISEASE

Hirschsprung disease, or congenital aganglionic megacolon, occurs in 1 in 5,000 children and results from the failure of the ganglion cells of the myenteric plexus to migrate down the developing colon. As a result, the abnormally innervated distal colon remains tonically contracted and obstructs the flow of feces. Hirschsprung disease is three times more common among boys and accounts for 20% of cases of neonatal intestinal obstruction. In 75% of cases, the aganglionic segment is limited to the rectosigmoid colon, whereas 15% extend beyond the splenic flexure.

Clinical Manifestations

The diagnosis should be suspected in any infant who fails to pass meconium within the first 24 to 48 hours of life or who requires repeated rectal simulation to induce bowel movements. In the first month of life, the neonate develops evidence of obstruction with poor feeding, bilious vomiting, and abdominal distention. In some cases, particularly those with short segment (less than 5 cm) involvement, the diagnosis goes undetected into childhood. In the older child, failure to grow may be seen, as well as intermittent bouts of intestinal obstruction, enterocolitis with bloody diarrhea, and, occasionally, bowel perforation, sepsis, and shock.

Stool that is palpable throughout the abdomen and an empty rectum on digital examination are most suggestive of the disease. Abdominal radiographs show distention of the proximal bowel and no gas or feces in the rectum. Contrast enema may demonstrate a transition zone between the narrowed abnormal distal segment and the dilated normal proximal bowel. However, a normal contrast enema does not rule out the diagnosis. Anal manometry demonstrates failure of the internal sphincter to relax with balloon distention of the rectum. Rectal biopsy reveals absence of ganglion cells, an abnormal pattern of acetylcholinesterase staining, and hypertrophied nerve trunks and is the diagnostic study of choice.

Treatment

Hirschsprung disease is often treated surgically in two stages. The first stage involves the creation of a diverting colostomy with the bowel that contains ganglion cells, thus permitting decompression of the ganglion-containing bowel segment. In the second stage, the aganglionic segment is removed and the ganglionic segment is anastomosed to the rectum. This procedure is often postponed until the infant is 12 months of age or delayed for 3 to 6 months when the disease has been diagnosed in an older child. The mortality rate for this disorder is low in the absence of enterocolitis; major complications include anal stenosis and incontinence.

GASTROINTESTINAL BLEEDING

GI bleeding may be acute or chronic, gross or microscopic, and may manifest as hematemesis, hematochezia, or melena. A plethora of disorders in childhood can cause GI bleeding.

Hematemesis refers to the emesis of fresh or old blood from the GI tract. Fresh blood becomes chemically altered to a ground-coffee appearance within 5 minutes of exposure to gastric acid. Hematochezia is the passage of fresh (bright red) or dark maroon blood from the rectum. The source is usually the colon, although upper GI tract bleeding that has a rapid transit time can also result in hematochezia. Melena describes shiny, jet black, tarry stools that are positive for occult blood. It usually results from upper GI bleeding and the color and consistency results from the blood being chemically altered during passage through the gut.

DIFFERENTIAL DIAGNOSIS

The differential diagnosis for GI bleeding is generally divided into upper and lower GI tract etiologies. Upper GI bleeding occurs at a site proximal to the ligament of Treitz, whereas lower GI bleeding occurs at a site distal to this ligament. Although hematemesis from upper GI bleeding can be seen in critically ill children from esophagitis or gastritis, or in children with portal hypertension from esophageal varices, most GI bleeding in children is from the lower tract and manifests as rectal bleeding. Table 8-3 lists the

■ **TABLE 8-3** Causes of Rectal Bleeding by Age of Patient			
Newborn	**Infant to 2 Yr**	**2 Yr to Preschool**	**Preschool to Adolescence**
Most frequent causes			
Vitamin K deficiency	Anal fissure	Infectious diarrhea	Infectious diarrhea
Ingested maternal blood	Cow/soy milk enterocolitis	Polyp	Polyp
Cow/soy milk enterocolitis	Infectious diarrhea	Anal fissure	IBD
Necrotizing enterocolitis	Intussusception	Meckel diverticulum	HSP
Hirschsprung disease	Meckel diverticulum		
Less frequent causes			
Volvulus	Duplication cyst	IBD	Anal fissure
Duplication cyst	Vascular malformation	Vascular malformation	Vascular malformation
Upper GI tract bleeding with rapid transit	Upper GI tract bleeding with rapid transit	Upper GI tract bleeding with rapid transit	Hemorrhoid

most common causes of rectal bleeding by age. Minor bleeding presents as stool streaked with blood and is usually caused by an anal fissure or polyp. Inflammatory diseases, such as IBD or infectious enterocolitis, result in diarrheal stool mixed with blood. In contrast, Meckel diverticulum typically results in a significant amount of bleeding without diarrhea. Table 8-4 lists the associated signs and symptoms of the major causes of GI bleeding.

CLINICAL MANIFESTATIONS

History

It is important to define the onset and duration of bleeding, color (bright red vs. dark maroon vs. tarry black), rate (brisk vs. gradual), and type of bleeding (hematochezia, hematemesis, melena, blood-streaked stool).

For upper GI bleeding, questions about forceful vomiting, ingestion of ulcerogenic drugs (salicylates, nonsteroidal anti-inflammatory drugs, steroids), and a history of liver disease or peptic ulcer disease are helpful. For lower GI tract bleeding, inquire about diarrhea, or constipation with large or hard stools and difficult or painful defecation.

Emesis of red fluid may not be blood and can be due to vomiting of ingested fluids or foods (sugared children's drinks, beets, red gelatin, acetaminophen elixir). Black stool is not always caused by blood in the stool; it can occur in children who have ingested iron, bismuth, or blackberries.

Physical Examination

The immediate priority when examining a child with GI bleeding is to determine if hypovolemia exists from an acute bleed. Vital signs should be examined for orthostatic changes or for evidence of shock (tachycardia, tachypnea, hypotension). The earliest sign of significant GI bleeding is a raised resting heart rate. A drop in blood pressure is not seen until at least 40% of the intravascular volume is depleted. Dermatologic abnormalities such as petechiae and purpura indicate coagulopathy, whereas cool or clammy skin with pallor is suggestive of shock or anemia. On abdominal examination, masses (e.g., in the right lower quadrant mass may be caused by Crohn disease or intussusception), tenderness (e.g., in the epigastrium suggests peptic ulcer disease), and splenomegaly or hepatosplenomegaly and caput medusae suggests evidence of portal hypertension and risk of varices.

■ **TABLE 8-4** Diagnosis of Gastrointestinal Bleeding		
Site	**Cause**	**Signs and Symptoms**
Upper	Medication	Ingestion of NSAIDs
	Varices	Splenomegaly or evidence of liver disease
	Esophagitis	Dysphagia, vomiting, dyspepsis
	PUD	Epigastric pain, meal related
Lower	Fissure	Bright red blood on surface of the stool
	Chronic polyps	Painless rectal bleeding on the surface of stool; may have some mucus admixed
	Cow's milk–soy enterocolitis	Blood mixed with stool; may have diarrhea, hypoalbuminemia, and edema
	Meckel diverticulum	Painless, often a large amount of blood
	IBD	Diarrhea, fever, abdominal pain, poor growth, associated systemic signs and symptoms
	Bacterial colitis	Diarrhea, abdominal pain, antecedent watery diarrhea, e.g., *E. coli* O157:H7 or antibiotic exposure, e.g., *C. difficile*
	HSP	Joint pain, abdominal pain, purpura
	Intussusception	Intermittent abdominal pain, pallor, currant jelly stools, right sided abdominal mass

HSP, Henoch-Schönlein purpura; IBD, inflammatory bowel disease; NSAID, nonsteroidal anti-inflammatory drug; PUD, peptic ulcer disease.

Capillary refill (thenar eminence in neonates and infants) should be assessed on the extremity examination. On rectal examination, the clinician may assess for anal fissure, which is best seen by spreading the buttocks and everting the anal canal (most fissures are located at the 6 and 12 o'clock positions), perform a stool test for occult blood, feel for hard stool, and look for a dilated rectum in children with chronic constipation or anal fissure.

DIAGNOSTIC EVALUATION

Unless the source of bleeding is clearly the nasopharynx, an anal fissure, or hemorrhoids, a complete blood count with differential and platelet count and usually coagulation studies should be sent. Hemodynamically significant GI bleeding is a medical emergency and requires careful monitoring, often in an intensive care unit with blood available for transfusion.

If the bleeding source is unclear and the patient is unstable, gastric lavage determines whether the bleeding is from the upper GI tract proximal to the ligament of Treitz. The stomach is lavaged with room-temperature normal saline. Esophageal varices are not an absolute contraindication to the placement of a nasogastric or orogastric tube. Return of clear lavage fluid makes the diagnosis of upper GI bleeding unlikely, although occasionally duodenal ulcers may bleed only distally. Return of bright red blood or "coffee grounds" that eventually clear indicates upper GI bleeding that has remitted. Persistent return of bright red blood indicates active bleeding and mandates aggressive intravenous fluid management and monitoring. A pediatric gastroenterologist should be consulted. A surgical consultation is often indicated although it is now uncommon to require surgery for an upper GI bleed in children.

In the stable patient, a thorough history and physical examination with consideration of the age-related causes usually leads to diagnosis. Gastric lavage is unnecessary in children with minor or nonacute GI bleeding. The precise diagnosis is often made by upper or lower endoscopy.

If there is bloody diarrhea, stool should be sent for culture. Bloody diarrhea following several days of non-bloody diarrhea is commonly seen in infection with *E. coli* O157:H7 which in 10% to 15% of patients can lead to hemolytic uremic syndrome. In the hospitalized neonate with bloody stool, necrotizing enterocolitis must be considered, and an abdominal film and evaluation for sepsis should be performed. When swallowed maternal blood is suspected as the cause of GI bleeding, the Apt red blood cell fragility test is performed on the child's stool or emesis to differentiate maternal blood from the blood of the neonate. A Meckel diverticulum should be considered when there is a large amount of painless rectal bleeding.

TREATMENT

The unstable child with severe bleeding or hypovolemia is evaluated by primary and secondary surveys as outlined in Chapter 1. A normal hemoglobin or hematocrit does not rule out severe acute bleeding; full hemodilution takes up to 12 hours in the acutely bleeding patient. Intravenous normal saline or Ringer lactate at 20 mL per kg boluses should be given until the vital signs are sufficiently improved. Type O-negative whole blood should be reserved for the unstable patient with acute bleeding that cannot quickly be brought under control. The most common error in management of the child with severe GI bleeding is inadequate volume replacement. Hypotension is a late finding; fluid resuscitation should be governed by the level of tachycardia. The stable child without heavy bleeding or signs of hypovolemia should be evaluated and treated according to the particular diagnosis.

Figure 8-1 illustrates a useful algorithm for the evaluation and management of GI bleeding. Three common causes of GI bleeding—Meckel diverticulum, ulcerative colitis, and Crohn disease—are discussed in the following sections.

MECKEL DIVERTICULUM

Meckel diverticulum, the vestigial remnant of the omphalomesenteric duct, is the most common anomaly of the GI tract. It is present in 2% to 3% of the population and is located within 100 cm of the ileocecal valve in the small intestine. The peak incidence of bleeding from the diverticulum is at 2 years of age. Heterotopic tissue, usually gastric, is ten times more common in symptomatic cases because of acid secretion and ulceration of nearby ileal mucosa.

Clinical Manifestations

The most common presentation of Meckel diverticulum is painless rectal bleeding. Eighty-five percent of patients with Meckel diverticulum have hematochezia, 10% develop intestinal obstruction from intussusception or volvulus, and 5% suffer from painful diverticulitis mimicking appendicitis. The diagnosis is made by performing a Meckel scan. The technetium-99

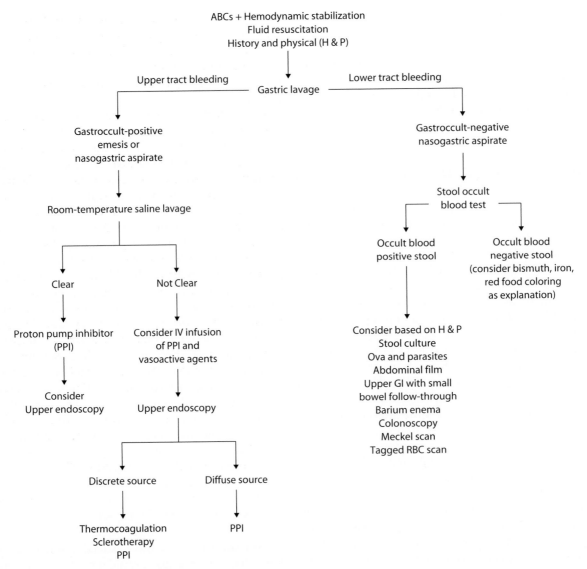

Figure 8-1 • Algorithm for evaluation and management of GI tract bleeding.

pertechne-tate scan, preceded by prepentagastrin stimulation or a histamine H2-receptor antagonist, identifies the ectopic acid-secreting cells that mediate the hemorrhage.

Treatment

Definitive treatment is surgical resection.

INFLAMMATORY BOWEL DISEASE

IBD is a generic term for **Crohn disease** and **ulcerative colitis**, which are chronic inflammatory disorders of the intestines.

Ulcerative colitis produces diffuse superficial colonic ulceration and crypt abscesses. It involves the rectum in 95% of patients, with or without contiguous extension higher in the colon. Ulcerative colitis does not affect the small intestine.

The pathology of Crohn disease involves transmural inflammation in a discontinuous pattern, which results in skip lesions. Crohn disease may involve any part of the GI tract (mouth to anus). In pediatric patients, the process is ileocolonic in 40% of cases, involves the small intestine alone in approximately 30% of cases, and is isolated to the colon in only 20% of cases. Crohn disease may result in transmural inflammation with fistula formation or perforation or fibrostenotic disease with stricture formation.

Although the exact etiology of these disorders is not known, a combination of genetic, immunologic, and environmental mechanisms is implicated. Most pediatric patients are adolescents, but both diseases are seen in infancy and in preschool children.

Clinical Manifestations

Crampy abdominal pain, recurrent fever, and weight loss are common manifestations in Crohn disease. Although diarrhea is common, it is not universal. Rectal bleeding is noted in only 35% of cases of Crohn disease. Abdominal pain tends to be more severe in Crohn disease than in ulcerative colitis, may be diffuse, and is frequently worse in the right lower quadrant. Perianal disease may produce skin tags, fissures, fistulas, or abscesses. Anorexia, poor weight gain, and delayed growth occur in 40% of patients.

Most children with ulcerative colitis exhibit bloody diarrhea with mucopus (100%), abdominal pain (95%), and tenesmus (75%). Ninety percent of patients exhibit mild to moderate disease. Mild disease is defined as less than six stools per day, no fever, no anemia, and no hypoalbuminemia, whereas moderate disease has greater than six stools per day, fever, anemia, and hypoalbuminemia. Severe disease may be fulminant, with high fever, abdominal tenderness, distention, tachycardia, leukocytosis, hemorrhage, severe anemia, and more than eight stools per day.

Toxic megacolon and intestinal perforation are rare complications. After 10 years of ulcerative colitis, there is a cumulative risk of 1% to 2% per year for the development of carcinoma.

Table 8-5 compares Crohn disease and ulcerative colitis.

Extraintestinal sequelae occur in both diseases, may precede or accompany GI symptoms, and include polyarticular arthritis, ankylosing spondylitis, primary sclerosing cholangitis, chronic active hepatitis, sacroiliitis, pyoderma gangrenosum, erythema nodosum, aphthous stomatitis, episcleritis, recurrent iritis, and uveitis. Patients with Crohn disease are also at increased risk for nephrolithiasis secondary to ileal disease and abnormal absorption of oxalate.

In the evaluation of suspected IBD in the pediatric patient, a full colonoscopy with ileoscopy is indicated to evaluate all affected areas and to attempt to differentiate between Crohn disease and ulcerative colitis. An upper endoscopy is often performed to assess for any microscopic inflammation in the upper GI tract. Even with a full evaluation, it is sometimes difficult to make a definitive diagnosis in patients with primary colonic disease. Visualization of the mucosa in ulcerative colitis reveals diffuse superficial ulceration and easy bleeding. In Crohn disease, deep ulcerations may be present, and diseased areas may be more focal.

Upper GI study with small bowel follow-through in Crohn disease often reveals ileal or proximal small bowel disease with segmental narrowing of the ileum

■ **TABLE 8-5** Comparison of Crohn Disease and Ulcerative Colitis		
Feature	**Crohn Disease**	**Ulcerative Colitis**
Malaise, fever, weight loss	Common	Sometimes
Rectal bleeding	Sometimes	Nearly always
Abdominal pain	Common	Common
Abdominal mass	Common	Rare
Perianal disease	Common	Rare
Ileal involvement	Common	Rare (backwash ileitis)
Stricture	Sometimes	Not seen
Fistula	Sometimes	Not seen
Skip lesions	Common	Rare
Transmural inflammation	Common	Not seen
Granulomas	Sometimes	Not seen
Long term risk of cancer	Increased	Greatly increased

(string sign) and longitudinal ulcers. A capsule endoscopy test may help identify small intestinal lesions in IBD.

Anemia is common and usually associated with iron deficiency. Megaloblastic anemia secondary to folate and vitamin B12 deficiency may also be present. An elevation in the erythrocyte sedimentation rate and the CRP is common but severe inflammation can be present without significant elevation of these inflammatory markers. Hypoalbuminemia can be seen with malnutrition or a protein losing enteropathy in Crohn disease. Serum aminotransferase levels are increased if hepatic inflammation is a complicating feature. Stool examination reveals blood and fecal leukocytes with a negative stool culture.

Differential Diagnosis

The differential diagnosis of IBD includes bacterial or parasitic causes of diarrhea (C. *difficile*, E. *coli* O157:H7, *Campylobacter jejuni*, *Yersinia enterocolitica*, amebiasis), appendicitis, HSP, eosinophilic gastrointestinal disease, and radiation enterocolitis.

Treatment

Treatment of IBD is aimed at control of inflammation and suppression of the immune system. Five-aminosalicylic compounds are a mainstay of anti-inflammatory treatment. Antibiotics have a role as anti-inflammatory agents in Crohn disease. Aggressive nutritional support (including tube feeding) is important for growth but also has an anti-inflammatory effect and improves symptom control in Crohn disease. Corticosteroids have both anti-inflammatory and immunosuppressive effects, and they remain a mainstay of early management. Other immunomodulatory treatments including mercaptopurine, azathioprine, and methotrexate are useful as steroid sparing agents. Biologic therapy with antitumor necrosis factor antibody is increasingly used in difficult to treat disease.

Because anorexia and increased nutrient losses in the stool are common in children with IBD, adequate calories and protein are essential. Oral supplements, nasogastric tube feedings, and, in some severe cases, central venous hyperalimentation are necessary. Vitamin and mineral supplementation, especially with iron, folate and B12, may be required.

Patients with ulcerative colitis for more than 10 years need annual colonoscopy and biopsy because of the high risk of colon cancer development. Studies have shown that patients with long-standing Crohn colitis are also at an increased risk for development of neoplasia.

Surgery is eventually needed in 25% of patients with ulcerative colitis and up to 70% of children with Crohn disease. Surgery is indicated in ulcerative colitis when there is fulminant colitis with severe blood loss or toxic megacolon, intractable disease with a high-dosage steroid requirement, steroid toxicity, growth failure, or colonic dysplasia. Because ulcerative colitis is restricted to the colon, colectomy is curative. Surgery is performed in Crohn disease when inflammation is not controlled with medical therapy, or when hemorrhage, obstruction, perforation, severe fistula formation, or ureteral obstruction is present. In general, conservative management is warranted because removal of the diseased bowel is not curative in Crohn disease. Recurrence rates of up to 50% have been reported after segmental resection.

KEY POINTS

- The history and physical examination help to determine whether abdominal pain is acute or chronic/recurrent and whether a medical, surgical, or nonorganic disorder is most likely. In the adolescent female, genitourinary pathology must be considered, and a pelvic examination should be performed.

- Appendicitis is the most common surgical indication for abdominal pain in childhood.

- Most intussusception results from invagination of the ileum into the colon of the ileocecal valve, which results in periodic episodes of irritability, colicky pain, and emesis.

- Most cases of emesis are caused by gastroesophageal reflux, acute gastroenteritis, or non-GI infectious disorders such as tonsillitis, otitis media, or urinary tract infection. However, intestinal obstruction, neurologic, metabolic, and drug-induced etiologies and nondigestive organ failure are important causes not to miss.

- Pyloric stenosis is an important cause of gastric outlet obstruction and emesis in the first 2 months of life.

- In most infants and older children with emesis, reflux, and heartburn, a history and physical examination are sufficient to reliably diagnose GERD, recognize complications, and initiate management.

- The most common cause of diarrhea in children is viral gastroenteritis.

- Most children with uncomplicated viral gastroenteritis or bacterial enterocolitis can be rehydrated orally; antidiarrheal medications are not indicated in children with acute diarrhea.

- Infants with diarrhea should be fed as close to their normal diet as possible. Recovery is faster than if a restricted diet is used.

- Constipation resulting from organic causes may be caused by decreased peristalsis, decreased expulsion, and anatomic malformation.

- Constipation is commonly associated with anal fissure in infancy and voluntary withholding or functional constipation in children and adolescents.

- Hirschsprung disease should be suspected in any infant who fails to pass meconium within the first 24 to 48 hours of life or who requires repeated rectal stimulation to induce bowel movements, or has poor feeding, bilious vomiting, and abdominal distention in the first month of life.

- The earliest sign of significant GI bleeding is a raised resting heart rate. A drop in blood pressure is not seen until at least 40% of the intravascular volume is depleted. Hemodynamically significant GI bleeding is a medical emergency and requires careful monitoring, often in an intensive care unit and blood available for transfusion.

- Meckel diverticulum is the most common anomaly of the GI tract, and presents with painless rectal bleeding.

- Ulcerative colitis produces diffuse superficial colonic ulceration and crypt abscesses. It involves the rectum in 95% of patients, with or without contiguous extension higher in the colon. Ulcerative colitis does not affect the small intestine.

- The pathology of Crohn disease involves transmural inflammation in a discontinuous pattern, which results in skip lesions. Crohn disease may involve any part of the GI tract (mouth to anus).

- Therapy for IBD is aimed at achieving maximum symptom control with minimum side effects.

9 Genetic Disorders

Bradley S. Marino • Emily Claybon

Structural birth defects are categorized as minor or major. Minor birth defects such as skin tags, inner epicanthal folds, and rudimentary polydactyly are of little physiologic significance. Approximately 15% of newborn infants have at least one minor anomaly; 0.5% of infants have three or more minor anomalies. In contrast, major birth defects such as cleft palate, myelomeningocele, and congenital heart disease have an adverse effect on the infant. Major birth defects occur in 2% to 3% of all newborns. The probability of having a major birth defect increases as the number of minor anomalies present increases (Table 9-1). Birth defects can be caused by environmental or genetic factors. Genetic defects may be chromosomal, single gene, imprinting, cytogenetic, or multifactorial disorders.

ENVIRONMENTAL FACTORS

Environmental factors are known to cause at least 10% of all birth defects. **Teratogens** are environmental agents that cause congenital developmental anomalies by interfering with embryonic or fetal organogenesis or growth. Exposure to a teratogen before implantation (days 7 to 10 postconception) can either have no effect or can result in loss of the embryo. To disrupt organogenesis, a teratogenic exposure typically occurs before 12 weeks' gestation. Any teratogenic exposure after 12 weeks' gestation predominantly affects growth and central nervous system development.

Teratogens include intra-uterine infections (Chapter 13), high-dosage radiation, maternal metabolic disorders (Chapter 13), mechanical forces, and drugs. The most common maternal metabolic disorder that has teratogenic potential is diabetes mellitus; 10% of infants of diabetic mothers have a birth defect. Abnormal intrauterine forces such as uterine fibroids or oligohydramnios may cause fetal constraint, resulting in club foot or hip dysplasia. Table 9-2 lists the most common teratogenic drugs and their effects.

GENETIC FACTORS

Genetic disorders can be classified as disorders of single genes, chromosomes, imprinting, and molecular cytogenetics. Advances in molecular genetics have blurred the distinction among these categories.

SINGLE-GENE DISORDERS

Normal human cells have 46 chromosomes (22 pairs of autosomes and 1 pair of sex chromosomes). Chromosomes contain genes, which occur in pairs at a single locus or site on specific chromosomes. These paired genes, called **alleles**, determine the genotype of an individual at that locus. If the genes at a specific locus are identical, the individual is **homozygous**; if they are different, the individual is **heterozygous**.

■ **TABLE 9-1** Incidence of Major Anomalies in the Presence of Minor Anomalies

Number of Minor Anomalies	Incidence of Major Anomalies (%)
0	<1
1	1
2	3
3	20

TABLE 9-2 Common Teratogenic Drugs

Drug	Results
Warfarin (Coumadin)	Hypoplastic nasal bridge, chondrodysplasia punctata
Ethanol	Fetal alcohol syndrome, microcephaly, CHD (septal defects, patent ductus arteriosus)
Isotretinoin (Accutane)	Facial and ear anomalies, CHD
Lithium	CHD (Ebstein anomaly, atrial septal defect)
Penicillamine	Cutis laxa syndrome
Phenytoin (Dilantin)	Hypoplastic nails, intrauterine growth retardation, cleft lip and palate
Radioactive iodine	Congenital goiter, hypothyroidism
Diethylstilbestrol	Vaginal adenocarcinoma during adolescence
Streptomycin	Deafness
Testosterone-like drugs	Virilization of female
Tetracycline	Dental enamel hypoplasia, altered bone growth
Thalidomide	Phocomelia, CHD (TOF, septal defects)
Trimethadione	Typical facies, CHD (TOF, TGA, HLHS)
Valproate	Spina bifida

CHD, congenital heart disease; HLHS, hypoplastic left heart syndrome; TGA, transpositions of the great arteries; TOF, tetralogy of fallot.

More than 3,000 different single-gene disorders have been described and are classified by their mode of inheritance (autosomal dominant, autosomal recessive, or X-linked).

AUTOSOMAL DOMINANT DISORDERS

Autosomal dominant disorders are expressed after alteration of only one gene in the pair (often coding for a structural protein). Homozygous disease states of autosomal dominant disorders are rare and are usually severe or lethal. A mutant gene is inherited from one parent with the same condition. The risk for the affected parents' offspring is 50% for each pregnancy. Sometimes an individual is the first person in a family to display a trait due to spontaneous mutation. When a spontaneous mutation has occurred in a fetus, the risk of recurrence in a subsequent pregnancy is the same as the chance of the spontaneous mutation occurring de novo. Autosomal dominant genes often cause conditions that manifest themselves with varying degrees of severity among affected individuals, a phenomenon known as **variable expressivity** or **variable penetrance**. Table 9-3 lists some important autosomal dominant diseases. Other chapters discuss some of these diseases in detail.

AUTOSOMAL RECESSIVE DISORDERS

Autosomal recessive disorders are only expressed after alteration of both the maternal and paternal genes of a gene pair (often coding for an enzyme). Because half of the normal enzyme activity is adequate under most circumstances, a person with only one mutant gene is not affected, whereas individuals who are homozygous for a defective gene have the disorder. Both parents of a child with an autosomal recessive disorder are usually heterozygous for that gene, and each child of such a couple has a 25% risk of inheriting the disorder. Table 9-4 lists the more common autosomal recessive disorders.

Most inborn errors of metabolism, with the exception of ornithine transcarbamylase (OTC) deficiency, are autosomal recessive disorders. Inborn errors of metabolism are discussed later in this chapter.

X-LINKED DISORDERS

X-linked disorders, which are usually recessive, occur when a male inherits a mutant gene on the X chromosome from his mother. The affected male, termed **hemizygous** for the gene, has only a single X chromosome and, therefore, a single set of X-linked

■ TABLE 9-3 Examples of Autosomal Dominant Diseases

Autosomal Dominant Disease	Frequency	Chromosome	Gene	Comments
Achondroplasia	1:25,000	4p	FGFR3	80% new mutations; proximal limb shortening
Adult polycystic kidney disease	1:1,200	16p	PKD1/PKD2	Renal cysts, intracranial aneurysm
Hereditary angioedema	1:10,000	11q	C1NH	Deficiency of C1 esterase inhibitor; episodic edema
Hereditary spherocytosis	1:5,000	8p, 14q	ANK1	See Chapter 10; some variants autosomal recessive
Marfan syndrome	1:20,000	15q	FBN1	Aortic root dilatation, tall stature
Neurofibromatosis	1:3,000	2p, 17q, 22q	NF1/NF2	50% new mutations; café au lait spots
Protein C deficiency	1:15,000	2q	Multiple genes	Hypercoagulable state
Tuberous sclerosis	1:30,000	9q, 12q, 16p	TSC1, TSC2, TSC3, TSC4	"Ash-leaf" spots; seizures
von Willebrand disease	1:100	12p	Multiple genes	See Chapter 10

p, short arm of chromosome; q, long arm of chromosome.

■ TABLE 9-4 Examples of Autosomal Recessive Diseases

Autosomal Recessive Disease	Frequency	Chromosome	Gene	Comments
Congenital adrenal hyperplasia	1:5,000 to 1:15,000; 1:700 in Yupik Eskimos	6p	CYP21A2, CYP11A1, CYP17, ACTHR	
Cystic fibrosis	1:2,000 (Caucasians)	7q, 19q	CFTR	See Chapter 20
Galactosemia disorder	1:60,000	9p	GALT	Carbohydrate metabolism
Gaucher disease	1:2,500 (Ashkenazi Jews)	1q	GBA	Lysosomal storage disorder
Infantile polycystic kidney	1:14,000	6p (or 16p = PKD1, TSC2)	PKD3	Renal and hepatic cysts, hypertension
Phenylketonuria	1:14,000	12q	PAH	Amino acid metabolism disorder
Sickle cell disease	1:625 (African Americans)	11p	HBB	See Chapter 10
Tay-Sachs disease	1:3,000 (Ashkenazi Jews)	15q	HEXA	Lysosomal storage disorder
Wilson disease	1:200,000	13q	ATP7B	Defective copper excretion

p, short arm of chromosome; q, long arm of chromosome.

genes. The mother of the affected individual is heterozygous for that gene, because she has both a normal X chromosome and a mutant one. She may be asymptomatic or demonstrate mild symptoms of the disorder due to lyonization, in which only one X chromosome is transcriptionally active in each cell. Recurrence risk for X-linked disorders differs depending on which parent has the abnormal gene. An affected father will pass the defective X chromosome on to his daughters, who are carriers for the disorder; his sons will not be affected. A mother with an abnormal X chromosome is a carrier, and there is a 50% chance she will pass the abnormal chromosome to her progeny. Daughters who receive the abnormal X chromosome will be carriers for the disease, and sons will have the disease. Table 9-5 lists the most common X-linked disorders.

CHROMOSOMAL DISORDERS

Chromosomal disorders are responsible for pregnancy loss, congenital malformation, and mental retardation. Although more than 50% of first-trimester pregnancy losses are due to chromosomal imbalances, only 0.6% of newborn infants have chromosomal abnormalities. Most chromosomal defects arise de novo during gametogenesis, so that an infant can be conceived with a chromosomal abnormality without any prior family history. Chromosomal abnormalities can also be passed from parent to offspring. In such cases, there is often a family history of multiple spontaneous abortions or a higher than chance frequency of children with chromosomal problems. Disorders of chromosome number may involve autosomes or sex chromosomes. Birth defects caused by autosomal abnormalities are generally more severe than those caused by sex chromosome abnormalities. Numeric defects of the autosomes include trisomy of chromosomes 21, 18, and 13. Examples of sex chromosome numerical abnormalities are Turner syndrome and Klinefelter syndrome.

Indications for obtaining chromosomal studies include: confirmation of a suspected chromosomal syndrome; multiple organ system malformations; significant developmental delay or mental retardation without an alternate explanation; short stature or extremely delayed menarche in girls; infertility or a history of multiple spontaneous abortions; ambiguous genitalia; or advanced maternal age. Fetal karyotyping may be accomplished through amniocentesis or chorionic villus sampling.

AUTOSOMAL TRISOMIES

Trisomy 21 (Down Syndrome)

Trisomy 21 is the most common autosomal chromosomal abnormality in humans, with an incidence of 1 per 700 live births. The risk of Down syndrome increases with advancing maternal age; it is 1 in 365 for mothers 35 years of age and 1 in 50 for those 45 or older. Of children with Down syndrome, 95% have three number 21 chromosomes (47 total

■ **TABLE 9-5** Examples of X-Linked Diseases		
X-Linked Disease	**Frequency**	**Comments**
Bruton agammaglobulinemia	1:100,000	Absence of immunoglobulins; recurrent infections
Chronic granulomatous disease	1:1,000,000	Defective killing by phagocytes; recurrent infections
Color blindness	1:100,000	
Duchenne muscular dystrophy	1:3,600	Proximal muscle weakness; Gower sign
Glucose-6-phosphate dehydrogenase	1:10 (African Americans)	Oxidant-induced hemolytic anemia deficiency
Hemophilias A and B	1:10,000	See Chapter 10
Lesch-Nyhan syndrome	1:100,000	Purine metabolism disorder; self-mutilation
Ornithine transcarbamylase deficiency	—	Urea cycle disorder; hyperammonemia

chromosomes), which results typically from chromosomal nondisjunction during maternal meiosis. Four percent have translocation of a third number 21 chromosome to another chromosome (46 total chromosomes). One-third of translocation cases are familial, meaning that one of the parents has a balanced translocation involving one number 21 chromosome and another chromosome. One percent of children with Down syndrome have chromosome mosaicism, with some cells having two number 21 chromosomes (46 total chromosomes) and some cells having three number 21 chromosomes (47 total chromosomes). The mosaicism results from a mitotic division error that occurred during embryonic development.

Common dysmorphic facial features include brachycephaly (flat occiput), flat facial profile, upslanted palpebral fissures, small ears, flat nasal bridge with epicanthal folds, and a small mouth with a protruding tongue. Anomalies of the hand include single palmar crease (simian creases), short, broad hands (brachydactyly) with an incurved fifth finger (clinodactyly) and hypoplastic middle phalanx, and an excessive gap between the first and second toes ("sandal sign"). Other features include short stature, generalized hypotonia, cardiac defects (endocardial cushion defects and septal defects are seen in 50% of cases), gastrointestinal anomalies (duodenal atresia and Hirschsprung disease), hypothyroidism, and mental retardation (IQ range 35 to 65). Leukemia is 20 times more common in children with trisomy 21 than in the general population. During the third and fourth decades, an Alzheimer-like dementia can develop. With improved medical, educational, and vocational management, life expectancy for patients with Down syndrome now extends well into adulthood.

Trisomy 18 (Edwards)

Trisomy 18 occurs in 1 per 8,000 live births. Eighty percent of cases are the result of meiotic nondisjunction, which is associated with advanced maternal age. The remaining 20% may be partial (involving only a portion of the chromosome) or mosaic, caused by mitotic nondisjunction in the zygote. Chromosome translocation as the cause of trisomy 18 is extremely rare, and its presence should prompt karyotyping of the parents to exclude an inherited defect. Clinical manifestations of trisomy 18 are shown in Table 9-6. The prognosis for patients with trisomy 18 is extremely poor: 30% die before reaching 1 month of age, and 90% die by 1 year of age.

■ TABLE 9-6 Key Features of Trisomy 13 and Trisomy 18		
	Trisomy 13	**Trisomy 18**
Head and neck	Microcephaly with sloping forehead	Prominent occiput
	Cutis aplasia of scalp	Narrow bifrontal diameter of forehead
	Microphthalmia	Low-set, malformed ears
	Cleft lip and palate	Micrognathia
Chest and abdomen	Congenital heart disease (VSD, ASD, PDA)	Congenital heart disease (VSD, ASD, PDA)
	Omphalocele	Short sternum
Extremities	Clenched hands with overlapping fingers	Clenched hands with overlapping fingers
	Polydactyly	Rocker-bottom feet
	Polycystic kidney or other renal defects	Horseshoe kidney
Other	Cryptorchidism	Lack of subcutaneous fat
	Agenesis of corpus callosum	
ASD, atrial septal defect; PDA, patent ductus arteriosus; VSD, ventricular septal defect.		

Trisomy 13 (Patau)

Trisomy 13 occurs in 1 per 10,000 live births but constitutes 1% of all spontaneous abortions. Approximately 75% of surviving cases are the result of meiotic nondisjunction, though the increased risk with advanced maternal age is much less than that for trisomy 21. Twenty percent of children with trisomy 13 have a translocation of a third chromosome 13 to another chromosome. One-fourth of translocation cases are familial, meaning that one of the parents has a balanced translocation involving one chromosome 13 and another chromosome. The remaining 5% of children with trisomy 13 have mosaicism; some cells have 46 chromosomes with two number 13 chromosomes, and some cells have 47 chromosomes with three number 13 chromosomes. The mosaicism results from a mitotic division error that occurrs during embryonic development. Clinical manifestations of trisomy 13 are shown in Table 9-6. Prognosis for patients with trisomy 13 is extremely poor: 50% die before reaching 1 month of age, and 90% die by 1 year of age.

SEX CHROMOSOME ABNORMALITIES

Sex chromosome anomalies involve abnormalities in the number or structure of the X or Y chromosomes or both.

Turner Syndrome

Turner syndrome occurs in 1 per 5,000 live births. Approximately 98% of fetuses with Turner syndrome expire in utero; only 2% are born. Therefore, the recurrence risk for parents who have a child with Turner syndrome is no higher than that of the general population.

Several genotypes can cause the Turner phenotype. In 60% of cases, the karyotype is 45,XO, in which the female lacks an X chromosome. Another 15% of individuals are mosaics with a genotype of 45,XO/46,XX; 45,XO/46,XX/47,XXX; or 45,XO/46,XY. Mosaic individuals may have fewer physical stigmata of Turner syndrome. In the remaining 25% of cases, there are two X chromosomes but the short (p) arm of one of the X chromosomes is missing.

Clinical Manifestations

Dysmorphic features include lymphedema of the hands and feet, a shield-shaped chest, widely spaced hypoplastic nipples, a webbed neck, low hairline, cubitus valgus (increased carrying angle), short stature, and multiple pigmented nevi. Additional abnormalities include gonadal dysgenesis, gonadoblastoma, renal anomalies, congenital heart disease, autoimmune thyroiditis, and learning disabilities. Gonadal dysgenesis, present in 100% of patients, is associated with primary amenorrhea and lack of pubertal development due to loss of ovarian hormones. The gonads are appropriately infantile at birth but regress during childhood and develop into "streak" ovaries by puberty. In mosaics with a Y chromosome in one of their cell lines, gonadoblastoma is common. Therefore, prophylactic gonadectomy is necessary in these patients. Renal anomalies, usually duplicated collecting system or horseshoe kidney, occur in 40% of those with Turner syndrome. Congenital heart disease occurs in 20% of patients; common defects include coarctation of the aorta, aortic stenosis, and bicuspid aortic valve. As a consequence of having only one functional X chromosome, females with Turner syndrome display the same frequency of sex-linked disorders as males. The diagnosis is made by karyotype and fluorescent in-situ hybridization. Because of their mosaicism, some girls suspected of having Turner syndrome have a 46,XX karyotype in the peripheral blood, and a skin biopsy may be necessary to make the diagnosis.

Short stature has been successfully treated using human growth hormone. Secondary sexual characteristics develop after estrogen and progesterone administration. As mentioned earlier, gonadectomy is indicated in patients with dysgenetic gonads and the presence of a Y chromosome. With the rare exception of a few mosaics, women with Turner syndrome cannot become pregnant.

Klinefelter Syndrome

Klinefelter syndrome, caused by an extra X chromosome, affects 1 in 1,000 newborn males, 20% of aspermic adult men, and 1 in 250 men over 6 ft tall. The karyotype is XXY in 80% of cases and mosaic (XY/XXY) in 20%. Recurrence risk is the same as the initial risk in the general population.

Clinical Manifestations

The physical stigmata of Klinefelter syndrome are not obvious until puberty, at which time males are incompletely masculinized. They have a female body habitus with decreased body hair, gynecomastia, and small phallus and testes. Infertility results from hypospermia or aspermia. Affected males are usually taller than average relative to their families and their arm span can be greater than their height. There is an increased incidence of learning difficulties, but the average IQ is 98. Gonadotropin levels are usually elevated because of inadequate testosterone levels.

Testosterone therapy during adolescence may improve secondary sexual characteristics and prevent gynecomastia.

IMPRINTING DISORDERS

Imprinting refers to different phenotypes resulting from the same genotype, depending on whether the abnormal chromosome is inherited from the mother or father. **Uniparental disomy** is the term used when both chromosomes of a pair have been inherited from only one parent. Prader-Willi and Angelman syndromes are examples of imprinting, and some cases are also examples of uniparental disomy.

Prader-Willi Syndrome

Prader-Willi syndrome occurs in 1 per 15,000 newborns and is associated with an interstitial deletion of the long arm of chromosome 15 (deletion of 15q11–13). Approximately 70% of those affected have a chromosome deletion in the paternally derived chromosome 15 and a normal maternal chromosome 15. Another 20% to 25% have a normal-appearing chromosome complement with two copies of maternal chromosome 15. This is known as **uniparental maternal disomy**, and the syndrome results from the lack of a paternal copy of chromosome 15. The remaining affected newborns have abnormalities of imprinting due to translocations narrowing the region. The recurrent risk for parents of an affected child is 1 in 100, unless the chromosome 15 deletion results from a parental translocation, which is extremely rare. The disorder is sporadic.

Clinical Manifestations

Dysmorphisms include narrow bifrontal diameter, almond-shaped eyes, a down-turned mouth, and small hands and feet. Short stature and hypogonadotropic hypogonadism with small genitalia and incomplete puberty are seen. These children suffer from severe hypotonia, which is associated with feeding difficulties and failure to thrive in infancy. By several years of age,

these children develop an uncontrollable appetite that leads to severe central obesity. These children eat constantly unless food is locked away. Obesity-related obstructive sleep apnea and cardiorespiratory complications (Pickwickian syndrome) may develop. There is mild mental retardation with characteristic impulse control problems.

For the average patient, strict dietary control is attempted but difficult to enforce. Although those affected can live normal life spans, complications of obesity such as obstructive sleep apnea and diabetes mellitus often lead to earlier death.

Angelman Syndrome

Approximately 60% of patients with Angelman syndrome have a microdeletion on the maternal chromosome 15 (deletion of 15q11–13) and a normal paternal chromosome 15. Five percent of cases result from **uniparental paternal disomy**, where two normal copies of paternally derived chromosome 15 are inherited. Five percent result from imprinting, and 5% are caused by a single gene mutation (UBE3A). Ten percent to 25% result from small subtelomeric deletions or translocations, or are of unknown etiology.

Clinical Manifestations

Dysmorphisms seen in Angelman syndrome include maxillary hypoplasia, large mouth, prognathism, and short stature. Patients are severely mentally retarded, with impaired or absent speech and inappropriate paroxysms of laughter. Jerky arm movements, ataxic gait, and tiptoe walk result in marionette-like movements, leading to its designation as the "happy puppet" syndrome. Many patients have seizures.

MOLECULAR CYTOGENIC DISORDERS

FRAGILE X SYNDROME

Fragile X, an X-linked form of mental retardation that occurs in 1 in 1,000 males, is an example of a trinucleotide repeat disorder. The gene involved, called FMR-1, is active in brain and sperm. In normal individuals, the DNA trinucleotide CGG is repeated about 30 times at the start of this gene. Those affected with fragile X have over 200 CGG repeats. The disorder received its name because a cytogenetically detectable breakage occurs at a specific fragile site on the X chromosome. Currently, Southern blot analysis and polymerase chain reaction (PCR) are used to determine the number of CGG repeats. Clinical manifestations may include macrosomia at birth, macroorchidism due to testicular edema, dysmorphic facial features (large jaw and large ears), perseverative speech, and mental retardation (90% of affected males have an IQ between 20 and 49). Some males with fragile X syndrome have mental retardation as the sole manifestation. Female carriers of the fragile X chromosome may have a subnormal IQ. Autism occurs more commonly in children with the fragile X chromosome than in the general population. There is no treatment for the syndrome.

CHROMOSOME 22Q11 DELETION SYNDROME

Microdeletion of 22q11.2 has been found in 90% of children with DiGeorge syndrome, in 70% of children with velocardiofacial syndrome, and in 15% of children with isolated conotruncal cardiac defects. Although the descriptive names of the above-mentioned disorders are still in use, the more general term **22q11.2 deletion syndrome** more appropriately encompasses the spectrum of abnormalities found in these children. Its prevalence in the general population is 1 per 4,000 live births. The deletion can be inherited (8% to 28% of cases), but more typically occurs as a de novo event. However, if a parent has the deletion, the risk to each child is 50%. The microdeletion can be detected using fluorescent in situ hybridization (FISH) probes. Classic cardiac features of this spectrum of disorders include conotruncal defects such as tetralogy of Fallot, interrupted aortic arch, and vascular rings. Other common findings are absent thymus, hypocalcemic hypoparathyroidism, T-cell mediated immune deficiency, and palate abnormalities. These children usually have feeding difficulties, cognitive disabilities, and behavioral and speech disorders.

OTHER MALFORMATIONS AND ASSOCIATIONS

Some syndromes without a detectable chromosomal abnormality have clinical features that suggest a chromosomal disorder. These syndromes often enter into the differential diagnosis of a suspected genetic disorder. CHARGE is an acronym for a nonrandom association of features including coloboma of the retina or iris; heart abnormalities; atresia of the choanae; retarded growth; genital hypoplasia in males; and ear abnormalities that can include deafness. Recently, CHARGE syndrome was found to result from a point mutation at gene CH7. VATER refers to the nonrandom association of vertebral and anal anomalies, tracheoesophageal fistula with esophageal atresia, and radial or renal abnormalities. Exposure to significant levels of serum alcohol results in a constellation of clinical features referred to as **fetal alcohol syndrome**. Typical findings include short palpebral fissures, smooth philtrum, and thin upper lip. Affected infants may also have hypotonia, poor growth, developmental delay, congenital heart disease, and renal anomalies.

METABOLIC DISORDERS

APPROACH TO METABOLIC DISORDERS

Although individual metabolic disorders are rare, collectively they are responsible for significant morbidity and mortality. Inborn errors of metabolism are genetic diseases that occur when a defective protein disrupts a metabolic pathway at a specific step. Precursors and toxic metabolites of excess precursors accumulate, and products needed for normal metabolism are deficient. Certain ethnic groups are at increased risk for specific metabolic errors.

Clinical presentation and age at onset vary. Urea cycle defects and organic acidemias present early in life with acute metabolic decompensation. Fatty acid oxidation and carbohydrate metabolism disorders usually present with lethargy, encephalopathy, and hypoglycemia after low carbohydrate intake or fasting. Lysosomal storage disorders are characterized by progressive hepatomegaly, splenomegaly, and, occasionally, neurologic deterioration. Findings that should increase suspicion for an inborn error of metabolism include emesis and acidosis after initiation of feeding, unusual odor of urine or sweat, hepatosplenomegaly, hyperammonemia, early infant death, failure to thrive, developmental regression, mental retardation, and seizures. Several important disorders are discussed here.

CARBOHYDRATE METABOLISM DISORDERS

Galactosemia

Galactosemia, the most common error of carbohydrate metabolism, is caused by a deficiency of the enzyme galactose-1-phosphate uridyltransferase, resulting in impaired conversion of galactose-1-phosphate to glucose-1-phosphate (which can undergo glycolysis). Galactose-1-phosphate accumulates in the liver, kidneys, and brain. The disorder occurs in 1 of 40,000 live births, and inheritance is autosomal recessive.

Clinical Manifestations

Clinical manifestations are noted within a few days to weeks after birth. Initial symptoms include evidence of liver failure (hepatomegaly, direct hyperbilirubinemia, disordered coagulation), renal dysfunction (acidosis, glycosuria, aminoaciduria), emesis, anorexia, and poor growth. Cataracts may develop by 2 months of age in untreated children. Infants with galactosemia are at increased risk of *Escherichia coli* sepsis. Older children can have severe learning disabilities, whether or not they were treated in infancy. Affected females have a high incidence of premature ovarian failure. Detecting reduced levels of erythrocyte galactose-1-phosphate uridyltransferase is diagnostic. Laboratory findings include a direct hyperbilirubinemia, elevated serum aminotransferase, prolonged prothrombin and partial thromboplastin times, hypoglycemia, and aminoaciduria. Galactose in the urine is detected by a positive reaction for reducing substances and no reaction with glucose oxidase on urine test strips.

Treatment

All formulas and foods containing galactose (including lactose-containing formulas and breast milk) must be eliminated from the child's diet.

GLYCOGEN STORAGE DISEASES

Glycogen is a highly branched polymer of glucose that is stored in liver and muscle. Glycogen storage diseases (GSDs) are a group of conditions that result from deficiency of enzymes involved in glycogen synthesis or breakdown. Because many different enzymes are involved in glycogen metabolism, the clinical manifestations of the GSDs are variable. Typical manifestations include growth failure, hepatomegaly, and fasting hypoglycemia. The most common GSDs are **type I**, **von Gierke disease**; **type II**, **Pompe disease**; and **type V**, **McArdle disease**. All are autosomal recessive disorders. Treatment is designed to prevent hypoglycemia while avoiding storage of even more glycogen in the liver.

AMINO ACID METABOLISM DISORDERS

Phenylketonuria

Phenylketonuria (PKU), the most common of these disorders, occurs in 1 in 10,000 live births. PKU results from a deficiency of phenylalanine hydroxylase, the enzyme that converts phenylalanine to tyrosine. With normal phenylalanine intake, patients develop high serum concentrations of toxic metabolites such as phenylacetic acid and phenyllactic acid.

Clinical Manifestations

Unlike most amino acid disorders, symptoms of untreated PKU develop in childhood rather than early infancy. Neurologic manifestations include moderate to severe mental retardation, hypertonia, tremors, and behavioral problems. Tyrosine is needed for the production of melanin, so the block in the conversion of phenylalanine to tyrosine results in a light complexion. The patient's urine smells mouse-like.

Treatment

Prevention of mental retardation in PKU is achieved by early and lifelong dietary restriction of phenylalanine. Most states include PKU detection on their mandatory neonatal screens. Pregnant women with PKU who do not restrict phenylalanine intake dramatically increase the risk of having a child with microcephaly, mental retardation, and congenital heart disease.

Homocystinuria

Homocystinuria is caused by a defect in the amino acid metabolic pathway that converts methionine to cysteine and serine. The incidence of the cystathionine synthase deficiency is 1 in 100,000 live births. The neonatal screen used by most states detects increased methionine levels in the blood.

Clinical Manifestations

There are no symptoms in infancy. Clinical manifestations observed during childhood include a Marfan-like body habitus (long thin limbs and digits, scoliosis, sternal deformities, and osteoporosis), dislocated eye lenses, mild to moderate mental retardation, and vascular thromboses that result in childhood stroke or myocardial infarction.

Treatment

Dietary management is extremely difficult because restriction of sulfhydryl groups leads to a very low-protein, foul-tasting diet. Approximately 50% of patients respond to large dosages of pyridoxine.

Ornithine Transcarbamylase Deficiency

Ornithine transcarbamylase (OTC) deficiency, a urea cycle defect, is one of the few inborn errors of metabolism with X-linked inheritance. Amino acid catabolism produces free ammonia that is detoxified to urea through a series of reactions known as the **urea cycle**. In the urea cycle, ornithine joins with carbamoylphosphate through the action of OTC to form citrulline within the mitochondria. When OTC levels are less than 20% of normal, the nitrogen-containing moiety in ornithine cannot be quickly converted to urea for excretion and, instead, forms ammonia, which results in severe hyperammonemia when the patient consumes protein. Milder forms of the condition are seen in heterozygous females and in some affected males.

Clinical Manifestations

Within 24 to 48 hours after the initiation of protein-containing feedings, the newborn becomes progressively lethargic and may develop coma or seizures as the serum ammonia level rises. Female carriers may develop headaches and emesis after protein meals and manifest mental retardation and learning disabilities. Diagnosis is aided by measuring the level of orotic acid, a by-product of carbamoylphosphate metabolism, in the urine.

Treatment

Treatment centers on an extremely low-protein diet and the exploitation of alternative pathways for nitrogen excretion using benzoic acid and phenylacetate. Early intervention may minimize deleterious effects, but management is complex and extremely difficult for parents to maintain.

LYSOSOMAL STORAGE DISORDERS

Deficiency of a lysosomal enzyme causes its substrate to accumulate in lysosomes of tissues that degrade it, creating a characteristic clinical picture. These "storage" diseases are classified as mucopolysaccharidoses (e.g., Hurler, Hunter, and Sanfilippo syndromes), lipidoses (e.g., Niemann-Pick, Krabbe, Gaucher, and Tay-Sachs diseases), or mucolipidoses (e.g., fucosidosis and mannosidosis), depending on the nature of the stored material.

Hurler Syndrome

Deficiency of α-iduronidase leads to accumulation of the dermatan and heparan sulfates in tissues and their excretion in urine. Typical features include coarse facies, corneal clouding, exaggerated kyphosis, hepatosplenomegaly, umbilical hernia, and congenital heart disease. Developmental regression begins in the first year of life. Most children with Hurler syndrome die in early adolescence.

Gaucher Disease

Gaucher disease is caused by deficiency of the enzyme β-glucosidase, leading to the accumulation of glucocerebroside. The classic form does not involve the central nervous system. Patients characteristically have hepatomegaly and splenomegaly. Storage of glucocerebroside in the bone marrow leads to anemia, leukopenia, thrombocytopenia, and recurrent episodes of bone pain. Radiologic changes include an Erlenmeyer flask shape of the distal femur. A low enzyme level in the white blood cells confirms the diagnosis. Recombinant enzyme therapy improves most symptoms.

KEY POINTS

- Environmental factors cause approximately 10% of birth defects.

- Infectious agents, high-dosage radiation, maternal metabolic disorders, mechanical forces, and drugs can all serve as teratogens.

- A teratogenic exposure before 12 weeks' gestation affects organogenesis and tissue morphogenesis, whereas an exposure thereafter usually retards fetal growth and affects central nervous system development.

- Single-gene defects are classified by their mode of inheritance into autosomal dominant, autosomal recessive, and X-linked disorders.

- In autosomal dominant disorders, the phenomenon of incomplete penetrance results in variable expression of the defective gene.

- Defective genes in autosomal dominant disorders typically code for structural proteins, whereas those in autosomal recessive disorders code for enzymes.

- Most inborn errors of metabolism (with the noted exception of ornithine transcarbamylase deficiency, and some mitochrondrial disorders) are autosomal recessive disorders.

- Approximately 50% of first trimester spontaneous abortions have chromosomal abnormalities.

- Birth defects caused by autosomal anomalies are generally more severe than those caused by sex chromosome abnormalities.

- Indications for obtaining chromosomal studies include confirmation of a suspected chromosomal syndrome, multiple organ system malformations, significant developmental delay or mental retardation not otherwise explained, short stature or extremely delayed menarche in girls, infertility or a history of multiple spontaneous abortions, ambiguous genitalia, or advanced maternal age.

10 Hematology

Vinod Balasa • Franklin O. Smith • Bradley S. Marino

ANEMIA

Anemia, defined as a hemoglobin concentration (or hematocrit) two or more standard deviations below the mean value for age and sex, is not a disease but rather a symptom of another disorder. The hemoglobin concentration is relatively high in the newborn but then declines, reaching a nadir known as **physiologic anemia** of infancy. This nadir occurs at approximately 6 weeks of age in the premature infant and 2 to 3 months of age in the term infant. Thereafter, the hemoglobin concentration rises gradually during childhood, reaching adult values after puberty.

DIFFERENTIAL DIAGNOSIS

Anemia results from decreased red cell production, increased red cell destruction, or blood loss. Decreased red cell production may have various etiologies including nutritional deficiencies, suppression or inhibition of bone marrow (by drugs, infections, autoimmune processes, toxin exposures, other medical conditions such as renal/liver disease or chronic inflammation), bone marrow replacement (leukemia, metastatic disease), and rarely congenital marrow failure conditions (dyserythropoietic anemias, Fanconi anemia, etc.). Increased red cell destruction results from hemolytic disease, which may be caused by extracorpuscular or intracorpuscular defects. Blood loss may be acute or chronic. Table 10-1 outlines the most common causes of anemia.

The adjusted reticulocyte count (ARC) is used to determine whether there has been an adequate erythropoietic response to the given anemia. The ARC is calculated as follows:

$$ARC = (\text{Measured Hematocrit/Expected Hematocrit}) \times \text{Reticulocyte Count}$$

An ARC less than two in an anemic patient signifies ineffective erythropoiesis. An ARC greater than two signifies effective erythropoiesis, suggesting hemolysis or chronic blood loss.

CLINICAL MANIFESTATIONS

History

In the young infant, perinatal history may reveal twin-to-twin or fetomaternal transfusion. In the older child, the dietary history may suggest risk factors for iron, vitamin B_{12}, or folate deficiency anemia. Both iron deficiency anemia and lead poisoning can manifest as pica. Signs of overt or occult bleeding include melena, hematochezia, hematuria, hematemesis, abnormal menses, or epistaxis. The patient's race/ethnicity and a family history of splenectomy or cholecystectomy may suggest an inherited hemolytic anemia. Poor weight gain should prompt consideration of anemia of chronic disease. Medications can cause either bone marrow suppression or hemolysis. Other questions should attempt to elicit a history of fever, weight loss, fatigue, rash, bruising, jaundice, and cough.

Physical Examination

A careful examination often suggests the severity of anemia. Important findings include pallor (skin,

TABLE 10-1 Differential Diagnosis of Common Anemias Defined by Mean Corpuscular Volume	
Anemia	**Differential Diagnosis**
Microcytic Anemias	Iron deficiency
	Severe lead poisoning
	Thalassemia syndromes
	Sideroblastic anemia
	Anemia of Chronic Disease*
Normocytic Anemias	
Blood Loss or Red Blood Cell (RBC)	Removal from the blood
	Acute blood loss
	Splenic sequestration
Decreased RBC Production	Anemia of Chronic Disease*
	Transient erythroblastopenia of childhood
	Chronic renal disease
	Malignant infiltration of the bone marrow
	Parvovirus B19 aplastic crisis
	Myelosupressive agent drug toxicity
Increased RBC Destruction	
Inherited hemolytic anemias	Abnormal hemoglobins
	Sickle cell disease
	Thalassemia
	Red blood cell enzyme disorders
	G6PD deficiency
	Pyruvate kinase deficiency
	Red blood cell membrane disorders
	Hereditary spherocytosis
	Hereditary elliptocytosis
Acquired hemolytic anemias	Antibody-mediated anemias
	Autoimmune hemolytic anemias
	Isoimmune hemolytic anemias
	Microangiopathic hemolytic anemias
	Hemolytic uremic syndrome
	Disseminated intravascular coagulation
	Paroxysmal nocturnal hemoglobinuria
Macrocytic Anemias	
Megaloblastic	Vitamin B_{12} deficiency
	Folate deficiency
	Orotic aciduria

■ **TABLE 10-1** Differential Diagnosis of Common Anemias Defined by Mean Corpuscular Volume *(continued)*

Anemia	Differential Diagnosis
Nonmegaloblastic	Aplastic anemia
	Diamond-Blackfan anemia
	Bone marrow infiltration
	Hypothyroidism
	Fanconi anemia
	Liver disease

*Seventy-five percent of anemias of chronic illness are normocytic; 25% are microcytic.

conjunctiva, mucosa) and loss of palmar crease pigmentation. Comparing the complexion of the patient and parents is also useful. Tachycardia and postural changes in heart rate and blood pressure are seen with acute blood loss. Other findings may provide evidence of congestive heart failure (hepatosplenomegaly, lower extremity edema, tachycardia); pancytopenia (petechiae, purpura); blood loss (positive stool guaiac or gastroccult, gross hematuria); hemolysis (scleral icterus, jaundice, urobilinogen in the urine); or infiltrative disorders (lymphadenopathy, hepatosplenomegaly). Table 10-2 lists physical findings that suggest a specific cause of anemia.

DIAGNOSTIC EVALUATION

The goal of testing is to determine whether the anemia results from decreased production, increased destruction, or blood loss. Initial laboratory tests needed to evaluate anemia include a complete blood count with manual differential and red blood cell indexes, reticulocyte count, and peripheral blood smear.

The mean corpuscular volume (MCV) and adjusted reticulocyte count categorize the disorder as microcytic, normocytic, or macrocytic anemia, with adequate or inadequate red blood cell production. Peripheral blood smear is used to assess the red and white blood cell morphology and the platelet number and size (Figs. 10-1 and 10-2). If hemolysis is suspected, electrolytes, lactate dehydrogenase, bilirubin, direct and indirect antiglobulin tests (DAT and IAT, previously called the Coombs test—direct and indirect), and serum haptoglobin should be obtained. Urobilinogen may be detected on urinalysis. A glucose-6-phosphate dehydrogenase (G6PD) assay should be performed in African American and Mediterranean populations who present with hemolytic anemia. Hemoglobin electrophoresis is used to diagnose suspected hemoglobinopathies. Newborn screening procedures to identify infants born with significant hemoglobinopathies, such as sickle cell disease and severe forms of thalassemia, are currently in place in almost every state in the United States. If iron deficiency anemia is high on the differential, then serum iron level, total iron-binding capacity, and serum ferritin level are needed for analysis. A lead level is indicated if lead poisoning is contemplated. Free erythrocyte protoporphyrin (FEP) levels can be obtained quickly and with a small amount of blood. Elevated FEP levels suggest the disordered heme incorporation seen with iron deficiency and lead poisoning. The erythrocyte sedimentation rate (ESR) is generally elevated in anemia of chronic disease. Positive heme tests of stool or gastric contents indicate gastrointestinal bleeding. If a macrocytic anemia is found, both vitamin B_{12} and red blood cell folate levels are needed.

TREATMENT

Treatment varies depending on the cause of the anemia.

MICROCYTIC ANEMIAS WITH DECREASED RED BLOOD CELL PRODUCTION

Hypochromic microcytic red blood cells indicate impaired synthesis of the heme or globin components of hemoglobin. Inadequate heme synthesis may be the result of iron deficiency, lead poisoning, chronic inflammatory disease, pyridoxine deficiency, or copper deficiency. Defective globin synthesis is characteristic

■ TABLE 10-2 Physical Findings in the Evaluation of Anemia

System	Observation	Significance
Skin	Hyperpigmentation	Fanconi anemia, dyskeratosis congenita
	Café au lait spots	Fanconi anemia
	Vitiligo	Vitamin B_{12} deficiency
	Partial oculocutaneous albinism	Chédiak-Higashi syndrome
	Jaundice	Hemolysis
	Petechiae, purpura	Bone marrow infiltration, autoimmune hemolysis with autoimmune thrombocytopenia, hemolytic uremic syndrome
	Erythematous rash	Parvovirus, Epstein-Barr virus
	Butterfly rash	SLE
Head	Frontal bossing	Thalassemia major, severe iron deficiency, chronic subdural hematoma
	Microcephaly	Fanconi anemia
Eyes	Microphthalmia	Fanconi anemia
	Retinopathy	Sickle cell disease
	Optic atrophy	Osteopetrosis
	Blocked lacrimal gland	Dyskeratosis congenita
	Kayser-Fleischer ring	Wilson disease
	Blue sclera	Iron deficiency
Ears	Deafness	Osteopetrosis
Mouth	Glossitis	B_{12} deficiency, iron deficiency
	Angular stomatitis	Iron deficiency
	Cleft lip	Diamond-Blackfan syndrome
	Pigmentation	Peutz-Jeghers syndrome (intestinal blood loss)
	Telangiectasia	Osler-Weber-Rendu syndrome (blood loss)
	Leukoplakia	Dyskeratosis congenita
Chest	Shield chest or widespread nipples	Diamond-Blackfan syndrome
	Murmur	Endocarditis: prosthetic valve hemolysis
Abdomen	Hepatomegaly	Hemolysis, infiltrative tumor, chronic disease, hemangioma, cholecystitis
	Splenomegaly	Hemolysis, sickle cell disease, (early) thalassemia, malaria, lymphoma, Epstein-Barr virus, portal hypertension
	Nephromegaly	Fanconi anemia
	Absent kidney	Fanconi anemia
Extremities	Absent thumbs	Fanconi anemia
	Triphalangeal thumb	Diamond-Blackfan syndrome
	Spoon nails	Iron deficiency
	Beau line (nails)	Heavy metal intoxication, severe illness
	Dystrophic nails	Dyskeratosis congenita

■ TABLE 10-2 Physical Findings in the Evaluation of Anemia *(continued)*

System	Observation	Significance
Rectal	Hemorrhoids	Portal hypertension
	Heme-positive stool	Intestinal hemorrhage
Nerves	Irritable, apathy	Iron deficiency
	Peripheral neuropathy	Deficiency of vitamins B_1, B_{12}, and E, lead poisoning
	Dementia	Deficiency of vitamins B_{12} and E
	Ataxia, posterior column signs	Vitamin B_{12} deficiency
	Stroke	Sickle cell disease, paroxysmal nocturnal hemoglobinuria

SLE, systemic lupus erythematosus.

of the thalassemia syndromes. Iron deficiency anemia, the thalassemia syndromes, and anemia of chronic disease are the most common causes of hypochromic microcytic anemias. Lead poisoning, which may cause a mild hypochromic microcytic anemia, is discussed in detail in Chapter 2.

IRON DEFICIENCY ANEMIA

Iron deficiency, the most common cause of anemia during childhood, is usually seen between 6 and 24 months of age but is not uncommon during adolescence. Nutritional iron deficiency develops when rapid growth and an expanding blood volume put excessive demands on iron stores. Dietary risk factors include extended exclusive breast-feeding (more

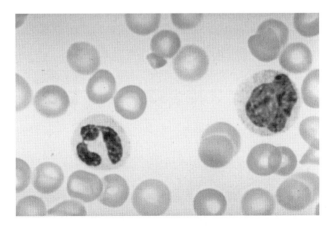

Figure 10-1 • Normal peripheral blood smear. The mature erythrocytes are of normal size and show central pallor. A neutrophil and monocyte are also present.
(From Rubin E, Farber JL. *Pathology*, 3rd ed. Philadelphia: Lippincott Williams & Wilkins, 1999.)

than 6 months) without iron supplementation, consumption of low-iron formula preparations, early institution of low-iron solids, excessive whole milk intake, and the absence of iron supplements. The iron present in breast milk is much more bioavailable than the iron in cow milk. Ascorbic acid enhances the absorption of nonheme iron, whereas tea decreases its absorption.

Iron deficiency anemia can occur as early as 3 months of age in the premature infant who has inadequate iron stores at birth. It can occur in the infant or toddler who receives a diet exclusively composed of milk or low-iron formula. Nutritional iron deficiency can also occur during adolescence when a rapid growth spurt coincides with a diet with suboptimal iron content. This is a particular problem in adolescent females because of iron loss during menses.

Iron deficiency caused by blood loss can also occur in young children. Prenatal iron loss can occur from fetomaternal transfusion or from twin-to-twin transfusion. Perinatal bleeding may result from obstetric complications such as placental abruption or placenta previa. Postnatal blood loss may occur from obvious sources such as surgery or trauma or may be occult, as occurs with idiopathic pulmonary hemosiderosis, parasitic infestations, and inflammatory bowel disease.

Clinical Manifestations

Mild iron deficiency is usually asymptomatic. With moderate iron deficiency (hemoglobin: 6 to 8 g per dL), the infant develops anorexia, irritability, apathy, and easy fatigability. On physical examination, the anemic infant may have skin and mucous membrane pallor, glossitis, angular stomatitis, and koilonychia (spoon nails). The child may also have tachycardia

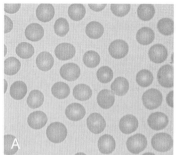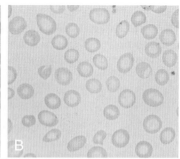

Figure 10-2 • A blood smear showing normal erythrocytes **(A)** compared with a blood smear revealing microcytic-hypochromic erythrocytes in a patient with iron deficiency anemia **(B)**.
(From Willis MC. *Medical Terminology: A Programmed Learning Approach to the Language of HealthCare.* Baltimore: Lippincott Williams & Wilkins, 2002.)

and a systolic ejection murmur at the left upper sternal border. The infant with severe anemia (hemoglobin less than 3 g per dL) shows signs of congestive heart failure, which include tachycardia, an S_3 gallop, cardiomegaly, hepatomegaly, distended neck veins, and pulmonary rales.

Table 10-3 lists the laboratory findings typical for the microcytic anemias. Bone marrow examination is not clinically indicated to confirm the diagnosis but when performed, it demonstrates micronormoblastic hyperplasia of the erythroid line. A response to appropriate iron supplementation is the best diagnostic test for iron deficiency.

Treatment

Mild to moderate iron deficiency anemia without evidence of congestive heart failure is treated with 3 to 6 mg/kg/day of elemental iron. The reticulocyte count increases within 2 to 3 days, and the hemoglobin increases at a rate of approximately 0.3 g/dL/day after 4 to 5 days. Therapy is continued for 8 weeks after the hemoglobin has returned to normal to replenish tissue stores. If the hemoglobin has not increased substantially after 1 month of therapy and compliance has been established, other causes of hypochromic microcytic anemia must be considered. Although infants can tolerate remarkable degrees of anemia, especially if the decline in hemoglobin is gradual, infants with severe anemia must be transfused very slowly with small (3 to 5 mL per kg) aliquots of packed red blood cells to avoid causing cardiac decompensation.

ALPHA AND BETA THALASSEMIA

Pathogenesis and Clinical Manifestations

The thalassemias are hereditary hemolytic anemias characterized by decreased or absent synthesis of one

■ **TABLE 10-3** Laboratory Findings for the Common Microcytic Anemias					
	Iron Deficiency	**Thalassemia Trait**	**Thalassemia Major**	**Plumbism**	**Chronic Disease**
RDW	↑	NL	↑	↑	NL
MCV	↓	↓	↓	↓	NL ↓
RBC no.	↓	NL	↓	↓	↓
FEP	↑	NL	NL	↑↑	↑
HgbA₂	↓	β-↑ α-NL	β-↑ α-NL	NL	NL
Iron	NL ↑	NL	↑	NL	↓
TIBC	↓	NL	NL ↑	NL	NL ↓
% saturation	↓	NL	↑	NL	↓
Ferritin		NL	↑	NL	

FEP, free erythrocyte protoporphyrin; hgb, hemoglobin; NL, normal; TIBC, total iron-binding capacity; ↑, increased; ↓, decreased.

or more globin subunits of the hemoglobin molecule. α-Thalassemia, caused by deletion of one or more of the four α-globin genes, leads to reduced synthesis of α-globin chains. β-Thalassemia is caused by errors in the transcription or translation of β-globin mRNA and leads to reduced synthesis of β-globin chains. Table 10-4 compares the thalassemia syndromes.

The number of deleted globin genes determines the hematologic consequences of α-thalassemia. These deletions can be cis or trans. Cis deletions occur when two α-globin genes are deleted from one chromosome, whereas trans deletions signify a single α-globin gene deletion on each of the two chromosomes. Different races and ethnicities have varying rates of both cis and trans deletions of α-globin genes in their population.

Homozygous α-thalassemia, or hemoglobin Bart disease, occurs when all four α-globin genes are deleted. Failure to produce any α-globin chains results in γ-globin tetramers (hemoglobin Bart). Hemoglobin Bart has a high affinity for oxygen and does not release it to the tissue. The result is severe anemia, tissue anoxia, heart failure, hepatosplenomegaly, generalized edema, and death in utero because of hydrops fetalis. The cis deletion is most prevalent in Southeast Asians.

Hemoglobin H disease results from deletion of three α-globin genes. γ-Globin chains are only produced in utero. In normal infants, fetal hemoglobin (which consists of two α-globin chains and two γ-globin chains) usually predominates at birth. In newborn infants with hemoglobin H disease, the dearth of α-globin leads to the formation of hemoglobin Bart, which accounts for 10% to 40% of the total hemoglobin. With the cessation of γ-globin synthesis and the onset of β-globin synthesis at birth, hemoglobin Bart diminishes and hemoglobin H (which consists of a β-globin tetramer) predominates after the first few months of life. Hemoglobin H eventually accounts for 30% to 40% of the total hemoglobin, and normal hemoglobin A accounts for approximately 60% to 70% of the total hemoglobin. This diagnosis is most common in children with

■ TABLE 10-4 Comparison of the Thalassemia Syndromes

Genetic Abnormality	Percentage Hemoglobin (Hb)			
	Hb A	Hb A$_2$	Hb F	Other
Normal αβ	90 to 98	2 to 3	2 to 3	—
Beta thalassemias				
Thalassemia major				
β-thal^0 β-thal^0	0	2 to 5	95	—
β-thal$^+$ β-thal$^+$	Very low	2 to 5	20 to 80	—
Thalassemia intermedia (varied genetic globin abnormalities)	Overlaps with thalassemia major			
Thalassemia minor				
β β-thal^0 or β β-thal$^+$	90 to 95	5 to 7	2 to 10	
Alpha thalassemias				
Homozygous α-thalassemia	—	—	—	Hb H (β4)
— — / — —				Hb Bart (γ4)
Hemoglobin H disease	60 to 70	2 to 5	2 to 5	Hb H 30 to 40
— — / — α				
Alpha thalassemia minor	90 to 98	2 to 3	2 to 3	
— α / — α				
α α / — —				
Silent carrier	90 to 98	2 to 3	2 to 3	
— α / α α				

Southeast Asian ancestry. α-Thalassemia trait, also known as α-thalassemia minor, results from the deletion of two α-globin genes. This defect manifests with mild anemia, hypochromia, and microcytosis. The α-thalassemia trait, present in 3% of U.S. blacks and 1% to 5% of those of Mediterranean descent, is often confused with mild iron deficiency. The hemoglobin electrophoresis is normal in these children, and the diagnosis is one of exclusion confirmed by documenting parental microcytosis.

Those with deletion of only one α-globin gene are considered silent carriers for α-thalassemia because they have a normal hemoglobin concentration and normal red blood cell indexes. The condition can be measured only by quantitative measurement of globin chain synthesis or by gene analysis. A carrier can produce offspring with α-thalassemia trait or hemoglobin H disease.

β-Thalassemia can be subdivided into homozygous (β-thalassemia major) and heterozygous forms (β-thalassemia minor). β-Thalassemia major results either from complete absence of β-globin synthesis (β^0/β^0 genotype) because of defective transcription of mRNA or from partial reduction of the gene product (B^+/B^+ genotype) because of translational errors. The child with β-thalassemia minor, the heterozygous form, has one normal β-globin gene and one abnormal β-globin gene.

Children with β-thalassemia major have severe hemolytic anemia and splenomegaly during the first year of life. If untreated, bone marrow hyperplasia and extramedullary hematopoiesis produce characteristic features such as tower skull, frontal bossing, maxillary hypertrophy with prominent cheekbones, and an overbite. Failure to thrive is prominent in this population. Death occurs within the first few years of life because of progressive congestive heart failure if the patient is not supported with blood transfusions. Despite severe anemia, there is reticulocytopenia, reflecting ineffective hematopoiesis. Peripheral blood smear reveals marked hypochromia, microcytosis, anisocytosis, and poikilocytosis. On hemoglobin electrophoresis, hemoglobin A is either markedly decreased (β^+/β^+ or β^+/β^0) or totally absent (β^0/β^0). On quantitative hemoglobin electrophoresis, hemoglobin F accounts for 95% in the β^0/β^0 genotype and 20% to 80% in the β^+/β^+ genotype. If the diagnosis is in question or the child's hemoglobin electrophoresis is equivocal, the parental complete blood counts, smears, and hemoglobin electrophoresis results may clarify the diagnosis.

Children with β-thalassemia minor have only mild hemolytic anemia. On blood smear, the hypochromia, microcytosis, and anisocytosis are disproportionately severe given the degree of anemia. Hemoglobin electrophoresis shows elevation of the hemoglobin A_2 level and sometimes a mild elevation of hemoglobin F.

Epidemiology

Thalassemia is most common in African, Southeast Asian, Mediterranean, and Middle Eastern populations. The most severe forms of α-thalassemia, three- and four-gene deletions, are seen in the Southeast Asian population because of the high prevalence of cis deletions. β-thalassemia is most often found in populations originating from the Mediterranean, Middle East, and India.

Treatment

Therapy for children with β-thalassemia major consists of frequent packed red blood cell transfusions to ameliorate the anemia and prevent congestive heart failure. These children require 10 to 20 mL per kg of leuco-depleted red blood cells every 3 to 5 weeks to maintain the hemoglobin count above 10 g per dL. This regimen eliminates an increased erythropoietic drive, allowing normal linear growth and bone development. Suppression of erythropoiesis also limits the stimulus for increased iron absorption, which helps minimize iron overload.

Splenectomy is considered when transfusion requirements exceed 250 mL/kg/year. Iron overload develops in children with β-thalassemia, whether they are transfused or not, because of hyperabsorption of dietary iron. When the bone marrow storage capacity for iron is exceeded, iron accumulates in the liver, heart, pancreas, gonads, and skin, producing symptoms of hemochromatosis. As a result, many thalassemic patients develop cardiomyopathy and congestive heart failure in their late teens. To minimize the morbidity associated with iron overload, patients are treated with chelating agents such as desferrioxamine or the new oral agent, deferasirox. Because of the constant state of increased erythropoiesis, folic acid supplementation is recommended for patients not maintained on chronic transfusion therapy in order to prevent folate deficiency and megaloblastic anemia. Bone marrow transplantation is curative, but because of its associated morbidity and mortality, this procedure is performed in only a few centers using HLA-matched sibling donors.

Principles of therapy for hemoglobin H disease are the same as those for β-thalassemia major. The need for transfusion and chelation therapy depends on the severity of the anemia.

No treatment is necessary for α- or β-thalassemia minor. Genetic counseling is recommended. Because the smear of iron deficiency anemia and α- and β-thalassemia minor are quite similar, the child with presumed iron deficiency anemia who does not respond to oral iron therapy and is believed to be compliant should have a hemoglobin electrophoresis to rule out β-thalassemia minor. The child with α-thalassemia trait has a normal hemoglobin electrophoresis (outside the neonatal period), whereas the electrophoresis of the child with β-thalassemia minor may show an elevated hemoglobin A_2 and hemoglobin F.

ANEMIA OF CHRONIC DISEASE

Anemia of chronic disease can result from chronic inflammatory diseases, such as inflammatory bowel disease and juvenile idiopathic arthritis (JIA); chronic infections, such as tuberculosis; and malignancy. Typically, anemia of chronic disease is normocytic; 25% of cases of anemia of chronic disease have microcytosis. Anemia of chronic disease results from an inability to mobilize iron from its storage sites in macrophages. The chronic inflammatory state triggers cytokines that result in reticuloendothelial blockade within the marrow. A modest decrease in the survival time of red blood cells and a relatively limited erythropoietin response also contribute to the anemia.

Clinical Manifestations

The anemia is mild in degree (hemoglobin: 8 to 10 g per dL). Table 10-3 notes the laboratory findings typical for anemia of chronic disease. As in iron deficiency anemia, the serum iron level is reduced; in contrast to iron deficiency anemia, the total iron-binding capacity is low, and the serum ferritin level is normal or increased. Bone marrow examination shows micronormoblastic hyperplasia and an increase in storage iron, but a decrease in the number of iron-containing erythroblasts.

Treatment

The anemia resolves when the underlying condition is treated adequately. Therapy with iron supplements is unnecessary unless true iron deficiency is also present.

NORMOCYTIC ANEMIAS WITH DECREASED RED CELL PRODUCTION

Normocytic anemias result from the failure of the bone marrow to produce adequate numbers of red blood cells because of systemic illness. Bone marrow function can be impaired by fibrosis, malignant infiltration, transient marrow failure, or failure to synthesize erythropoietin (chronic renal disease). Transient marrow failure states include transient erythroblastopenia of childhood, parvovirus B_{19}-induced aplastic crisis, and drug toxicity from myelosuppressive agents. A normocytic anemia also occurs with acute blood loss. Re-equilibration of the total blood volume before erythropoiesis results in the anemia. Chronic inflammatory states result in anemia of chronic disease, which can be normocytic (75%) or microcytic (25%).

TRANSIENT ERYTHROBLASTOPENIA OF CHILDHOOD

Transient erythroblastopenia of childhood (TEC) is an acquired pure red cell aplasia caused by transient bone marrow suppression. The resulting anemia is normocytic. Although a specific etiology has not been identified, TEC is usually preceded by a viral infection. TEC occurs between 6 months and 5 years of age, with a peak incidence at 2 years of age. In contrast to Diamond-Blackfan syndrome, which is a congenital macrocytic pure red cell aplasia, 85% of cases of TEC occur after 1 year of age, there are no other associated anomalies, and fetal hemoglobin and i antigen are not present.

Clinical Manifestations

The history and physical examination are unremarkable except for the gradual onset of pallor over the course of weeks. Peripheral smear is normal other than reticulocytopenia. Bone marrow examination reveals few erythroid precursors and normal myeloid and platelet precursors.

Treatment

The hemoglobin is usually at its nadir at the time of diagnosis. Spontaneous recovery occurs within 1 to 2 months of diagnosis. Red blood cell transfusions are necessary only if the patient has signs or symptoms of congestive heart failure.

NORMOCYTIC ANEMIAS WITH INCREASED RED CELL PRODUCTION

HEMOLYTIC ANEMIA

Normocytic anemias with increased red cell production are most commonly caused by hemolytic anemias. The red blood cell destruction and anemia are sensed by the kidneys, which release erythropoietin to stimulate bone marrow erythropoiesis. Hemolytic anemias are caused by factors extrinsic to the red cell (extracorpuscular) or by defects intrinsic to the red cell (intracorpuscular). In general, extrinsic defects are acquired and intrinsic defects are hereditary.

Extracorpuscular anomalies are divided into isoimmune, autoimmune, and nonimmune hemolytic anemias. Isoimmune hemolytic anemia results from antibodies produced by one individual against the red blood cells of another individual of the same species. ABO or minor antigen incompatibility is an example of isoimmune hemolytic anemia (see Chapter 13). In autoimmune hemolytic anemia, abnormal antibodies directed against red blood cells are produced by the patient. Autoimmune hemolytic anemias can be idiopathic, postinfectious (*Mycoplasma pneumoniae*, Epstein-Barr virus), drug induced (penicillin, quinidine, a-methyldopa), or may result from a chronic autoimmune disease (systemic lupus erythematosus) or malignancy (nonHodgkin lymphoma). Therapy for autoimmune hemolytic anemia varies depending on the etiology of the hemolysis and the clinical condition of the patient. In general, treatment is supportive, with the careful use of packed red blood cell transfusions and corticosteroids. Autoantibodies react with virtually all red blood cells, making crossmatching difficult. In some severe chronic cases, intravenous immunoglobulin, immunosuppressive pharmacotherapy, and splenectomy may be indicated.

The antibodies that cause isoimmune and autoimmune hemolytic anemias may be of the IgG or IgM classes. IgG antibodies tend to be warm reactive (maximal activity at 37°C) and are considered incomplete antibodies. They coat the surface of the red blood cells and fix early complement components but cannot agglutinate red blood cells or activate the complement cascade through the entire hemolytic sequence. Hemolysis occurs extravascularly because of the trapping of the opsonized red blood cells by macrophages in the reticuloendothelial system. IgG antibodies are associated with autoimmune diseases, lymphomas, and viral infections. These antibodies are identified by the direct antiglobulin (Coombs) test. IgM antibodies are usually cold reactive (maximal activity at low temperatures) and are deemed complete antibodies. They agglutinate red blood cells and activate the complement sequence through C9, causing lysis of red blood cells. Hemolysis occurs intravascularly. IgM antibodies are associated with *Mycoplasma pneumoniae*, Epstein-Barr virus, and transfusion reactions.

Nonimmune hemolytic anemias can be microangiopathic (disseminated intravascular coagulation, thrombotic thrombocytopenic purpura, hemolytic uremic syndrome, malignant hypertension, giant hemangioma, preeclampsia, renal graft rejection) or can be caused by damage from nonendothelialized surfaces (artificial heart valve, arteriovenous malformation, Kasabach-Merritt syndrome), hypersplenism, abetalipoproteinemia, toxins (snake venom, copper, and arsenic), malaria, or burns.

Intracorpuscular defects include intrinsic membrane defects such as hereditary spherocytosis, hereditary elliptocytosis, hereditary stomatocytosis, and paroxysmal nocturnal hemoglobinuria (PNH). PNH is the only intracorpuscular disorder that is not inherited. Hemoglobinopathies (sickle cell disorders) and enzyme disorders (G6PD deficiency, pyruvate kinase deficiency) are also intracorpuscular disorders. Following this section are discussions of hereditary spherocytosis, sickle cell anemia, and G6PD deficiency, three of the most common intracorpuscular defects.

HEREDITARY SPHEROCYTOSIS

Hereditary spherocytosis is caused by a defect in red blood cell membrane-supporting proteins (spectrin, ankyrin, or band 3 protein). The defect leads to a loss of membrane fragments without a proportional loss of volume. Therefore, microspherocytes (small spherical red blood cells with a high volume-to-surface ratio) form. Microspherocytes are less deformable than normal red blood cells, so they are trapped and destroyed in the microvasculature of the spleen. Inheritance is usually autosomal dominant, but 25% of cases are caused by new mutations or autosomal recessive forms.

Clinical Manifestations

Hereditary spherocytosis varies greatly in clinical severity, ranging from an asymptomatic, well-compensated, mild hemolytic anemia discovered incidentally to a severe hemolytic anemia with growth failure, splenomegaly, and chronic transfusion requirements in infancy necessitating early splenectomy. The newborn with this disorder may present with severe unconjugated hyperbilirubinemia caused by hemolysis. Occasionally, patients present with aplastic crisis after parvovirus B_{19} infection. Because of chronic hemolysis, teenagers develop gallstones and cholecystitis. Physical examination reveals pallor, scleral icterus, and mild to moderate splenomegaly. Laboratory studies demonstrate mild normocytic anemia, reticulocytosis, and indirect hyperbilirubinemia. During an aplastic crisis, the anemia becomes severe and reticulocytopenia occurs. Diagnosis is confirmed by a positive osmotic fragility test.

Treatment

Treatment includes folic acid supplementation to meet the needs of increased red blood cell turnover and red blood cell transfusions during an aplastic crisis. Splenectomy alleviates anemia, reticulocytosis, and scleral icterus, although microspherocytes persist. Splenectomy should be deferred until after 6 years of age because of the higher risk of sepsis from encapsulated organisms in young children.

SICKLE CELL DISEASE

Pathogenesis

Sickle cell disease is an autosomal recessive disorder that results from a valine-for-glutamine substitution in the sixth amino acid position of the β-globin chain. This substitution alters the structure of the hemoglobin molecule, which, under conditions of deoxygenation, promotes aggregation of hemoglobin into long polymers that distort the red blood cell into a sickle shape. Sickling shortens red blood cell survival time and results in a chronic hemolytic anemia. Sickled cells also cause microvascular obstruction, which leads to tissue ischemia and infarction. The sickling phenomenon is accentuated by hypoxia, acidosis, increased or decreased temperature, and dehydration. If only one of the two β-globin genes is affected, the individual has sickle cell trait, which is the heterozygous state without clinical consequence. If both β-globin genes have the genetic substitution, the patient is homozygous for hemoglobin S and has sickle cell disease. Sickling disorders of varying severity also result from hemoglobin S existing in combination with other abnormal hemoglobins (hemoglobin C, $D_{Los\ Angeles}$, O_{Arab}) or thalassemias (β^+ or β^0 thalassemia).

Epidemiology

Sickle cell disease affects 1 in 625 African Americans, making it the most common autosomal recessive disorder in that population. It also occurs in those of Greek, Italian, and Saudi Arabian descent.

Clinical Manifestations and Management

Children with sickle cell trait are generally asymptomatic. Rarely, an individual exhibits painless hematuria and inability to properly concentrate the urine (isosthenuria). Patients with sickle cell trait occasionally have sickle cells on peripheral blood smear, but hemoglobin electrophoresis provides the definitive diagnosis. Typically, hemoglobin electrophoresis reveals 55% to 60% hemoglobin A, 40% to 45% hemoglobin S, and 2% to 3% hemoglobin A_2. It is important to detect the trait for genetic counseling.

Unlike sickle cell trait, sickle cell disease causes severe morbidity and mortality. Quantitative hemoglobin electrophoresis shows 0% hemoglobin A, 80% to 95% hemoglobin S, 2% to 3% hemoglobin A_2, and up to 15% hemoglobin F. In most cases, diagnosis is made from newborn screening tests. The highly variable clinical manifestations of sickle cell disease result from anemia, infection, and vaso-occlusion (Table 10-5).

At approximately 4 months of age, when the percentage of hemoglobin F diminishes and the percentage of hemoglobin S rises, the child with sickle cell disease develops a progressive hemolytic anemia. The anemia of sickle cell disease is a chronic, well-compensated, severe anemia that is rarely transfusion dependent. Common manifestations of the anemia include pallor, jaundice, and splenomegaly in infancy, a systolic ejection murmur, and delayed sexual development and growth. Splenic sequestration, aplastic crisis, and hyperhemolytic crisis all superimpose acute life-threatening declines in hemoglobin concentration on the chronic compensated anemia of sickle cell disease. In splenic sequestration, rapid splenic engorgement caused by trapping of red blood cells may lead to hypovolemic shock. Sequestration typically occurs between 6 months and 2 years of age. Viral suppression of red blood cell precursors in the bone marrow, most often by parvovirus B_{19}, precipitates aplastic crisis. Exposure of a patient with sickle cell disease and concomitant G6PD deficiency to an oxidative

TABLE 10-5 Clinical Manifestations of Sickle Cell Anemia*

Manifestation	Comments
Anemia	Chronic, onset 3 to 4 mo of age; requires folate therapy for chronic hemolysis
Aplastic crisis	Parvovirus infection; may require transfusion
Sequestration crisis	Massive splenomegaly, shock; treat with transfusion
Hemolytic crisis	May be associated with G6PD deficiency
Dactylitis	Hand-foot swelling in early infancy
Pain crisis	Microvascular painful, vaso-occlusive infarcts of muscle, bone, lung, intestines
Cerebral vascular accidents	Large- and small-vessel sickling and thrombosis (stroke); requires chronic transfusion
Acute chest syndrome	Infection and/or infarction, severe hypoxemia, infiltrate, dyspnea, rales
Chronic lung	Pulmonary fibrosis, restrictive lung disease, cor pulmonale disease
Priapism	May causes eventual impotence; treat with pseudoephedrine, venous, drainage, transfusion oxygen, or corpora cavernosa-to-spongiosa shunt
Ocular	Retinopathy
Gallbladder disease	Bilirubin stones; cholecystitis
Renal	Hematuria, papillary necrosis, renal-concentrating deficit; nephropathy
Cardiomyopathy	Heart failure (fibrosis)
Infections	Functional asplenia; increased risk of invasive infection due to encapsulated bacteria such as *S. pneumoniae*, *H. influenzae*, and *N. meningitidis*; *Salmonella* and *Staphylococcus aureus* osteomyelitis; severe *Mycoplasma pneumoniae*; transfusion-acquired infections
Growth failure, delayed puberty	May respond to nutritional supplements

*Clinical manifestations with sickle cell trait are rare but include renal papillary necrosis (hematuria), sudden death on exertion, intraocular hyphema extension, and sickling in unpressurized airplanes.
CMV, cytomegalovirus; EBV, Epstein-Barr virus; G6PD, glucose-6-phosphate dehydrogenase.

stress results in acute hemolysis superimposed on a chronic hemolytic anemia (hyperhemolytic crisis). Medications or infection usually cause the acute hemolysis. Splenic sequestration, aplastic crisis, and hyperhemolytic crisis are often treated with red blood cell transfusion. Because of the presence of chronic hemolytic anemia, gallstone formation and cholecystitis are common during adolescence.

As the sickled cells traverse the spleen, they cause microvascular obstruction, infarction, and fibrosis of the spleen. This process, known as autoinfarction, causes the spleen to regress in size gradually; by 4 years of age, the spleen is no longer palpable. More important, **autoinfarction** diminishes the capability of the spleen to filter encapsulated bacterial organisms and places the infant at great risk for overwhelming infection from *Streptococcus pneumoniae* or *Haemophilus influenzae*. Any infant or child who has

sickle cell disease and fever (temperature greater than 38.5°C) must be evaluated immediately. Although the child likely has a benign viral infection, invasive bacterial infection must be excluded. To minimize the risk of life-threatening infection, children with sickle cell disease start penicillin prophylaxis at approximately 4 months of age and receive vaccinations. Both the *H. influenzae* type b (Hib) and heptava-lent pneumococcal conjugate (Prevnar) vaccines are given at the 2-, 4-, and 6-month visits and then again between 12 months and 15 months of age. The 23-valent pneumococcal polysaccharide vaccine (PPV) should be administered at 2 years of age and then again at 4 to 6 years of age. Penicillin prophylaxis is continued until at least 5 years of age.

Vaso-occlusive crises result from microvascular infarcts, may occur in any organ or tissue of the body, and are commonly precipitated by infection, cold exposure, dehydration, venous stasis, and acidosis. Dactylitis, or hand-foot syndrome, is symmetrical painful swelling of the dorsal surface of the hands and feet caused by avascular necrosis of the metacarpal and metatarsal bones. Dactylitis occurs at 4 to 6 months of age and is the earliest clinical manifestation of vaso-occlusive disease in the sickle cell patient. In older children, pain crises most often localize to the long bones of the arms and legs, vertebral column, and sternum. Pain crises last from 2 to 7 days and are treated with nonsteroidal anti-inflammatory drugs and narcotics. Hydroxyurea maintenance therapy decreases the number and severity of vaso-occlusive crises. Avascular necrosis of the femoral head, another vaso-occlusive manifestation in bone, typically occurs in the adolescent population.

Microvascular obstructive disease can also occur in the lungs, central nervous system, penis, myocardium, and intestine. Acute chest syndrome, a vaso-occlusive crisis within the lungs, is often caused by pulmonary infection and infarction. Patients present with hypoxia, respiratory distress, and pulmonary infiltrates. Oxygen, analgesia, antibiotics, and exchange transfusion are used to maximize respiratory status and minimize further pulmonary damage. Similarly, occlusion of the large cerebral vessels results in stroke. Patients present with mental status changes, seizures, and focal paralysis. Because of the high risk of recurrence, children who have had a stroke are placed on chronic red blood cell transfusion protocols to minimize the risk of future stroke. Priapism typically occurs in males between 6 and 20 years of age. The child develops sudden painful engorgement of the penis that will not subside. Acute chest syndrome, stroke, and priapism are treated by exchange transfusion to decrease the percentage of hemoglobin S to below 30% in an attempt to minimize vaso-occlusion.

By adolescence, the effects of chronic myocardial microvascular obstruction and infarction are evident by an enlarged hypertrophic heart. Many adults eventually succumb to congestive heart failure from progressive myocardial damage. Abdominal crisis results from microvascular obstruction of the intestinal circulation. Patients present with ileus and rebound tenderness, mimicking an acute abdomen. The pain may be familiar to the patient and readily recognized as "crisis pain." Abdominal pain consistent with the child's normal pain constellation during crisis may warrant a period of observation with hydration and analgesic administration. If the abdominal pain is not typical for the patient during a vaso-occlusive crisis, surgical consultation should be obtained.

GLUCOSE-6-PHOSPHATE DEHYDROGENASE DEFICIENCY

G6PD deficiency, the most common red blood cell enzyme defect, is transmitted as an X-linked recessive trait. The lack of this enzyme in the hexose monophosphate shunt pathway results in depletion of nicotinamide adenine dinucleotide phosphate (NADPH) and the inability to regenerate reduced glutathione, which is needed to protect the red blood cell from oxidative stress.

The most common forms of G6PD deficiency are the A^+ and Mediterranean variants. The A^+ variant, found in approximately 10% of African Americans in the United States, is associated with an isoenzyme that deteriorates rapidly, with a half-life of 13 days. The Mediterranean variant occurs predominantly in persons of Greek and Italian descent; its isoenzyme is extremely unstable, with a half-life of several hours.

When there is an oxidative stress on the red blood cell, exposed sulfhydryl groups on the hemoglobin are oxidized, leading to dissociation of heme and globin moieties, with the globin precipitating as **Heinz bodies** (Fig. 10-3). Damaged red cells are removed from circulation by the reticuloendothelial system; severely damaged cells may lyse intravascularly. Known oxidants include sulfonamides, nitrofurantoin, primaquine, and dimercaprol. Hemolysis may also be precipitated by fava beans and infection.

Clinical Manifestations

The classic course of G6PD deficiency is episodic stress- or drug-induced hemolytic anemia. Patients with the A^- variant have a limited hemolysis confined to the older red blood cell population. Recovery occurs as young red blood cells with enzyme activity sufficient to resist oxidative stress emerge from the bone marrow. Hemolysis is most common in males who possess a single abnormal X chromosome. Heterozygous females who have randomly inactivated a higher percentage of the normal gene may become symptomatic, as may homozygous females with the A^- variant. One percent of African American females are A^- variant homozygous. Patients with the Mediterranean variant have hemolysis that destroys most of their red cells and may require transfusions until the drug is eliminated from their bodies. The neutrophils of patients with the most severe degrees of G6PD deficiency demonstrate defective oxidative killing because of the

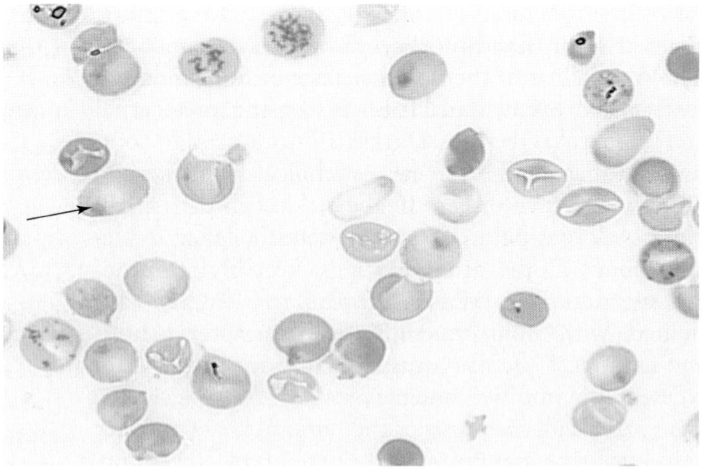

Figure 10-3 • Heinz bodies. Round, refractile inclusions found on the periphery of the cell when stained with a supravital dye; consists of denatured globin produced by the destruction of hemoglobin; they may occur in multiple numbers.
(From Anderson SC, Poulsen KB. *Anderson's Atlas of Hematology*. Baltimore: Lippincott Williams & Wilkins, 2003.)

depletion of NADPH, which serves as an electron donor to the membrane-bound oxidase that produces bactericidal oxygen species.

On peripheral blood smear, the red cells appear to have "bites" taken out of them (blister cells). The bitten areas result from phagocytosis of Heinz bodies by splenic macrophages. During hemolytic episodes, physical examination reveals jaundice and dark urine (caused by hemoglobinuria and high levels of urobilinogen). Laboratory tests reveal elevated indirect bilirubin and lactate dehydrogenase and low haptoglobin. Initially, the hemolysis exceeds the ability of the bone marrow to compensate, so the reticulocyte count may be low for the first 3 to 4 days.

The diagnosis of G6PD deficiency is made by finding deficient NADPH formation on G6PD assay. G6PD levels may be normal in the setting of acute, severe hemolysis because most of the deficient cells have been destroyed. Repeating the test at a later time when the patient is in a steady-state condition, testing the mother of males with suspected G6PD deficiency, and performing electrophoresis to identify the precise variant, all facilitate diagnosis.

Treatment

Patients with G6PD deficiency associated with acute severe hemolysis need to avoid drugs that initiate hemolysis. Treatment is supportive, including packed red blood cell transfusion during significant cardiovascular compromise and vigorous hydration and urine alkalinization to protect the kidneys against damage from precipitated free hemoglobin.

MACROCYTIC ANEMIAS WITH DECREASED RED CELL PRODUCTION

Macrocytic anemias are subdivided according to the presence or absence of megaloblastosis, a marker of ineffective DNA synthesis within a red blood cell precursor. Causes of megaloblastic anemia include vitamin B_{12} and folate deficiency, drugs that interfere with folate metabolism (phenytoin, methotrexate, trimetho-prim), and metabolic disorders (orotic aciduria, methylmalonic aciduria, Lesch-Nyhan syndrome). Macrocytic anemias without megaloblastosis result from bone marrow failure and include bone marrow failure syndromes (Diamond-Blackfan syndrome, Fanconi anemia, idiopathic aplastic anemia, preleukemia); drug-induced anemias (azidothymidine, valproic acid, carbamazepine); chronic liver disease; and hypothyroidism.

MEGALOBLASTIC MACROCYTIC ANEMIAS

Vitamin B_{12} Deficiency

Vitamin B_{12}, a coenzyme for 5-methyl-tetrahydrofolate formation, is needed for DNA synthesis. It is found in meat, fish, cheese, and eggs. Dietary vitamin B_{12} deficiency is rare in developed countries except in the breast-fed infant whose mother is a vegan with poor attention to dietary sources of vitamin B_{12}. Another cause of vitamin B_{12} deficiency is selective or generalized malabsorption. Vitamin B_{12} combines with intrinsic factor, which is produced by gastric parietal cells, and absorbed in the terminal ileum. Transcobalamin II then transports vitamin B_{12} to the liver for storage. The availability of vitamin B_{12} is reduced by any condition that alters intrinsic factor production, interferes with intestinal absorption, or reduces transcobalamin II levels. Disorders such as congenital pernicious anemia (absent intrinsic factor), juvenile pernicious anemia (autoimmune destruction of intrinsic factor), and transcobalamin II deficiency result in vitamin B_{12} deficiency. Other causes include ileal resection, small bowel bacterial overgrowth, and infection with the fish tapeworm *Diphyllobothrium latum*.

Clinical Manifestations

The effects of vitamin B_{12} deficiency include glossitis, diarrhea, and weight loss. Neurologic sequelae include paresthesias, peripheral neuropathies, and, in the most severe cases, dementia, ataxia, and/or posterior column spinal degeneration. Vitiligo is the main dermatologic manifestation.

Megaloblastic changes on peripheral blood smear include ovalocytosis, neutrophils with hypersegmented nuclei (more than four per cell), nucleated red blood cells, basophilic stippling, and Howell-Jolly bodies. The mean corpuscular volume is usually greater than 100 fL. Intramarrow hemolysis results in elevated levels of serum lactate dehydrogenase, indirect bilirubin, and serum iron. In severe cases, megaloblastic anemia may be accompanied by leukopenia and thrombocytopenia.

Diagnosis is confirmed by a subnormal serum level of vitamin B_{12}. In nondietary deficiency, the **Schilling test** helps delineate pernicious anemia from bacterial overgrowth. In this test, an oral dosage of radiolabeled vitamin B_{12} is given, and its absorption is checked by urinary excretion. If urinary excretion is minimal, an oral dosage of intrinsic factor is given. Normal urinary excretion after intrinsic factor confirms the diagnosis of pernicious anemia. Inadequate urinary excretion after intrinsic factor suggests bacterial overgrowth. Antibiotics are given, and if vitamin B_{12} urinary excretion then increases, the patient has bacterial overgrowth.

Treatment

Treatment for most forms of vitamin B_{12} deficiency, with the exception of bacterial overgrowth and fish tapeworm, is monthly intramuscular vitamin B_{12}.

The erythropoietic response is rapid, with marrow megaloblastosis improving within hours, reticulocytosis appearing by day 3 of therapy, and anemia resolving within 1 to 2 months.

Folate Deficiency

Folate is found in liver, green vegetables, cereals, and cheese and converted to tetrahydrofolate, which is required for DNA synthesis. Because folate stores are relatively small, deficiency may develop within 1 month and anemia within 4 months of deprivation. Etiologies include inadequate dietary intake, impaired absorption of folate, increased demand for folate, and abnormal folate metabolism. Dietary deficiency of folic acid is unusual in developed countries. Children at risk are infants fed goat milk, evaporated milk, or heat-sterilized milk or formula; each has inadequate folate content. Malabsorptive states of the jejunum, such as inflammatory bowel disease and celiac sprue, can cause folate deficiency. Increased demand for folate occurs with an increased rate of red blood cell turnover (hyperthyroidism, pregnancy, chronic hemolysis, malignancy). Relative folate deficiency may develop if the diet does not provide adequate folate to meet these needs. Certain anticonvulsant drugs (phenytoin, phenobarbital) interfere with folate metabolism.

Clinical Manifestations

Specific symptoms are often absent, although pallor, glossitis, malaise, anorexia, poor growth, and recurrent infection may be seen. Unlike vitamin B_{12} deficiency, neurologic disease is not associated with folate deficiency.

Laboratory findings include low red blood cell folate and normal serum vitamin B_{12} levels. Megaloblastic changes on peripheral blood smear and bone marrow aspirate are the same as those noted with vitamin B_{12} deficiency.

Treatment

It is imperative not to misdiagnose B_{12} deficiency as folate deficiency because treatment with folate may result in hematologic improvement and allow for progressive neurologic deterioration. Treatment with 1 mg of folate given orally each day for 1 to 2 months treats the anemia and replenishes body stores. Clinical response is rapid, following a time course similar to that of vitamin B_{12} replacement therapy. Children with chronic hemolytic conditions require continued folate supplementation.

NONMEGALOBLASTIC MACROCYTIC ANEMIAS

Diamond-Blackfan Syndrome

Diamond-Blackfan syndrome is a congenital pure red cell aplasia. Both autosomal dominant and recessive patterns are reported. Twenty-five percent of patients have a mutation in the ribosomal protein S19 gene (RPS19).

Clinical Manifestations

The anemia develops shortly after birth but is not usually detected until later, when symptoms develop; 90% of cases are observed within the first year of life. Infants present with mild macrocytosis and reticulocytopenia. On hemoglobin electrophoresis, there is an elevated hemoglobin F, and fetal i antigen is present on the red cells. Twenty-five percent of patients have associated congenital anomalies that include short stature, web neck, cleft lip, shield chest, and triphalangeal thumb. These children are at high risk for leukemia later in life.

Treatment

Seventy-five percent of patients respond to high-dosage corticosteroids but must receive therapy indefinitely. Those who do not respond to steroid treatment are transfusion dependent and at-risk for the complications of iron overload. Bone marrow transplantation with a matched sibling donor is an option for some patients.

Severe Aplastic Anemia

Severe aplastic anemia is an acquired failure of the hematopoietic stem cells that results in pancytopenia. The disorder may result from exposure to chemicals (benzene, phenylbutazone), drugs (chloramphenicol, sulfonamides), infectious agents (hepatitis virus), or ionizing radiation. Often an etiologic agent is not identified, and the case is classified as idiopathic.

Clinical Manifestations

These patients suffer from pancytopenia, and bone marrow aspirate reveals a hypocellular marrow.

Treatment

The treatment of choice is a bone marrow transplant with a matched sibling donor. In patients who do not have a donor, antithymocyte or antilymphocyte globulin in combination with corticosteroids and growth factors (G-CSF) may be effective. Cyclosporin A and high-dosage cyclophosphamide have also been used. Without treatment, 80% of patients die within 3 months of diagnosis from bleeding or infection. If transplantation is considered, it is important to minimize transfusions to reduce exposure to potentially sensitizing blood products. Neutropenic patients are at risk for serious bacterial infection and usually require antibiotics when they develop fever.

Fanconi Anemia

Fanconi anemia is an autosomal recessive disorder that results in pancytopenia. Some forms may also be inherited in an X-linked recessive manner. Mutations in 13 known genes can cause Fanconi anemia. Commonly associated conditions include pigmentary changes and skeletal, renal, and developmental abnormalities. The disorder results from defective DNA repair mechanisms that lead to excessive chromosomal breaks and recombinations. These chromosomal anomalies are found in all cells of the body, not just the hematopoietic stem cells. The mean age at onset of pancytopenia is 8 years.

Clinical Manifestations

Common signs include hyperpigmentation and café au lait spots, microcephaly, microphthalmia, short stature, horseshoe or absent kidney, and absent thumbs. Hematologic manifestations include progressive pancytopenia. Macrocytosis is universal even before the onset of anemia, and hemoglobin F is seen on hemoglobin electrophoresis. Approximately 10% of children with Fanconi anemia develop leukemia during adolescence.

Diagnosis is confirmed by demonstrating increased chromosomal breakage with exposure to diepoxybutane (DEB) or other agents that damage DNA.

Treatment

Patients frequently require red blood cell transfusions and antibiotics to treat anemia and infections. Some patients transiently respond to androgens. Corticosteroids are often given with the androgens to counterbalance androgen-induced growth acceleration. Bone marrow transplantation is the treatment of choice if an HLA-matched donor can be found. Because of chromosomal sensitivity, the preparative radiation and chemotherapy dosages must be reduced because normal protocols used for the transplantation of non-Fanconi anemia patients result in severe morbidity and mortality.

WHITE BLOOD CELL DISORDERS

White blood cells (WBC), or leukocytes, are the primary systemic defense mechanisms against infections. The total white blood cell count and the differential count often provide valuable clues for the diagnosis and treatment of various disorders. The leukocytes are broadly categorized as granulocytes (neutrophils, eosinophils, and basophils), lymphocytes, and mononuclear phagocytes (monocytes). Granulocytes are so named because of the presence of intracytoplasmic granules on microscopic examination. Neutrophils are the largest population of granulocytes and are also referred to as *segs* that denote segmented neutrophils, the mature form. Bands (or stabs) refer to an immature form of the circulating neutrophil. An increase in neutrophil count is often seen in the presence of inflammation and chemotactic factor productions, such as bacterial infections. Neutrophils and monocytes are strong phagocytes. In addition, monocytes also function as antigen presenting cells. An increase in eosinophil counts is often seen in chronic allergic reactions and parasitic infections. Basophils are the least numerous of the leukocytes and may also be involved in allergic responses. Lymphocytes are a critical component of the immune system, and are responsible for both humoral and cellular immune responses.

When a child with a suspected WBC dysfunction is encountered, a thorough medical history including the past and family history should be obtained along with a detailed physical examination. In particular, a history of medications, toxin or other environmental exposures, and frequency and severity of prior infections is absolutely critical. A family history of other similarly affected individuals with a history of early childhood or in utero deaths and any delays in umbilical cord separation should also be obtained. Recurrent fevers and infections of the skin and mucous membranes (especially of the perianal region) are particularly indicative of WBC disorders. White blood cell disorders may be broadly classified into abnormalities of the WBC number (leukopenia or low count and leukocytosis or an elevated WBC count) and of WBC function (leukocyte function disorders).

Leukopenia is generally defined as a total WBC count of less than 4,000 cells/cu mm. The most common causes of transient leukopenia are infections (bacterial or viral) and drugs. In these cases, the mechanism of leukopenia could be variable and include antibody-mediated destruction, bone marrow suppression, or a shift into the storage or marginated compartments. Since leukopenia may be due to suppression of one of more types of WBCs, one must pay close attention to the differential count and obtain microscopic confirmation. Neutropenia is the most common type of leukopenia and is also the most serious, and depending on the severity, may warrant institution of parenteral antibiotic therapy and hospitalization. Transient neutropenia secondary to the above causes usually resolves spontaneously and any prolonged neutropenia or concomitant decreases in other cell types should prompt consideration of a bone marrow evaluation. A decrease in other white blood cell types is much less common. A marked decrease in lymphocytes, especially in young infants, should prompt further evaluation for an underlying immune disorder after ruling out steroid therapy, which can be associated with lymphocytopenia.

An increase in the WBC count above the normal range is called leukocytosis and is most often encountered in response to inflammatory stimuli such as infection, allergy, or malignancy. Leukocytosis is a normal physiologic finding in the newborn period, during stress, and in pregnancy. Leukocytosis is commonly seen in association with bacterial and viral infections and in chronic inflammatory states. An increase in neutrophils or lymphocytes is the most common cause for leukocytosis. Rarely, an increase in eosinophils (eosinophilia) is also encountered. Disorders associated with eosinophilia include allergy and drug hypersensitivity, parasitic infestations, skin and connective tissue disorders, gastrointestinal disorders, and idiopathic hypereosinophilic syndrome.

Disorders of leukocyte function are extremely rare and may involve abnormalities in one or more of the normal physiologic functions which include motility and migration, chemotaxis, opsonization, and bacterial killing. Highly specialized testing is required for their diagnosis and if these are suspected, a referral to the pediatric hematologist is warranted.

DISORDERS OF HEMOSTASIS

Normal hemostasis requires the integrity of the blood vessels, platelets, and soluble clotting factors. Bleeding derangements can result from abnormal hemostatic plug formation, which occurs in platelet disorders; aberrant clot formation, which is noted in defects of the coagulation cascade; or with vascular abnormalities.

Examples of vascular anomalies that result in bleeding include hereditary defects of collagen synthesis

(Ehlers-Danlos syndrome), acquired disorders of collagen production (vitamin C deficiency, scurvy), and vasculitis (Henoch-Schönlein purpura, or HSP). HSP is associated with abdominal pain, arthritis, nephritis, and purpura classically distributed over the buttocks and lower extremities.

PLATELET DISORDERS

Platelet disorders can be either quantitative or qualitative and result in abnormal hemostatic plug formation. Quantitative abnormalities are detected by the platelet count or platelet estimate on peripheral blood smear, whereas qualitative disorders are detected by the bleeding time or platelet aggregation studies. **Thrombocytopenia**, defined as a platelet count below 150,000/mm^3, is the most common cause of abnormal bleeding. A low platelet count can result from inadequate production or increased destruction of platelets. Platelet production is evaluated by assessing the number of megakaryocytes in the bone marrow aspirate.

Decreased platelet production can result from failure of the bone marrow or bone marrow suppression. Bone marrow failure states causing thrombocytopenia include disorders resulting in pancytopenia (Fanconi anemia, idiopathic aplastic anemia, leukemia); thrombocytopenia-absent radius (TAR) syndrome; and Wiskott-Aldrich syndrome. TAR syndrome, also known as congenital megakaryocytic hypoplasia, is an autosomal recessive disorder in which thrombocytopenia develops in the first few months of life and then resolves spontaneously after 1 year of age. Transient leukocytosis is common and often suggests leukemia. Deformity of the radii is pathognomonic. Wiskott-Aldrich syndrome is an X-linked disorder characterized by hypogammaglobulinemia, eczema, and thrombocytopenia. Bone marrow transplantation is curative. Etiologies of thrombocytopenia caused by bone marrow suppression include chemotherapeutic agents; acquired viral infections (human immunodeficiency virus [HIV], Epstein-Barr virus, measles); congenital infections, including toxoplasmosis, syphilis, rubella, cytomegalovirus, and parvovirus B19; and certain drugs (anticonvulsants, sulfonamides, quinidine, quinine, and thiazide diuretics). Acquired postnatal infections (with the exception of HIV) and drug reactions usually cause transient thrombocytopenia, whereas congenital infections may produce prolonged suppression of bone marrow function.

Thrombocytopenia caused by shortened platelet survival is much more common than thrombocytopenia caused by inadequate production. Platelet destruction is most commonly immune-mediated. Thrombocytopenia in the newborn can result from isoimmune or autoimmune antibodies. Isoimmune IgG antibodies are produced against the fetal platelets when the fetal platelet crosses the placenta and presents itself to the maternal immune system. If there is an antigen on the fetal platelet that does not exist on the maternal platelet, it is recognized as foreign and isoimmune antibodies are created against the antigen. Maternal antiplatelet antibodies then cross the placenta, causing destruction of the fetal platelet. This disorder is known as **neonatal isoimmune thrombocytopenic purpura**. The maternal antiplatelet antibody does not produce maternal thrombocytopenia. Autoimmune IgG antibodies are transferred to the fetus through the placenta when the mother has idiopathic thrombocytopenic purpura, systemic lupus erythematosus, or drug-induced thrombocytopenia. In all three cases, maternal autoantibodies cross the placenta and attack the fetal platelets. In contrast to isoimmune antibodies, autoimmune antibodies also result in maternal thrombocytopenia. After birth, infants with severe isoimmune or autoimmune thrombocytopenia may be treated with corticosteroids or intravenous immunoglobulin until the maternal antiplatelet antibodies dissipate. A detailed discussion of childhood idiopathic thrombocytopenia purpura (ITP) appears later in this chapter.

Microangiopathic hemolytic anemias also cause thrombocytopenia by decreasing platelet survival. Microangiopathic disorders include disseminated intravascular coagulation (DIC), hemolytic-uremic syndrome (HUS), and thrombotic thrombocytopenic purpura (TTP). DIC is discussed later. HUS, characterized by a microangiopathic hemolytic anemia, renal cortical injury, and thrombocytopenia, is a major cause of acute renal failure in children. Verotoxin-producing gram-negative organisms (such as *Escherichia coli* O157:H7) that bind to endothelial cells cause HUS. Because of endothelial cell injury, there is localized clotting and platelet activation. Microangiopathic hemolytic anemia results from mechanical injury to red cells as they pass through the injured vascular endothelium, and thrombocytopenia results from platelet adhesion to the damaged endothelium. An estimated 60% to 80% of patients with HUS transiently require dialysis. Most children survive the acute phase and recover normal renal function. In TTP, there is a lack of the von Willebrand factor cleaving protease (ADAMTS 13) with a resultant increase in the large multimeric forms of von Willebrand factor. These large multimers have an increased affinity for platelet aggregation which leads to thrombocytopenia. Other associated symptoms in TTP include a hemolytic anemia, fever, renal involvement, and neurological findings.

Diminished platelet survival can also result from platelet trapping, as seen with giant hemangiomas and hypersplenism. Hypersplenism most commonly occurs secondary to sickle cell anemia, thalassemia syndromes, Gaucher disease, and portal hypertension. Table 10-6 lists the common causes of thrombocytopenia during the neonatal, infant, and childhood periods.

Idiopathic Thrombocytopenic Purpura

Idiopathic thrombocytopenic purpura (ITP) refers to a thrombocytopenia for which a cause is not apparent. ITP results from the development of antiplatelet antibodies that bind to the platelet membrane. These antibody-coated platelets are then destroyed in the reticuloendothelial system. Rarely, ITP may be the presenting symptom of an autoimmune disease, such as systemic lupus erythematosus or HIV infection.

Clinical Manifestations

Children typically present 1 to 4 weeks after a viral illness with abrupt onset of petechiae and ecchymoses on the skin and bleeding of the mucous membranes. Severe bleeding occurs after trauma. Spontaneous internal hemorrhage, although rare, has been noted with platelet counts below 10,000/mm^3.

Other than thrombocytopenia, the complete blood count is normal. Large platelets are seen on peripheral blood smear, and serology reveals antiplatelet antibodies. Diagnosis of ITP does not require a bone marrow aspirate. However, if there are atypical findings on the complete blood count or the peripheral blood smear, marrow examination is indicated to exclude leukemia and idiopathic aplastic anemia. In ITP, bone marrow aspiration reveals normal myeloid and erythroid elements and an increased number of megakaryocytes.

Treatment

Approximately 80% of the cases of acute ITP resolve spontaneously within 6 months. Some cases, however, become relapsing or chronic.

Clinically significant bleeding or severe thrombocytopenia (platelet count less than 20,000) is treated with high-dosage steroids, intravenous immunoglobulins (IVIG), or antiD immune globulin (in Rh-positive children). These measures all decrease the duration of severe thrombocytopenia by decreasing the rate of clearance of antibody-coated platelets in the reticuloendothelial system, but do not diminish the

■ TABLE 10-6 Causes of Thrombocytopenia

Neonate
Maternal ITP,* SLE, drugs, preeclampsia
Isoimmune*
Congenital megakaryocytic hypoplasia (thrombocytopenia absent radius)
Giant hemangioma
Sepsis*
DIC
Congenital infections

Infant
Wiskott-Aldrich syndrome
Viral infections*
Medications
Malignancies (leukemia, neuroblastoma)
Hemolytic-uremic syndrome
Sepsis
ITP

Childhood
ITP*
Medications*
Aplastic anemia
Leukemia*
Hypersplenism (thalassemia, Gaucher disease, portal hypertension)
Sepsis
SLE
Virus-induced hemophagocytic syndrome
ITP with autoimmune hemolytic anemia (Evan syndrome)
AIDS

*Common.
AIDS, acquired immunodeficiency syndrome; DIC, disseminated intravascular coagulation; ITP, idiopathic thrombocytopenic purpura; SLE, systemic lupus erythematosus.

production of antiplatelet antibodies. None of these measures affects the long-term outcome of ITP.

Chronic ITP, defined as thrombocytopenia continuing for more than 6 months after an acute ITP episode, is treated with IVIG and/or splenectomy. Repeated treatments with IVIG have been effective in delaying splenectomy. Splenectomy induces remission in 70% to 80% of cases of chronic ITP. Rituximab (antiCD20 antibody) may also be effective. In refractory cases, immunosuppression with azathioprine or cyclophosphamide and plasmapheresis may be indicated. Aminocaproic acid (Amicar), a drug that inhibits fibrinolysis, may be helpful for oral bleeding.

Disseminated Intravascular Coagulation

Normal homeostasis is a balance between hemorrhage and thrombosis. In DIC, this balance is altered by severe illness so the patient has activation of both coagulation (thrombin) and fibrinolysis (plasmin). Endothelial injury, release of thromboplastic procoagulant factors into the circulation, and impairment of clearance of activated clotting factors directly activate the coagulation cascade. Intravascular activation of the coagulation cascade leads to fibrin deposition in the small blood vessels, tissue ischemia, release of tissue thromboplastin, consumption of clotting factors, and activation of the fibrinolytic system. Coagulation elements, especially platelets, fibrinogen, and clotting factors II, V, and VIII, are consumed, as are the anticoagulant proteins, especially antithrombin III, protein C, and plasminogen. Acute and chronic conditions associated with DIC include sepsis, burns, trauma, asphyxia, malignancy, and cirrhosis.

Clinical Manifestations

The bleeding diathesis is diffuse, with bleeding from venipuncture sites and around indwelling catheters. Gastrointestinal and pulmonary bleeding can be severe, and hematuria is common. Thrombotic lesions affect the extremities, skin, kidneys, and brain. Both ischemic and hemorrhagic strokes can occur.

The diagnosis of DIC is a clinical one bolstered by laboratory evidence. Thrombocytopenia is evident, along with prolonged prothrombin time (PT) and partial thromboplastin time (PTT). Fibrin split products and d-dimers are elevated. Fibrinogen and factor V and VIII levels are low. The peripheral blood smear reveals schistocytes, which are classically seen with microangiopathic disease.

Treatment

The treatment of DIC is supportive. The disorder that caused DIC must be treated, and hypoxia, acidosis, and perfusion abnormalities need to be corrected. If bleeding persists, the child should be treated with platelets and fresh-frozen plasma, which replaces depleted clotting factors. Heparin may be useful in the presence of significant arterial or venous thrombotic disease unless sites of life-threatening bleeding coexist.

DEFECTS OF THE COAGULATION CASCADE

Coagulation disorders can be inherited or acquired. The most common inherited defects are hemophilia A and B and von Willebrand disease, whereas vitamin K deficiency is an important acquired coagulation defect.

Hemophilia A and B

Hemophilia A is caused by deficiency of **factor VIII** and occurs in 1 in 5,000 males, whereas hemophilia B results from **factor IX** deficiency and is found in 1 in 25,000 males. Both are X-linked recessive disorders. All other clotting factors are coded on autosomal chromosomes and are therefore inherited in an autosomal fashion. The lack of factor VIII or IX causes a delay in the production of thrombin, which catalyzes the formation of the primary fibrin clot by the conversion of fibrinogen to fibrin and stabilizes the fibrin by activating factor XIII.

Clinical Manifestations

Other than their factor replacement regimens, hemophilia A and B are indistinguishable clinically, and the severity of each disorder is determined by the degree of factor deficiency. Children with mild hemophilia (5% to 49% of normal factor) require significant trauma to induce bleeding, and spontaneous bleeding does not occur. Patients with moderate hemophilia (1% to 5% of normal factor) require moderate trauma to induce bleeding episodes. Severe hemophiliacs (children with less than 1% of normal factor) may have spontaneous bleeding and bleed with very minor trauma. Mild hemophilia may go undiagnosed for many years, whereas severe hemophilia manifests itself during infancy. Hemophilia is characterized by spontaneous or traumatic hemorrhages, which can be subcutaneous, intramuscular, or within joints (hemarthroses). Life-threatening internal hemorrhage may follow trauma or surgery. In newborns with hemophilia, there may be intracranial bleeding secondary to traumatic delivery or after circumcision; otherwise, bleeding complications are uncommon in the first year of life. Circumcision should be avoided in boys with a family history of hemophilia.

In both forms of hemophilia, the PTT is prolonged. In hemophilia A, factor VIII coagulant activity (VIII:c) is low, whereas in hemophilia B, factor IX activity is low. Table 10-7 compares hemophilia A, hemophilia B, and von Willebrand disease.

Treatment

The goal of therapy is to prevent long-term crippling orthopedic injuries caused by hemarthroses. Most patients require periodic infusions of factor VIII or IX to raise their factor levels high enough to stop the bleeding. Many patients with severe hemophilia receive regular infusions of factor to prevent bleeding episodes (prophylaxis). Whereas plasma-derived factors were used in the past, recombinant factors VIII and IX are now available. For mild-to-moderate bleeding episodes, such as hemarthroses, a 40% factor level is appropriate. For life-threatening bleeding, levels of 80% to 100% of normal factors VIII and IX are necessary. Desmopressin acetate (DDAVP), a synthetic vasopressin analogue, releases factor VIII from endothelial cells. When administered, it triples or quadruples the initial factor VIII level of a patient with hemophilia A but has no effect on factor IX levels. If adequate hemostatic levels of factor VIII can be achieved with DDAVP, it is the initial treatment of bleeding for those afflicted with mild to moderate hemophilia A. Because DDAVP is an antidiuretic hormone analogue, hemophiliacs who frequently use DDAVP should be monitored for hyponatremia caused by water retention. Mild acute bleeding episodes can be treated in the home once the patient has attained the appropriate age and the parents have learned how to administer recombinant factor VIII or IX or DDAVP. Bleeding associated with surgery, trauma, or dental extraction can be anticipated, and excessive bleeding can be prevented with appropriate replacement therapy. Aminocaproic acid (Amicar), an inhibitor of fibrinolysis, may help treat oral bleeding after a dental procedure. It is generally given before and after the procedure.

Testing of blood products for HIV and hepatitis viruses did not begin until the mid-1980s, and as a result, many hemophiliacs contracted the viruses. Between 1979 and 1984, 90% of hemophiliacs who received plasma-derived factor products became HIV seropositive. Acquired immunodeficiency syndrome

■ **TABLE 10-7** Comparison of Hemophilia A, Hemophilia B, and von Willebrand Disease			
	Hemophilia A	**Hemophilia B**	**von Willebrand Disease**
Inheritance	X-linked	X-linked	Autosomal dominant
Factor deficiency	Factor VIII	Factor IX	von Willebrand factor and VIII:C
Bleeding site(s)	Muscle, joint, surgical	Muscle, joint, surgical	Mucous membranes, skin, surgical, menstrual
PT	Normal	Normal	Normal
APTT	Prolonged	Prolonged	Prolonged or normal
Bleeding time	Normal	Normal	Prolonged or normal
Factor VIII coagulant activity (VIII:C)	Low	Normal	Low or normal
vWF:Ag	Normal	Normal	Low
vWF:Act	Normal	Normal	Low
Factor IX	Normal	Low	Normal
Ristocetin-induced platelet agglutination	Normal	Normal	Normal or low
Platelet aggregation	Normal	Normal	Normal

(AIDS) is the most common cause of death in older patients with hemophilia. Newer pooled concentrates are safer, and all recombinant preparations are safe from viral agents.

Another significant complication of therapy is the formation of inhibitors, which are IgG antibodies directed against transfusion factors VIII and IX. Inhibitors arise during therapy in 15% of patients with factor VIII deficiency and in 1% of those with factor IX deficiency. The treatment of bleeding patients with an inhibitor is difficult. For low-titer inhibitors, options include continuous factor VIII infusions or administration of porcine factor VIII. For high-titer inhibitors, it usually is necessary to administer a product that bypasses the inhibitor, such as activated prothrombin complex concentrates or recombinant factor VIIa. The use of frequent high dosages of prothrombin complex concentrates, and especially of the activated products, paradoxically increases the risks of thrombosis, which has resulted in fatal myocardial infarction and stroke in adults. Induction of immune tolerance with continuous antigen exposure with or without immunosuppression may be beneficial.

von Willebrand Disease

von Willebrand disease is caused by deficiency of von Willebrand factor (vWF), an adhesive protein that connects subendothelial collagen to activated platelets and also binds to circulating factor VIII, protecting it from rapid clearance. von Willebrand disease is classified on the basis of whether vWF is quantitatively reduced but not absent (type 1), qualitatively abnormal (type 2; dysproteinemia), or absent (type 3).

Clinical Manifestations

The clinical manifestations of von Willebrand disease are similar to those of thrombocytopenia and include mucocutaneous bleeding, epistaxis, gingival bleeding, cutaneous bruising, and menorrhagia. In severe von Willebrand disease, factor VIII deficiency may be profound and the patient may also have manifestations similar to those of hemophilia A. If there is little or no vWF in the blood to bind factor VIII, factor VIII is cleared quickly from the circulation, resulting in factor VIII deficiency. Approximately 85% of patients with von Willebrand disease have classic type 1 disease, which results in mild to moderate deficiency of vWF.

Laboratory testing includes measurement of the amount of protein, usually accomplished by immunologic detection of vWF antigen (vWF:Ag) and vWF activity (vWF:Act). vWF activity is measured functionally by the ristocetin cofactor assay (vWF:RCoF), which uses the antibiotic ristocetin to induce vWF to bind to platelets. The patient typically has a prolonged bleeding time because of the effect of vWF deficiency on platelet activity, and a prolonged PTT, which results from the effect of vWF deficiency on factor VIII activity. The PFA-100 (Platelet Function Analyzer) test is a new test of platelet function and is increasingly used in place of the bleeding time. This test measures the time taken for blood, drawn through a fine capillary, to block a membrane coated with collagen and epinephrine (CEPI) or collagen and ADP (CADP). This is referred to as the *closure time* and is measured in seconds and is abnormally prolonged in von Willebrand disease and in some platelet function disorders. Table 10-7 compares the findings in classic von Willebrand disease with those in hemophilia A and B.

Treatment

The treatment of von Willebrand disease depends on the severity of bleeding. DDAVP, which stimulates the release of vWF from endothelial cells, is the treatment of choice for bleeding episodes in most patients with type I vWD. Patients with type 3 disease (who have no vWF to release), or with severe bleeding not responding to DDAVP, can be treated with a virally attenuated vWF-containing concentrate (Humate P). Cryoprecipitate may also be used, but it cannot be virally attenuated. Hepatitis B vaccine should be given before exposure to plasma-derived products. As in all bleeding disorders, medications that alter platelet function, such as aspirin, should be avoided.

Vitamin K Deficiency

Coagulation factors (factors II, VII, IX, and X) and antithrombotic factors (protein C and protein S) are synthesized in the liver and depend on vitamin K for their activity. When vitamin K is deficient, coagulation is impaired. Vitamin K deficiency often occurs because of malabsorption, especially with cystic fibrosis and with antibiotic-induced suppression of intestinal bacteria that produce vitamin K. Overdose of warfarin, a drug that interferes with vitamin K metabolism, causes deficiency of vitamin K-dependent factors. Similarly, maternal use of warfarin or anticonvulsant therapy (phenobarbital, phenytoin) may also result in vitamin K deficiency in the newborn. The most common disorder resulting from vitamin K deficiency is hemorrhagic disease of the newborn, which occurs in neonates who do not receive intramuscular vitamin K at birth.

Clinical Manifestations

Although most newborn infants are born with reduced levels of vitamin K-dependent factors, only a few develop hemorrhagic complications. Because breast milk is a poor source of vitamin K, breast-fed infants who do not receive prophylactic vitamin K on the first day of life are at the highest risk for hemorrhagic disease. Peak incidence is at 2 to 10 days of life. The recommended preventive dose of vitamin K is 1.0 mg given intramuscularly. The disorder is marked by generalized ecchymoses, gastrointestinal hemorrhage, and bleeding from the circumcision site and umbilical stump. Affected neonates are at risk for intracranial hemorrhage.

Both the PTT and PT are prolonged in vitamin K deficiency because factors of both extrinsic and intrinsic pathways are affected. Prolongation of the PT is a more sensitive test for vitamin K deficiency because most infants have transient prolongation of the PTT at birth. The coagulopathy seen with hemorrhagic disease may be confused with liver disease or DIC, both of which have a prolonged PT and decreased factor VII level. Table 10-8 differentiates vitamin K deficiency, liver disease, and DIC by laboratory data.

Treatment

Nutritional disorders and malabsorptive states respond to parenteral administration of vitamin K.

■ TABLE 10-8 Differentiation of Vitamin K Deficiency, Liver Disease, and DIC

Laboratory Test	Vitamin K Deficiency	Liver Disease	DIC
PT	↑	↑	↑
Platelets	nl	↓ to nl	↓
Fibrinogen	nl	↓↓	
Factor VIII	nl	nl to ↑	↓
Fibrinogen degradation products	nl	nl to ↑	↑
Factor VII	↓	↓	↓ to nl
Factor V	nl	low	Low

nl, normal.

Fresh-frozen plasma or prothrombin complex concentrate, which is a mixture of coagulation factors II, VII, IX, and X, is indicated for severe bleeding.

Deep Vein Thrombosis, Pulmonary Embolism, and Anticoagulation Therapy

Venous thrombosis is rare in children but the incidence is rapidly rising with advances in pediatric tertiary care. The estimated risk for thrombosis in children in the general populations is 0.07/10,000 and about 5.3/10,000 in hospitalized children. The rate of venous thrombosis in children is only one-tenth of that in adults. Thrombosis in infants and teenagers accounts for 70% of the cases seen in children. Venous thrombosis usually develops under conditions of slow blood flow and is augmented by further retardation and stagnation of flow. In neonates, thrombosis is usually related to umbilical catheters and may present as a white, pulseless limb in the initial stages, and can progress to a black, necrotic extremity if left untreated. In older children, unilateral acute limb swelling, with pain and discoloration, and distended superficial veins should make one suspect a deep vein thrombosis. Childhood thrombosis is usually multifactorial in etiology and is precipitated by the concurrence of multiple risk factors. The various risk factors for childhood venous thromboembolism are listed in the Table 10-9.

The presence of central venous devices is the most common thrombotic risk factor encountered in pediatrics. Several genetic mutations have been identified that are associated with an increased risk of thrombosis. The most common mutations in the Caucasian population are the factor V Leiden mutation and the prothrombin gene 20210A mutations. In addition, hereditary deficiencies in the natural anticoagulant factors, protein C, protein S, and antithrombin are also associated with an increased risk for thrombosis. Diabetes, obesity, and nephrotic syndrome are some examples of concurrent medical illnesses that also increase this risk. The most important complication of venous thrombosis is pulmonary embolism, which occurs when a thrombus or other substance (i.e., fat, air, bone marrow) enters the pulmonary circulation and causes vascular obstruction. Pulmonary embolism may lead to significant ventilation-perfusion mismatch and respiratory distress. The lung parenchyma affected by the embolism can undergo necrosis leading to pulmonary infarction. Anticoagulation with various forms of heparin (unfractionated or standard heparin, low molecular weight heparin) or with vitamin K

■ TABLE 10-9 Risk Factors for Venous Thromboembolism

- Central venous catheterization
- Previous VTE
- Inherited or acquired thrombophilia
- Surgery
- Trauma (major or lower extremity)
- Immobility, paresis
- Obesity
- Malignancy
- Cancer therapy (hormonal, chemotherapy, or radiotherapy)
- Increasing age
- Estrogen-containing oral contraception or hormone replacement therapy
- Acute medical illness
- Heart or respiratory failure
- Inflammatory bowel disease
- Nephrotic syndrome
- Smoking

VTE, venous thromboembolism.

antagonists such as warfarin are used as standard therapy for the treatment of venous thrombosis and pulmonary embolism. In specific cases, thrombolytic therapy with tissue plasminogen activator (tPA) may be indicated to dissolve the clot or surgical embolectomy may be needed to remove the clot.

BLOOD PRODUCT TRANSFUSION AND REACTIONS TO TRANSFUSIONS OF BLOOD PRODUCTS

Transfusion of blood products should be performed only when strict clinical and laboratory criteria for their requirement are met. Packed red blood cells (PRBCs) and platelets are the most commonly transfused blood products. Transfusion of granulocytes, whole blood, fresh frozen plasma (FFP), and cryoprecipitate may be warranted in special circumstances. PRBC transfusions are generally recommended when the hemoglobin has fallen to 8 g/dL or less in patients with cardiopulmonary compromise or active bleed-

ing. PRBC transfusions increase the oxygen carrying capacity in anemic patients and help to ensure adequate tissue oxygenation. Fresh PRBCs have better oxygen carrying capacity and are preferable in neonates and in patients with cardiopulmonary disease. One unit of PRBCs derived from a routine blood donation is equivalent to 250 to 300 mL of red blood cells. Administration of 10 to 15 mL/kg of PRBCs usually raises the hemoglobin level by 2 to 3 g/dL. This volume can safely be administered over 3 to 4 hours except in severely anemic (hemoglobin <5 g/dL) patients or those at risk for cardiac failure, where the rate of transfusion has to be much slower. Platelet transfusions are normally indicated to prevent or stop bleeding in patients with thrombocytopenia or platelet function disorders. Platelet transfusions are indicated when the platelet count drops below 20,000/mm^3 in stable patients, or below 50,000/mm^3 in patients with bleeding symptoms. Platelet transfusions are usually not indicated in patients with ITP irrespective of the platelet count, except with life-threatening hemorrhage. Platelet concentrates are stored at room temperature and have a maximum shelf life of 5 days, while PRBCs are stored between 3° to 6°C and have a shelf life of 35 to 42 days, depending on the preservative used. Fresh frozen plasma infusions are indicated for replacement of missing coagulation factors (when the specific factor concentrate is unavailable) or for plasma exchange. Cryoprecipitate is a rich source of coagulation factors VIII and XIII and fibrinogen. Granuloctye infusions are usually used in the neonate or infant with prolonged neutropenia and life-threatening sepsis unresponsive to other therapies. Whole blood transfusions are rarely used these days, except during exchange transfusions in neonates and in autologous blood transfusions.

Blood product transfusion is associated with significant risks and complications, although current monitoring and testing procedures have markedly reduced their incidence. The most commonly encountered transfusion reactions include:

1. Allergic reactions: occur in 1% to 2% of PRBC transfusions and are associated with pruritus, rash, and urticaria typically beginning minutes after the infusion is started. The transfusion should be paused, and antihistamines should be administered.
2. Febrile reactions: are due to preformed antibodies to incompatible leukocytes present in PRBC and platelet transfusions and can be prevented by the use of leukocyte filters or leukocyte-depleted blood

products. If they occur, the transfusion should be paused, a blood bank transfusion work-up should be started, and antipyretics administered.

3. Hemolytic reactions: are most commonly due to clerical error resulting in administration of the wrong unit or to the wrong patient. These reactions are characterized by a sudden onset of fever, chills, tachycardia, tachypnea, and vomiting, and may progress to severe hemolysis resulting in multi-organ failure, shock, and DIC unless the transfusion is immediately stopped and necessary supportive care given.

4. Infections: are extremely rare secondary to the intensive screening of donors and testing of products. The current estimated risk of transmission of HIV infection is less than one in two million, less than 1 in 500,000 for hepatitis C virus, and less than 1 in 200,000 for hepatitis B virus.

5. Graft versus Host disease (GVHD): occurs due to the transfusion of immunocompetent lymphocytes contained in a cellular component that engraft in a recipient whose immune system cannot reject them. Irradiation of blood products can prevent this complication.

KEY POINTS

- Anemia results from decreased red cell production, increased red cell destruction, or blood loss. The mean corpuscular volume and adjusted reticulocyte count categorize the disorder into a microcytic, normocytic, or macrocytic anemia, with adequate or inadequate red blood cell production.

- Iron deficiency anemia, the thalassemia syndromes, and anemia of chronic disease are the most common causes of hypochromic microcytic anemias.

- Transient erythroblastopenia of childhood is a normocytic anemia caused by bone marrow suppression, and has a peak incidence at 2 years of age.

- Normocytic anemias with increased red cell production are most commonly caused by hemolytic anemias.

- Hemolytic anemias are caused by extracorpuscular factors and intracorpuscular defects. In general, extracorpuscular defects are acquired, and intracorpuscular defects are hereditary. Extracorpuscular anomalies are divided into isoimmune, autoimmune, and nonimmune hemolytic anemias. Intracorpuscular defects include intrinsic membrane defects, hemoglobinopathies, and enzymopathies.

- Hereditary spherocytosis is caused by an intrinsic membrane defect in the major supporting proteins of the red blood cell membrane.

- Sickle cell disease results from an abnormal β-globin chain in the hemoglobin molecule, which, under conditions of deoxygenation, promotes aggregation of hemoglobin into long polymers that distort the red blood cell into a sickle shape. The clinical manifestations of sickle cell anemia result from anemia, infection, and vaso-occlusion.

- Glucose-6-phosphate dehydrogenase (G6PD) deficiency, is the most common red blood cell enzyme defect.

- Megaloblastic macrocytic anemias reflect ineffective DNA synthesis and can result from vitamin B_{12} or folate deficiency, drugs that interfere with folate metabolism, and some rare metabolic disorders.

- Macrocytic anemias without megaloblastosis result from bone marrow failure and include bone marrow failure syndromes (Diamond-Blackfan syndrome, Fanconi anemia, idiopathic aplastic anemia, preleukemia), drug-induced anemias, chronic liver disease, and hypothyroidism.

- Platelet disorders can be either quantitative or qualitative, and result in abnormal hemostatic plug.

- Thrombocytopenia is the most common cause of abnormal bleeding in children. Thrombocytopenia caused by shortened platelet survival is much more common than thrombocytopenia caused by inadequate production and is caused by isoimmune antibodies, autoimmune antibodies, and microangiopathic hemolytic anemias.

- Idiopathic thrombocytopenic purpura (ITP) results from autoimmune antibody formation against host platelets.

- Disseminated intravascular coagulation (DIC) results from severe illness, causing activation of both coagulation (thrombin) and fibrinolysis (plasmin).

- Hemophilia A results from a deficiency of factor VIII, and hemophilia B results from a lack of factor IX. Both types of hemophilia are characterized by spontaneous or traumatic hemorrhages, which can be

KEY POINTS *(continued)*

subcutaneous, intramuscular, or within joints (hemarthroses). Life-threatening internal hemorrhage may follow trauma or surgery.

- von Willebrand disease is caused by deficiency of vWF, an adhesive protein that connects subendothelial collagen to activated platelets and also binds to circulating factor VIII, protecting it from rapid clearance, and is characterized by mucocutaneous bleeding, epistaxis, gingival bleeding, cutaneous bruising, and menorrhagia.

- The most common disorder resulting from vitamin K deficiency is hemorrhagic disease of the newborn, which occurs in neonates who do not receive vitamin K at birth.

Immunology, Allergy, and Rheumatology

Claas Hinze • Robert A. Colbert • Marc E. Rothenberg • Katie S. Fine

IMMUNOLOGY

The immune system, composed of specialized cells and molecules, is responsible for recognizing and neutralizing foreign antigens. Specific complex interactions produce adaptive inflammatory responses and defend against infection. **Immunodeficiency syndromes** increase susceptibility to infection, malignancy, and autoimmune disorders (Table 11-1). Table 11-2 lists clinical criteria that should prompt an evaluation for immunodeficiency.

DISORDERS OF HUMORAL IMMUNITY

B cells produce antibodies, the primary effectors of humoral immunity. Antibodies are a vital component of the immune system, particularly in defense against extracellular pathogens such as encapsulated bacteria. A variety of antibodies activate complement, serve as opsonins, inhibit microbial adherence to mucous membranes, and neutralize various toxins and viruses. As a group, **antibody (humoral) deficiency syndromes** are the most common immunodeficiency diseases encountered in pediatric practice.

Clinical Manifestations

History and Physical Examination

A history of recurrent infections with **encapsulated** organisms such as *Haemophilus influenzae* and *Streptococcus pneumoniae* and failure to respond to appropriate antibiotic therapy are suggestive of a primary B-cell deficiency. In addition, there is often a history of frequent upper respiratory tract infections beginning after 6 months of age, including otitis media, sinusitis, and pneumonia.

Differential Diagnosis

X-linked agammaglobulinemia (XLA; also termed Bruton tyrosine kinase deficiency or Bruton disease) occurs in boys and appears after 6 months of age as maternally derived antibody levels fall. These patients do not produce antibodies and have virtually no mature B-cells. In addition to their susceptibility to encapsulated organisms, individuals with this disorder are prone to severe, often life-threatening enterovirus infections.

Common variable immunodeficiency is an inherited disorder of hypogammaglobulinemia (particularly IgG and IgA) with equal distribution between the genders. In addition, antibody formation may be defective. Infections are usually less severe; however, the incidences of lymphoma and autoimmune disease are increased in these patients.

Selective IgA deficiency is the mildest and most common immunodeficiency syndrome. Serum levels of the other antibody classes are usually normal. Patients react normally to viral infections but are more susceptible to bacterial infections of the respiratory, gastrointestinal, and urinary tracts.

Diagnostic Evaluation

Quantitative measurement of total and fractionated serum immunoglobulin levels is an important screening test for specific deficiencies and for

■ TABLE 11-1 Causes, Characteristics, and Evaluation of Immune Component Deficiencies

Condition	Mechanism	Sequelae	Laboratory Tests
Disorders of humoral immunity	—Impaired opsonization —Inability to lyse, agglutinate bacteria —Inability to neutralize bacterial toxins	—Frequent, recurrent pyogenic infections with extracellular encapsulated organisms —Frequent bacterial otitis media, sinusitis, and pneumonia infections	—Quantitative total, fractionated immunoglobulin levels —Vaccination antibody titers
Disorders of cell-mediated immunity	—Inability of T-cells to direct B-cell antibody synthesis to T-cell-specific antigens	—Frequent, recurrent infections with opportunistic/low-grade organisms and viruses —Increased incidence of autoimmune disorders and malignancies —Anergy	—Absolute lymphocyte count (ALC) —Abnormal mitogen stimulation response —Delayed hypersensitivity skin testing
Phagocytic disorders (neutropenia)	—Insufficient number of neutrophils	—Cellulitis, skin abscesses, furunculosis —Stomatitis, gingivitis, rectal inflammation —Pneumonia, sepsis	—Absolute neutrophil count —Blood smear examination for blasts —Antineutrophil antibodies
Phagocytic disorders (chronic granulomatous disease)	—Inability to kill intracellular bacteria secondary to failure to generate oxygen metabolites such as the superoxide anion	—Increased susceptibility to infections with catalase-positive bacteria and fungi —Chronic lymphadenitis, abscesses, granulomas, osteomyelitis	—Nitroblue tetrazolium test —DHR conversion test
Complement disorders	—Impaired opsonization	—Recurrent bacterial infections with encapsulated, extracellular organisms —Increased susceptibility to meningococcal, gonnococcal disease —Increased incidence of autoimmune disease	—Total hemolytic complement (CH_{50}) —Assays of the classical and alternative pathways

■ TABLE 11-2 Clinical Criteria for Evaluation for Immunodeficiency Syndromes

Two serious/systemic bacterial infections within 1 year
Any bacterial or fungal infection which recurs despite or does not respond to appropriate therapy
Infection by an unusual* or opportunistic pathogen
Infection at an unusual site (e.g., brain or liver abscess)
Chronic gingivitis

*Including Aspergillus, Serratia marcescens, Nocardia species, and Burkholderia cepacia.

panhypogammaglobulinemia. Antibody titers generated against tetanus, diphtheria, and pneumococci after immunization assess B-cell function.

Treatment

The mainstays of therapy are appropriate antibiotic use and periodic gammaglobulin administration. **Intravenous immunoglobulin** (IVIG) and/or intramuscular gammaglobulin provide antibody replacement and have revolutionized the treatment of humoral immunodeficiency syndromes.

TRANSIENT HYPOGAMMAGLOBULINEMIA OF INFANCY

Although maternal IgG is actively transported across the placenta and is protective throughout the first few months of life, neonates are considered relatively immunocompromised. All serum immunoglobulin classes are present at birth, but most do not reach adult levels until early to middle childhood. Over the first 6 to 8 weeks of life, maternally derived immunoglobulins decrease and are replaced by the child's growing production. Thus, infants are particularly susceptible to infection at ages 6 to 12 weeks, their immunologic nadir.

Transient hypogammaglobulinemia of infancy is a recognized disorder in which the acquisition of normal infant immunoglobulin levels is delayed. Although some of these patients are subsequently diagnosed with other primary immunodeficiencies, most eventually develop normal immunity.

DISORDERS OF CELL-MEDIATED IMMUNITY

T-cells modulate most immune responses, primarily through the secretion of interleukins. In addition, they are major effectors of cell-mediated immunity, important in the defense against intracellular and opportunistic infections. Certain subclasses are capable of killing tumor and viral-infected cells. Patients with dysfunctional T-cells are at increased risk for autoimmune disorders. T-cell diseases generally impart significantly greater morbidity and mortality to their victims than humoral disorders alone. Chromosome 22q11 deletion (DiGeorge) syndrome, a congenital disorder, and human immunodeficiency virus, an acquired one, both represent **T-cell immunodeficiencies**.

Clinical Manifestations

History and Physical Examination

T-cell abnormalities predispose patients to infections with intracellular pathogens, including viruses and mycobacteria. Patients with near-total thymic hypoplasia are highly susceptible to opportunistic infections from organisms such as fungi and *Pneumocystis jiroveci*.

Children with DiGeorge syndrome present early in infancy with disease unrelated to the immune system (e.g., congenital heart disease, hypocalcemic tetany from thymic hypoplasia). Other structures and organs derived from the branchial pouches during embryogenesis may be malformed as well, including the ears and face. The severity of the immunodeficiency is extremely variable.

Diagnostic Evaluation

Absolute lymphocyte counts (calculated by multiplying the percentage of lymphocytes by the total white blood cell count) are normal or moderately decreased. T-cell function, measured by in vitro mitogen stimulation and intradermal delayed hypersensitivity testing, is absent or significantly compromised. No thymic shadow is seen on chest x-ray in patients with DiGeorge syndrome. Fluorescent in situ hybridization (FISH) testing of chromosome 22 detects the 22q11.2 deletion.

Treatment

The immunodeficiency of chromosome 22q11.2 deletion (DiGeorge) syndrome has been successfully treated with both thymic and bone marrow transplantation. Initial therapy should be aimed at repairing associated congenital heart defects and maintaining normocalcemia.

Human immunodeficiency virus is discussed in detail in Chapter 12.

COMBINED IMMUNODEFICIENCY SYNDROMES

Combined humoral and cell-mediated immunodeficiencies tend to be inherited and manifest a wide range of clinical severity. Affected patients display increased susceptibility to both traditionally virulent and opportunistic infections.

Severe combined immunodeficiency disease (SCID) is a devastating disorder characterized by substantial deficits in both humoral and cell-mediated immunity. The disease may be X-linked, autosomal recessive, or spontaneous. Patients are susceptible to a wide range of infections and usually present with multiple illnesses (pneumonia, sepsis, meningitis) in the first few months of life. An absolute lymphocyte count, noted on a routine CBC, is less than 2,800. T-cell response to stimulation is abnormal, and immunoglobulin levels are extremely low. Bone marrow and cord blood transplantation have been curative; gene therapy is now being studied as a possible alternative treatment.

Ataxia-telangiectasia is an extremely rare autosomal recessive disorder characterized by variable humoral and cell-mediated immune deficits, cerebellar ataxia, and oculocutaneous telangiectasia (small dilated vessels easily visible along the bulbar conjunctiva and skin surface). The incidence of malignancy, especially non-Hodgkin lymphoma and gastric carcinoma, is increased. No specific therapy is currently available; most patients are wheelchair-bound by puberty and die prematurely.

Wiskott-Aldrich syndrome is an X-linked recessive disorder of (primarily) B- and (usually) T-cell immunity, atopic dermatitis, and thrombocytopenia. Specifically, the host's antibodies do not respond normally to carbohydrate antigens. Survival to adulthood is rare because of bleeding, infections, and associated malignancies.

DISORDERS OF PHAGOCYTIC IMMUNITY

Phagocytes are responsible for removing particulate matter from the blood and tissues by ingesting and destroying microorganisms. These cells must be able to adhere to the endothelium, move through the tissues to their site of action, engulf the harmful matter, and kill it intracellularly. Phagocytic disorders are due to an insufficient number of normal neutrophils (neutropenia) or to phagocytic cell dysfunction. **Neutropenia** may result from infection (particularly viruses), medication administration (penicillin, sulfonamides, anticonvulsants), circulating antineutrophil antibodies, malignancy in the bone marrow, or aplastic anemia. **Chronic granulomatous disease** (CGD), the most common inherited disorder of phagocytic immunity, occurs when neutrophils and monocytes are unable to kill certain organisms after ingesting them due to a failure to generate superoxide.

Clinical Manifestations

History and Physical Examination

Patients with neutropenia generally do not experience serious or life-threatening infections unless the neutropenia is both *severe* (absolute neutrophil count (ANC) $<0.5 \times 10^3/\mu L$) and *chronic* (lasting longer than 2 to 3 months). Typical complaints include gingivitis, skin infections, rectal inflammation, otitis media, pneumonia, and sepsis. Patients are often infected with *Staphylococcus aureus* and gram-negative organisms. Of note, patients with neutropenia are unable to mount a sufficient inflammatory response, so typical signs of infection such as erythema, warmth, and swelling may be absent even the presence of significant involvement.

CGD is characterized by chronic or recurrent pyogenic infections caused by bacterial and fungal pathogens that produce catalase (*Staphylococcus aureus, Candida albicans, Aspergillus*), and most gram-negative enteric bacteria. Both X-linked and autosomal inheritance occur. Abscesses and granuloma formation occur in the lymph nodes, liver, spleen, lungs, skin, and gastrointestinal tract. Failure to thrive, chronic diarrhea, and persistent candidiasis of the mouth and diaper area are common. Affected individuals are also at increased risk for opportunistic infections, disseminated viral illnesses, and inflammatory bowel disease.

Diagnostic Evaluation

Severe neutropenia is defined as an ANC $<0.5 \times 10^3/\mu L$. Serial complete blood counts will reveal a leukoerythroblastic response unless the condition is chronic. Bone marrow examination is required if malignancy or aplastic anemia is a consideration.

In CGD, the white blood cell count typically ranges between 10,000 and 20,000/μL with 60% to 80% polymorphonuclear cells. Leukocyte chemotaxis is normal. The hallmark abnormality is the inability of affected cells to produce an oxidative burst resulting in hydrogen peroxide. The **nitroblue tetrazolium test** (NBT) and the dihydrorhodamine reduction (DHR) test are laboratory studies performed to detect the inability to perform this reduction reaction.

Treatment

Children with acute neutropenia need no special treatment. Patients with chronic neutropenia and those with infectious complications may respond to recombinant human granulocyte-colony stimulating factor (rhG-CSF) injections. All patients with CGD should receive prophylactic trimethoprim-sulfamethoxazole and gamma-interferon therapy. Judicious antibiotic therapy during infections is critical. Bone marrow transplantation is not as successful as in other immunodeficiency syndromes. Gene therapy is a promising area of research.

DISORDERS OF COMPLEMENT IMMUNITY

Although quantitative deficiencies of virtually all complement components have been described, they are less common than the immunodeficiencies mentioned earlier. The primary mechanism of disease is impaired opsonization. Patients with **complement disorders** have increased susceptibility to bacterial infections and a higher incidence of rheumatologic disease. In particular, deficiencies of the terminal complement components C5 to C8 increase the likelihood of *Neisseria meningitidis* infections.

ALLERGY

An **allergic reaction** is an undesirable immune-mediated response to an environmental stimulus. Allergies have been implicated as a contributing factor in anaphylaxis, asthma, allergic rhinitis, and atopic dermatitis. Allergic reactions range from mild to life-threatening and are *never* considered adaptive.

The **allergic triad** of atopic disease consists of allergic rhinitis, asthma, and atopic dermatitis (eczema). Children with one known atopic disease are likely to suffer from a second atopic condition.

ALLERGIC RHINITIS

Pathogenesis

Allergic rhinitis is a type 1 hypersensitivity immune response to environmental allergens including airborne pollens, animal dander, dust mites, and molds. The offending allergen binds to IgE on mast cells in the upper respiratory tract, with subsequent release of inflammatory mediators. This localized inflammation results in nasal congestion, rhinorrhea and/or postnasal drainage, sneezing, and occasionally itching. Allergic rhinitis is the most frequent cause of chronic or recurrent clear rhinorrhea in the pediatric population.

Epidemiology

It is estimated that 40% of children are affected by allergic rhinitis by the time they are 6 years of age. Seasonal allergic rhinitis, or **hay fever**, is limited to months of pollination and is uncommon before 5 years of age. Tree pollens are common during early spring, followed by grass pollens, which are detected until the early summer. Ragweed season starts in the late summer and persists until the first frost. Perennial disease persists year round, usually in response to household allergens (molds, dust mites).

Risk Factors

Atopy and genetic predisposition are the major risk factors. Maternal smoking in the first year of life also increases the likelihood of subsequent disease. Paradoxically, heavy exposure to animal dander early in life may reduce the risk of subsequent atopic disease.

Clinical Manifestations

History

Patients with allergic rhinitis are plagued with nasal congestion, profuse watery rhinorrhea, and sneezing. Associated allergic conjunctivitis is common. Unrelenting postnasal drip produces frequent coughing and/or throat clearing. Patients may also complain of drowsiness because of recurrent brief awakenings at night. As a group, children with untreated allergic rhinitis have been shown to have decreased school performance when compared with their peers.

Physical Examination

On examination, the nasal mucosa appears boggy and bluish. Two characteristic features of allergic rhinitis are **allergic shiners** (dark circles that develop under the eyes secondary to venous congestion) and the **allergic salute** (a horizontal crease across the middle of the nose due to a constant upward wiping motion with the hand). Because of the severe congestion, patients may become obligate mouth breathers, and a gaping mouth and palatal arching may be seen on physical exam. Children with allergic rhinitis are also prone to recurrent sinusitis and otitis media with effusion.

Differential Diagnosis

Infectious rhinitis is much more common than allergic rhinitis in infants and toddlers and is often mucopurulent. *Sinusitis* causes chronic rhinorrhea and postnasal drip associated with facial tenderness, cough, and/or headache. When a *nasal foreign body* is present, the discharge is usually unilateral, thick, and foul-smelling. Other possible diagnoses include *vasomotor (idiopathic nonallergic) rhinitis*, which appears to be due to an exaggerated vascular response to irritants, and *rhinitis medicamentosa*, which results from overuse of topical decongestants.

Diagnostic Evaluation

Usually, a careful history confirms the diagnosis. Patients who do not respond favorably to a trial of second-generation (nonsedating) antihistamines may require further workup. Elevated nasopharyngeal eosinophil levels may support the diagnosis; however, a serum radioallergosorbant (RAST) test or direct skin testing is the preferred method for specific allergy testing.

Treatment

The most effective treatment for any allergic condition is **allergen avoidance**. Switching to air-conditioning in the summer (rather than keeping the windows open) affords some protection to patients with pollen allergies. Limiting the amount of humidity in the home can decrease the presence of dust mites and various fungi. Eliminating animal dander and limiting exposure to cigarette smoke are also helpful.

Pharmacotherapy is an important adjunct if avoidance is not possible. **H₁-histamine blockers** (oral or intranasal) are the mainstay of treatment. They are now available in nonsedating formulations approved for use in children greater than 2 years of age. Intranasal cromolyn is helpful as a preventive medication if taken prior to the onset of symptoms. Nasal topical steroids are very effective treatments with minimal side effects. Oral leukotriene receptor antagonists may be beneficial in some patients. Topical and inhaled sympathomimetics (the most popular being pseudoephedrine) are useful for short-term therapy only and, if taken improperly, may result in severe rebound congestion. Allergy immunotherapy (shots) are painful, time-consuming, and expensive; they are indicated only for severe symptoms not controlled with conventional pharmacotherapy.

Recent studies suggest that children with seasonal allergies who are appropriately treated at a young age have a lower risk of developing subsequent atopic disease than those who are left untreated.

ASTHMA

Asthma is discussed in detail in Chapter 20. A significant proportion of cases of asthma is allergic in nature. Allergens frequently associated with asthma exacerbations include mold, dust mites, and pet dander. Allergen avoidance is the first step in effective treatment. Other therapies are discussed in Chapter 20.

ATOPIC DERMATITIS

Atopic dermatitis is a chronic, relapsing and remitting inflammatory skin reaction to specific allergens, including specific foods and environmental allergens. Eczema usually appears in infancy and affects upwards of 10% of the pediatric population. Genetic predilection is the highest risk factor. About half of patients with atopic dermatitis later develop asthma.

Clinical Manifestations

The typical rash consists of a pruritic, erythematous, weeping papulovesicular reaction that progresses to scaling, hypertrophy, and lichenification. In infants younger than 2 years, the eruption involves the extensor surfaces of the arms and legs, the wrists, the face, and the scalp; the diaper area is invariably spared. Flexor areas predominate in older age groups, as well as the neck, wrists, and ankles. The diagnosis of atopic dermatitis is primarily clinical, based on history, physical examination, and response to treatment. The differential diagnosis includes contact dermatitis and psoriasis, a chronic nonallergic skin disorder (see Chapter 5).

Treatment

The goal of treatment is termination of the itch-scratch-itch cycle. Patients should try to keep their skin well hydrated by avoiding hot water and strong or fragrant soaps. Tight clothing and heat may precipitate exacerbations and should be avoided. Moisturizers are the mainstay of treatment, followed by the use of **topical corticosteroids** for areas of inflammation. Pimecrolimus cream, a cytokine blocker, has recently been approved for patients over 24 months of age who cannot tolerate topical steroids or have resistant disease. Topical tacrolimus is another immunomodulator that may be used in more severe cases. Severe chronic eczema may be complicated by bacterial superinfection.

URTICARIA AND ANGIOEDEMA

Urticaria and angioedema are classic type 1 hypersensitivity reactions. **Urticaria** describes the typical raised edematous hives on the skin or mucous membranes resulting from vascular dilation and increased permeability. The lesions itch, blanch, and generally resolve within a few hours to days. **Angioedema** is a similar process confined to the lower dermis and subcutaneous areas; the depth results in a well-demarcated area of swelling devoid of pruritus, erythema, or warmth. Although acute urticaria and angioedema occur frequently in the pediatric population, chronic forms are rare.

Clinical Manifestations

The diagnosis is based on a detailed history of recent exposures or changes in the patient's environment. The multiple allergens and conditions associated with urticaria and angioedema include foods, medications, infections, and some systemic illnesses. Clinical manifestations may be delayed as long as 48 hours after the initial encounter. Hereditary forms exist; patients with hereditary angioedema have an inherited **C1 esterase** inhibitor deficiency. Greater than 50% of the time, the inciting trigger remains a mystery.

Treatment

Treatment depends on severity, which ranges from mild to life-threatening (i.e., swelling around the airway). Subcutaneous epinephrine is the treatment of choice in emergency situations, followed by intravenous diphenhydramine and steroids. Oral antihistamines, sympathomimetics, and occasionally oral steroids are appropriate in milder cases.

FOOD ALLERGIES

Pathogenesis

Food allergy is an immune-mediated response to a specific food protein. It is important to distinguish between food intolerance (an undesirable nonimmunologic reaction) and true food hypersensitivity, which is mediated by immune mechanisms. Examples of nonimmunologic adverse food reaction include caffeine-induced tachycardia and lactose intolerance.

Epidemiology

Eighty percent of all food allergies present during the first year of life. The overall prevalence of food allergies is also higher in children (5% to 8%) than in adults (1% to 2%). Relatively few foods are represented; **peanuts, eggs, milk proteins, soy, wheat, and fish** account for over 90% of reported cases. Exclusive breastfeeding may delay presentation unless the mother is ingesting the offending proteins regularly. One-third of patients with atopic dermatitis and 10% of those with asthma also have a food allergy.

Clinical Manifestations

History and Physical Examination

A detailed history, including daily records of intake and symptoms, is essential for the diagnosis. True food allergies can present with isolated cutaneous reactions, gastrointestinal symptoms, respiratory symptoms, and life-threatening anaphylaxis. Symptoms that develop during weaning are particularly suggestive of food allergies.

Diagnostic Evaluation

Skin testing has a low positive predictive value; it is more helpful for ruling out specific food proteins as causative IgE triggers. A RAST test will identify IgE antibodies to specific foods in the serum. The **double-blind, placebo challenge–food challenge** is the current gold standard. Several foods are eliminated from the patient's diet for a period before testing. Then the foods are disguised and tested, alternating with placebos, over several days. A challenge is considered positive if signs and symptoms recur after ingestion. Such testing must be performed in a hospital setting, as anaphylaxis is a possible complication.

Treatment

Treatment entails eliminating the offending food from the diet. Patients and their caregivers should be educated in the use of an autoinjectable epinephrine pen. In children with severe, widespread allergies, elemental hypoallergenic formulas are available. Cow milk, soy, egg, and wheat allergies are usually outgrown after avoidance of the offending food. Oral challenges can be conducted safely to reintroduce the food. However, nut and fish allergies usually persist. Breastfeeding coupled with delay in the introduction of solid foods until after age 4 to 6 months may prevent the development of certain food allergies.

RHEUMATOLOGY

The modern concept of **rheumatic diseases** encompasses a large number of **autoimmune** and **autoinflammatory** conditions. In autoimmune disorders,

■ TABLE 11-3 Clinical Manifestations and Laboratory Findings of Rheumatic Disease

Sign/Symptom	Suggested Rheumatic Disease	Sign/Symptom	Suggested Rheumatic Disease
Dry eyes, dry mouth	Sjögren syndrome	Thrombocytosis	Systemic JIA
Oral/nasal ulcers	SLE	**Laboratory findings**	
	Wegener granulomatosis	Leukocytosis	Systemic JIA
	Behçet disease		Kawasaki disease
Chest pain/pleuritis	SLE	Markedly elevated ESR	Systemic JIA
	Systemic JIA		Kawasaki disease
Arthritis (joint swelling, morning stiffness)	JIA		Vasculitis
	SLE	Proteinuria/hematuria	SLE (lupus nephritis)
Muscle weakness	Juvenile dermatomyositis		Small-vessel vasculitis
Skin tightening/ thickening	Systemic sclerosis		Henoch-Schönlein purpura
	Linear scleroderma	Sterile pyuria	Kawasaki disease
Raynaud phenomenon	SLE	Elevated muscle-related enzymes	Juvenile dermatomyositis
	Systemic sclerosis		Juvenile polymyositis
Purpura	Henoch-Schönlein purpura	Antinuclear antibody (ANA)	SLE and related disorders (scleroderma, Sjögren syndrome)
	Small- and medium-vessel vasculitis		JIA (not systemic)
Malar rash	SLE	Anti-dsDNA, anti-Smith	SLE
	Juvenile dermatomyositis	Antiphospholipid antibodies	SLE
Gottron papules (extensor surface rash)	Juvenile dermatomyositis	Anti-ssDNA	Linear scleroderma
Nailfold capillary changes	SLE	Rheumatoid factor	Rheumatoid factor-positive polyarticular JIA
	Juvenile dermatomyositis	Low complement C3, C4	SLE
	Systemic sclerosis		
	Kawasaki disease		

JIA, juvenile idiopathic arthritis; SLE, systemic lupus erythematosus.

autoantibodies and self-reactive T-cells result in loss of self-tolerance, leading to inflammation and target organ damage. As a group, autoimmune disorders are not uncommon in pediatrics; examples include most juvenile idiopathic arthritis (JIA), systemic lupus erythematosus (SLE), and juvenile dermatomyositis (JDM). In contrast, autoinflammatory disease develops when the innate immune system is stimulated, often due to genetic predisposition. Most are quite rare, with the exceptions of systemic JIA and Crohn disease. Some rheumatic diseases are chronic (SLE, rheumatoid arthritis); others are self-limited (HSP, Kawasaki disease, acute rheumatic fever). The manifestations of rheumatic disease in childhood are protean, and typical presenting signs and symptoms are often seen in nonrheumatic conditions as well. Particularly common are constitutional symptoms such as malaise, fatigue, or fever. Clinical manifestations and laboratory abnormalities associated with specific disorders are noted in Table 11-3.

JUVENILE IDIOPATHIC ARTHRITIS

Pathogenesis

Juvenile idiopathic arthritis (JIA) is an umbrella term for the classification of chronic arthritis (>6 weeks) occurring in individuals under 16 years of age. Other causes of arthritis must be excluded before the diagnosis of JIA can be applied. In the past, childhood arthritis was called "juvenile rheumatoid arthritis" and classified according to slightly different criteria. The etiology of JIA is unclear, but genetic and environmental factors are likely both involved. Certain human leukocyte antigen (HLA) types are associated with increased risk of disease. The underlying pathophysiology in most forms of chronic inflammatory arthritis is **synovitis** (inflammation and hypertrophy of the synovium), a term that is often used interchangeably with *arthritis*.

Epidemiology

JIA has a prevalence of at least 1:1,000 children in the United States. The most common subtype is oligoarticular (~45%), followed by polyarticular (~25%), systemic (~10%), psoriatic (~5%) and enthesitis-related arthritis (~15%).

Clinical Manifestations

History and Physical Examination

Arthritis is defined as swelling within a joint, painful or limited movement, and/or joint tenderness. Morning stiffness is particularly common and typically lasts >30 minutes. Any synovial joint can be affected; often overlooked is the temporomandibular joint. The presence of severe joint pain suggests an alternate diagnosis (infectious or reactive arthritis, mechanical disorders). JIA subtypes are classified by number and location of joints involved, physical findings, associated diseases or family history, and extra-articular manifestations (Table 11-4).

Oligoarticular JIA is the most common subtype. The typical patient is a young girl 2 to 4 years of age. Large joints (knee, ankle) are most commonly involved. Long-standing arthritis can result in contractures, muscle atrophy, and increased extremity growth in the affected limb (leading to limb length discrepancy). Up to 75% of patients have a positive

---

■ **TABLE 11-4** Clinical Manifestations of JIA

JIA Subtype	Joint Findings	Extra-articular Findings/Complications
Oligoarticular JIA	• Fewer than five joints involved • Most commonly involves knee, ankle, wrist	• Chronic anterior uveitis
Polyarticular JIA (rheumatoid factor-negative)	• Five or more joints involved	• Chronic anterior uveitis
Polyarticular JIA (rheumatoid factor-positive)	• Five or more joints involved • Most commonly distal symmetric arthritis	• Rheumatoid nodules
Systemic JIA	• Can involve large and small joints	• Quotidian fevers • Intermittent rash • Hepatosplenomegaly • Lymphadenopathy • Serositis
Psoriatic JIA	• Large and small joint arthritis • Often dactylitis	• Psoriasis • Nail changes (pitting)
Enthesitis-associated JIA	• Sacroiliitis • Spondylitis • Lower extremity large joint arthritis • Enthesitis	• Enthesitis • Acute anterior uveitis* • Aortitis • Colitis

* In contrast to the chronic, nongranulomatous anterior uveitis seen in other forms of JIA, *acute anterior uveitis* manifests with eye redness, severe pain, and photophobia. Miosis and perilimbic conjunctival injection are present on ocular examination.

antinuclear antibody (ANA) test. The majority of patients with oligoarticular JIA experience remission after several years of active arthritis; late recurrences can occur.

Chronic, nongranulomatous anterior uveitis (iridocyclitis) is detected in up to a third of patients with oligoarticular JIA. A positive ANA test is associated with the development of this condition. Chronic anterior uveitis is typically asymptomatic but can be appreciated on slit lamp examination. Due to the risk of visual impairment and blindness, routine screening is indicated in JIA patients at risk for this complication.

Polyarticular JIA, the next most common subtype, and can be subdivided into rheumatoid factor (RF)+ and RF− disease. RF+ JIA resembles adult rheumatoid arthritis, with erosive, predominantly distal, symmetric small joint arthritis (wrist, hand, fingers), and rheumatoid nodules. RF+ JIA typically has its onset in adolescence and takes a chronic course. RF− JIA usually presents in early childhood, may have both have large and small joint involvement, and carries a better prognosis than RF+ disease.

In **systemic JIA**, extra-articular manifestations are prominent and often precede the onset of arthritis. Systemic JIA presents with intermittent high fevers that occur once or twice daily, with normal temperatures in the interval. The patient appears toxic and suffers from profound malaise during the fever episodes; a faint, evanescent, nonpruritic salmon-colored rash is often present as well. Hepatosplenomegaly, lymphadenopathy, and signs of serositis (pericarditis) may be noted on physical examination. The arthritis can involve both large and small joints and often is destructive. There is a marked acute phase reaction, including leukocytosis, thrombocytosis, anemia, elevated ESR and CRP, and (characteristically) very elevated ferritin. Neither ANA nor rheumatoid factor is present.

A common manifestation of **enthesitis-related arthritis** (ERA) is spondyloarthritis, i.e., inflammation of the axial skeleton (sacroiliac joints, small intervertebral joints) and the large weight-bearing joints of the lower extremities. In addition, *enthesitis* (inflammation and tenderness at the site of tendon insertion) is often present in the Achilles tendon, plantar fascia, patellar tendon insertion, and anterior superior iliac spines. ERA is associated with HLA-B27 and occurs predominantly in boys >6 years of age. Extra-articular manifestations include acute anterior uveitis, colitis, and/or aortitis.

Psoriatic arthritis is defined as arthritis in the setting of psoriasis (see Chapter 5) in the patient or a first-degree relative. Findings of psoriasis such as nail pitting or onycholysis may be quite subtle. Dactylitis, a typical finding in psoriatic arthritis, is due to flexor tendon tenosynovitis.

Differential Diagnosis

The differential diagnosis of JIA is extensive. Reactive or postinfectious arthritis (including acute rheumatic fever), other systemic inflammatory conditions (inflammatory bowel disease, connective tissue diseases, Henoch-Schönlein purpura), and infection (septic arthritis, viral arthritis, Lyme disease) can present with bona fide arthritis. Malignancy (leukemia, neuroblastoma, bone tumors), benign tumors, and musculoskeletal trauma may mimic arthritis.

Diagnostic Evaluation

Laboratory assessment is primarily used to supplement the clinical evaluation. Evidence of a mild acute phase reaction is typically present (excepting the impressive response in systemic JIA), but nonspecific. ANA is often present, as is rheumatoid factor, an autoantibody directed against a portion of the IgG molecule; however, these autoantibodies are invariably absent in systemic JIA and ERA. The presence of the HLA-B27 allele is useful for classification; however, it should not be considered a diagnostic test since it is present in 7% to 8% of the healthy population. Synovial fluid analysis yields a white blood cell count >2,000/mm^3 with predominantly mononuclear cells.

Treatment

Treatment consists of medical management, physical therapy, and rarely surgery. Single large joint arthritis is often best managed with intra-articular corticosteroid injection. When multiple inflamed joints are present, a disease-modifying drug (e.g., methotrexate) is frequently necessary. In recent years, more potent "biologic" therapies have been developed which target specific cytokines (anti-TNF-α, anti-IL-1) or immune cell interactions. Currently, only etanercept, a TNF-α antagonist, is approved for use in children.

Prognosis and Complications

The prognosis of JIA varies. Generally, the more joints involved in the first 6 months, the more likely the disease course will be chronic. Complications of arthritis include bony erosions, deformities, and growth disturbances (limb overgrowth, growth failure).

SYSTEMIC LUPUS ERYTHEMATOSUS

Pathogenesis

Systemic lupus erythematosus (SLE) is a chronic autoimmune disease characterized by widespread inflammation that can affect multiple organs. The pathophysiology is complex, but a predominant factor is the generation of multiple autoantibodies that cause immune-complex disease and antibody-mediated cellular cytotoxicity, with subsequent target organ injury. Autoantibodies are often directed against components of the cell nucleus (antinuclear antibodies). The etiology of SLE is multifactorial. Individuals with deficiencies of early complement components (C1q, C2, C4) are more prone to develop SLE.

Epidemiology

Pediatric SLE is usually diagnosed in late childhood or adolescence and is far more common in females. Asians, African Americans, and Hispanics have a higher incidence than Caucasians.

Differential Diagnosis

Given its ability to affect so many organ systems, SLE is considered a "great masquerader." Adding to diagnostic uncertainty is the fact that overlap conditions can result in a mixed clinical picture when the patient has features of two or more rheumatic diseases at the same time.

Clinical Manifestations

History and Physical Examination

The diagnosis of SLE is based on the American College of Rheumatology (ACR) classification criteria (Table 11-5). Fever, malaise, fatigue, and weight loss are very common. Mucocutaneous findings include painless oral ulcers, malar rash, discoid lupus, and photosensitivity. The arthritis in SLE is nonerosive but otherwise can mimic JIA. **Lupus nephritis** (LN), glomerulonephritis precipitated by immune-complex deposition, is one of the most severe organ manifestations of SLE and is often present at diagnosis. Renal involvement is described as class I (normal light microscopy), class II (mesangial proliferation), class III (focal proliferative), class IV (diffuse proliferative), or class V (membranous). Renal failure is most common in class IV LN. **CNS lupus** can present with psychosis, depression, confusion, or seizures.

■ **TABLE 11-5** Systemic Lupus Erythematosus: Classification Criteria

Four of the following must be present:
Malar rash
Discoid rash
Photosensitivity
Oral ulcers
Arthritis
Serositis
Renal disorder (hematuria, proteinuria)
Neurologic disorder
Hematologic disorder (anemia, leukopenia, thrombocytopenia)
Antinuclear antibody (ANA)
Immunologic disorder (anti-Smith, anti-dsDNA, antiphospholipid antibodies)

From American College of Rheumatology 1982, revised 1997.

Diagnostic Evaluation

Anemia, leukopenia (most commonly lymphopenia), and thrombocytopenia are characteristic. The ESR is elevated during a disease flare, but C-reactive protein is usually normal. A Coombs test is often positive. Complement levels, including C3, C4, and CH_{50}, are generally depressed or falling, especially during active disease. The ANA is virtually always positive, but this finding alone is insufficient for diagnosis. Antiphospholipid antibodies (including lupus anticoagulant and anticardiolipin antibodies) are associated with an increased risk of arterial and venous thromboses and Libman-Sacks endocarditis. More specific autoantibodies against nuclear components include anti-Smith (Sm), anti-double-stranded DNA (dsDNA), anti-RNP, anti-Ro, and anti-La antibodies. Elevation in anti-dsDNA is associated with renal involvement. Anti-Sm is very specific for lupus, but only is present in a third of affected patients. Circulating anti-Ro and anti-La antibodies in an SLE-affected mother may cause congenital heart block in her fetus.

Treatment

Although SLE has historically been associated with high morbidity and mortality, prognosis and quality of life are improving. With appropriate therapy, a majority of patients have good long-term survival and normal function. Treatment depends on which organ systems are involved. General considerations include avoidance of sun exposure and use of sunscreen; associated photosensitivity can trigger not only skin rashes but also systemic SLE flares. The antimalarial drug hydroxychloroquine is particularly helpful in treating mucocutaneous disease manifestations. Mild cases of SLE with predominantly musculoskeletal involvement are addressed with NSAIDs or disease-modifying drugs if necessary. Renal and CNS involvement requires more aggressive treatment. In severe cases, immunosuppressive therapy is necessary. Daily oral or intermittent intravenous pulse corticosteroid administration is often employed. In severe target organ disease, drugs such as cyclophosphamide, mycophenolate mofetil, or azathioprine may be necessary. In the future, biologic therapies (e.g., B-cell depletion) may offer additional benefits to patients with SLE.

DERMATOMYOSITIS

Pathogenesis

Juvenile dermatomyositis (JDM) is a multisystem autoimmune disease predominantly involving skin and skeletal muscles. The gastrointestinal tract is less commonly involved. The primary disease process occurs in the small blood vessels (vasculopathy) and is humorally mediated. Immune complex deposition, complement activation, and infiltration with CD4 lymphocytes in the musculature lead to subsequent capillary and muscle injury. The etiology of JDM is unclear but likely includes genetic and environmental factors. HLA B8/DR3 and HLA DQalpha1*0501 are associated with higher risk for disease. The condition seems to be associated with viral illnesses in some cases.

Epidemiology

JDM is rare (annual incidence ~3/1,000,000). Girls are affected more commonly than boys, with age at presentation typically between 5 and 10 years.

Differential Diagnosis

Polymyositis, an inflammatory muscular condition without skin findings, has a similar clinical presentation but is less common in children. The pathologic features are distinct from those of JDM; in polymyositis, CD8 lymphocytes infiltrate the muscle fascicles and attack muscle fibers directly.

Clinical Manifestations

History and Physical Examination

Since it predominantly affects the limb girdle musculature, JDM produces characteristic proximal muscle weakness with relative sparing of distal strength. Activities such as climbing stairs, doing sit-ups, and lifting the hands over the head become difficult. Patients often report a history of malaise, fatigue, weight loss, and intermittent fevers. The muscle weakness is accompanied by the pathognomonic **violaceous** dermatitis of the eyelids (heliotrope), hands, elbows, knees, and ankles. **Gottron papules** are characteristic lesions resembling scaly erythematous papules on the extensor surfaces of the metacarpophalangeal and interphalangeal joints of the fingers, the elbows, and the knees. Nailfold capillary changes are common. The weakness may advance to involve bulbar muscle groups used for swallowing and phonation. Long-standing inflammation eventually may result in calcium deposits in the skin and muscle (calcinosis cutis), scarring, and significant muscle atrophy.

Diagnostic Evaluation

The most striking laboratory abnormality is marked elevation of **serum creatine phosphokinase,** an enzyme released during muscle breakdown (as well as other muscle enzymes such as aldolase, aspartate aminotransferase, and lactic dehydrogenase). Von Willebrand factor is typically elevated, presumably secondary to active endothelial inflammation. MRI permits good visualization of muscle inflammation; electromyography is less frequently employed. Definitive diagnosis rests on characteristic muscle biopsy findings, including perivascular inflammatory infiltrate, perifascicular atrophy, loss of capillaries, focal necrosis, and muscle fiber regeneration.

Treatment

Treatment consists of pharmacologic management and physical therapy. The major component of the medical regimen is corticosteroid therapy, either in the form of daily oral prednisone or intermittent pulse (high-dose) methylprednisolone therapy. Corticosteroid-sparing agents such as methotrexate are often given from the onset of treatment. Important second-line agents include intravenous immunoglobulin (IVIG) and cyclosporine. Hydroxychloroquine is thought to be effective in treating the cutaneous manifestations of JDM. Physical therapy is essential and should be tailored to the individual patient based on disease activity and course.

Prognosis

Patients with a limited (monocyclic) disease course generally have a good long-term outcome; those with a more chronic course may suffer from significant disability. Spontaneous perforation of the bowel, although rare, is the leading cause of death.

OTHER CONNECTIVE TISSUE DISORDERS

Other connective tissue disorders are quite rare in childhood. Presentations are similar, and clinical differentiation may be difficult.

Systemic sclerosis is characterized by fibrous thickening of the skin (scleroderma), particularly involving the distal extremities and face, and fibrotic disease of internal organs (i.e., esophagus, intestinal tract, heart, lungs, kidneys). Early clinical findings include *Raynaud phenomenon*, the triphasic discoloration of the fingers and toes from white (ischemia) to purple (cyanosis) to red (reactive hyperemia), and *hand and foot edema*, which later progresses to frank sclerodactyly. Mortality risk is related to degree of cardiopulmonary involvement (pulmonary fibrosis), pulmonary arterial hypertension, and renal disease (systemic hypertension).

Linear scleroderma and **morphea** are characterized by discrete areas of linear streaks (linear scleroderma) or patchy lesions (morphea). The affected skin initially appears erythematous, later becoming indurated, with thickening and hardening of the skin and underlying soft tissues. Internal organ disease is very rare. Disability can result if the sclerodermatous lesions occur over joints, involve the face, or are large enough to restrict growth.

Sjögren syndrome is characterized by the lymphocytic infiltration of exocrine glands, most commonly the salivary and lacrimal glands, resulting in dry mouth (*xerostomia*) and dry eyes (*xerophthalmia*). Affected individuals may develop chewing and swallowing difficulties and are at risk for severe dental caries. Anti-Ro (SS-A) and anti-La (SS-B) antibodies are often detected. Secondary Sjögren syndrome may be a consequence of other connective tissue diseases.

PRIMARY SYSTEMIC VASCULITIS

Vasculitis is an inflammatory process of the vessel wall. A number of primary disorders, including Henoch-Schönlein purpura and Kawasaki disease, present with vasculitis as the primary manifestation. In **Henoch-Schönlein purpura** (HSP), IgA-containing immune complexes are found within vessel walls. The annual incidence of HSP is approximately 1:5,000, but is as high as 1:1,400 in children ages 4 to 6 years. HSP is somewhat more common in boys. **Kawasaki disease** occurs in about 1:10,000 children annually in the United States, is more common in boys, and has a peak age of onset between 2 and 3 years of age.

Clinical Manifestations and Treatment

HSP typically presents with symptoms of skin, joint, gastrointestinal, and kidney disease. Incidence peaks in the winter months, and the condition is often preceded by an upper respiratory infection (most commonly group A *Streptococcus*). The classic rash consists of nonthrombocytopenic purpura localized to dependent areas of the body (lower extremities, buttocks). Distribution of the rash may be atypical (primarily facial) in children less than 2 years of age. Other common findings, particularly early in the disease, consist of scrotal edema and extremity swelling. When present, acute arthritis may be exquisitely painful, even rendering a child immobile. Gastrointestinal involvement is usually significant, including colicky abdominal pain, vomiting, and upper and lower tract bleeding. Bowel wall thickening and intussusception can occur. Glomerulonephritis is present in up to 40% of patients. It is usually mild; however, up to 5% of children with HSP-associated glomerulonephritis will develop end-stage renal disease. Demonstration of IgA deposition in the vessel wall by direct immunofluorescence is pathognomonic. HSP usually requires only supportive treatment. Spontaneous resolution occurs in the majority of patients in less than 4 weeks, although symptoms may persist for up to 12 weeks. Musculoskeletal pain responds to treatment with NSAIDs. Systemic glucocorticoids are reserved for severe gastrointestinal manifestations and significant renal involvement (which may require cyclophosphamide). Fifteen percent of patients experience recurrence of their disease.

The diagnosis of Kawasaki disease rests on the presence of guidelines established by the American Heart Association in 2004 (Table 11-6). The sequential (rather than simultaneous) appearance of disease manifestations may initially result in misdiagnosis. The disease progresses in phases. During the *acute phase* (first 1 to 2 weeks), the typical diagnostic features accompanied by extreme irritability. Characteristic laboratory findings include leukocytosis, significantly elevated erythrocyte sedimentation rate and C-reactive protein, elevated liver transaminases, and sterile pyuria. Defervescence marks transition to the *subacute phase*, lasting several weeks. Clinical findings subside, but significant thrombocytosis carries a high risk for the development of coronary artery aneurysms; about 25% of untreated patients develop this complication. Aneurysms constitute the most significant cause of morbidity and mortality due to rupture or thrombosis. Current treatment recommendations consist of IVIG (2 g/kg) and high-dose aspirin therapy (80 to 100 mg/kg/day) in four divided doses during the acute stage, followed by low-dose aspirin therapy (3 to 5 mg/kg/day) until the end of the *convalescent phase* (several months later). IVIG typically results in rapid and profound improvement, and administration significantly reduces the risk of formation of coronary artery aneurysms. Repeated IVIG treatment may become necessary if fevers recur or persist. Second-line treatment regimens incorporate high-dose corticosteroids and possibly TNF inhibitors (infliximab), although the latter remain experimental. Anticoagulant therapy may be indicated in patients with documented coronary aneurysms.

■ TABLE 11-6 Clinical Criteria for Diagnosis of Kawasaki Disease

Fever persisting for 5 days or more, together with four of the following clinical criteria (by history or physical examination):

1. Changes in extremities
   - Acute (erythema of palms/soles, swelling of hands/feet)
   - Chronic (periungual peeling of fingers/toes)
2. Polymorphous exanthem
3. Bilateral bulbar conjunctival injection
4. Changes on lips and/or oral cavity (erythema, cracked lips, diffuse injection of oral mucosa)
5. Cervical lymphadenopathy >1.5 cm (usually unilateral)

 KEY POINTS

- Humoral immunodeficiency predisposes patients to infection with encapsulated organisms. Common infections include otitis media, pneumonia, and sinusitis. Quantitative immunoglobulin studies and antibody titers against vaccine antigens are abnormal in patients with humoral immune dysfunction. Gammaglobulin therapy (intravenous or intramuscular) provides antibodies to patients with humoral immunodeficiency.

- Patients with cell-mediated immune dysfunction are susceptible to autoimmune disorders, intracellular organisms, and opportunistic infections from organisms such as *Pneumocystis jiroveci*.

- Persistent hypocalcemic tetany and/or aortic arch anomalies coupled with absence of the thymic shadow and cell-mediated immunodeficiency suggest chromosome 22q11 deletion (i.e., DiGeorge) syndrome.

- Severe neutropenia, defined as an ANC $<0.5 \times 10^3/\mu L$, may result from infection, certain medications, circulating antineutrophil antibodies, malignancy, or bone marrow dysfunction. Typical signs of infection (erythema, warmth, swelling) are often absent in the presence of neutropenia.

- Chronic granulomatous disease is characterized by chronic or recurrent infections due to catalase-producing bacteria or fungi. In particular, patients develop frequent skin infections and abscesses. The nitroblue tertrazolium test and the dihydrorhodamine reduction (DHR) test are laboratory studies which are useful for detecting CGD. Patients with CGD should receive daily prophylactic trimethoprim-sulfamethaxazole and gamma-interferon.

- Allergic rhinitis may be seasonal or perennial. Nonsedating H_1-histamine blockers and nasal topical steroids are the mainstays of treatment. Peanuts, eggs, milk, soy, wheat, and fish account for the overwhelming majority of food allergies.

- Signs and symptoms of food allergy in infants include irritability, diarrhea, and failure to thrive.

- Juvenile idiopathic arthritis is characterized by chronic synovitis and classified by the number and location of joints involved, physical findings, associated diseases or family history, and extra-articular manifestations.

- SLE consists of widespread connective tissue inflammation and vasculitis. The diagnosis of SLE is clinical. Lupus nephritis is the most common clinical manifestation, resulting in significant morbidity. Typical laboratory findings include falling complement levels, a positive antinuclear antibody titer, and a positive double-stranded DNA antibody titer.

- Dermatomyositis is an inflammatory disease of the skin, striated muscle, and occasionally the gastrointestinal tract. Weakness begins in the proximal extremity muscle groups and is accompanied by a characteristic violaceous dermatitis. Serum creatine kinase levels are markedly elevated.

- Henoch-Schönlein purpura is characterized by abdominal pain, vomiting, gastrointestinal bleeding, and palpable, nonthrombocytopenic purpura over dependent regions.

- Kawasaki disease presents with high fever, lymphadenopathy, and mucocutaneous lesions. High-dose IVIG reduces the risk of coronary artery aneurysms in Kawasaki disease.

Infectious Disease

Rebecca C. Brady • David I. Bernstein • Katie S. Fine

Remarkable advances in the diagnosis, management, and prevention of infectious diseases have occurred during the past century. Specific treatment of bacterial illnesses began with the introduction of sulfonamides in the 1930s and penicillin in the 1940s. Newer classes of antibacterial agents include semisynthetic penicillins, tetracyclines, macrolides, fluoroquinolones, aminoglycosides, carbapenems, and four generations of cephalosporins. Antifungal, antiviral, and antiparasitic agents have also been developed. Other anti-infective agents include specific antibodies, intravenous immunoglobulin, phagocyte stimulating factors, and interferons. Vaccines have led to a dramatic decline in certain infectious diseases. Smallpox was eradicated worldwide in 1977, and indigenous poliomyelitis was eliminated from the United States in 1979. The annual incidence of measles, mumps, rubella, diphtheria, and *Haemophilus influenzae* type b meningitis has decreased by more than 98% because of vaccine use in the United States.

Unfortunately, new pathogens continue to emerge. Severe acute respiratory syndrome (SARS) appeared early in the new millennium, caused by a previously unknown coronavirus. Health organizations all over the world are concerned about the possibility of a bird flu mutation that would allow the disease to be spread among humans. Equally disconcerting is the rapid emergence of resistance to known antibiotics (e.g., methicillin-resistant *Staphylococcus aureus* and penicillin-resistant *Streptococcus pneumoniae*). Thus, after 100 years of progress against infectious diseases, the current challenges are every bit as formidable as at the beginning of the last century.

VACCINATIONS

ROUTINE IMMUNIZATIONS

Active immunization involves stimulating an individual's immune system to develop a rapid protective response that mimics that of natural infection but that usually presents little or no risk to the recipient. A vaccine contains all or part of either a weakened or nonviable form of the organism. Table 12-1 contains a simplified version of the current U.S. recommended immunization schedule for children ages 0 to 6 years. Periodically, the Centers for Disease Control and Prevention releases additional vaccine recommendations which can be accessed at http://www.cdc.gov/vaccines/recs/acip/default.htm.

Recently, vaccinations have been added to the recommended immunization schedule for adolescents. The tetanus and diphtheria toxoids and acellular pertussis vaccine (Tdap) is recommended for administration starting at age 11 to 12 years for those who have completed the recommended childhood DTaP vaccination series and have not received a tetanus and diphtheria toxoids (Td) booster dose. The meningococcal conjugate vaccine may be administered to adolescents age 11 to 12 years and previously unvaccinated adolescents at high school entry (approximately 15 years of age). It is also recommended for previously unvaccinated college freshman living in dormitories. A human papillomavirus (HPV) vaccine is licensed for administration to females 9 to 26 years of age as a three-dose series over 6 months.

■ TABLE 12-1 Childhood Immunization Schedule (0 to 6 Years of Age)

Age	Immunizations						
	Hepatitis vaccines					*Live viral vaccines*	
Birth to 2 mo	HBV (1)[c]						
2 mo	HBV (2)	DTaP (1)	Hib (1)	IPV (1)	PCV (1)		Rota (1)
4 mo		DTaP (2)	Hib (2)	IPV (2)	PCV (2)		Rota (2)
6 mo[a]		DTaP (3)	Hib (3)		PCV (3)		Rota (3)
6 to 18 mo	HBV (3)			IPV (3)			
12 to 15 mo			Hib (4)		PCV (4)	MMR (1) Varicella (1)	
>12 mo	HAV (1)						
15 to 18 mo		DTaP (4)					
18 to 23 mo	HAV (2)[d]						
4 to 6 yr		DTaP (5)[b]		IPV (4)		MMR (2) Varicella (2)	

The numbers in parentheses indicate the number in the sequence of immunizations. DTaP, diphtheria, tetanus, and acellular pertussis vaccine; HBV, hepatitis B virus vaccine; HAV, hepatitis A virus vaccine; Hib, *Haemophilus influenzae* type b vaccine; IPV, inactivated polio virus vaccine; MMR, measles, mumps, rubella vaccine; PCV, conjugated seven-valent pneumococcal vaccine; and Rota, rotavirus vaccine.
[a]Influenza vaccine also is recommended annually for all children aged 6 months to 59 months and for all children ≥59 months with chronic pulmonary, cardiovascular, metabolic, sickle cell, or HIV disease. The trivalent inactivated influenza vaccine (TIV) is licensed for use in children 6 months of age and older. The live attenuated influenza vaccine (LAIV) is only licensed for use in healthy children 24 months of age and older.
[b]Tetanus-diphtheria vaccine (either as Td or Tdap) is given at age 11 years and then every 10 years thereafter.
[c]Children who were not vaccinated against hepatitis B in infancy should receive 3 doses of the vaccine.
[d]The two doses in the HAV vaccine series should be administered at least 6 months apart.

Despite their long history of safe use and impressive cost-to-benefit ratio, vaccines should be held or delayed in certain circumstances. Table 12-2 lists absolute and relative contraindications to vaccine administration and some common misconceptions.

ADDITIONAL VACCINATIONS

Children with congenital, iatrogenic, or functional (e.g., sickle cell anemia) asplenia should receive the polysaccharide pneumococcal and polysaccharide meningococcal vaccines at 2 years of age. A yearly influenza vaccine is recommended for children over 59 months of age who have certain chronic diseases (including asthma, diabetes mellitus, HIV, cystic fibrosis, sickle cell anemia, and cardiac conditions) or are receiving immunosuppressive therapy.

FEVER OF UNKNOWN ORIGIN

The phrase *fever of unknown origin* (FUO) implies fever of prolonged duration (≥14 days), documented temperature greater than 38.3°C (101°F) on multiple occasions, and uncertain etiology.

DIFFERENTIAL DIAGNOSIS

FUO in the pediatric population is usually a common disorder presenting in an uncommon manner. Overall, infectious etiologies are more common than rheumatologic ones, which are more common than oncologic illnesses as a source for FUO. Diagnostic considerations include the following:

- **Infection:** Sinusitis, hepatitis, cytomegalovirus (CMV), Epstein-Barr virus (EBV), parasites, cat-scratch disease, Rocky Mountain spotted fever, endocarditis, septic arthritis, osteomyelitis, intraabdominal abscess, enteric fever, tuberculosis, HIV, opportunistic infection
- **Connective tissue disease:** Systemic juvenile idiopathic arthritis, systemic lupus erythematosus
- **Malignancy:** Leukemia, lymphoma, neuroblastoma

■ TABLE 12-2 Absolute and Relative Contraindications Regarding Vaccination

Absolute Contraindications	Precautions (Relative Contraindications)	Not Contraindications
Severe allergic reaction (e.g., anaphylaxis) after a previous vaccine dose	Shock/hyporesponsive episode ≤48 hours after previous dose of DTaP*	Mild illness with or without low-grade fever
Known severe immune deficiency (MMR; varicella, rotavirus, and live attenuated influenza vaccine)	Fever ≥40.5°C (104.8°F) within 48 hours of previous dose of DTaP*	Current antibiotic
Encephalopathy within 7 days of administration of the previous dose (DTaP)*	Seizure ≤3 days after previous dose of DTaP*	Positive tuberculin skin test
Pregnancy (MMR; varicella)	Moderate to severe acute illness with or without fever	Prematurity[a]

*Applies to DTaP only.
[a]Premature infants should be vaccinated according to chronologic age. Hepatitis B vaccine may be delayed until up to 30 days of age if the infant weighs less than 2,000 g at birth and the mother is HBsAg negative.
DTaP, diphtheria, tetanus, and acellular pertussis vaccine; HBsAg, hepatitis B surface antigen; MMR, measles, mumps, rubella vaccine.

- **Other:** Inflammatory bowel disease, Kawasaki disease, drug fever, thyrotoxicosis, sarcoidosis, and factitious fever

CLINICAL MANIFESTATIONS

History

The age and gender of the patient narrow the differential diagnosis. Inflammatory bowel disease and connective tissue disorders are uncommon in younger children. Autoimmune disorders occur more frequently in girls. Sexual history, travel history, current medications, exposure to animals, tick bites, antecedent illness, trauma, associated symptoms, and family history are important areas of inquiry. Different fever patterns (constant, recurrent, cyclical) occasionally suggest particular diagnoses. A thorough history and physical examination (usually after repeated encounters) will reveal the diagnosis in more than half of the children in whom a cause of the fever is found.

Physical Examination

Conjunctivitis, lymphadenopathy, joint tenderness, oral ulcers, thrush, heart murmurs, organomegaly, masses, abdominal tenderness, cutaneous manifestations (rash, hyperpigmentation, etc.), joint findings, and mental status changes may suggest a specific cause and guide further evaluation.

DIAGNOSTIC EVALUATION

The initial evaluation can be performed in the outpatient setting in older, well-appearing children. Neonates and ill-appearing children require hospitalization.

Screening laboratory tests include CBC and differential, serum electrolytes, BUN and creatinine levels, LFTs, alkaline phosphatase, and UA. Bacterial cultures should be obtained from specimens of blood, urine, stool, and possibly cerebrospinal fluid (CSF). Additional tests to consider include ESR, C-reactive protein, and specific serologic tests such as antibody studies for cat-scratch disease and EBV. A chest radiograph and skin testing for tuberculosis are often performed. More expensive and invasive studies may be warranted based on screening results. Usually, children recover without sequelae even if no etiology is determined.

BACTEREMIA AND SEPSIS

Bacteremia is the presence of bacteria in the blood. Bacteremia is further described as **occult** if it occurs in a well-appearing child without any obvious source of infection. From studies in the 1990s, the risk of occult bacteremia was highest (1.5% to 2.5%) in children between 2 and 24 months of age with a fever greater than 39.0°C and leukocytosis. Most episodes were caused by *Streptococcus pneumoniae* and resolved spontaneously. Rarely, localized infection (e.g., meningitis, pneumonia) occurred. Since 2000, when the conjugated seven-valent pneumococcal vaccine was recommended for routine use in infants, the incidence of all invasive pneumococcal infections has decreased by 80% for children younger than 24 months of age.

In contrast, **sepsis** implies bacteremia with evidence of a systemic response (tachypnea, tachycardia, etc.) and altered organ perfusion. Affected children appear quite toxic and may develop shock. The cause of sepsis varies by age. In neonates, group B streptococci, enteric gram-negative bacilli, and *Listeria monocytogenes* are most prevalent. In older children up to 5 years of age, *S. pneumoniae* predominates, followed by *Neisseria meningitidis*. *Staphylococcus aureus* is a common pathogen in children ≥5 years of age. Less common causes include *Salmonella* species, *Pseudomonas aeruginosa*, and viridans streptococci.

The evaluation of the child with suspected sepsis includes cultures from the blood, urine, and CSF (if meningitis is a concern). A chest radiograph is obtained if respiratory signs or symptoms are present. Initial empiric antimicrobial therapy is selected based on the age of the child, the likely etiologic agents, and any identified foci of infection.

ACUTE OTITIS MEDIA

Pathogenesis

Suspected or confirmed acute infection of the middle ear accounts for more physician visits than any other pediatric illness. The middle ear is normally sterile; a patent but collapsible eustachian tube allows fluid drainage from the middle ear into the nasopharynx but normally prevents the retrograde entry of upper respiratory flora. In children, the angle of entry, short length, and decreased tone of the tube (eustachian tube dysfunction) increase susceptibility to infection. When the eustachian tube is further narrowed by edema from a concurrent viral upper respiratory infection (URI), a relative vacuum is created, drawing secretions (and bacteria) from the nasopharynx into the middle ear.

Epidemiology

Acute otitis media (AOM) is most common in children 6 to 24 months of age. By 2 years of age, 90% of all children in the United States have had at least one episode of otitis media (OM), and 50% have had at least three episodes. Viruses (respiratory syncytial virus, parainfluenza virus, and influenza viruses) are a common cause of AOM, which may be complicated by bacterial superinfection. Common bacterial causes include *S. pneumoniae* (40%), nontypeable *Haemophilus influenzae* (25%), and *Moraxella catarrhalis* (10%). Unfortunately, approximately 50% of *S. pneumoniae* isolates are resistant to penicillin, and many species of *H. influenzae* and *M. catarrhalis* exhibit beta-lactamase activity.

Risk Factors

Caretaker smoking, bottle feeding, day-care attendance, allergic disease, craniofacial anomalies, immunodeficiency, genetic tendencies, and pacifier use all predispose children to AOM.

Clinical Manifestations

History and Physical Examination

Children may have local or systemic complaints or both, including ear pain, fever, and fussiness. AOM is frequently preceded by symptoms of URI (cough, rhinorrhea, congestion). On physical examination, the affected tympanic membrane appears bulging, opaque, and erythematous with an aberrant light reflex. Pneumatic otoscopy reveals decreased tympanic membrane mobility. The diagnosis of AOM should only be made when there is an acute history of symptoms and a bulging, poorly or nonmobile tympanic membrane is noted in the presence of signs of local or systemic inflammation.

Differential Diagnosis

Otitis media with effusion (OME) is diagnosed when there is apparent fluid behind the tympanic membrane (reduced mobility on pneumatic otoscopy) but no evidence of inflammation (tympanic membrane translucent/gray, no fever, no evidence of ear pain). **Myringitis** is inflammation of the eardrum accompanied by normal mobility. This condition often accompanies a viral URI. **Otitis externa** (inflammation of the external ear canal) also causes ear pain; however, the tympanic membranes should appear normal on physical examination. The pain of otitis externa is exacerbated by manipulation of the external ear. A tympanic membrane that is erythematous without any other signs of disease may be caused by vigorous crying and should not be considered AOM.

Treatment

Because more antibiotics are prescribed for AOM than any other pediatric condition, and because antibiotic resistance is a growing concern, the Centers for Disease Control has issued consensus recommendations relating to the treatment of AOM. Patients younger than 24 months of age, patients thought to be at risk for poor follow-up, ill-appearing patients, and any patients with chronic illnesses (including immunodeficiencies) or recurrent, severe, or perforated AOM should be prescribed antibiotics. High-dose amoxicillin is the recommended first-line treatment. Patients who have been treated with antibiotics within the last month and those who have not improved within 48 hours are eligible for second-line therapy with amoxicillin/clavulanic acid, an oral second- or third-generation cephalosporin, or IM ceftriaxone. Children older than 24 months with less severe disease may be offered the choice of immediate antibiotic therapy versus pain control and watchful waiting. Those children who initially have antibiotics withheld should receive a prescription to fill 48 hours later if there has been no improvement. Patients with perforated tympanic membranes in addition to AOM should receive oral (and possibly topical) antibiotics at initial diagnosis. Most spontaneous perforations caused by AOM resolve within 24 to 72 hours.

The most common complication of AOM is OME, which follows virtually all cases of AOM and takes a variable amount of time to resolve. Children with OME that persists longer than 3 months should be referred for possible tympanostomy tube placement. Chronic OME increases the risk of delay of language acquisition and hearing loss. Tympanostomy tubes should also be considered for patients with at least 4 episodes of AOM within 6 months or 5 episodes within 12 months. Complications of frequent episodes of AOM include excessive scarring (tympanosclerosis), cholesteatoma formation, and chronic suppurative AOM.

Mastoiditis (infection of the mastoid bone of the skull) is a potentially severe but uncommon complication of AOM characterized clinically by high fever, tenderness of the mastoid bone, and anterior displacement of the external ear. Mastoiditis is treated with intravenous antibiotics; surgical drainage may also be required.

SINUSITIS

The maxillary and ethmoid sinuses are present at birth; the sphenoid and frontal sinuses develop later in childhood. The spectrum of pathogens responsible for sinusitis is virtually identical to that for OM. Sinusitis is often difficult to diagnose in a young child because the classic symptoms of headache, facial pain, and sinus tenderness may be absent or difficult to articulate. Acute bacterial sinusitis has two common clinical presentations: (a) persistent respiratory symptoms (>10 to 14 days) without improvement, including either nasal discharge (clear or purulent) or a daytime cough, and (b) severe symptoms including high fever and purulent nasal discharge for at least 3 days. The differential diagnosis includes viral URIs, allergic rhinitis, and nasal foreign body. Sinusitis is primarily a clinical diagnosis. Radiologic studies of the sinuses may be useful in older children when there is a poor response to therapy and the diagnosis is in doubt. Sinus aspiration may be needed for recurrent or recalcitrant disease. Antibiotic coverage is similar to that for OM, although treatment should continue longer (14 to 21 days). Complications are uncommon but include bony erosion, orbital cellulitis, and intracranial extension. Children with recurrent or chronic sinusitis should be evaluated for cystic fibrosis, ciliary dyskinesia, or primary immune deficiency.

HERPANGINA

Herpangina is a symptom complex caused by enteroviruses (including groups A and B coxsackieviruses and other enterovirus serotypes). It is typically diagnosed during the summer and fall in younger children. Initially, the patient develops a high fever and very sore throat. On examination, characteristic vesicular lesions that progress to ulcers are scattered over the soft palate, tonsils, and pharynx. Primary herpetic gingivostomatitis (caused by herpes simplex virus [HSV]) presents in a similar manner, although the lesions are generally more widespread over the gums, lips, and mucosa. Herpangina is self-limited (5 to 7 days) and requires no specific therapy. When similar lesions are noted on the palms and soles (and occasionally on the buttocks), the more inclusive name **hand-foot-and-mouth disease** is used.

STREPTOCOCCAL PHARYNGITIS

Pathogenesis

Group A beta-hemolytic streptococci (group A *Streptococcus* [GAS]; *Streptococcus pyogenes*) are the most important cause of bacterial infection of the throat. Antimicrobial therapy for streptococcal disease is recommended because of the frequency of **suppurative (peritonsillar abscess, retropharyngeal abscess)** and **nonsuppurative (rheumatic fever, post-streptococcal glomerulonephritis)** complications.

Epidemiology

Strep throat most commonly afflicts school-aged children and adolescents. The organism is spread person to person through infected oral secretions. At any one point in time, approximately 10% to 15% of well children carry GAS as part of their normal oral flora.

Clinical Manifestations

History and Physical Examination

Classic symptoms include sore throat, fever, headache, malaise, nausea, and occasionally abdominal pain. Physical examination reveals enlarged, erythematous, exudative tonsils, and tender anterior cervical lymphadenopathy. Petechiae may be present on the soft palate. Rhinorrhea, hoarseness, and coughing, the hallmarks of viral URIs, are notably absent. The diagnosis of **scarlet fever** is made when a characteristic erythematous, "sandpaper-like" rash accompanies the fever and pharyngitis. The rash commonly begins on the neck, axillae, and groin, spreads to the extremities, and may desquamate 10 to 14 days later.

Differential Diagnosis

Differentiating viral pharyngitis and infectious mononucleosis from streptococcal pharyngitis may be impossible based on clinical symptoms; definitive diagnosis requires either throat culture or antigen detection test for GAS.

Diagnostic Evaluation

Therapeutic decisions should be based on throat culture or rapid antigen detection test results. The specificity of most rapid antigen tests is greater than 95% (compared with throat culture), so false-positive test results are rare. The sensitivity of rapid antigen tests is more variable and is highly dependent on the quality of the throat swab specimen. Therefore, a negative rapid antigen test should be confirmed by a throat culture.

Treatment

Patients with documented group A streptococcal pharyngitis should receive a 10-day course of oral penicillin (or a single dose of IM benzathine penicillin G) to hasten symptom resolution, decrease transmissibility, and prevent acute rheumatic fever. A clinical isolate of GAS resistant to penicillin never has been documented. Erythromycin, azithromycin, and clindamycin are acceptable alternatives for children allergic to penicillin. The treatment of scarlet fever is identical to that for streptococcal pharyngitis.

Acute rheumatic fever (ARF) occurs about 3 weeks after streptococcal pharyngitis in a small percentage of untreated patients. ARF is an inflammatory condition involving connective tissues of the heart (carditis, valvular destruction), joints (migratory polyarthritis), and CNS (transient chorea). Diagnosis rests on fulfilling the Jones criteria (Table 12-3). Initially, fever, dyspnea, chest pain, cardiac

---

■ TABLE 12-3 Revised Jones Criteria for the Diagnosis of Acute Rheumatic Fever

Major Manifestations	Minor Manifestations	Supporting Evidence of Antecedent GAS Infection
Carditis	*Clinical*	Positive throat culture for GAS or
Polyarthritis	Fever	Positive rapid antigen test or
Sydenham chorea	Arthralgia	Increased streptococcal antibody titer*
Erythema marginatum		
Subcutaneous nodules	*Laboratory*	
	Elevated ESR or	
	C-reactive protein	
	Prolonged P-R interval on ECG	

Diagnosis of acute rheumatic fever requires two major or one major and two minor criteria plus supporting evidence of antecedent group A streptococcal infection.
*Antibody tests include antistreptolysin-O (ASO), anti-DNase B, antihyaluronidase, or antistreptokinase.

murmur, and arthritis predominate; long-term morbidity results from valvular destruction with consequent mitral or aortic valve insufficiency or stenosis. Acute episodes respond favorably to antibiotics, anti-inflammatory drugs, and cardiac management. ARF may recur after the initial episode; thus, individuals diagnosed with ARF should receive prophylactic penicillin therapy to prevent recurrent ARF.

Acute poststreptococcal glomerulonephritis may follow either group A streptococcal pharyngitis or skin infection (cellulitis) and is not prevented by timely antibiotic therapy. Clinical manifestations follow infection by approximately 10 days and include hematuria, edema, oliguria, and hypertension. Complement (C3) levels are low. Treatment consists of penicillin therapy and diuretics; steroids are rarely indicated. In contrast to affected adults, the majority of affected children recover without renal sequelae.

INFECTIOUS MONONUCLEOSIS

Pathogenesis

Infectious mononucleosis (IM) is a disease that occurs in older children and adolescents when they develop a primary EBV infection. Other pathogens, notably cytomegalovirus and *Toxoplasma gondii*, can result in a similar clinical picture.

Epidemiology

Transmission occurs by mucosal contact with infected saliva (hence the term "kissing disease") or genital fluids. A majority of people are infected with EBV and seroconvert in early childhood. Such early infections are generally asymptomatic or mild in immunocompetent hosts, although the mononucleosis syndrome can occur in younger children as well.

Clinical Manifestations

History and Physical Examination

The predominant symptom is usually a severe, exudative pharyngitis. Fever, generalized lymphadenopathy, and profound fatigue occur. Although the pharyngitis usually resolves within 1 to 2 weeks, the malaise may persist for several weeks. Other manifestations include hepatosplenomegaly, palatal petechiae, jaundice, and rash. Patients infected with EBV who are misdiagnosed with a bacterial infection and receive amoxicillin or ampicillin are much more likely to manifest the rash, which involves the face and trunk and is generally maculopapular.

Differential Diagnosis

Classic mononucleosis caused by EBV accounts for most cases. Other infectious agents that cause similar symptoms include CMV, *Toxoplasma gondii*, human herpesvirus 6, adenovirus, and HIV. Pharyngitis caused by GAS is difficult to distinguish from that of viruses without laboratory studies. Pancytopenia in the presence of the clinical manifestations listed previously suggests malignancy.

Diagnostic Evaluation

Leukocytosis or leukopenia may be present; lymphocytes account for more than 50% of leukocytes, and usually at least 10% are **atypical lymphocytes**. A heterophile antibody test allows rapid detection of EBV-associated mononucleosis in the outpatient setting; however, it has limited sensitivity in younger patients (<4 years of age) because they do not typically produce detectable heterophile antibodies. Specific serologic antibody testing is available for EBV (Fig. 12-1) and CMV. Other laboratory findings may include thrombocytopenia and elevated hepatic transaminase levels.

Treatment

The disorder is typically self-limited, requiring only supportive care. Activity restrictions (i.e., no contact sports) are advised until any associated splenomegaly resolves because of the possibility of splenic rupture.

Rare but serious complications include upper airway obstruction (treated with corticosteroids), splenic rupture, and meningoencephalitis. Immuno-compromised individuals are at risk for severe disseminated disease and lymphoproliferative disorders.

CROUP

Acute laryngotracheobronchitis, commonly called **croup**, refers to virus-induced inflammation of the laryngotracheal tissues, resulting in a syndrome of upper airway obstruction. Croup usually is caused by a parainfluenza virus but can also result from other viruses, such as influenza and respiratory syncytial virus (RSV). It is most pronounced in young children (6 to 36 months of age) because of the narrow caliber

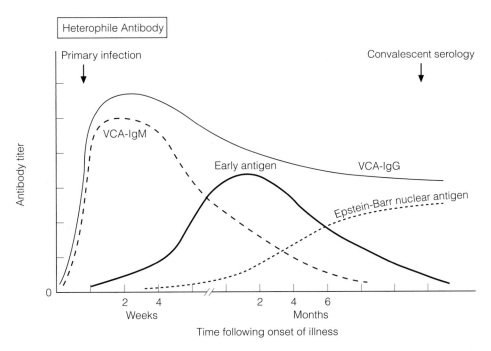

Figure 12-1 • Appearance of antibodies during EBV infection.

of the airway below the vocal cords (subglottic region). Incidence peaks during the late fall and winter. At its most severe, the disease progresses to partial or total airway obstruction.

Clinical Manifestations

History and Physical Examination

Children typically experience the sudden onset of a hoarse voice, barky (seal-like) cough, and inspiratory stridor, which may progress to respiratory distress. There is often a prodrome consisting of low-grade fever and rhinorrhea 12 to 24 hours prior to the onset of stridor. Respiratory compromise varies from minimal stridor with agitation to severe distress with tachypnea, hypoxia, nasal flaring, retractions, and impending airway obstruction.

Diagnostic Evaluation

The diagnosis usually is made on the basis of clinical findings. If obtained, anteroposterior neck and chest radiographs may reveal a tapered, narrow subglottic airway (steeple sign) (Fig. 12-2). However, this finding is present in less than 50% of cases and does not correlate with disease severity.

Differential Diagnosis

The differential diagnosis of upper airway obstruction (see Chapter 20) includes epiglottitis, bacterial tracheitis, foreign body aspiration, anaphylaxis, and angioneurotic edema. **Epiglottitis** consists of inflammation and edema of the epiglottis and aryepiglottic folds. It is considered a life-threatening emergency because of the propensity of the swollen tissues to result in sudden and irreversible airway occlusion. Most cases occur during the winter months in children 3 to 5 years of age. Fever, sore throat, hoarseness, and progressive stridor develop over 1 to 2 days. On examination, the child appears toxic, drools, and leans forward with chin extended to maximize airway patency. Lateral neck radiographs show "thumbprinting" of the epiglottis (Fig. 12-3). Although radiographs may aid in diagnosis, they are not recommended because they delay appropriate care. The child with suspected epiglottitis requires timely transport to the operating room and emergent endotracheal intubation. Emergency cricothyroidotomy may be performed if an endotracheal airway cannot be secured in the face of rapidly progressive obstruction. Intravenous ampicillin-sulbactam or a third-generation cephalosporin provides appropriate empirical coverage until the organism is identified by culture and sensitivities are known. The incidence of epiglottitis has decreased

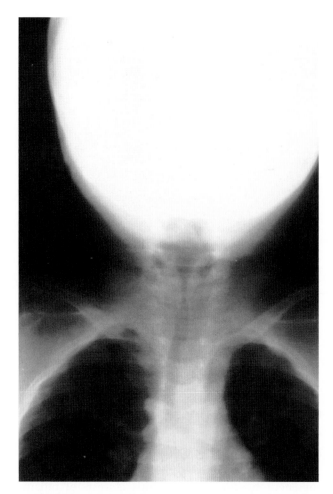

Figure 12-2 • Croup in a 3-year-old child. Note the "steeple sign" indicative of subglottic narrowing.

markedly since the advent of routine administration of the *Haemophilus influenzae* type b (Hib) vaccine in the late 1980s. Cases caused by *S. pneumoniae*, GAS, and *Staphylococcus aureus* are also reported. Failure to maintain current Hib shots is the biggest risk factor for developing epiglottitis.

Treatment

Most children with croup never become symptomatic enough to prompt a visit to the pediatrician. Cough and stridor respond well to cool night air or humidity, and the disease resolves over 4 to 7 days. In the emergency department, stridulous infants receive cool mist, nebulized racemic epinephrine, and oral, intravenous, or IM corticosteroids. Impending respiratory failure and airway obstruction constitute medical emergencies and are addressed accordingly (see Chapter 1).

BRONCHIOLITIS

Pathogenesis

Bronchiolitis is an acute viral lower respiratory tract infection that results in inflammatory obstruction of the peripheral airways. There is a predominantly lymphocytic infiltrate into the peribronchial and peribronchiolar epithelium that promotes submucosal edema. Intraluminal mucous plugs and cellular debris accumulate because of impaired mucociliary clearance.

Epidemiology

Respiratory syncytial virus (RSV) causes the majority of cases; parainfluenza, influenza, human metapneumovirus, and adenovirus are also responsible viruses. Bronchiolitis typically occurs between November and

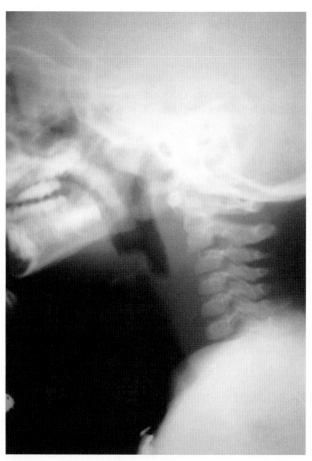

Figure 12-3 • Epiglottitis in a 4-year-old child with massive edema of the epiglottis, thickened aryepiglottic folds, and effacement of the valleculae.

April. At least half of all children are infected with RSV before 1 year of age, and recurrent infections throughout life are common. About 1% of young children with bronchiolitis require hospitalization.

Risk Factors

Children with chronic lung disease, congenital heart disease, and congenital or acquired immunodeficiencies are more susceptible to severe disease. Hospitalization rates peak between 2 and 5 months of age. Predictors of severe illness include a respiratory rate greater than 70 per minute, hypoxia, atelectasis on chest radiograph, and a history of preterm birth.

Clinical Manifestations

History

The acute illness lasts for 5 to 10 days, followed by gradual recovery over the next 1 to 2 weeks. Infected neonates may develop life-threatening **apnea**. Infants initially present with fever, cough, and rhinorrhea followed by progressive respiratory distress. Household contacts usually have upper respiratory symptoms.

Physical Examination

Physical findings include fever, tachypnea, and mild to severe respiratory distress. Wheezing, rhonchi, crackles, and accessory muscle use during respiration (tugging) may be noted. Ill infants may be restless or lethargic. Hypoxia is common in severely affected patients.

Differential Diagnosis

The wheezing associated with bronchiolitis may be difficult to distinguish from asthma or airway foreign body in older infants. Causes of recurrent episodes of wheezing include vascular rings, cystic fibrosis, and ciliary dyskinesia.

Diagnostic Evaluation

Rapid assays exist for RSV and influenza detection. Most respiratory viruses may be cultured from nasal secretions. Chest radiographs should be obtained for ill or hypoxic patients and for those with recurrent or unexplained wheezing. Findings consistent with bronchiolitis include lung hyperinflation, peribronchial thickening ("cuffing"), and increased interstitial markings.

Treatment

Hypoxic or ill-appearing children require hospitalization. Children with oxygen saturations greater than 94%, minimal respiratory distress, good fluid intake, reliable caretakers, and good follow-up may be treated as outpatients.

Most hospitalized infants require only supportive care (oxygen, fluid support) for their self-limited illness. Corticosteroids are not effective and are not indicated. Beta-adrenergic agents are not recommended for routine care of first-time wheezing associated with bronchiolitis. Nebulized ribavirin has antiviral activity against RSV but its use is not routinely recommended because it is expensive and does not decrease the duration of hospitalization.

RespiGam, an intravenous polyclonal immunoglobulin with high RSV antibody concentration, and **palivizumab**, an intramuscular RSV monoclonal antibody, provide passive prophylaxis and are recommended during the winter months for patients younger than 2 years of age who are at risk for severe disease (former premature infants and children with bronchopulmonary dysplasia who require oxygen). Palivizumab is currently preferred because it is easier to administer and is not a blood product.

The mortality rate for hospitalized patients is approximately 1%. Children with congenital heart defects, chronic lung disease, and immunodeficiency fare particularly poorly. Patients with documented RSV bronchiolitis may have more airway hyperresponsiveness later in life than the general population.

PERTUSSIS

Infection with *Bordetella pertussis* causes a URI and persistent cough in adults but may result in life-threatening respiratory disease in neonates and infants. The organism is spread via aerosolized droplets expelled during intense coughing. The agent is highly infective among unimmunized hosts. The vaccine is 95% effective against severe disease, but immunity wanes significantly within several years.

Clinical Manifestations

History and Physical Examination

Patients with pertussis are almost invariably afebrile. The classic presentation in young children is "whooping cough." The **catarrhal phase** follows a 7- to 10-day incubation period and consists of 1 to 2 weeks of low-grade fever, cough, and coryza. Then comes a 2- to 6-week **paroxysmal phase** characterized by intense spasms of coughing followed by sudden inhalation, which produces the characteristic whoop. Posttussive emesis is common. Facial petechiae and scleral hemorrhages often develop due to forceful coughing. Most symptoms remit during the **convalescent phase**, but the cough may persist for 2 to 8 weeks. Infants with severe disease may present with apnea or the typical paroxysmal cough followed by choking and progressive cyanosis. The characteristic whoop is absent in very young infants because they cannot generate sufficient negative inspiratory force.

Adolescents and adults can also be infected with pertussis and usually present with nonspecific upper respiratory symptoms and a protracted cough.

Diagnostic Evaluation

Laboratory evaluation usually reveals significant leukocytosis with a predominance of lymphocytes. Nasopharyngeal secretions contain the organism, which may be detected by fluorescent antibody staining, PCR, or culture. The chest radiograph usually is normal, but nonspecific infiltrates may be seen.

Treatment

Young infants with severe disease should be hospitalized to manage apnea, cyanosis, hypoxia, and feeding difficulties. Erythromycin estolate (and other macrolides) shortens the duration of illness *if given early in the catarrhal phase.* After the coughing paroxysms begin, antibiotics do not affect the course of illness but are recommended to decrease the period of infectivity. A 14-day course of erythromycin completely eradicates the organism from the nasopharynx and respiratory tract. Household and other close (daycare) contacts require chemoprophylaxis with erythromycin regardless of immunization status.

PNEUMONIA

Pathogenesis

Pneumonia refers to an acute inflammatory process occurring in the lungs. It may be infectious or noninfectious. Inflammation can occur in the alveolar space (lobar pneumonia), the alveolar walls (interstitial pneumonia), and/or the bronchi.

Epidemiology

The age of an immunocompetent child suggests an etiologic organism (Table 12-4). Viruses are the most common cause of pneumonia in young children. *Chlamydia trachomatis* pneumonia manifests at 2 to 3 months of age in infants born to women with untreated genital *C. trachomatis* infection. *S. pneumoniae* should be considered in any community-acquired lower respiratory tract infection. *Mycoplasma pneumoniae* pneumonia is uncommon in children younger than 5 years but, along with *Chlamydophila* (formerly *Chlamydia*) *pneumoniae*, becomes a more frequent and important pathogen in school-age children and adolescents. Less common bacterial causes include nontypeable *H. influenzae*, *M. catarrhalis*, *S. aureus*, *N. meningitidis*, and GAS.

Risk Factors

Conditions associated with an increased risk of bacterial pneumonia include the following:

- Chronic lung disease, including cystic fibrosis and asthma
- Neurologic impairment (swallowing dysfunction or neuromuscular disease)
- Gastroesophageal reflux with aspiration of gastric contents
- Upper airway anatomic defects (tracheoesophageal fistula, cleft palate)
- Hemoglobinopathies (including sickle cell anemia)
- Immunodeficiency or immunosuppressive therapy

Clinical Manifestations

History

Viral pneumonia develops gradually over 2 to 4 days. It is usually preceded by upper respiratory symptoms such as cough, rhinorrhea, postnasal drip, coryza, and low-grade fever. Infants with pneumonia caused by *C. trachomatis* are afebrile and have conjunctivitis and a staccato cough. Infants and young children with bacterial pneumonia may present with nonspecific constitutional complaints, including fever, irritability, poor feeding, vomiting, abdominal pain, and lethargy. Abrupt onset of fever, chills, dyspnea, and chest pain is typical. Productive cough is more common in older patients. *M. pneumoniae* and *C. pneumoniae* pneumonia present initially with fever, headache, and myalgia. These symptoms gradually subside over 5 to 7 days, whereas coughing increases and persists for 2 weeks or more.

TABLE 12-4 Causes of Infectious Pneumonia by Age

<1 Month	1 to 6 Months	6 Months to 5 Years	School Age/Adolescent
Group B streptococci	Streptococcus pneumoniae[a]	Streptococcus pneumoniae[a]	Mycoplasma pneumoniae
Escherichia coli/gram-negative enteric bacilli	Staphylococcus aureus	Moraxella catarrhalis	Chlamydophila pneumoniae
Haemophilus influenzae	Moraxella catarrhalis	Haemophilus influenzae	Streptococcus pneumoniae[a]
Streptococcus pneumoniae	H. influenzae	Staphylococcus aureus	H. influenzae
Group D streptococci	Bordetella pertussis	Neisseria meningitidis	S. aureus
Listeria monocytogenes	Chlamydia trachomatis[b]	Mycoplasma pneumoniae	Mycobacterium tuberculosis
Anaerobes	Ureaplasma urealyticum[b]	Group A streptococci	Viruses[c]
Cytomegalovirus	Cytomegalovirus[b]	Mycobacterium tuberculosis	
Herpes simplex virus	Viruses[c]	Viruses[c]	
Ureaplasma urealyticum			
Staphylococcus aureus			

[a]Most common cause of bacterial pneumonia in this age group.
[b]Although acquired perinatally, these infections often do not present as pneumonia until after 1 month of age.
[c]Including respiratory syncytial virus, influenza, parainfluenza, and adenovirus.

Physical Examination

Any indication of respiratory distress can signal pneumonia, although tachypnea and dyspnea are most common. Tachypnea out of proportion to fever is an important clue to pneumonia in the young child. Diffuse wheezing and crackles suggest involvement of multiple areas of the lung, characteristic of viral or atypical (M. pneumoniae, C. pneumoniae, C. trachomatis) pneumonia. Focal findings such as focal crackles or decreased breath sounds, dullness to percussion, egophony, and bronchophony suggest pneumonia of bacterial origin. Pneumonia can also present with only fever and tachypnea in the absence of chest findings.

Cyanosis is uncommon except in severe disease. Approximately 10% of patients with M. pneumoniae infection develop a rash, usually macular and erythematous or urticarial; erythema multiforme has also been reported.

Differential Diagnosis

Pneumonia is much more common in the pediatric population than are other conditions with similar presentations, including congestive heart failure (CHF), chemical pneumonitis, pulmonary embolism, sarcoidosis, and primary or metastatic malignancy.

Diagnostic Evaluation

A thorough history and physical examination usually suggest the diagnosis. Sputum culture is not likely to be helpful because pediatric patients typically do not produce adequate sputum samples. Chest radiograph remains an excellent test for defining the extent and pattern of involvement and assessing related complications (i.e., pleural effusion, pneumatocele). Bacterial pneumonia usually causes lobar consolidation. Diffuse interstitial infiltrates suggest viral or atypical pneumonia, although children with Mycoplasma pneumonia may have lobar consolidation. Aspiration pneumonia is typically located in the right middle or right upper lobe. C. trachomatis pneumonia is diagnosed by direct fluorescent antibody testing of conjunctival or nasopharyngeal specimens. M. pneumoniae can be noted by PCR of specimens obtained by nasopharyngeal swab or by specific antimycoplasmal IgM antibody determination. However, these IgM antibodies persist in serum for several months and may not represent current infection. Cold-agglutinin titers are elevated not only in *M. pneumoniae* infections but also in many cases of viral (and some cases of bacterial) pneumonia.

Treatment

Therapy depends on the most likely pathogen. In the outpatient setting, amoxicillin (high-dose) or amoxicillin/clavulanic acid is appropriate for most cases of bacterial pneumonia when antibiotics are thought to be necessary. Erythromycin, clarithromycin, or azithromycin is recommended for so-called walking pneumonia caused by *M. pneumoniae* or *C. pneumoniae*. Erythromycin or azithromycin is used to treat infants with pneumonia caused by *C. trachomatis*.

Any child with persistent hypoxia (which necessitates oxygen therapy), moderate to severe respiratory distress, and/or hemodynamic instability requires hospitalization. Intravenous antibiotic options for bacterial pneumonia include ampicillin/sulbactam, clindamycin, cefuroxime, ceftriaxone, azithromycin, and vancomycin depending on the suspected pathogens and community susceptibility patterns. Neonates with suspected bacterial pneumonia receive additional workup (lumbar puncture) and are started on ampicillin and cefotaxime (or gentamicin if the CSF is sterile). Most viral infections are self-limited. Patients with severe disease (bacterial or viral) may require supportive therapy and intubation.

The most frequent complication is development of a pleural effusion large enough to compromise respiratory effort. Although virtually any infectious agent can cause an effusion, large effusions are much more likely to result from *S. aureus*. Pleurocentesis (with possible chest tube placement) provides rapid relief. Empyema results when purulent fluid from an adjacent lung infection drains into the pleural space. Lung abscesses may complicate anaerobic infections.

MENINGITIS

Pathogenesis

Almost any pathogen can infect the leptomeninges and CSF. Viral meningitis is typically an acute, self-limited illness; bacterial meningitis is a life-threatening condition associated with substantial morbidity and mortality. The term **aseptic meningitis** refers to meningeal inflammation caused by an antigenic stimulus other than pyogenic bacteria (e.g., enterovirus or *Borrelia*).

Epidemiology

The likely etiology of meningitis depends on age (Table 12-5). Beyond the neonatal period, viral meningitis is much more common than bacterial meningitis. Both infants and older children are at risk for meningitis caused by enteroviruses (the most common cause of viral meningitis). Enteroviruses primarily circulate in the late summer and early fall. Overall, *S. pneumoniae* and *N. meningitidis* are the most common bacterial pathogens. Neonates and children younger than 3 years are at highest risk for bacterial meningitis. Hib vaccine has nearly eliminated *H. influenzae* type b meningitis in the United States. Lyme meningitis, caused by *Borrelia burgdorferi*, usually

■ **TABLE 12-5** Causes of Meningitis by Age			
<1 Month	**1 to 2 Months**	**2 Months to 6 Years**	**School Age/Adolescent**
Group B streptococci	*Escherichia coli*	*Streptococcus pneumoniae*	*S. pneumoniae*
Escherichia coli	*S. pneumoniae*	*Neisseria meningitidis*	*N. meningitidis*
Other gram-negative bacilli	Enteroviruses	Enteroviruses	Enteroviruses
Herpes simplex virus	*Haemophilus influenzae* type b[a]	*Borrelia burgdorferi*	*B. burgdorferi*
Listeria monocytogenes	Group B streptococci	*H. influenzae* type b[a]	
Streptococcus pneumoniae			
[a]Rare in immunized populations.			

affects school-age children and adolescents. Rare causes of meningitis and meningoencephalitis include EBV, *Bartonella henselae* (cat-scratch disease), *M. tuberculosis*, and *Cryptococcus neoformans*.

Risk Factors

Risk factors for bacterial meningitis are the same as those for sepsis, because most cases result from hematogenous seeding. Direct invasion occurs as a result of trauma, mastoiditis, sinusitis, and anatomic defects in the scalp or skull. In the neonate, low birth weight, prolonged rupture of membranes, and chorioamnionitis predispose to septicemia and meningitis; myelomeningocele also increases the risk.

Clinical Manifestations

History

Classic symptoms of meningitis include nausea, vomiting, photophobia, irritability, lethargy, headache, and stiff neck. Viral meningitis is preceded by a nonspecific prodrome of fever, malaise, sore throat, and myalgias. Unless complicated by encephalitis, symptoms of most viral CNS infections generally resolve over 2 to 4 days and may improve after LP. In bacterial meningitis, the prodromal phase is absent and the fever is generally quite high. Mental status changes, focal neurologic signs, ataxia, seizures, and shock are not uncommon. Lyme meningitis is characterized by low-grade fever, headache, stiff neck, and photophobia developing over the course of 1 to 2 weeks. Cranial nerve palsies may occur.

Physical Examination

Patients with bacterial meningitis often appear toxic and may be hypertensive, bradycardic, and even apneic. In older children, signs of increased intracranial pressure include cranial nerve palsies and papilledema. Nuchal rigidity and positive **Kernig** (flexion of the leg at the hip with subsequent pain on knee extension) and **Brudzinski** (involuntary leg flexion on passive neck flexion) **signs** are markers for meningeal irritation. These findings are rarely present in children younger than 1 year. Infants may present with a bulging fontanelle. A rash is often present with *N. meningitidis* (petechial or purpuric) and Lyme (erythema migrans) CNS infections.

Differential Diagnosis

The differential diagnosis includes encephalitis, which may develop concurrently or subsequently (see Chapter 15). Other conditions that may present with a similar clinical picture include drug intoxication or side effects, recent anoxia or hypoxia, primary or metastatic CNS malignancy, bacterial endocarditis with septic embolism, intracranial hemorrhage/hematoma, malignant hypertension, and demyelination disorders.

Diagnostic Evaluation

CSF analysis is diagnostic. Tests include cell counts and differential, Gram stain, glucose and protein levels, and culture. Bacteria are detected on Gram stain in approximately 80% of cases of bacterial meningitis. PCR assays for CSF HSV and enteroviruses are available and are highly sensitive and specific. Table 12-6 describes CSF findings that suggest a specific etiology. Because of the potential for brainstem herniation, LP should not be attempted in a child with focal neurologic deficits and/or increased intracranial pressure until an expanding mass lesion is excluded

---

■ TABLE 12-6 Cerebrospinal Fluid Findings Suggesting a Specific Etiology for Meningitis in Childhood

CSF Parameter	Bacterial	Viral	Lyme
White blood cells (per mm^3)	>1,000	<500	<100
Neutrophils	>75%	<50%[a]	<30%
Protein	↑↑	Normal or ↑	Normal or ↑
Glucose	↓ or ↓↓	Normal	Normal

[a]Neutrophils may predominate early in the course of viral meningitis; mononuclear cells usually predominate in Lyme meningitis.
↑, mild increase; ↑↑, moderate or severe increase; ↓, mild decrease; ↓↓, moderate or severe decrease.

by CT or MRI. Other contraindications include cardiopulmonary instability and skin infection overlying the LP site.

Treatment

When the diagnosis of uncomplicated viral meningitis is unequivocal, hospitalization is generally not necessary. If bacterial meningitis cannot be excluded, the patient should be hospitalized for intravenous antibiotic therapy.

Vancomycin plus a third-generation cephalosporin (cefotaxime or ceftriaxone) achieves therapeutic levels in the CSF and provides broad-spectrum coverage of the most likely pathogens in infants and older children. Neonates should be treated with ampicillin to treat group B streptococci and *L. monocytogenes*; cefotaxime is added to cover gram-negative pathogens. Once an organism and its susceptibility pattern are known, antibiotic coverage may be adjusted. The course of therapy for bacterial meningitis is usually 10 to 14 days. Exceptions include meningococcal meningitis (5 to 7 days), Lyme meningitis (14 to 28 days), and neonatal meningitis (14 to 21 days).

The current mortality rate for bacterial meningitis is up to 30% for neonates and less than 10% for infants and older children. However, 10% to 20% of patients experience some persistent neurologic deficit, most commonly hearing loss, developmental delay, motor incoordination, seizures, and hydrocephalus.

GASTROENTERITIS

Pathogens cause diarrhea by a variety of mechanisms. For example, some bacteria invade intestinal tissue directly, whereas others secrete injurious toxins before or after ingestion. Viruses, parasites, and protozoa also are capable of inflicting disease. Excessive stooling causes dehydration, inadequate nutrition, and electrolyte abnormalities, all of which are poorly tolerated in infants and small children.

Clinical Manifestations

History

The history should include information about symptoms in other family members, recent travel, medication use, immune status, daycare attendance, source of drinking water, contact with animals, duration of symptoms, fever, and number, color, and character of stools.

The most common bacterial causes of gastroenteritis include *Salmonella* species, *Shigella* species, *Escherichia coli*, *Yersinia enterocolitica*, and *Campylobacter jejuni*; *Vibrio cholerae* may be acquired during travel to developing nations and from eating undercooked Gulf Coast shellfish. Patients with bacterial diarrhea present with fever, significant abdominal cramping, malaise, and tenesmus; vomiting is less common. The stools contain mucus and may be guaiac positive or streaked with blood. Occasionally, children with shigellosis present with **neurologic** manifestations (lethargy, seizures, mental status changes). *Salmonella* species are capable of invading the bloodstream and causing extraintestinal disease, including meningitis and osteomyelitis (particularly in children with sickle cell anemia). *Shigella dysenteriae* and *E. coli* O157:H7 produce an enterotoxin (Shiga or Shigalike toxin) associated with **hemolytic uremic syndrome**, a serious complication consisting of microangiopathic hemolytic anemia, nephropathy, and thrombocytopenia. Up to 30% of individuals infected with *Y. enterocolitica* develop subsequent **erythema nodosum**. In some patients, particularly those with *Yersinia*, severe pain localizes to the right lower quadrant, creating a "pseudoappendicitis" picture.

In cholera, the stools quickly become colorless and flecked with mucus, termed "rice-water" stools. Severe diarrhea leading to hypovolemic shock may develop in hours to a few days.

Rotavirus is the major cause of nonbacterial gastroenteritis in infants and toddlers in the Western world. Infections peak between January and April. Complaints include profuse diarrhea, vomiting, and low-grade fever. Severe diarrhea may lead to significant dehydration, acidosis, and electrolyte disturbances.

Giardiasis is the most commonly reported intestinal parasitic disease in the United States. More water-related outbreaks of diarrhea are caused by *Giardia lamblia* than any other organism. The illness presents with frequent, foul-smelling, watery stools that rarely contain blood or mucus; abdominal pain, nausea, vomiting, anorexia, and flatulence often accompany the diarrhea. Symptoms generally resolve within 5 to 7 days, although some cases linger for more than a month. Patients with chronic giardiasis are at risk for failure to thrive resulting from ongoing malabsorption.

Physical Examination

The main goals of the physical examination are estimating the degree of dehydration (see Chapter 7), judging the stability of the patient's condition, identifying findings that may point to a specific infectious or noninfectious etiology, and ruling out a surgical condition.

Differential Diagnosis

Acute diarrhea in childhood is usually caused by infection. Other conditions associated with diarrhea include malabsorption, celiac disease, antibiotic use, cystic fibrosis, and inflammatory bowel disease.

Diagnostic Evaluation

Electrolyte and renal function studies (Na^+, K^+, Cl^-, HCO_3^-, BUN, creatinine) guide replacement therapy in significantly dehydrated children (see Chapter 7). Abdominal radiographs, if obtained, are generally normal or nonspecific. Blood, mucus, and fecal leukocytes suggest a bacterial origin for the illness. Blood culture should be performed at the time of initial evaluation if bacterial disease is suspected. Bacterial stool culture results take several days but are helpful in determining the need for antibiotics. If there is a history of antibiotic use, stool should be tested for *Clostridium difficile* toxins A and B. Rapid antigen testing is available for rotavirus. If *G. lamblia* infection is suspected, multiple stool samples from different times should be examined for cysts. Immunofluorescent antibody detection in stool can also be used to diagnose *G. lamblia* infection. Endoscopic biopsy may be indicated if the diarrhea becomes chronic and no etiology has been identified.

Treatment

Treatment incorporates oral rehydration whenever possible; aggressive parenteral therapy may be required in severe cases. Antidiarrheal agents are to be avoided in children.

Unless the patient is a febrile infant younger than 3 months or appears toxic, antibiotics should generally be withheld pending culture results. Antibiotic therapy prolongs *Salmonella* shedding and should be reserved for bacteremia or extraintestinal dissemination and for high-risk patients with noninvasive gastroenteritis, including infants less than 3 months of age and immunocompromised persons. Antibiotics may enhance the likelihood of development of hemolytic uremic syndrome among patients with diarrhea caused by *E. coli* O157:H7. Trimethoprim-sulfamethoxazole is often effective in treating shigellosis. Erythromycin is the treatment of choice for C. *jejuni*. Patients with C. *difficile* enterocolitis usually improve with suspension of antibiotic therapy, but if treatment is warranted, metronidazole is the medication of choice. Patients with giardiasis are also treated with oral metronidazole.

As long as the patient does not develop hypovolemic shock, prognosis for full recovery is excellent. Even in life-threatening cases, appropriate management often prevents permanent sequelae.

HEPATITIS

Pathogenesis

Acute hepatic inflammation in children can be caused by a large number of infectious and noninfectious viruses. Primary hepatotropic viruses include hepatitis A virus (HAV), hepatitis B virus (HBV), hepatitis C virus (HCV), hepatitis D virus (HDV, formerly delta hepatitis), and hepatitis E virus (HEV). Table 12-7 compares features of HAV, HBV, and HCV.

Epidemiology

HAV and HEV are acquired via fecal-oral transmission. Hepatitis A is the most common infectious cause of jaundice in children. HBV, HCV, and HDV are transmitted by percutaneous or mucosal exposure to infectious body fluids and by vertical transmission from an infected mother to her infant. HDV, or delta antigen, consists of single-stranded RNA. It is a "defective" virus in that it requires the presence of an active HBV infection to replicate. HBV and HCV can persist for many years following acute infection. This "carrier state" is associated with development of hepatocellular carcinoma. The incidence of hepatitis B infection is decreasing in the pediatric population because of routine vaccination against hepatitis B in infancy.

Risk Factors

Intravenous drug users, those who have unprotected sex with multiple partners, and those who receive blood transfusions are at increased risk of contracting HBV, HCV, and HDV. Risk factors for HAV and HEV include foreign travel, poor sanitation, and contact with other children in day care.

■ **TABLE 12-7** Viruses Responsible for Hepatitis: Comparison and Summary

Feature	Hepatitis A	Hepatitis B	Hepatitis C
Virus type	RNA	DNA	RNA
Incubation (days)	15 to 45	45 to 180	14 to 180
Period of infectivity	Late incubation to early symptomatic state	When HBsAg seropositive	Unknown
Fulminant hepatitis	<1%	1% to 3%	1%
Chronic hepatitis	No	5% to 10% of adults; 25% to 50% of infants; 90% of neonates whose mothers are HBeAg positive	50%
Diagnostic evaluation	Anti-HAV IgM	HBsAg, HBeAg, anti-HBs, anti-HBc, anti-HBe	Anti-HCV antibody, HCV PCR

anti-HBc, total antibody to hepatitis B core antigen; anti-HBe, total antibody to hepatitis B e antigen; anti-HBs, total antibody to hepatitis B surface antigen; HAV, hepatitis A virus; HBeAg, hepatitis B e antigen; HBsAg, hepatitis B surface antigen; HCV, hepatitis C virus.

Clinical Manifestations

History

Perinatally infected infants are usually asymptomatic. Clinical signs of acute hepatitis include anorexia, nausea, malaise, vomiting, jaundice, dark urine, abdominal pain, and low-grade fever. Children with HAV and HEV may also have diarrhea. However, a wide range of severity exists, and as many as 30% to 70% of infected children are asymptomatic. HBV and HCV infection are usually silent, in that the patient complains of no symptoms unless chronic infection has caused significant hepatic damage.

Physical Examination

Scleral icterus and jaundice may or may not be present. Other possible signs and symptoms include hepatomegaly and right upper-quadrant tenderness. A benign-appearing rash may appear early in the course of hepatitis B.

Differential Diagnosis

EBV, CMV, enterovirus, and other viral infections can also cause hepatitis, but other organ systems are usually involved. Jaundice may also result from autoimmune hepatitis, metabolic liver disease, biliary tract disorders, and drug ingestions.

Diagnostic Evaluation

Liver enzymes are uniformly elevated in hepatitis. Because the clinical manifestations are so similar, spe-cific serologic tests are indispensable for securing an accurate diagnosis. The presence of anti-HAV IgM antibody confirms HAV infection (Fig. 12-4). Tests are also available to detect antibodies to the delta antigen.

Three different particles may be found in the serum of patients infected with HBV. The Dane particle is the largest, made up of a core antigen (HBcAg) and envelope antigen (HBeAg) surrounded by a spherical shell of HBsAg ("surface") particles. Figure 12-5 and Table 12-8 present the clinical course and serologic markers important in diagnosing HBV disease stage. Anti-HBs heralds resolution of the illness and confers lifelong immunity.

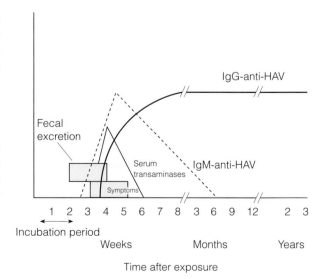

Figure 12-4 • Typical course of acute hepatitis A.

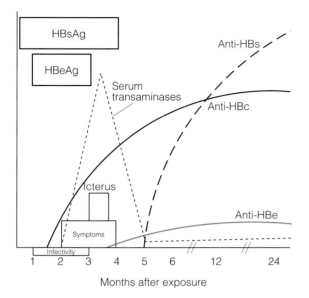

Figure 12-5 • The course of acute hepatitis B.

HCV antibody is present in both acute and chronic infection. HCV RNA can be detected by PCR within 1 week of infection, whereas the "window period" from infection to antibody response for HCV may be as long as 12 weeks. Therefore, the presence of HCV RNA in the absence of an antibody response indicates acute infection. Recovery is characterized by the disappearance of HCV RNA from the blood.

Prevention

Both active and passive forms of immunization are available, depending on the source of infection. HAV immunization is recommended for all infants in the United States. Immune globulin prevents hepatitis A clinical disease when administered within 14 days of exposure. The HBV vaccine series is also recommended for all infants in the United States. Infants of infected mothers should receive both the vaccine and the HBV immunoglobulin at delivery to prevent the disease and development of the carrier state.

Prognosis

The prognosis for patients with hepatitis depends on the virus responsible.

- HAV: Very few patients develop fulminant hepatitis, but the mortality rate among those who do is almost 50%.
- HBV: HBV may persist as chronic hepatitis, and the course may be relatively benign or more severe. Chronic persistent hepatitis B is characterized by little cellular inflammation and usually resolves within one year. Chronic active hepatitis is more aggressive, progressing to cirrhosis and increasing the risk of hepatocellular carcinoma. Chronic infection is more likely among infected children than adults.
- HDV: When HDV and HBV are acquired simultaneously, the recipient is at greater risk for more severe chronic hepatitis B and fulminant hepatitis associated with a higher mortality rate. When an individual is infected with HDV on top of preexisting HBV, acute exacerbation and an accelerated course result. The risk of progressing to cirrhotic liver disease is also increased when HDV is present.
- HCV: Half of those infected with HCV develop chronic hepatitis, with an increased risk for cirrhosis.
- HEV: HEV does not appear to result in chronic hepatitis.

■ TABLE 12-8 Comparisons of Disease States in Hepatitis B Virus			
Test	**Acute HBV**	**Resolved HBV**	**Chronic HBV**
HBsAg	+	−	+
Anti-HBs	−	+	−
Anti-HBc	+	+	+
HBeAg	±	−	±
Anti-HBe	−	+	±
anti-HBc, total antibody to hepatitis B core antigen; anti-HBe, total antibody to hepatitis B e antigen; anti-HBs, total antibody to hepatitis B surface antigen; HBeAg, hepatitis B e antigen; HBsAg, hepatitis B surface antigen; HBV, hepatitis B virus.			

SYPHILIS

Pathogenesis

Syphilis is primarily a sexually transmitted disease (STD) resulting from infection with the spirochete *Treponema pallidum*.

Epidemiology

Syphilis in the pediatric population may be acquired transplacentally (congenital syphilis) or through sexual contact. The incidence of syphilis has increased sharply over the past few decades. Coinfection with other STDs is common.

Risk Factors

Neonates born to a mother with untreated infection are at risk for congenital syphilis. Adolescents and adults who have unprotected sex with an infected partner or multiple partners are at risk for primary syphilis.

Clinical Manifestations

History and Physical Examination

Approximately half of infants with congenital syphilis die shortly before or after birth. Those who survive are often asymptomatic at birth but develop symptoms within 1 month if untreated. Infants with congenital syphilis may have hepatomegaly, splenomegaly, mucocutaneous lesions, jaundice, lymphadenopathy, and the characteristic **snuffles** (a bloody, mucopurulent nasal discharge). Long-term sequelae include deafness and retardation.

Syphilis acquired through sexual contact progresses through three stages. After a 2- to 4-week incubation period, infected individuals enter the **primary** stage of syphilis, characterized by the classic **chancre** at the inoculation site: a well-demarcated, firm, strangely painless genital ulcer with an indurated base (Color Plate 17). Because the lesion heals spontaneously within 3 to 6 weeks, patients with primary syphilis often do not seek medical attention.

About one-third of untreated patients develop **secondary** syphilis, manifested by widespread dermatologic involvement coinciding with dissemination of the spirochete throughout the body. Onset follows the primary stage directly, often while the chancre is still present. The typical rash consists of generalized (including the soles and palms) erythematous macules (3 to 10 mm) that progress to papules (Color Plate 18). Some patients also develop systemic symptoms including fever, malaise, pharyngitis, mucosal ulcerations, and generalized lymphadenopathy; patchy alopecia and thinning of the lateral third of the eyebrow are also associated with secondary syphilis. Symptoms of secondary syphilis resolve in 1 to 3 months.

Tertiary syphilis develops years after primary exposure and is rare in the pediatric population. Granulomatous lesions called **gummas** destroy surrounding tissues, especially in the skin, bone, heart, and CNS. Unfortunately, tertiary syphilis may occur without any previous primary or secondary manifestations.

Differential Diagnosis

Syphilis is one of the great masqueraders, a disease with a wide spectrum of presentations. The presence of the rash, if characteristic, greatly aids in diagnosis.

Diagnostic Evaluation

Chancre scrapings (and mucosal secretions in infected neonates) demonstrate rapidly mobile organisms moving in a corkscrewlike motion under dark-field microscopy. Aspiration of enlarged lymph nodes may also yield the organism. Both the VDRL (developed by the Venereal Disease Research Laboratory of the U.S. Public Health Service) and the RPR (Rapid Plasma Reagin) are excellent blood screening tests for high-risk populations, providing rapid, inexpensive, quantitative results. Both are nontreponemal tests for antibodies to a lipoidal molecule rather than the organism itself. Both are considered highly sensitive when titers are high or when the test is complemented by historical or physical evidence of the disease. However, infectious mononucleosis, connective tissue disease, endocarditis, and tuberculosis may all result in false-positive VDRL and RPR results. By contrast, treponemal tests, such as the fluorescent treponemal antibody absorption (FTA-ABS) and microhemagglutination assay for *T. pallidum* (MHA-TP), are much less likely to produce false positives. A positive screening VDRL or RPR coupled with a positive FTA-ABS in a newborn or sexually active adolescent is virtually diagnostic of untreated syphilis. Nontreponemal tests may become negative after treatment, whereas treponemal studies remain positive for life.

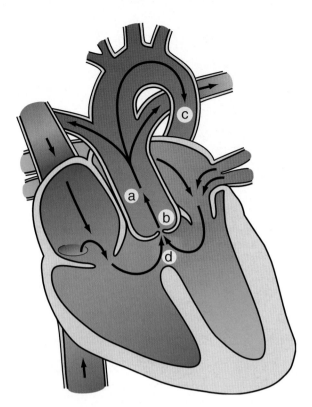

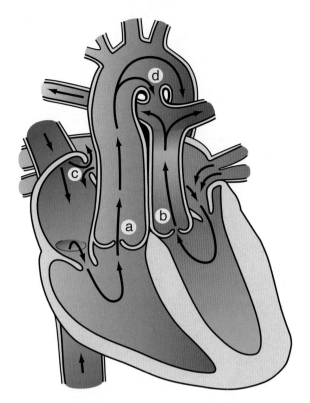

Color Plate 1 • Truncus arteriosus. Typical anatomic findings include (A) a single truncal vessel arising from the heart giving off the coronary arteries, pulmonary arteries, and aortic arch; (B) abnormal truncal valve; (C) left aortic arch shown (right aortic arch occurs in 30% of cases); (D) ventricular septal defect. (Illustration by Patricia Gast.)

Color Plate 2 • Transposition of the great arteries with an intact ventricular septum, a large patent ductus arteriosus, and an atrial septal defect. Note the following: (A) aorta arises from the morphologic right ventricle; (B) pulmonary artery arises from the morphologic left ventricle; (C) mixing occurs across the atrial septal defect; (D) shunting from the aorta to the pulmonary artery via the ductus arteriosus. (Illustration by Patricia Gast.)

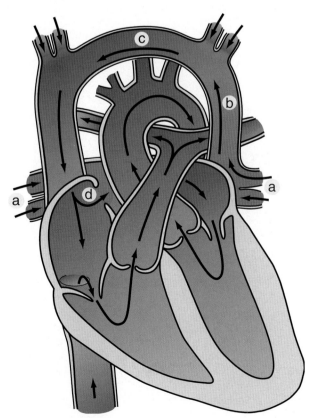

Color Plate 3 • Supradiaphragmatic total anomalous pulmonary venous connection. Note the following: (A) pulmonary veins join into a confluence; (B) the confluence joins a vertical vein which ascends to connect with the (C) innominate vein and then drains via the SVC into the right atrium; (D) venous return must cross the PFO to fill the left atrium. (Illustration by Patricia Gast.)

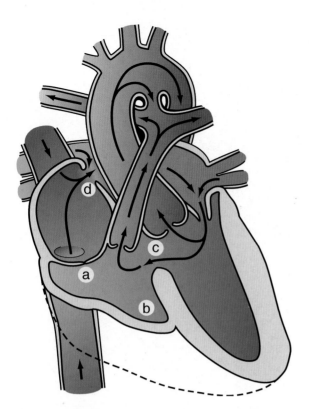

Color Plate 4 • Tricuspid atresia with normally related great arteries and a patent ductus arteriosus. Typical anatomic findings include (A) atresia of the tricuspid valve; (B) hypoplasia of the right ventricle; (C) ventricular septal defect; (D) patent foramen ovale (PFO). Note: All systemic venous return must pass through the PFO to reach the left atrium and left ventricle. (Illustration by Patricia Gast.)

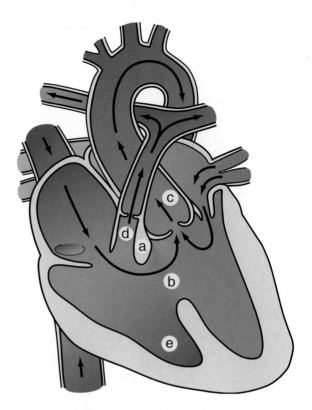

Color Plate 5 • Tetralogy of Fallot. Typical anatomic findings include (A) an anteriorly displaced infundibular septum, resulting in subpulmonary stenosis; (B) large anterior malalignment VSD; (C) overriding of the aorta over the muscular septum; (D) hypoplasia of the pulmonary valve and main pulmonary artery; (E) right ventricular hypertrophy, secondary to right ventricular outflow tract obstruction. (Illustration by Patricia Gast.)

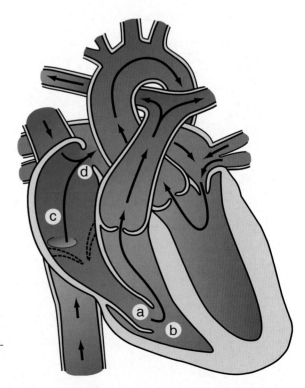

Color Plate 6 • Ebstein anomaly. Typical anatomic findings include (A) inferior displacement of the tricuspid valve into the right ventricle (the normal placement of the tricuspid valve is noted in dashed lines); (B) small right ventricle; (C) marked enlargement of the right atrium because of "atrialized" portion of right ventricle as well as tricuspid regurgitation; (D) right-to-left shunting at the atrial level. (Illustration by Patricia Gast.)

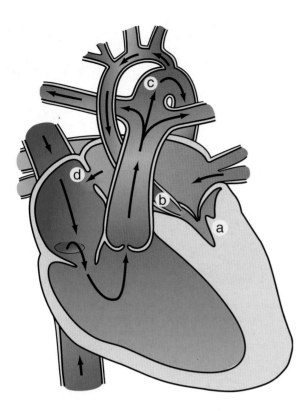

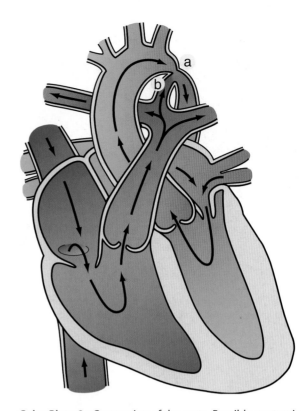

Color Plate 7 • Hypoplastic left heart syndrome. Typical anatomic findings include (A) atresia or hypoplasia of the mitral valve and hypoplasia of the left ventricle; (B) aortic atresia or stenosis and a diminutive ascending aorta and transverse aortic arch; (C) patent ductus arteriosus supplying systemic blood flow; (D) patent foramen ovale, with a left to right shunt.
(Illustration by Patricia Gast.)

Color Plate 8 • Coarctation of the aorta. Possible anatomic findings include (A) narrowing distal to the left subclavian artery; (B) patent ductus arteriosus supplying systemic flow to descending aorta.
(Illustration by Patricia Gast.)

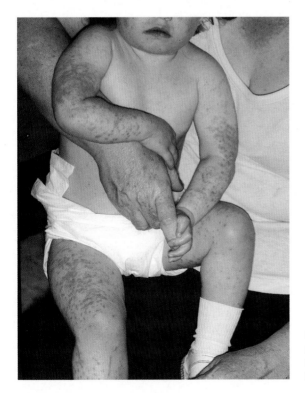

Color Plate 9 • A toddler with erythematous, edematous papules concentrated on the extremities and strikingly sparing the trunk that are typical of this condition. It appears to be a reaction to a viral infection.
(Image courtesy of Anne W. Lucky, MD.)

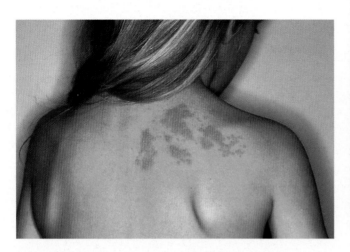

Color Plate 10 • Tender grouped papulovesicles on an erythematous base involving the upper right back in a dermatomal distribution.
(Image courtesy of Anne W. Lucky, MD.)

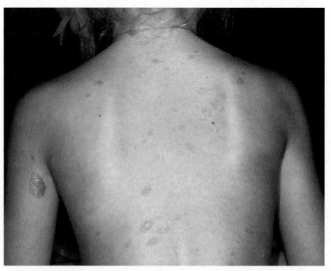

Color Plate 11 • A salmon-pink annular patch with a collarette of scale developed on the back of the patient's left arm followed several days later by an eruption of smaller salmon-colored lesions in a "Christmas-tree" distribution on the trunk.
(Image courtesy of Anne W. Lucky, MD.)

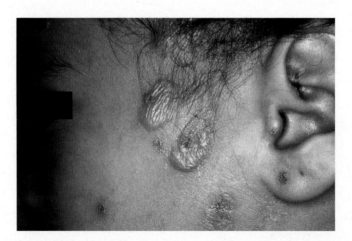

Color Plate 12 • Intact fluid-filled thin bullae with scale peripherally and a hemorrhagic crust centrally that can be mistaken for cigarette burns especially following bullae rupture. Toxin–producing *S. aureus* is causative.
(Image courtesy of Anne W. Lucky, MD.)

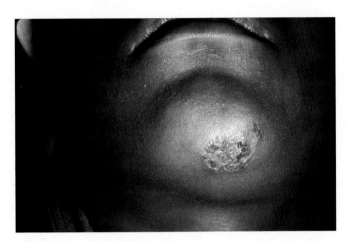

Color Plate 13 • Non-bullous impetigo has a honey-colored crust on an erythematous ulcerated base. *Streptococcus* or *Staphylococcus* species can usually be cultured from the lesion. (Image courtesy of Anne W. Lucky, MD.)

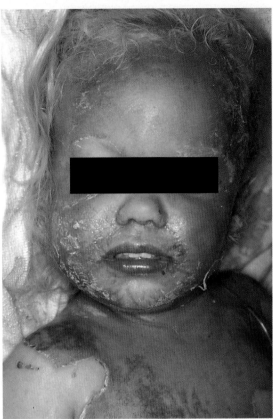

Color Plate 14 • Diffuse areas of erythema with superficial flaccid vesicles and ruptured bullae associated with significant pain and fevers are seen in SSSS due to a toxin-producing strain of *S. aureus*.
(Image courtesy of Anne W. Lucky, MD.)

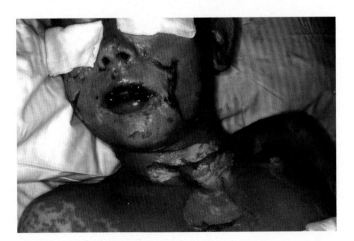

Color Plate 15 • Typical inflammatory hemorrhagic bullae of the oral mucosa noted in SJS.
(Image courtesy of Anne W. Lucky, MD.)

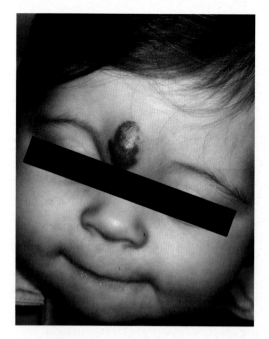

Color Plate 16 • A hemangioma with superficial and deep components involving the glabella.
(Image courtesy of Anne W. Lucky, MD.)

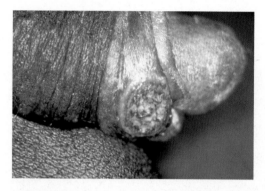

Color Plate 17 • Chancre of primary syphilis.
(From Goodheart HP. *Goodheart's Photoguide of Common Skin Disorders*, 2nd ed. Philadelphia: Lippincott Williams & Wilkins, 2003.)

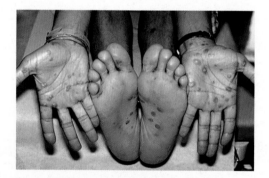

Color Plate 18 • Typical lesions of secondary syphilis (palms, soles).
(From Goodheart HP. *Goodheart's Photoguide of Common Skin Disorders*, 2nd ed. Philadelphia: Lippincott Williams & Wilkins, 2003.)

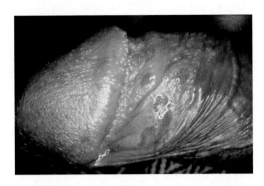

Color Plate 19 • Genital herpes (multiple erythematous ulcerations).
(From Goodheart HP. *Goodheart's Photoguide of Common Skin Disorders*, 2nd ed. Philadelphia: Lippincott Williams & Wilkins, 2003.)

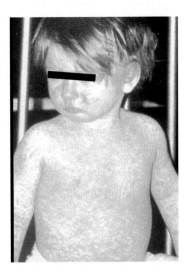

Color Plate 20 • A child with measles.
(Photo courtesy of Centers for Disease Control and Prevention.)

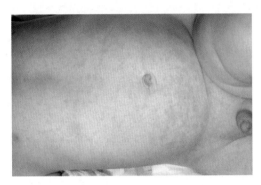

Color Plate 21 • Typical roseola exanthem.
(From Goodheart HP. *Goodheart's Photoguide of Common Skin Disorders*, 2nd ed. Philadelphia: Lippincott Williams & Wilkins, 2003. Image courtesy of Bernard Cohen, MD.)

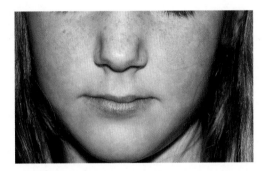

Color Plate 22 • "Slapped cheeks" of erythema infectiosum (fifth disease).
(From Goodheart HP. *Goodheart's Photoguide of Common Skin Disorders*, 2nd ed. Philadelphia: Lippincott Williams & Wilkins, 2003.)

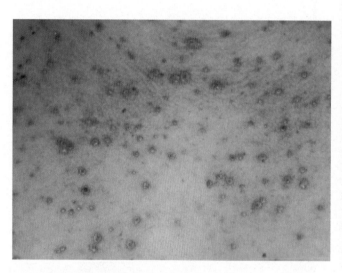

Color Plate 23 • Typical varicella lesions.
(From Sweet RL, Gibbs RS. *Atlas of Infectious Diseases of the Female Genital Tract*. Philadelphia: Lippincott Williams & Wilkins, 2005.)

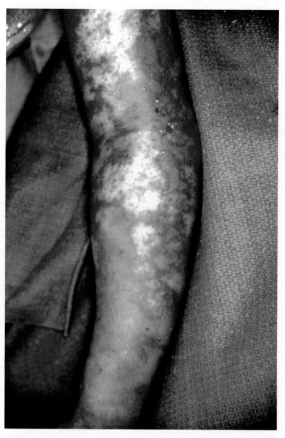

Color Plate 24 • Petechial lesions of Rocky Mountain spotted fever.
(Image from E Rubin, MD, and JL Farber, MD. *Pathology*, 3rd ed. Philadelphia: Lippincott Williams & Wilkins, 1999.)

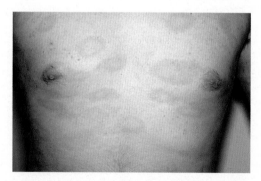

Color Plate 25 • Lyme disease (erythema migrans).
(From Goodheart HP. *Goodheart's Photoguide of Common Skin Disorders*, 2nd ed. Philadelphia: Lippincott Williams & Wilkins, 2003.)

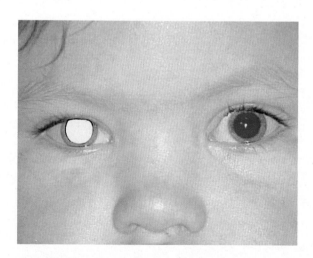

Color Plate 26 • Leukokoria due to advanced intraocular retinoblastoma of right eye.
(From Tasman W, Jaeger E. *The Wills Eye Hospital Atlas of Clinical Ophthalmology*, 2nd ed. Philadelphia: Lippincott Williams & Wilkins, 2001.)

Neonates with suspected congenital syphilis require lumbar puncture. Cerebrospinal fluid pleocytosis and elevated protein suggest neurosyphilis. A positive CSF VDRL is diagnostic. Untreated infants may develop anemia, thrombocytopenia, and radiographic abnormalities of the long bones.

Treatment

Parenteral penicillin G (IM or intravenous) remains the treatment of choice for any stage of infection and fully eradicates the organism from the body.

GENITAL HERPES SIMPLEX VIRUS INFECTION

Genital herpes usually results from infection with herpes simplex virus (HSV) type 2. Small mucosal tears or skin cracks are inoculated with the virus during sexual activity. Herpes is one of the most common sexually acquired diseases; about 20% of adults have a history suggestive of prior genital herpes infection. Transmission of HSV from mother to infant at the time of birth may result in devastating infection in the newborn.

Clinical Manifestations

History and Physical Examination

After a variable incubation period (5 to 14 days), genital burning and itching progress to vesicular, often pustular, lesions. These burst to form painful shallow ulcers that heal without scarring (Color Plate 19). Fever, pharyngitis, headache, and malaise may accompany the primary episode. After acquisition, the virus ascends peripheral nerves to dorsal root ganglia, where it may lie latent or recur periodically. Recurrences have fewer symptoms than the primary episode, and asymptomatic shedding occurs.

Diagnostic Evaluation

Giant multinucleated cells with intranuclear inclusions are found in scrapings from the ulcer base (Tzanck testing). HSV may be cultured from the active lesions in 1 to 4 days; direct fluorescent antibody staining and PCR testing are also available.

Treatment

Oral antiviral agents (including acyclovir) diminish the length of both symptoms and shedding but do not eradicate HSV. They have limited efficacy in recurrent episodes. Continued prophylactic use of oral acyclovir prevents or reduces the frequency of recurrences.

PELVIC INFLAMMATORY DISEASE

Pathogenesis

Pelvic inflammatory disease (PID) is a constellation of symptoms and signs related to the ascending spread of pathogenic organisms from the lower female genital tract (vagina, cervix) to the endometrium, fallopian tubes, and contiguous structures.

Epidemiology

PID is generally polymicrobial, with *Chlamydia trachomatis* and *Neisseria gonorrhoeae* the most commonly isolated organisms. Other potential causes of PID include anaerobes and enteric gram-negative bacilli. Barrier contraceptive methods are protective. *N. gonorrhoeae* or genital *C. trachomatis* infection in a prepubertal child strongly suggests sexual abuse.

Risk Factors

Adolescence is a period of increased risk for development of PID because of the presence of cervical ectopy and the increased incidence of high-risk behavior during the teenage years. Risk factors also include sexual intercourse with multiple partners, unprotected intercourse, and a preexisting mucosal sexually transmitted infection.

Clinical Manifestations

The clinical diagnosis of PID is based on the presence of at least one of the two **minimum criteria.** **Additional criteria** are often used to support the diagnosis of PID.

- Minimum criteria: cervical motion tenderness or uterine or adnexal tenderness
- Additional criteria:
  - Oral temperature greater than 38.3°C (101°F)
  - Elevated ESR and/or C-reactive protein
  - Presence of WBCs on saline microscopy of vaginal secretions

- Abnormal cervical or vaginal discharge
- Intracellular gram-negative diplococci found on endocervical smear
- Laboratory evidence of cervical infection with *N. gonorrhoeae* or *C. trachomatis*

History and Physical Examination

Other symptoms include cramping, vaginal discharge or bleeding, nausea/vomiting, and malaise. The physical examination may be positive for peritoneal signs if the disease is severe.

Diagnostic Evaluation

Nucleic acid amplification tests are sensitive and specific for both gonorrhea and chlamydia. If a patient is suspected of having PID, she should be offered testing for syphilis, HIV, and other sexually transmitted infections. Often, a specific pathogen responsible for PID is not identified, because PID is an upper genital tract disease, whereas samples are routinely obtained from the lower tract.

Differential Diagnosis

Other gynecologic conditions and intra-abdominal pathology are included in the differential diagnosis:

- Gynecologic: mucopurulent cervicitis, ectopic pregnancy, ruptured ovarian cyst, septic abortion, endometriosis
- Nongynecologic: appendicitis, pyelonephritis, inflammatory bowel disease

Patients with suspected PID should always receive a pregnancy test because treatment may need to be altered and because ectopic pregnancy is a life-threatening condition that must be ruled out.

Treatment

Patients with clinical PID should be treated for both *N. gonorrhoeae* and *C. trachomatis*. Coverage against anaerobes (such as metronidazole and clindamycin) and other gram-negative organisms is often added. A single dose of a long-acting parenteral third-generation cephalosporin, such as ceftriaxone or cefotaxime, is sufficient to eradicate *N. gonorrhoeae*. A 14-day course of oral doxycycline eradicates *C. trachomatis*. An alternative treatment for both organisms consists of oral ofloxacin or levofloxacin for 14 days.

Significant infections require more extensive courses of therapy. All patients who are released for outpatient treatment should return for a follow-up visit within 72 hours. Sexual contacts need to be treated to avoid reinfection.

Indications for hospitalization include severe illness, vomiting, pregnancy, blood pressure instability, or a possible surgical condition. These patients should receive intravenous antibiotics, including cefotetan or cefoxitin plus doxycycline. An alternative regimen consists of clindamycin and gentamicin.

Twenty percent of infected women become infertile after a single episode of PID. Other gynecologic complications include increased risks for ectopic pregnancy, dyspareunia, chronic pelvic pain, and adhesions.

N. gonorrhoeae is capable of invading the bloodstream and thus any organ system. Joint involvement is most common. The arthritis may affect only one joint or may be polyarticular and migratory with associated tenosynovitis and skin lesions. Although *C. trachomatis* seldom causes systemic illness, untreated individuals may go on to develop **Reiter syndrome** (a constellation of urethritis, conjunctivitis, and arthritis). **Fitz-Hugh-Curtis syndrome**, a form of perihepatitis, is a known complication of infection with either organism.

VULVOVAGINAL INFECTIONS

Trichomoniasis, bacterial vaginosis, and *Candida* vaginitis are all bothersome but relatively benign vaginal infections collectively manifested by changes in the amount and character of vaginal secretions. All three are easily diagnosed during the office visit by examination of vaginal fluid samples.

Clinical Manifestations and Treatment

Trichomoniasis

Trichomoniasis results from sexually transmitted *Trichomonas vaginalis*, a mobile flagellated protozoan. Most infected individuals remain asymptomatic. Typical symptoms in women include a malodorous, frothy gray discharge and vaginal discomfort. Some patients also develop dysuria and vague lower abdominal pain. The cervix and vaginal mucosa may be either normal or visibly irritated and inflamed. A fresh wet preparation of the vaginal fluid reveals polymorphonuclear leukocytes and the characteristic motile trichomonads. Oral metronidazole twice daily for 7 days is the treatment of choice for patients and their sexual partners.

Bacterial Vaginosis

Bacterial vaginosis, long thought to be harmless, is now known to increase the risks of PID, chorioamnionitis, and premature birth. Its microbiologic cause has not been clearly delineated, but concentrations of *Gardnerella vaginalis*, *Mycoplasma hominis*, and various anaerobic organisms are increased in the vagina. The epidemiology of the disease suggests sexual transmission. Infection is usually asymptomatic except for a thin, white, foul-smelling discharge that emits a fishy odor when mixed with potassium hydroxide. The clinical diagnosis is based on patient history (much more common in sexually active females), the appearance and odor of discharge, a vaginal pH greater than 4.5, and characteristic clue cells on the wet prep (squamous epithelial cells with smudged borders caused by adherent bacteria). Oral metronidazole twice daily for 7 days effectively cures the infection. Concurrent antibiotic treatment of male partners seems to have no effect on recurrence rates.

Vaginal Candidiasis

Vulvovaginal candidiasis is not an STD. All women are colonized with *Candida*; however, factors such as antibiotic use, pregnancy, diabetes, immunosuppression, and oral contraceptive use predispose women to candidal overgrowth (moniliasis). Signs and symptoms include a thick white vaginal discharge with vaginal itching and burning. Yeast and pseudohyphae are evident on wet preparation treated with potassium hydroxide. Over-the-counter topical antifungal creams are safe and generally effective. A single dose of oral fluconazole is an alternative.

URETHRITIS

Urethritis is inflammation of the urethra caused by infection with an STD. It occurs much more commonly in adolescent males than females. *N. gonorrhoeae* and *C. trachomatis* are the most important pathogens. Symptoms include urethral discharge, itching, dysuria, and urinary frequency. Asymptomatic infections are common. The disease is diagnosed by notation of at least one of the following: mucoid or purulent urethral discharge; positive leukocyte esterase test or WBCs on microscopic examination of a first-void urine; or gram-negative intracellular diplococci on Gram stain. Patients with suspected urethritis should be offered testing for other STDS including syphilis and HIV. If gonorrhea is ruled out, the patient may be treated with 1 dose of oral azithromycin or 7 days of oral doxycycline. If *N. gonorrhoeae* is a consideration, IM ceftriaxone should be given in the office. Complications are rare.

HIV AND AIDS

Pathogenesis

HIV is a retrovirus that infects $CD4^+$ T-lymphocytes. HIV produces a wide range of clinical manifestations in children, the most severe of which is AIDS. A child is defined as having AIDS when an AIDS-defining illness occurs (see later) or when the $CD4^+$ lymphocyte count is less than a defined number for age (e.g., <200 per mm^3 for children older than 12 years).

Epidemiology

The disease is more common in urban populations, lower socioeconomic classes, and racial minorities. Most infections in children are acquired in utero or perinatally ($>90\%$). The risk of HIV transmission from an untreated seropositive mother to her fetus is approximately 25%. Treatment of infected pregnant women with zidovudine (AZT; a reverse transcriptase inhibitor) alone or in combination with other antiretrovirals during the second and third trimesters, followed by treatment of the infant for the first 6 weeks of life, reduces the vertical transmission rate to approximately 2%. Asymptomatic HIV-positive women may not realize they are infected, and therefore they often do not receive therapy.

As a group, the adolescent population has the most rapidly increasing rate of HIV infection in the United States.

Risk Factors

Risk factors include birth to an HIV-positive mother, birth to a woman who uses intravenous drugs and shares needles, and birth to a woman with multiple sexual partners who does not practice safe sex. Other groups at risk include patients who received multiple units of blood products (e.g., hemophiliacs) before 1985, victims of sexual abuse, and adolescents who engage in high-risk behaviors (intravenous drug use or unprotected sexual activity with multiple partners).

Clinical Manifestations

History and Physical Examination

HIV may present in infants and children with any one or several of the following signs and symptoms: generalized lymphadenopathy, hepatomegaly, splenomegaly, failure to thrive, recurrent or chronic diarrhea, oral candidiasis, parotitis, and developmental delay. Respiratory manifestations include lymphoid interstitial pneumonia (LIP) and *Pneumocystis jiroveci* pneumonia (PCP). Regression in developmental milestones and progressive encephalopathy may occur. Recurrent, often severe, bacterial and opportunistic (fungal, disseminated HSV or CMV, and *Mycobacterium avium*) infections are the hallmark of the acquired helper T-lymphocyte immunodeficiency.

A significant percentage of infected adolescents presents with a mononucleosis-type syndrome within 6 weeks of HIV acquisition. Symptoms and signs include sore throat, fatigue, fever, rash, and cervical or diffuse lymphadenopathy.

PCP and LIP are two of several AIDS-defining illnesses in the pediatric population. When any of these conditions occurs, the child is considered to have AIDS regardless of the absolute CD4$^+$ T-lymphocyte count.

Differential Diagnosis

HIV has become known as a "great masquerader" because of its variable presentation; the virus can affect any organ system, and symptoms are often nonspecific. A high degree of suspicion is required to diagnose the disease at an early stage when it is most easily contained.

Diagnostic Evaluation

Infants born to HIV-positive mothers are seropositive for maternally derived IgG antibodies to the virus (i.e., ELISA and Western blot testing are positive); these tests are not helpful in children younger than 18 months. If the mother is HIV positive, HIV DNA PCR of the infant's blood should be performed at birth. If this test is positive on two separate occasions, the infant is considered HIV positive. Negative tests should be repeated at regular intervals (1 and 4

months of age). Almost all HIV-infected infants have positive HIV DNA PCR results by 1 month of age.

Treatment

The standard of care consists of nucleoside analogue reverse transcriptase inhibitor drugs such as AZT (zidovudine) and 3TC (lamivudine), nonnucleoside analogue reverse transcriptase inhibitors (NNRTIs), and protease inhibitors. Trimethoprim-sulfamethoxazole provides prophylaxis against PCP, the most common opportunistic infection. New pharmacologic therapies have drastically improved the chances of converting HIV infection from disease of near-certain death to a chronic lifelong condition.

VIRAL INFECTIONS OF CHILDHOOD

Viral infections are quite common in the infant and young child but decrease with age due to acquired immunity. Many of these present with characteristic rashes that permit reliable clinical diagnosis. Live attenuated vaccines are routinely administered to prevent measles, mumps, rubella, and varicella (chickenpox). Roseola and erythema infectiosum are generally benign in children. Table 12-9 describes the typical presentations and complications of these viral illnesses in children, which are discussed further in Chapter 5.

ROCKY MOUNTAIN SPOTTED FEVER

Pathogenesis

Rocky Mountain spotted fever (RMSF) is a tick-borne disease caused by *Rickettsia rickettsii*, a gram-negative intracellular bacterium. Rickettsiae are introduced into the skin by a tick bite and subsequently spread via the lymphatics and blood vessels. They invade and multiply within the endothelial cells of blood vessels, causing thrombosis and increasing vascular permeability (vasculitis).

Epidemiology

RMSF occurs more often between April and September in tick-infested areas of the south Atlantic states (but has been reported year round). Despite the name, none of the top 10 states reporting RMSF is near the Rocky Mountains. Tick vectors include the wood tick, dog tick, and lone star tick.

■ TABLE 12-9 Presentations and Complications of Childhood Viral Illnesses

Virus	Exanthem	Other Features	Complications
Measles	Confluent, erythematous maculopapular rash that starts on head and progresses caudally (color plate 12–4)	Coryza, cough, conjunctivitis, Koplik spots (on buccal mucosa early in disease)	Pneumonia, myocarditis, encephalitis; rare: subacute sclerosing panencephalitis
Mumps	None	Swollen salivary glands, especially parotid glands	Orchitis, pancreatitis; rare: meningitis, encephalitis
Rubella	Similar to measles but does not coalesce	Suboccipital and posterior auricular lymphadenopathy	Polyarticular arthritis or arthralgias; rare: encephalitis
Roseola (human herpesvirus 6)	Maculopapular (color plate 12–5)	High fever resolves as rash appears	Febrile seizures; rare: meningoencephalitis
Erythema infectiosum (fifth disease; parvovirus B19)	Facial erythema giving "slapped cheeks" appearance followed by spread to extremities in reticular pattern (color plate 12–6)	Transient aplastic crisis in child with hemoglobinopathy	Arthritis; rare: encephalitis
Chickenpox (varicella)	Pruritic, erythematous macules evolve to vesicles and then crust over; begins on face and spreads to extremities (color plate 12–7)	As initial lesions resolve, new crops form so that lesions in different stages are observed simultaneously	Secondary bacterial infection; rare: pneumonia, cerebellar ataxia, encephalitis, hepatitis

Risk Factor

The most significant risk factor is residence in or travel to an endemic area during times of the year when ticks are most active.

Clinical Manifestation

History and Physical Examination

The classic presentation of RMSF includes fever, headache, and rash. Symptoms develop approximately 7 days after a tick bite. Initial symptoms often are nonspecific and include fever, chills, headache, malaise, nausea, vomiting, and myalgias. The rash begins on the second to fifth day and consists of blanching, erythematous, macular lesions that progress to form petechiae or purpura (Color Plate 20). It characteristically appears initially on the wrists and ankles and spreads proximally to involve the trunk and head over several hours. Typically, the palms and soles are involved as well. The rash is absent in up to 20% of patients. Children may have some impairment of mental status.

Diagnostic Evaluation

Although immunofluorescent staining of skin biopsies taken from rash sites may demonstrate the organism, there is no reliable diagnostic test that becomes positive early enough in the course of the disease to guide therapy. Thus, the clinician must maintain a high suspicion for the disease. Antibodies to confirm the clinical diagnosis are detectable approximately 10 days after symptom onset. Key laboratory features include thrombocytopenia and hyponatremia; however, these are present in only a minority of patients.

Differential Diagnosis

RMSF is essentially indistinguishable from ehrlichiosis (another tick-borne illness) and meningococcemia. Because approximately half of patients with RMSF and ehrlichiosis do not remember being bitten by a tick, initial antibiotic therapy for patients with these suspected illnesses and no tick history should include coverage for *N. meningitidis* as well. Atypical measles may present in a similar fashion; knowledge of a local outbreak should clarify this diagnosis.

Treatment

Treatment with doxycycline is effective in all age groups. Cefotaxime or ceftriaxone should be added if meningococcemia is a possibility. If RMSF is suspected, antibiotics must not be withheld pending laboratory results. Mortality is higher when treatment is delayed.

LYME DISEASE

Pathogenesis

Lyme disease is a tick-borne illness resulting from infection with the spirochete bacterium *Borrelia burgdorferi*. The pathogen lives in deer ticks (eastern United States) and western black-legged ticks (Pacific states).

Epidemiology

Although cases have been reported across the country, most occur in southern New England, southeastern New York, New Jersey, eastern Pennsylvania, Maryland, Delaware, Minnesota, and Wisconsin. The incidence of Lyme disease is highest among children 5 to 9 years of age. Most cases occur between April and October.

Risk Factors

Individuals with increased occupational or recreational exposure to tick-infested woodlands in endemic areas are at highest risk of Lyme disease. An infected tick must feed for more than 48 hours to transmit *B. burgdorferi*.

Clinical Manifestation

History

Most patients do not recall a tick bite. The clinical manifestations depend on the stage of the disease: early localized, early disseminated, or late. **Erythema migrans**, the manifestation of **early localized** disease, appears at the site of the tick bite 3 to 30 days after the bite. The rash begins as a red macule or papule and progressively enlarges to form a large, annular, erythematous lesion with central clearing (resembling a bull's-eye) up to 10 cm in diameter. The skin

lesion often is accompanied by fever, malaise, headache, arthralgias, and myalgias. **Early disseminated** Lyme disease (days to weeks after the tick bite) may manifest as multiple erythema migrans lesions (Color Plate 21), cranial nerve palsy, meningitis, and carditis (heart block). The most common manifestation of **late** Lyme disease (>6 weeks after tick bite) is arthritis, usually involving the knee.

Physical Examination

Children with early disseminated Lyme disease may have multiple erythema migrans lesions, facial nerve palsy, or signs of meningitis. Late disease may present with swollen and tender joints.

Differential Diagnosis

The differential diagnosis depends on the presentation. When the rash is atypical, it may be confused with erythema multiforme or erythema marginatum (seen in acute rheumatic fever). The differential diagnosis of arthritis also includes juvenile idiopathic arthritis, reactive arthritis, and Reiter syndrome. The differential diagnosis of Lyme meningitis includes other causes of aseptic meningitis.

Diagnostic Evaluation

Testing for Lyme disease in the presence of vague or nonspecific complaints is not helpful; false-positive test results can occur, especially with ELISA (enzyme-linked immunosorbent assay) or immunofluorescent antibody testing. For the most part, early localized Lyme disease is a clinical diagnosis, based on suggestive history and the characteristic rash on physical examination. Lyme IgM titer is elevated several weeks after the tick bite. Antibodies to *B. burgdorferi* cross-react with other infectious agents, particularly other spirochetes (including syphilis). The VDRL and RPR tests remain negative in patients with Lyme disease. The Western blot is specific for antibodies to *B. burgdorferi* but does not usually become positive early enough in the course of disease to guide therapy. Cardiac involvement, usually in the form of conduction abnormalities, is rare but can be diagnosed by ECG in conjunction with supporting history and antibody studies.

Treatment

Treatment of early localized Lyme disease prevents early disseminated and late disease, including meningitis and arthritis. Younger children can be treated with oral amoxicillin or cefuroxime. Children older than 8 years should receive oral doxycycline. Patients with vomiting, persistent arthritis, cardiac disease, or neurologic involvement warrant parenteral therapy with high-dose penicillin G or ceftriaxone. A small minority of patients continues to experience low-grade, chronic symptoms despite appropriate therapy; long-term antibiotic treatment is not helpful in this population.

 KEY POINTS

- The three most common bacteria implicated in acute otitis media (AOM) are *S. pneumoniae*, nontypeable *H. influenzae*, and *M. catarrhalis*. In AOM, the tympanic membrane is bulging, opaque, and erythematous, with diminished mobility. Symptom onset is acute. High-dose amoxicillin is the appropriate first-line treatment for most cases of AOM. Tympanostomy tubes should be considered for children with recurrent episodes of AOM. Chronic effusions and recurrent infection predispose to permanent conductive hearing loss and language delay.

- Children with pharyngitis should not be treated with antibiotics empirically because most episodes are caused by viruses. Therapeutic decisions should be based on throat culture or rapid antigen detection test results. Penicillin is the antibiotic of choice for GAS pharyngitis.

- Classic infectious mononucleosis is caused by EBV. Clinical manifestations include exudative pharyngitis, generalized lymphadenopathy, fever, and profound fatigue. Helpful laboratory findings include lymphocytosis with a high percentage (10%) of atypical lymphocytes and a positive heterophile antibody test.

- Children with croup develop a hoarse voice, barky ("seal-like") cough, and stridor, which may progress to respiratory distress. Infants with severe stridor are treated with corticosteroids and nebulized epinephrine. The typical patient with epiglottitis, a life-threatening emergency, has a toxic appearance, with drooling and severe, progressive respiratory distress. When epiglottitis is suspected, the child should be transported to the operating room for endotracheal intubation and direct visualization under general anesthesia.

- The classic presentation of bronchiolitis includes fever, wheezing, tachypnea, rhinorrhea, and respiratory distress. Apnea is a frequent presentation in neonates. Prophylactic administration of palivizumab, an intramuscular RSV monoclonal antibody, is indicated during the winter months for patients younger than 24 months who were premature infants or who have chronic lung disease (bronchopulmonary dysplasia) requiring oxygen.

- *S. pneumoniae* is the most common cause of bacterial pneumonia in most age groups. *M. pneumoniae* and *C. pneumoniae* should be considered in older children and adolescents. The majority of large pleural effusions complicating pneumonia are caused by *S. aureus* pneumonia.

- Meningitis may be septic (bacterial) or aseptic. LP is invaluable in the diagnosis and development of a treatment strategy for meningitis. Appropriate empirical antibiotic choices for presumed bacterial meningitis are ampicillin and cefotaxime (in the neonate) and vancomycin and a third-generation cephalosporin (in the child).

- Infectious diarrhea may be bacterial, viral, parasitic, or toxin mediated. Children with shigellosis may present with mental status changes. *S. dysenteriae* and *E. coli* O157:H7 are associated with hemolytic uremic syndrome.

- Clinical signs of acute hepatitis include anorexia, nausea, malaise, vomiting, jaundice, dark urine, abdominal pain, and low-grade fever. However, a wide range of severity exists, and as many as 30% to 70% of infected children are asymptomatic. HAV and HEV are spread via fecal-oral transmission. HBV, HCV, and HDV are transmitted through infected bodily fluids. Liver enzymes are uniformly elevated in hepatitis. Because the clinical manifestations are so similar, specific serologic tests are indispensable for securing an accurate diagnosis.

- Syphilis may be transmitted transplacentally or sexually. Neonates with congenital syphilis present with snuffles, hepatosplenomegaly, mucocutaneous lesions, jaundice, and lymphadenopathy. The VDRL and RPR are excellent screening tests but may produce false positives. Parenteral penicillin G is the treatment of choice.

- The diagnosis of PID is clinical, based on history, physical examination, and supporting laboratory results.

KEY POINTS *(continued)*

- *C. trachomatis* and *N. gonorrhoeae* are the most commonly isolated organisms in PID. A single dose of a parenteral cephalosporin (for *N. gonorrhoeae*) and 14 days of oral doxycycline (for *C. trachomatis*) are appropriate outpatient therapy for mild PID.

- Most HIV infections in children are acquired in utero or perinatally. Infants born to HIV-positive mothers are seropositive for maternally derived IgG antibodies to HIV; thus, the ELISA and Western blot are not helpful in children younger than 18 months. The HIV DNA PCR should be used in this population.

- The classic presentation of RMSF includes fever, headache, and rash. The disease is rapidly progressive, and there is no laboratory test that becomes abnormal soon enough in the disease to guide therapy. Treatment (doxycycline) should be started based on clinical suspicion alone.

- The classic rash of Lyme disease is erythema migrans. Lyme disease is treated with oral amoxicillin in children younger than 8 years and with oral doxycycline in older children. Lyme meningitis requires intravenous ceftriaxone.

Neonatology

Bradley S. Marino • *Katelyn Mellion* • *James M. Greenberg*

BIRTH

NEONATAL MORTALITY

The late fetal and early neonatal period is the time of life exhibiting the highest mortality rate of any pediatric age interval. The **perinatal mortality rate** refers to fetal deaths occurring from the 20th week of gestation until the 7th day after birth. Intrauterine fetal death (i.e., stillbirth) represents 40% to 50% of the perinatal mortality rate.

The **neonatal mortality rate** includes infants who die between birth and 28 days of life. Modern neonatal intensive care has delayed the mortality of many newborn infants who have life-threatening diseases, so that they survive beyond the neonatal period only to die of their original diseases or of complications of therapy sometime after the 28th day of life. This delayed mortality occurs during the **postneonatal** period, which begins after 28 days of life and extends to the end of the first year of life.

The **infant mortality rate** includes both the neonatal and the postneonatal periods and is expressed as the number of deaths per 1,000 live births. The infant mortality rate in the United States declined in 2004 to 6.8 per 1,000 live births. The rate for African American infants in 2004 remained a distressing 13.2 per 1,000 live births. There were 28 countries with lower infant mortality rates than the United States in 2004.

APGAR SCORING

The Apgar score at 1 minute is reflective of the interuterine environment and birth process, whereas the 5-minute Apgar is more indicative of the neonate's success at transitioning. Table 13-1 shows the Apgar scoring system. At 1 and 5 minutes after birth, each of five physiologic parameters is evaluated. Full-term infants with a normal cardiopulmonary transition have a total score of 8 to 9 at 1 and 5 minutes. An Apgar score of 0 to 3 indicates either cardiorespiratory arrest or a condition resulting from metabolic acidosis, hypoventilation, and/or central nervous system (CNS) depression. Most low Apgar scores are caused by difficulty in establishing adequate ventilation, severe perinatal depression, or preexisting fetal problems such as hydrops, infection, or congenital malformations.

BIRTH TRAUMA

CEPHALOHEMATOMA

A cephalohematoma is a traumatic subperiosteal hemorrhage (usually involving the parietal bone) that does not cross suture lines. The scalp hematoma is characteristically fluctuant without discoloration of overlying skin and may not become apparent until hours to days after delivery. Predisposing factors include large head size, prolonged labor, vacuum extraction, and forceps delivery. Spontaneous resolution occurs over several weeks. Two percent of hematomas organize, calcify, and form a central depression in the calvarium. Cephalohematoma dissolution may promote an indirect hyperbilirubinemia requiring phototherapy, especially in a premature infant.

CAPUT SUCCEDANEUM

A caput succedaneum is a diffuse, edematous, and often dark swelling of the soft tissue of the scalp that

■ **TABLE 13-1** Apgar Scoring System

Physical Exam Evaluated at 1 and 5 Minutes	0 Points	1 Point	2 Points
Heart rate	Absent	<100	>100
Respiratory effort	Absent	Irregular, weak cry	Vigorous cry
Color	Pale, cyanotic	Cyanotic extremities	Pink throughout
Muscle tone	Absent	Weak, slightly flexed extremities	Active
Reflex irritability	Absent	Grimace	Active cry and avoidance

extends across the midline and/or suture lines and is commonly found in infants who are delivered vaginally in the customary occiput-anterior position. Pressure induced from overriding parietal and frontal bones against their respective sutures causes the molding associated with the caput. The caput is commonly seen after prolonged labor in both full-term and premature infants.

FRACTURED CLAVICLE

A fractured clavicle is found in 2% to 3% of vaginal deliveries. The right clavicle is two times more likely to fracture than the left. This predilection exists because the right shoulder must move beneath the pubic symphysis during normal delivery and may become entrapped. Predisposing factors include large size, shoulder dystocia, and traumatic delivery. On examination, there may be swelling and fullness over the fracture site, crepitus, and decreased arm movement. Of affected neonates, 80% have no symptoms and only minimal physical findings. The injury is often diagnosed when a callus is detected at 3 to 6 weeks of age. Radiographs are not indicated, and no specific treatment is necessary. The parents should be advised to avoid tension on the affected arm.

ERB PALSY

Injury to nerves of the brachial plexus results from excessive traction on the neck, producing paresis. Erb palsy results from stretching of the fifth and sixth cervical nerves. The infant's arm is held in the "waiter's tip" position, with the arm extended and internally rotated and the wrist flexed. When there is an absent Moro reflex in the right arm and the right hand grasp is intact, Erb palsy should be suspected.

Ninety percent of these lesions resolve spontaneously by 4 months of age, but if the deficit persists, nerve grafting may be beneficial.

PREMATURITY

Low-birth-weight (LBW) infants, defined as those having birth weights less than 2,500 g, represent a disproportionately large percentage of neonatal and infant deaths. Although these infants make up only 7% of all births, they account for two-thirds of all neonatal deaths. **Very low-birth-weight** (VLBW) infants, weighing less than 1,500 g at birth, represent approximately 1% of all births but account for 50% of neonatal deaths.

In contrast to the improvements in the overall infant mortality rate, there has not been improvement in the rate of LBW *births*. This is one reason that the infant mortality rate of the United States is the worst of the large, modern, industrialized countries. If birth-weight mortality rates are calculated, the United States has one of the highest survival rates, but because of the large number of LBW infants, the total infant mortality rate remains relatively high.

LBW is caused by premature birth or intrauterine growth retardation. Maternal factors associated with having an LBW infant include previous LBW birth, low socioeconomic status, low level of educational achievement, lack of prenatal care, maternal age younger than 16 years or older than 35 years, a short time interval between pregnancies, unmarried status, low prepregnancy weight (less than 100 lb), poor weight gain during pregnancy (less than 10 lb), maternal substance use, and African American race. Table 13-2 lists specific medical causes of preterm birth.

■ **TABLE 13-2** Medical Causes of Preterm Birth
Fetal
Fetal distress
Multiple gestations
Erythroblastosis fetalis
Nonimmune hydrops fetalis
Congenital anomalies
Placental
Placenta previa
Abruptio placenta
Uterine
Bicornuate uterus
Incompetent cervix
Maternal
Preeclampsia
Chronic medical illness
Infection (chorioamnionitis)
Drug abuse (esp. cocaine)
Other
Premature rupture of membranes
Polyhydramnios
Trauma
Diethylstilbestrol exposure

POSTMATURITY

Infants whose gestation exceeds 42 weeks are considered postmature and are at risk for the syndrome of postmaturity. The cause of prolonged pregnancy is not known in most cases.

Clinical Manifestations

The syndrome of postmaturity is characterized by normal length and head circumference but decreased weight. Infants with this syndrome are distinct from small for gestational age infants in that they were doing well until they went beyond 42 weeks' gestation and became nutritionally deprived from placental insufficiency. Common symptoms include dry, cracked, peeling, loose, and wrinkled skin and a malnourished appearance with decreased amounts of subcutaneous tissues. Conditions that appear more

commonly in postmature infants include meconium aspiration and depression at birth, persistent pulmonary hypertension of newborn (PPHN), hypoglycemia, hypocalcemia, and polycythemia.

Treatment

Fetal well-being can be monitored closely by ultrasound (US), biophysical profile, and nonstress tests. Induction of labor may be indicated if fetal well-being is compromised. Optimal intrapartum management requires delivery room preparation for management of an infant with perinatal depression and meconium aspiration. Early feeding to reduce the risk of hypoglycemia and evaluation for the conditions noted encompass postpartum treatment.

INTRAUTERINE PROBLEMS

SMALL FOR GESTATIONAL AGE

Pathogenesis and Clinical Manifestations

Infants who are **small for gestational age** (SGA) have birth weights below the 10th percentile for gestational age. The term "small for gestational age" is merely descriptive and includes normal infants who followed a stable growth curve through fetal development and infants who suffered intrauterine growth retardation (IUGR) at some point in utero. Two broad categories of IUGR are described: early onset and late onset. A third of LBW neonates—infants weighing less than 2,500 g—are SGA.

Early-onset (**symmetrical**) IUGR is thought to result from an insult that begins before 28 weeks' gestation. The early insult results in a neonate whose head circumference and height are proportionately sized and whose weight-for-height ratio is relatively normal. This pattern is seen in infants whose mothers have severe vascular disease with hypertension and renal disease or in infants with congenital malformations or chromosomal abnormalities.

Late-onset, or asymmetric, IUGR starts after 28 weeks' gestation. These infants usually have a normal head circumference with a reduced length and weight. The weight-for-height ratio is low, and the infant appears long and emaciated. In this type of IUGR, the neonate initially follows a normal percentile line, then falls off the curve late in gestation when placental function fails to keep up with fetal requirements for growth.

Risk Factors

Potential causes of IUGR are delineated in Table 13-3.

Delivery of SGA infants should take place at a center with a high-risk nursery because infants who are very small for gestational age are at risk for life-threatening problems at the time of delivery. The delivery team should be prepared for perinatal asphyxia and/or depression, and hypothermia. Examination of the placenta after delivery for pathology consistent with congenital infection or infarction may be helpful in determining the cause of the IUGR. The newborn that is small for gestational age should be monitored for hypothermia, hypoglycemia, hypocalcemia, hyponatremia, polycythemia, pulmonary hemorrhage, and persistent pulmonary hypertension. Commencing feedings as soon as possible minimizes hypoglycemia.

LARGE FOR GESTATIONAL AGE

Infants whose weights are greater than 2 standard deviations above the mean or above the 90th percentile are defined as **large for gestational** age (LGA). Neonates at risk for being LGA are those of diabetic mothers (class A, B, or C); postmature infants; and neonates with transposition of the great vessels, erythroblastosis fetalis, or Beckwith-Wiedemann syndrome. Most LGA infants are constitutionally large (from large parents or a family with a predilection for large infants). After birth, the infant should be evaluated for the disorders described previously, as well as birth trauma, which is more common in LGA neonates. The blood sugar of the LGA infant should be monitored and the child fed early because LGA infants are prone to hypoglycemia. A hematocrit should be obtained because LGA neonates have an increased incidence of polycythemia.

Macrosomic neonates have birth weights greater than 4,000 g. All macrosomic infants are LGA, but not all LGA neonates are macrosomic. Macrosomic infants have an increased risk of shoulder dystocia and other birth trauma. Conditions such as maternal diabetes mellitus, obesity, and postmaturity are associated with an increased incidence of macrosomia.

■ TABLE 13-3 Causes of IUGR	
Fetal causes	Multiple gestation
	Congenital viral infections
	Chromosomal abnormalities (trisomies or Turner syndrome)
	Congenital malformation syndromes (especially CNS)
Placental causes	Chorionic villitis
	Chronic abruption placentae
	Twin-twin transfusion
	Placental tumor
	Placental insufficiency secondary to maternal vascular disease
Maternal causes	Severe peripheral vascular diseases that reduce uterine blood flow
	Chronic hypertension
	Diabetic vasculopathy
	Preeclampsia
	Sickle cell anemia
	Cardiac disease
	Renal disease
	Reduced nutritional intake
	Alcohol or drug abuse
	Cigarette smoking
	Uterine anomalies
	Uterine constraint (noted in mothers of small stature and reduced weight gain during pregnancy)

POLYHYDRAMNIOS

Polyhydramnios is defined as an amniotic fluid volume greater than 2 L; it occurs in 1 in 1,000 births. Acute polyhydramnios is associated with premature labor, maternal discomfort, and respiratory compromise. More often polyhydramnios is chronic, seen with gestational diabetes, immune or nonimmune hydrops fetalis, abdominal wall defects (omphalocele and gastroschisis), multiple gestations, trisomy 18 or 21, neural tube defects, and certain congenital anomalies of the GI tract. Anencephaly and meningomyelocele are neural tube defects that impair fetal swallowing, whereas esophageal or duodenal atresia, diaphragmatic hernia, and cleft palate interfere with swallowing and GI fluid dynamics.

OLIGOHYDRAMNIOS

Oligohydramnios is associated with IUGR, amniotic fluid leak, postmaturity, and congenital anomalies of the fetal kidneys. Bilateral renal agenesis results in **Potter syndrome**, characterized by clubbed feet, compressed facies, low-set ears, scaphoid abdomen, and diminished chest wall size accompanied by pulmonary hypoplasia. Uterine compression in the absence of amniotic fluid retards lung growth. Patients with this condition expire of respiratory failure rather than renal insufficiency. Oligohydramnios increases the risk of fetal distress during labor. This risk may be reduced by normal saline amnioinfusion during labor.

CONGENITAL INFECTIONS

Infections of the fetus during the first, second, or early third trimester are referred to as **congenital infections**. There are many similarities in the congenital syndromes, so focusing on the differences can help refine the evaluation. Table 13-4 summarizes disease, causative agent, clinical manifestations, diagnostic evaluation, and treatment.

NEONATAL INFECTION

NEONATAL SEPSIS

Neonatal sepsis is generally divided into early-onset, late-onset, and nosocomial sepsis. **Early-onset** sepsis, occurring from birth to 3 days, can be an overwhelming multiorgan systemic disease manifested by respiratory failure, shock, meningitis (30%), dis-

seminated intravascular coagulation (DIC), and acute tubular necrosis. Early-onset sepsis is caused by infection with bacteria residing in the mother's genitourinary tract. Organisms causing early-onset sepsis include group B streptococcus, *Escherichia coli* (*E. coli*), *Klebsiella* species, and *Listeria monocytogenes*. Administration of intrapartum penicillin to a colonized mother can reduce the risk of early-onset group B streptococci disease. Predisposing factors for early-onset sepsis include prolonged rupture of the membranes (>24 hours), chorioamnionitis, maternal fever or leukocytosis, fetal tachycardia, and preterm birth. African American race and male sex are unexplained additional risk factors for neonatal sepsis.

Late-onset sepsis, occurring between days 3 and 28, often occurs in a full-term infant who was discharged in good health from the normal newborn nursery. Bacteremia leads to hematogenous seeding that results in focal infections such as meningitis (75%, usually caused by group B streptococci or *E. coli*); osteomyelitis (group B streptococci and *Staphylococcus aureus* [*S. aureus*]); arthritis (*Neisseria gonorrhoeae*, *S. aureus*, *Candida albicans*, gram-negative bacteremia); and urinary tract infection (gram-negative bacteremia).

Nosocomially acquired sepsis (occurring between day 3 and discharge) occurs predominantly among premature infants in the newborn intensive care unit (NICU) because many of these infants have been colonized with the multidrug-resistant bacteria indigenous to the NICU. Frequent treatment with broad-spectrum antibiotics for sepsis and the presence of central venous indwelling catheters, endotracheal tubes, umbilical vessel catheters, and electronic monitoring devices increase the risk for such serious bacterial or fungal infections. The most common pathogens are *S. aureus*, *Staphylococcus epidermidis*, gram-negative bacteria, and *Candida albicans*.

The incidence of group B streptococcal disease has dramatically decreased since the institution of maternal screening protocols and intrapartum antibiotic regimens in culture-positive mothers. Group B streptococci are recovered from the vaginal cultures of approximately 20% of American women at the time of delivery.

Clinical Manifestations

Most infants with early-onset sepsis present with nonspecific cardiorespiratory signs such as grunting, tachypnea, and cyanosis at birth. As a result, it is often hard to differentiate early-onset sepsis from respiratory distress syndrome (RDS) in the preterm

TABLE 13-4 Congenital and Neonatal Infections

Disease / Causative Agent	Clinical Manifestations During the Neonatal Period	Diagnostic Evaluation	Treatment	Miscellaneous
Toxoplasmosis *Toxoplasma gondii*	Maculopapular rash Generalized lymphadenopathy Hepatosplenomegaly Jaundice Thrombocytopenia Secondary to in utero meningoencephalitis: Hydrocephalus with generalized calcifications Microcephaly Chorioretinitis Seizures	Congenital infection confirmed by persistently positive IgG and IgM antibody titres in the infant Ophthalmologic, auditory, neurologic examinations with lumbar puncture and head CT	Pyrimethamine and sulfadiazine Corticosteroids (for ocular and CNS disease)	Infected cats excrete toxoplasma oocytes in their stool, resulting in fecal–oral transmission to humans Only primary infection of the mother, which is usually asymptomatic, results in congenital infection. Infants with congenital infection are asymptomatic in 70% to 90% of cases **Prevention:** Ingestion of well-cooked meat Avoidance of cat defecation
Syphilis *Treponema pallidum*	Hepatosplenomegaly Persistent rhinitis (snuffles) Lymphadenopathy Mucocutaneous lesions Osteochondritis and pseudoparalysis Eczematoid skin rash Hemolytic anemia Thrombocytopenia	Nontreponemal test such as RPR or VDRL, supported by treponemal test such as IgM FTA-ABS	Penicillin	Syphilis results from transplacental transmission of *Treponema pallidum* in utero Syphilis in the untreated pregnant woman may be transmitted to the fetus at any time, but fetal transfer is more likely during the first year of maternal infection
Rubella *Rubella virus*	Ophthalmologic: Cataracts Pigmentary retinopathy Microphthalmia Congenital glaucoma Auditory: Sensorineural hearing impairment Cardiac: Patent ductus arteriosus Peripheral pulmonary artery stenosis	Presence of *Rubella*-specific IgM or rising IgG titre Ophthalmologic, Auditory, cardiac, dermatologic examination	No specific antiviral chemotherapy Appropriate treatment of specific defects is recommended	Congenital rubella syndrome results from transplacental transmission of Rubella virus Congenital rubella syndrome has become rare, reflecting the success of the rubella vaccine Vaccination should not be given during pregnancy (inadvertent administration carries a very low risk of fetal disease) Infants considered contagious until 1 year of age

	Skin: Dermal Erythropoiesis "Blueberry muffin" spots; Intrauterine growth retardation; Hepatomegaly; Thrombocytopenia; Interstitial pneumonitis; Radiolucent bone disease			
Neonatal Cytomegalovirus Infection *Cytomegalovirus (CMV)*	Central nervous system (CNS): Microcephaly; Intracerebral calcifications; Retinitis; Intrauterine growth retardation; Jaundice; Thrombocytopenia; Hepatosplenomegaly	CMV culture positive from urine, stool, respiratory tract secretions, or CSF obtained within 3 weeks of birth; Positive CMV-specific IgM; Neurologic evaluation with head CT and brain MRI is recommended	Although ganciclovir has been used to treat some infected neonates and infants, it is not routinely recommended because of insufficient efficacy data; Newborn hearing screening by brainstem auditory evoked responses is important; Repeated evaluations are imperative; Pregnant healthcare workers should not take care of infected infants	Neonatal cytomegalovirus (CMV) infection is common, and results from transplacental transmission, inoculation during passage through the vaginal canal, or via the ingestion of infected breast milk. It occurs in 1% of newborns in the United States; Most cases of congenital CMV are asymptomatic with no sequelae; Approximately 10% of the infants with congenital CMV manifest significant infection with neurological morbidity
Neonatal Herpes Simplex Virus (HSV) Infection	Disseminated disease involving multiple organs, most prominently liver and lungs	Positive viral cultures from CSF, skin vesicles, conjunctivae, urine, blood, mouth, nasopharynx, and/or rectum	Antiviral therapy with acyclovir	Most neonatal HSV infection is caused by HSV-2 because it accounts for the majority of genital herpes
Herpes Simplex Virus –1.	Localized CNS disease with or without seizures			The child is infected as he or she moves through the vaginal canal. The majority of neonatal herpes is therefore a result of perinatal infection, and true congenital herpes is rare
Herpes Simplex Virus –2.	Localized disease to the skin, eye, and mouth	Positive HSV PCR of CSF		The risk of HSV infection at delivery for an infant born vaginally to a mother with primary genital infection is estimated to be 33% to 50%
	Approximately 1/3 of patients present with disseminated disease, 1/3 with localized CNS disease, and 1/3 with localized skin, eye, and mouth disease			

continues

■ TABLE 13-4 Congenital and Neonatal Infections *(continued)*

Disease Causative Agent	Clinical Manifestations During the Neonatal Period	Diagnostic Evaluation	Treatment	Miscellaneous
				The risk of HSV infection at delivery for an infant born vaginally to a mother shedding HSV as a result of reactivation infection is less than 5%.
				Most neonatal herpetic infection is severe with a high mortality and morbidity rate
Varicella-zoster infection (congenital varicella syndrome and neonatal chickenpox)	Congenital varicella syndrome (<20 weeks gestation - varicella embryopathy) Limb hypoplasia Cutaneous scarring Eye abnormalities CNS damage	Tissue culture using vesicular fluid, CSF, or biopsy tissue PCR using vesicular swabs, scabs from lesions, biopsy tissue or CSF	Infants with congenital varicella do not require isolation Infants with neonatal varicella should be placed in strict isolation for at least 7 days after the onset of rash	Varicella virus infection in the neonate results from transplacental transmission of varicella-zoster virus in utero The incidence of congenital varicella syndrome among infants born to mothers with varicella infection before 20 weeks gestation is 1% to 2%
Varicella-zoster virus (VZV)	Neonatal chickenpox (≥20 weeks gestation) Generalized, pruritic, vesicular rash Bacterial superinfection of skin lesions Pneumonia CNS involvement (cerebellar ataxia and encephalitis) Thrombocytopenia		Infants born to mothers with onset of varicella 5 or more days before delivery require no specific treatment other than isolation, if kept in the hospital Infants whose mothers have onset of varicella within 5 days before delivery, or within 2 days after delivery, should receive varicella-zoster immune globulin (VZIG), preferably at birth or within 96 hours Infants with acute varicella in the first week of life should receive acyclovir for 10 days	Varicella exposure during the second 20 weeks of gestation may result in inapparent varicella and subsequent zoster later in life, without having any extrauterine varicella manifestations Ninety percent of women of childbearing age are immune to varicella-zoster virus (VZV), so congenital and neonatal varicella are rare

				Infants who are exposed to VZV infection as a result of contact with nursery personnel should have their immune status verified and, if susceptible, they should receive VZIG within 96 hours of exposure
Human immunodeficiency virus infection *Human immunodeficiency virus (HIV)*	HIV infection of the infant is generally asymptomatic during the neonatal period	The preferred test is HIV-1 PCR assay of DNA extracted from peripheral blood mononuclear cells	Antiretroviral therapy. Consultation with an expert. Treatment strategies that may decrease mother-to-child transmission of HIV in two-thirds of cases include: 1. Oral administration of zidovudine to pregnant women with HIV infection beginning at 14 to 34 weeks' gestation and continuing throughout pregnancy 2. Intravenous administration of zidovudine during labor until delivery 3. Oral administration of zidovudine to the infant for the first 6 weeks of life	Human immunodeficiency virus infection in the neonate results from transplacental transmission of HIV in utero Eighty percent of pediatric AIDS cases result from maternal transmission. Postnatal transmission of HIV from infected mothers through breast milk to infants who were not infected perinatally occurs in 15% of infants HIV may cause acquired immunodeficiency syndrome HIV is particularly tropic for cells expressing CD4 including helper T cells, monocytes, and macrophages. It is the infection and destruction of these cells that cause immunodeficiency

neonate. Because of this difficulty, most premature infants with RDS receive broad-spectrum antibiotics. Common signs and symptoms of early sepsis include poor feeding, emesis, lethargy, apnea, ileus, and abdominal distention. Petechiae and purpura are noted when DIC is present. Meningitis is present in 25% of neonates with late-onset sepsis.

Infants with suspected early-onset sepsis should have blood and CSF sent for culture. CSF should also be tested for Gram stain, cell count and differential, and protein and glucose levels. A white blood cell count less than 5,000 or greater than 40,000, a total neutrophil count under 1,000, and a ratio of bands to neutrophils of greater than 20% all correlate with an increased risk of bacterial infection. Thrombocytopenia may also be seen. The chest radiograph is used to determine the presence of pneumonia. Arterial blood gases (ABGs) may be indicated to manage hypoxemia and metabolic acidosis associated with shock. Blood pressure, urine output, central venous pressure, and peripheral perfusion are monitored to determine the need to treat septic shock with fluids and vasopressor agents.

The clinical manifestations of late-onset sepsis are nonspecific and include lethargy, poor feeding, hypotonia, apathy, seizures, bulging fontanelle, fever, and direct hyperbilirubinemia. The evaluation for late-onset sepsis is similar to that for early-onset sepsis, with special attention given to examination of the bones, the laboratory values, and urine culture obtained by sterile suprapubic aspiration or urethral catheterization. Late-onset sepsis may be caused by the same pathogens as early-onset sepsis or those usually found in the older infant (*Streptococcus pneumoniae, Neisseria meningitidis*).

The initial clinical manifestations of nosocomial infection in the premature neonate may be subtle and include apnea and bradycardia, temperature instability, abdominal distention, and poor feeding. In the later stages, there may be severe metabolic acidosis, shock, DIC, and respiratory failure.

Treatment

A combination of ampicillin and gentamicin for 10 to 14 days remains the most effective treatment against most organisms responsible for early sepsis. Once an organism is identified and antibiotic sensitivities are determined, antibiotic therapy may be tailored to treat the infecting organism. If meningitis is present, the treatment is extended, and a third-generation cephalosporin is recommended for improved penetration across the blood–brain barrier. Cefotaxime and an aminoglycoside antibiotic such as amikacin (for synergy) are used to treat *E. coli* or *Klebsiella* meningitis. Sepsis resulting from group B streptococcal meningitis or *Listeria* is treated with ampicillin and gentamicin (for synergy). The treatment of late-onset neonatal sepsis and meningitis is the same as that for early-onset sepsis.

The treatment of nosocomially acquired sepsis depends on the indigenous microbiologic flora of the particular hospital and their antibiotic sensitivities. Because *S. aureus* (sometimes methicillin-resistant), coagulase-negative *Staphylococcus* species (usually methicillin-resistant), and gram-negative pathogens are the most common bacterial nosocomial infections, a combination of vancomycin and gentamicin may be warranted. Persistent signs of infection despite antibacterial treatment suggest candidal (fungal) sepsis, which is treated with amphotericin B.

CHLAMYDIA INFECTION

Chlamydia trachomatis is transmitted from the genital tract of infected mothers to their newborn infants. Acquisition occurs in approximately 50% of infants born vaginally to infected mothers. Of the infants who acquire *C. trachomatis*, the risk of conjunctivitis is 25% to 50%, and the risk of pneumonia is 5% to 20%. The nasopharynx is the most commonly infected anatomic site. A symptomatic infection of the conjunctiva, pharynx, rectum, or vagina of the infant can persist for more than 2 years. Prevalence among pregnant women varies between 6% and 12% in most populations.

Clinical Manifestations

In neonatal chlamydial conjunctivitis, ocular congestion, edema, and discharge develop a few days to several weeks after birth and last for 1 to 2 weeks.

Pneumonia in young infants caused by *C. trachomatis* is usually an afebrile illness that presents between 3 and 19 weeks after birth. A repetitive, staccato cough and tachypnea are characteristic but not always present. Crackles can be present, whereas wheezing is less likely. Hyperinflation on chest radiograph is prominent. Untreated disease can linger or recur.

Treatment

Topical erythromycin may be instilled into the eye at birth to prevent gonococcal ophthalmia, but this treatment will not reliably prevent neonatal chlamydial pneumonia. Chlamydial conjunctivitis and pneumonia in young infants are treated with oral erythromycin for 14 days. Topical treatment of conjunctivitis is ineffective and unnecessary. The efficacy of erythromycin therapy is only 80%, so a second course is sometimes required. A specific diagnosis of *C. trachomatis* infection in the infant should prompt treatment of the mother and evaluation of her sexual partner.

NEONATAL RESPIRATORY DISEASE

RESPIRATORY DISTRESS SYNDROME

Pathogenesis

Respiratory distress syndrome (RDS), or hyaline membrane disease, is the most common cause of respiratory failure in newborn infants. It occurs predominantly in premature infants who are born with immature lungs. In the average child, lung maturity is attained at 32 to 43 weeks' gestation, when pulmonary **surfactant**, a complex phospholipid and protein mixture that lines the alveoli, is produced by the type II pneumocytes. RDS is caused by a deficiency of surfactant. The major function of surfactant is to decrease alveolar surface tension and increase lung compliance. Surfactant prevents alveolar collapse at the end of expiration and allows for opening of the alveoli at low intrathoracic pressures.

Surfactant deficiency causes poor compliance, leading to progressive atelectasis, intrapulmonary shunting, hypoxemia, and cyanosis. The forces generated by mechanical ventilation, oxygen exposure, and alveolar capillary leak result in formation of a hyaline membrane. This membrane, composed of protein and sloughed alveolar epithelium, lines the alveolar ducts. The incidence of RDS increases with decreasing gestational age. Measurement of amniotic fluid lecithin-to-sphingomyelin ratio and phosphatidylglycerol content can be used to predict lung maturity.

The production of surfactant is accelerated by maternal antenatal steroid administration. Prolonged rupture of fetal membranes, maternal narcotic addiction, preeclampsia, chronic fetal stress, maternal hyperthyroidism, and theophylline are also associated with accelerated lung maturation. The production of surfactant is delayed by combined fetal hyperglycemia and hyperinsulinemia, as occurs in maternal diabetes.

Clinical Manifestations

Affected premature infants characteristically present with tachypnea, grunting, nasal flaring, chest wall retractions, and cyanosis in the first few hours of life. There is poor air entry on auscultation. The amniotic fluid lecithin-to-sphingomyelin ratio is less than 2, and phosphatidylglycerol is absent in the amniotic fluid. Diagnosis is confirmed by chest radiograph that reveals a uniform **reticulonodular or ground-glass** pattern and air bronchograms that are consistent with diffuse atelectasis.

The natural course is a progressive worsening over the first 24 to 48 hours of life. After the initial insult to the airway lining, the epithelium is repopulated with type II alveolar cells, which produce surfactant. Subsequently, there is increased production and release of surfactant, so there is a sufficient quantity in the air spaces by 72 hours of life. This results in improved lung compliance and resolution of respiratory distress, which is frequently heralded by an increase in urine output.

Acute complications associated with RDS include pulmonary interstitial emphysema, pneumothorax, pneumomediastinum, and pneumopericardium. Rupture of the alveolar epithelial lining produces pulmonary interstitial emphysema as air dissects along the interstitial spaces and the peribronchial lymphatics. Extravasation of gas into the lung parenchyma reduces lung compliance and worsens respiratory failure.

Treatment

Surfactant is the primary therapy for RDS; respiratory support is necessary but adjunctive. Therapy with artificial surfactant improves RDS dramatically and significantly decreases the rate of neonatal mortality in premature infants. After surfactant administration, the FiO_2 may be lowered to nontoxic levels ($<60\%$ FiO_2). As surfactant therapy improves the compliance of the lungs ventilator parameters may be weaned to avoid overdistention and ventilator-induced lung injury. When amniotic fluid assessment of the premature infant reveals fetal lung immaturity and preterm delivery cannot be prevented, administration of corticosteroids to the mother 48 hours before delivery can induce or accelerate the production of fetal surfactant and minimize the incidence of RDS. Conventional respiratory therapy for the infant with RDS includes support with oxygen via nasal cannula, continuous positive airway pressure (CPAP), and/or mechanical ventilation. CPAP is useful in treating apnea that is unresponsive to nasal cannula stimulation and during the weaning process after extubation.

Very premature neonates who require mechanical ventilation for long periods of time are at risk for alveolar rupture and the development of pulmonary interstitial emphysema, pneumothorax, pneumomediastinum, and/or pneumopericardium. The risk of lung injury increases as the duration of mechanical ventilation, mean airway pressure, and the intermittent mandatory ventilation rate increase. When RDS is very severe, pulmonary hypertension may occur, causing a right-to-left shunt at the patent foramen ovale and the ductus arteriosus. Infants with respiratory distress deserve evaluation for sepsis and pneumonia which may mimic RDS on clinical presentation and chest radiograph. Until blood culture results are known, antibiotics are recommended. Intraventricular hemorrhage and necrotizing enterocolitis (NEC) are more likely to occur in the neonate with RDS.

Bronchopulmonary dysplasia (BPD), which is also referred to as chronic lung disease of prematurity, is the most common chronic lung disease of childhood. BPD most commonly affects those infants with very low birth weight born at less than 26 weeks' gestation. Infants meet diagnostic criteria for BPD if they require oxygen therapy for at least 28 days and fail a room air challenge test at 36 weeks postmenstrual age. Depending on the oxygen requirement and the need for ventilatory support, patients are classified as having mild, moderate, or severe BPD. The etiology of BPD is multifactorial. The major abnormality is **arrested alveolar development** resulting in a decreased number of alveoli or "alveolar hypoplasia." Alveoli are large and mature appearing but are decreased in number. Factors that may contribute to the diminished number of alveoli include host susceptibility and genetic predisposing factors, oxygen toxicity, chronic inflammation, neonatal infection, ventilation with volutrauma, the pulmonary edema associated with a patent ductus arteriosus, and poor nutrition. Complications include chronic respiratory insufficiency, requiring home use of continuous oxygen therapy, diuretics, and bronchodilators; right-sided congestive heart failure secondary to pulmonary hypertension; and pneumothorax. Weaning the infant off oxygen to room air can take several months. Reactive airway disease is a common long-term sequela of BPD and can be severe. Sudden infant death syndrome (SIDS) is more common in infants

with BPD. Lower respiratory infections caused by usually benign viral agents, most notably RSV, may cause severe respiratory distress. Some infants recover fully, but the healing process takes years.

MECONIUM ASPIRATION

Pathogenesis

The clinical significance of meconium-stained amniotic fluid and the pathogenesis of meconium aspiration syndrome have evolved over time. Meconium is present in the fetal intestine by the second trimester. Maturation of intestinal smooth muscle and the myenteric plexus progresses through the third trimester. Thus intrauterine passage of meconium is unusual before 36 weeks, and does not typically occur for several days following preterm delivery. The potential for intrauterine meconium passage increases with each week of gestation thereafter. The physiologic stimuli for passage of meconium are still incompletely understood. Clinical experience and epidemiologic data suggests that a stressed fetus can also pass meconium prior to birth. Infants born through meconium-stained amniotic fluid have lower pH and are likely to have nonreassuring fetal heart tracings. Meconium-stained amniotic fluid at delivery is common with a reported incidence ranging from 12% to 15% of all deliveries. In addition to post-term gestation, African-American infants have a higher incidence.

Meconium aspiration syndrome is a clinical diagnosis that, by definition, includes delivery through meconium-stained amniotic fluid along with respiratory distress and a characteristic chest radiograph (air trapping and patchy atelectasis). Meconium aspiration syndrome ranges in severity. The hallmark of severe disease is that it requires management with positive pressure ventilation and is complicated by pulmonary hypertension. Severe meconium aspiration is associated with significant mortality and morbidity risk, including air leak, chronic lung disease, and developmental delay.

Over the past decade, the supposed pathophysiologic relationship between meconium-stained amniotic fluid and meconium aspiration syndrome has been called into question. Several controlled studies have failed to demonstrate the value of time-honored interventions such as tracheal suctioning and amnioinfusion to reduce the incidence of meconium aspiration syndrome in infants born through meconium-stained amniotic fluid.

Risk Factors

The risk of meconium aspiration is markedly increased in postmature infants and neonates who suffer from IUGR. Both have placental insufficiency as a common pathway for fetal hypoxia.

Clinical Manifestations

Meconium aspiration syndrome is characterized by tachypnea, hypoxia, and hypercapnia. Diagnosis is established by the presence of meconium in the tracheal or amniotic fluid, combined with symptoms of respiratory distress and a chest radiograph that reveals a pattern of diffuse infiltrates with hyperinflation. However, identical symptoms have been observed in infants born through clear amniotic fluid. Of infants with severe meconium aspiration syndrome, 10% develop pneumothoraces.

Treatment

In pregnancies in which uteroplacental insufficiency is either documented or suspected, tests of fetal well-being, such as the nonstress test, biophysical profile, fetal monitoring, and scalp pH sampling, help identify those infants at high risk for meconium aspiration.

When meconium is noted, the obstetrician suctions the oropharynx before delivery of the thorax (and the first intake of breath). After delivery, the infant who appears vigorous immediately upon delivery does not require intubation, but should have routine suctioning of the oropharynx.

If meconium or other material obstructs the airway, suctioning should be employed. However, suctioning of the oropharynax and/or trachea in the unobstructed airway, thereby delaying initiation of effective ventilation, may be deleterious. After suctioning the infant with poor respiratory effort, bag-valve mask should be initiated with or without intubation of the trachea.

If aspiration has occurred and the infant is in distress, therapy consists of administration of oxygen and/or mechanical ventilation. Because meconium inactivates endogenous surfactant, surfactant administration may be beneficial. Although the exact mechanism is unclear, surfactant administration reduces ventilation-perfusion mismatch and probably reduces the risk of ventilator-associated lung injury. The severity of disease is related to the amount of meconium the infant has aspirated and the severity of the related pulmonary hypertension. For persistent hypoxia (PaO_2 <50 mm Hg) or severe hypercapnia (PCO_2 >60 mm Hg), intubation and mechanical ventilation are indicated. Some neonates with severe PPHN and hypoxemia may require high-frequency oscillation and/or extracorporeal membrane oxygenation (ECMO).

Treatment of severe meconium aspiration syndrome has dramatically improved in recent years, leading to decreases in morbidity and mortality. The most significant advance centers on the treatment of pulmonary hypertension with selective pulmonary vasodilators (e.g., inhaled nitric oxide). These agents not only improve oxygenation, but also allow less injurious ventilator strategies with less subsequent morbidity from air leak and chronic lung disease. Exogenous surfactant administration is another useful treatment modality.

PERSISTENT PULMONARY HYPERTENSION OF THE NEWBORN

Pathogenesis

PPHN, or persistent fetal circulation, is a disorder of term or post-term infants who have experienced acute or chronic hypoxia in utero. The primary abnormality is the failure of the pulmonary vasculature resistance to fall with postnatal lung expansion and oxygenation. At birth, the systemic vascular resistance normally rises as a result of cessation of blood flow through the placenta, and pulmonary vascular resistance decreases after the first few breaths. With persistence of the fetal circulation, the pulmonary vascular resistance continues to be high and may in fact exceed the systemic resistance. This results in shunting of the deoxygenated blood, which is returning to the right atrium, away from the lungs. The right-to-left shunt can occur at the foramen ovale, the ductus arteriosus, or both. Because the lungs are bypassed, the blood is not oxygenated and hypoxemia ensues. The hypoxemia and acidosis caused by the right-to-left shunt only worsens the baseline pulmonary arteriolar hypertension, resulting in a vicious cycle of increasingly severe pulmonary arteriolar hypertension and cyanosis culminating in cardiopulmonary failure.

Risk Factors

PPHN is associated with meconium aspiration, severe RDS, diaphragmatic hernia, pulmonary hypoplasia, neonatal pneumonia sepsis, and Down syndrome.

Clinical Manifestations

The diagnosis is suggested by a history of perinatal hypoxia and rapidly progressive cyanosis associated with mild to severe respiratory distress. Often the clinical severity of pulmonary insufficiency is greater than the findings on chest radiograph; the chest radiograph may be normal or abnormal depending on the specific cause of the PPHN. Echocardiography reveals absence of structural heart disease, evidence of increased pulmonary vascular resistance, and the presence of right-to-left shunting at the foramen ovale, ductus arteriosus, or both. The severity varies from mild disease with spontaneous resolution to death from intractable hypoxemia. Pulmonary hypertension usually resolves within 3 to 7 days after birth.

Treatment

Treatment focuses on maximizing oxygen delivery and decreasing pulmonary arteriolar hypertension.

Conditions that potentiate PPHN include hypoxia, acidosis, hypoglycemia, hyperviscosity, anemia, and systemic hypotension. The therapies used to treat PPHN combat the conditions that worsen pulmonary hypertension and include supplemental oxygen, hyperventilation, and administration of sodium bicarbonate, pulmonary vasodilators, and support of systemic blood pressure.

Inhaled nitric oxide is now the cornerstone of treatment for PPHN. Nitric oxide relaxes pulmonary arteriolar smooth muscle cells leading to pulmonary vasodilatation. Sedation facilitates relaxation of the infant and pulmonary vasodilatation. The overall mortality rate associated with PPHN is 25% in term infants. Infants who require very high ventilator settings have a high mortality rate and may benefit from ECMO, which improves outcomes in the group of most severely ill patients.

NEONATAL GASTROINTESTINAL DISEASE

HYPERBILIRUBINEMIA

Bilirubin is a bile pigment formed from the degradation of heme that is derived from red blood cell (RBC) destruction and ineffective erythropoiesis. Figure 13-1 illustrates normal bilirubin metabolism. Abnormalities in any step in the process may result in hyperbilirubinemia.

Hyperbilirubinemia manifests as jaundice—a yellowing of the skin, mucous membranes, and sclera. Jaundice becomes clinically apparent when serum bilirubin levels are greater than 5 mg/dL in neonates and greater than 2 mg/dL in children and adolescents. The two types of hyperbilirubinemia are **unconjugated** (indirect), which can be physiologic or pathologic in origin, and **conjugated** (direct), which is always pathologic. Conjugated hyperbilirubinemia exists when the direct fraction of bilirubin in the blood exceeds 2 mg/dL or 15% of the total bilirubin.

Neonatal hyperbilirubinemia is monitored with great care, because elevated levels of unconjugated bilirubin cause kernicterus. Unconjugated bilirubin is normally bound tightly to albumin in the blood, but at high levels the unconjugated bilirubin exceeds the binding capacity of albumin, allowing free bilirubin to cross the blood–brain barrier. In premature infants, much lower levels of bilirubin may result in kernicterus because the blood–brain barrier is more permeable. Kernicterus is characterized by a yellow staining of the basal ganglia and hippocampus, resulting in widespread cerebral dysfunction. Clinical features include lethargy and irritability, hypotonia, opisthotonos, seizures, mental retardation, cerebral palsy, and hearing loss.

Most full-term and preterm neonates develop a transient, unconjugated hyperbilirubinemia during the first week of life. This **physiologic jaundice** is caused by an elevated bilirubin load (secondary to an increased RBC volume, decreased RBC survival time, and increased enterohepatic circulation); limited hepatic uptake of bilirubin; inadequate bilirubin conjugation caused by decreased UDP glucuronyltransferase activity; and reduced bilirubin excretion. Physiologic jaundice begins after 24 hours of life, is associated with a peak of 12 to 15 mg/dL at 3 to 5 days of life, and returns to normal levels by 10 to 14 days of life. Risk factors for developing more severe physiologic jaundice include prematurity, maternal diabetes, and Asian or Native American ancestry, male gender, exclusive breastfeeding, and diminished intake.

The mechanism of **breast milk jaundice**, which is also quite common, is not completely understood. Some researchers have theorized that it is caused by an increase in enterohepatic circulation from an unknown maternal factor in breast milk. The infant's peak bilirubin level tends to be higher and lasts longer than that found with physiologic jaundice.

Infants who develop jaundice in the first 24 hours of life, have an increase in serum bilirubin greater than 0.5 mg/dL/hr, have risk factors noted earlier,

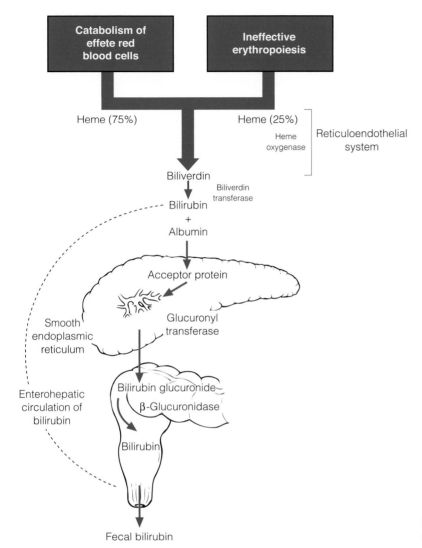

Figure 13-1 • Bilirubin metabolism in the neonate.

have prolonged jaundice (more than 1 week in the full-term infant or more than 2 weeks in the premature neonate), or have conjugated hyperbilirubinemia need to be evaluated. The differential diagnosis of hyperbilirubinemia is delineated in Table 13-5.

Clinical Manifestations

History

Feeding history, including breast or formula feeding, volumes taken per feed, and duration of feeding are key points. Other important clues include a family history of red cell structural defects, hemoglobinopathies, or enzyme deficiencies, or a previous child who had ABO incompatibility. Prenatal screens should be reviewed for possible indications of congenital infection. The length of time the jaundice has

been present, whether it is worsening or improving, and associated GI or constitutional symptoms should be explored. Also, it is important to ask whether the stool color has changed (to a gray color) or the urine has darkened.

Physical Examination

In neonates, jaundice tends to progress in a cephalopedal sequence. Therefore, those infants with clinically apparent jaundice below the umbilicus are likely to have higher levels than those with only facial jaundice.

Diagnostic Evaluation

Infants with clinical jaundice should have a serum bilirubin measurement. Maternal and infant blood

■ TABLE 13-5 Differential Diagnosis of Hyperbilirubinemia

Unconjugated hyperbilirubinemia	Physiologic jaundice
	Hemolytic process
	Immune etiology
	ABO/Rh incompatibility
	Erythroblastosis fetalis
	Drug reaction (penicillin, sulfonamides, oxytocin)
	Red cell defects
	Structural (spherocytosis, elliptocytosis)
	Hemoglobinopathy (sickle cell, α-thalassemia)
	Enzyme deficiency (G6PD or pyruvate kinase deficiency)
	DIC
	Polycythemia
	Extravascular blood loss
	Bruising from birth trauma (petechiae, cephalohematoma)
	Hemorrhage (pulmonary, cerebral)
	Increased enterohepatic circulation
	Intestinal obstruction (pyloric stenosis, duodenal stenosis or atresia, annular pancreas)
	Hirschsprung disease
	Meconium ileus and/or meconium plug syndrome
	Drug-induced paralytic ileus (magnesium)
	Breast milk jaundice
	Disorders of bilirubin metabolism:
	Gilbert syndrome
	Crigler-Najjar syndrome
	Lucey-Driscoll syndrome
	Endocrine disorders
	Hypothyroidism
	Infants of diabetic mothers
	Hypopituitarism
	Bacterial sepsis
Conjugated hyperbilirubinemia	Extrahepatic obstruction
	Biliary atresia
	Choledocholithiasis
	Choledochal cyst
	Common duct stenosis
	Inspissated bile syndrome from cystic fibrosis
	Extrinsic bile duct compression
	Pancreatitis

TABLE 13-5 Differential Diagnosis of Hyperbilirubinemia *(continued)*
Persistent intrahepatic cholestasis
Paucity of intrahepatic ducts
Benign recurrent intrahepatic cholestasis
Arteriohepatic dysplasia
Acquired intrahepatic cholestasis
Neonatal hepatitis
Bacterial sepsis
Congenital infections
Hepatitis A, B, and C
Varicella zoster
Epstein-Barr virus
Echovirus
Coxsackievirus
Tuberculosis
Leptospirosis
Amoebiasis
Idiopathic
Drug-induced cholestasis
Total parenteral nutrition cholestasis
Cirrhosis
Drug or metal toxicity
Neoplasms (hepatoblastoma, secondary liver metastases)
Genetic and metabolic disorders
Disorders of bilirubin metabolism (Dubin-Johnson syndrome, Rotor syndrome, hypothyroidism)
Disorders of carbohydrate metabolism (galactosemia, fructosemia)
Disorders of amino acid metabolism (tyrosinemia, hypermethioninemia)
Disorders of lipid metabolism (Niemann-Pick disease, Gaucher disease)
Chromosomal disorders (trisomy 18 and 21)
Metabolic liver disease (Wilson disease, α-antitrypsin deficiency)

types should be determined. Some centers are now using transcutaneous measurement devices as screening tools. Those with pathologic bilirubin levels should be further evaluated with a CBC. If a hemolytic process is suspected, a Coombs test, reticulocyte count, and examination of the peripheral smear are useful. Recent studies demonstrate the utility of using nomograms to plot hour-specific bilirubin measurements to facilitate subsequent management. These are increasingly used in newborn nurseries in the United States. Figure 13-2 shows an algorithm for the evaluation of hyperbilirubinemia.

Treatment

The goal in treating unconjugated hyperbilirubinemia is to avoid kernicterus or sublethal bilirubin encephalopathy. The two modalities used to decrease

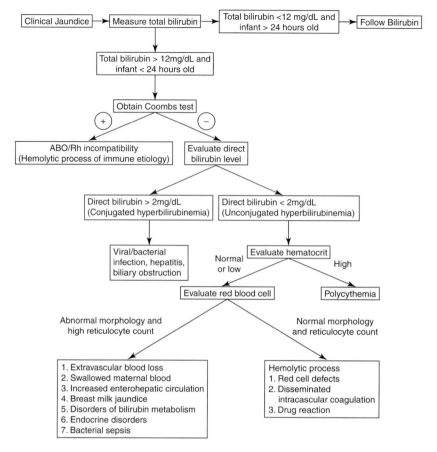

Figure 13-2 • Algorithm for the evaluation of hyperbilirubinemia in the neonate.

unconjugated bilirubin are phototherapy and exchange transfusion. When to use these treatments depends on the birth weight of the neonate. Given a specific LBW, Table 13-6 provides a general guide for treatment at different levels of unconjugated hyperbilirubinemia. When to use phototherapy in the full-term neonate is quite controversial. No studies show evidence of encephalopathic damage from unconjugated hyperbilirubinemia peak levels less than 25 mg dL in the full-term healthy neonate with uncomplicated physiologic jaundice. As a result, there is much debate among pediatricians as to when to begin phototherapy. However, because kernicterus continues to be a problem in the United States, the American Academy of Pediatrics released a policy statement in 2004 recommending that every infant have a bilirubin level checked before discharge. The statement includes treatment recommendations differentiating among infants of low, moderate, and high risk. Phototherapy converts the unconjugated bilirubin into several water-soluble photoisomers that can be ex-

creted without conjugation, so it is important to optimize the infant's hydration status. Exchange transfusion directly removes the bilirubin from the intravascular space as well as maternal immunoglobulin that may be contributing to a hemolytic process. Exchange transfusion is usually reserved for the bilirubin levels above 25 in the setting of hemolytic disease.

Treatment of conjugated hyperbilirubinemia is directed at the underlying cause of the hyperbilirubinemia. Phototherapy of conjugated bilirubin is not effective and causes bronzing of the skin that takes months to resolve.

NECROTIZING ENTEROCOLITIS

Pathogenesis

Necrotizing enterocolitis (NEC) refers to a process of transluminal and mucosal necrosis that is seen in premature infants. The cause is unknown but likely

■ **TABLE 13-6** Hyperbilirubinemia in Low-Birth-Weight Neonates

Weight (g)	Bilirubin Level (mg/dL)	
	Consider Phototherapy	**Consider Exchange Transfusion**
<1,000	5 to 7	12 to 15
1,000 to 1,500	7 to 10	15 to 18
1,500 to 2,500	10 to 15	8 to 20
>2,500	>15	>20

involves a component of ischemia or reperfusion injury, followed by translocation of bacteria into the wall of the intestine. Most cases of NEC are sporadic. Occasional clusters of NEC suggest that infection could have a primary role in some instances. **Pneumatosis intestinalis** results from bacterial gas production in the bowel wall. It can be detected on abdominal radiography and is pathognomonic for NEC.

NEC occurs primarily in premature infants and is ultimately diagnosed in almost 5% to 10% of very low-birth-weight infants (<1,500 g). Prenatal factors associated with NEC include maternal age greater than 35, maternal infection requiring antibiotics, premature rupture of membranes (PROM), and cocaine exposure. Perinatal factors include maternal anesthesia, depressed Apgar score at 5 minutes, birth asphyxia, RDS, and hypotension. Postnatal factors include patent ductus arteriosus, congestive heart failure, umbilical vessel catheterization, polycythemia, and exchange transfusion. Although previously thought to be significant, feeding practices and osmotic load of feedings probably do not contribute to the pathogenesis of NEC.

Clinical Manifestations

The presentation varies from mild to fulminant. The earliest signs are feeding intolerance with bilious aspirates and abdominal distention. The patient may develop occult blood in the stool, which can become grossly bloody. Extreme abdominal tenderness with discoloration, hypo- or hyperglycemia, severe metabolic acidosis, sepsis, shock, DIC, temperature instability, and ineffective respiratory effort (caused by severe abdominal distention) requiring mechanical ventilation are seen in the more severe cases.

Long-term complications include intestinal strictures, which may be demonstrated by contrast study. Laboratory findings include leukocytosis, neutropenia, thrombocytopenia, and metabolic acidosis.

Treatment

If NEC is suspected, feeds should be discontinued immediately and a nasogastric (NG) tube should be placed to suction. Systemic antibiotics should be started and blood cultures sent. Abdominal radiographs are obtained at least every 6 hours to monitor for **pneumatosis intestinalis**, portal air, and free peritoneal air. Intravenous fluids are administered to prevent shock. If free air is seen in the peritoneal cavity or intestinal necrosis is suspected, surgical intervention is indicated. If there is no free air, a 10- to 14-day course of bowel rest and broad antibiotic treatment generally leads to full recovery, although mortality rates remain high for this disease.

NEONATAL HEMATOLOGIC DISORDERS

POLYCYTHEMIA

Pathogenesis

Polycythemia is defined as a greater than normal number of RBCs with hyperviscosity. Neonatal polycythemia (defined as a central venous hematocrit >70%) is almost always a consequence of fetal hypertransfusion. A significantly elevated hematocrit leads to hyperviscosity of the blood, resulting in vascular stasis, microthrombi, hypoperfusion, and tissue ischemia. Neonatal erythrocytes are less filterable and deformable than adult erythrocytes, further contributing to hyperviscosity. Although a central venous hematocrit of greater than 65% occurs in 3%

to 5% of infants, few of these develop hyperviscosity syndrome.

Risk Factors

Infants at risk for polycythemia are post term and small for gestational age neonates; infants of diabetic mothers; infants with delayed cord clamping (maternal–fetal transfusion); and infants suffering from neonatal hyperthyroidism, adrenogenital syndrome, the trisomies (13, 18, and 21), twin–twin transfusion (recipient), or Beckwith-Wiedemann syndrome. In some infants, polycythemia reflects a compensation for prolonged periods of fetal hypoxia from placental insufficiency; these infants have increased erythropoietin levels at birth.

Clinical Manifestations

Polycythemic infants appear ruddy and plethoric. Irritability, lethargy, poor feeding, emesis, tremulousness, and seizures all reflect abnormalities of the microcirculation of the brain. Acute renal failure results from inadequate renal perfusion. Hepatomegaly and hyperbilirubinemia are caused by poor hepatic circulation and the increased amount of hemoglobin that is metabolized into bilirubin. Because of stasis in the pulmonary vessels, pulmonary vascular resistance increases, and PPHN may result. Other complications include NEC and hypoglycemia. Vascular impairment in the penis can cause **priapism**, and the formation of microthrombi may result in thrombocytopenia. If ischemia is severe enough, both the EEG and the ECG may be abnormal. Chest radiograph often reveals cardiomegaly, increased vascular markings, pleural effusions, and interstitial edema.

Long-term complications from neonatal polycythemia are more likely in the symptomatic child, particularly if hypoglycemia is present. Neurodevelopmental abnormalities include mild deficits in speech, hearing, and coordination. If cerebral infarction occurs, cerebral palsy and mental retardation are likely.

Treatment

Long-term complications may be prevented by treatment of symptomatic infants with **partial exchange transfusion** after birth. A partial exchange transfusion removes whole blood and replaces it with normal saline or albumin.

This intervention should be reserved for patients with hematocrits greater than 70% or symptomatic infants. Hematocrits should be determined from free-flowing venous specimens rather than capillary blood samples.

ANEMIA

Anemia in the neonate can result from blood loss, hemolysis, decreased RBC production, or (physiologic) decreased erythropoiesis (Table 13-7).

Clinical Manifestations

A complete family history, including questions about anemia, jaundice, cholestatic disease, and splenectomy, may give important clues to newborn disease. The obstetric history may identify blood loss as the cause of the anemia. The physical examination can usually differentiate acute blood loss, chronic blood loss, and hemolytic disease. Manifestations of acute blood loss include shock, tachypnea, tachycardia, low venous pressure, weak pulses, and pallor. Chronic blood loss is manifested by extreme pallor and a low hematocrit. These infants are typically normovolemic and may have congestive heart failure or hydrops fetalis. Chronic hemolysis is associated with pallor, jaundice, and hepatosplenomegaly.

Neonatal anemia may be classified by evaluation of the reticulocyte count, bilirubin level, Coombs test, and RBC morphology (Table 13-8). The **Apt test** helps identify maternal blood that has been swallowed by the neonate, and the **Kleihauer-Betke preparation** determines if fetomaternal transfusion has occurred. US of the head is used to define an intracranial bleed. Laboratory tests on the parents help determine the likelihood of a hemolytic process. If a congenital infection is suspected as the cause of the anemia, diagnostic tests such as bone marrow aspiration may be indicated.

Treatment

Healthy, term, asymptomatic newborns self-correct a mild anemia, provided that iron intake is adequate. Although nonbreastfeeding infants are sent home on iron-fortified formulas, iron supplementation is not required until 2 months of age, when reticulocytosis resumes.

If the neonate has acute blood loss at birth, immediate access should be obtained, and blood must be

■ **TABLE 13-7** Causes of Anemia

Causes	Manifestation	Etiology
Blood loss	Hematocrit is often normal	Obstetric causes
	Reticulocyte count is normal	Abruptio placentae
		Placenta previa
		Incision of the placenta during cesarean delivery
		Rupture of anomalous placental vessels
		Hematoma or rupture of the cord
		Occult blood loss may result from
		Fetomaternal bleeding
		Fetoplacental bleeding
		Twin-to-twin transfusion
		Bleeding in the neonatal period may be caused by
		Intracranial bleeding
		Massive cephalohematoma
		Retroperitoneal bleeding
		Ruptured liver or spleen
		Adrenal or renal hemorrhage
		GI bleeding
		Bleeding from the umbilicus
		*Excessive blood loss may result from blood sampling with inadequate replacement.
Hemolysis	Decreased hematocrit	Immune mechanisms
	Increased reticulocyte count	Rh incompatibility
	Increased bilirubin level	ABO incompatibility
		Minor blood group incompatibility (c, E, Kell, Duffy)
		Maternal hemolytic anemia from systemic lupus erythematosus
		Hereditary red cell disorders
		RBC membrane defects (spherocytosis)
		Enzymopathies (G6PD deficiency, pyruvate kinase deficiency)
		Hemoglobinopathies (sickle cell disease, α and β-thalassemias)
		Acquired hemolysis
		Bacterial or viral infection
		DIC
		Microangiopathic hemolytic anemia
Diminished	Decreased hematocrit	Diamond-Blackfan syndrome
RBC	Decreased reticulocyte count	Fanconi anemia
production	Normal bilirubin level	Congenital leukemia
		Infections (especially rubella and parvovirus)
		Drug-induced RBC suppression
		Physiologic anemia*

continues

TABLE 13-7 Causes of Anemia *(continued)*

Causes	Manifestation	Etiology
		Anemia of prematurity
		*Physiologic anemia of the full-term or premature neonate is caused by physiologically decreased erythropoiesis. Full-term infants have a nadir of the hemoglobin level at 6 to 12 weeks, LBW infants have a nadir at 5 to 10 weeks, and VLBW neonates have a nadir at 4 to 8 weeks when the infant's oxygen demand increases, erythropoietin will increase; if iron stores are adequate, the reticulocyte count will increase and the hemoglobin level will rise

sent for typing and cross-matching. If present, hypovolemic shock (manifested by decreased venous pressure, pallor, tachycardia) is treated as detailed in Chapter 1. Chronic blood loss is usually well tolerated; these infants should not be transfused unless congestive heart failure is present and symptomatic.

Anemia of prematurity is tempered by iron administration in premature formulas. Otherwise healthy premature infants tolerate hemoglobins as low as 6.5 to 8.0 g/dL. The level itself is not an indication for transfusion. Transfusion should occur if another condition exists that requires increased oxygen-carrying

TABLE 13-8 Classification of Anemia in the Newborn

Reticulocytes	Bilirubin	Coombs Test	RBC Morphology	Diagnostic Possibilities
Normal or decreased	Normal	Negative	Normal	Physiologic anemia of infancy or prematurity; congenital hypoplastic anemia; other causes of decreased production
Normal or increased	Normal	Negative	Normal Hypochromic microcytes	Acute hemorrhage (fetomaternal, placental, umbilical cord, or internal hemorrhage)
				Chronic fetomaternal hemorrhage
Increased	Increased	Positive	Spherocytes	Immune hemolysis (blood group incompatibility or maternal autoantibody)
Normal or increased	Increased	Negative	Spherocytes	Hereditary spherocytosis
			Elliptocytes	Hereditary elliptocytosis
			Hypochromic microcytes	α- or γ-thalassemia syndrome
			Spiculated RBCs	Pyruvate kinase deficiency
			Schistocytes and RBC fragments	DIC; other microangiopathic processes
			Bite cells (Heinz bodies with supravital stain)	Glucose-6-phosphate dehydrogenase deficiency
			Normal	Infections; enclosed hemorrhage (cephalohematoma)

capacity, such as sepsis, NEC, pneumonia, chronic lung disease, and apnea.

NEONATAL CENTRAL NERVOUS SYSTEM DISORDERS

APNEA OF PREMATURITY

Pathogenesis

Apnea in the premature infant is defined as a cessation of breathing for longer than 20 seconds or a shorter pause associated with cyanosis, pallor, hypotonia, or a heart rate of less than 100 beats per minute (bpm). Apnea in the full-term neonate (apnea of infancy) is discussed in Chapter 20. In the premature infant, apneic episodes may be caused by central, obstructive, or mixed mechanisms. In central apnea, there is a complete cessation of air flow and respiratory effort with no chest wall movement, whereas in obstructive apnea, there is respiratory effort and chest wall movement but no air flow. Apnea of prematurity usually has a mixed central and obstructive picture. Periodic breathing, which must be differentiated from apnea, is defined as pauses of 5 to 10 seconds followed by a short period of rapid breathing. Periodic breathing is normal in neonates and infants.

Epidemiology

Apnea occurs in most infants of less than 28 weeks' gestation, approximately 50% of infants 30 to 32 weeks' gestation, and in less than 7% of infants 34 to 35 weeks' gestation.

Clinical Manifestations

Apnea of prematurity is associated with bradycardia, which is a heart rate less than 80 bpm. Bradycardia and cyanosis are usually present after 20 seconds of apnea but may occur more rapidly in the small, premature infant. After 30 to 40 seconds, pallor and hypotonia are also seen, and the infant may be unresponsive to tactile stimulation. A neonate may rouse itself and stop the apneic spell, but more symptomatic apnea is apparent if a caregiver must touch the infant to discontinue the apnea. With hypotonia and pallor, bag-mask ventilation is required to return the child to a normal breathing pattern.

A diagnosis of apnea of prematurity is made after excluding other causes of apnea, which can be grouped into the following broad categories: hypoxemia, diaphragmatic fatigue, respiratory center depression, infection, vagal stimulation, airway obstruction, and inappropriate environmental temperature. Hypoxemia may result from anemia, hypovolemia, and congenital heart disease, whereas RDS and pneumonia can cause diaphragmatic fatigue. Respiratory center depression can occur with metabolic abnormalities (hypoglycemia, hypocalcemia, hyponatremia), drugs, seizures, or intraventricular hemorrhage (IVH). Infectious processes such as sepsis, NEC, and meningitis all can cause apnea, whereas gastroesophageal reflux, suctioning of the oropharynx, and NG tube passage can cause vagally mediated depression of the respiratory center. Excessive oral secretions, anatomic obstruction, or malposition may result in obstructive apnea.

Treatment

Treatment for apnea of prematurity includes maintenance of a skin-core temperature gradient in the incubator, supplemental oxygen, tactile stimulation, and administration of respiratory stimulants such as caffeine. Apnea of prematurity may also be managed by increasing the mean airway pressure through the use of CPAP or intermittent assisted ventilation. For the other causes of apnea, treatment of the underlying disorder usually leads to cessation of the apneic episodes.

Many centers consider an infant ready for discharge when the infant reaches 34 to 35 weeks' postconceptional age, is tolerating feeds orally, and has not had an apneic or bradycardiac episode for 7 days. The apnea monitor sent home with the patient can be discontinued when the infant has been apnea free for a period of time.

INTRAVENTRICULAR HEMORRHAGE

Pathogenesis

Intraventricular hemorrhage (IVH) is seen almost exclusively in preterm infants and results from bleeding of the germinal matrix, an area of immature vasculature. Changes in cerebral blood flow or pressure have been proposed as a contributing mechanism. IVH is very common among VLBW infants, and the risk decreases as gestational age increases. IVHs that are confined to the germinal matrix (grade I) or are associated with a small amount of blood in the ventricle (grade II) often resolve without sequelae. Large IVHs that are associated with ventricular dilatation (grade III) or with extension into the brain parenchyma (grade IV) are associated with permanent functional impairment, neurodevelopmental delay, and hydrocephalus.

Posthemorrhagic hydrocephalus is a consequence of obstruction of the ventricular outlets (obstructive hydrocephalus) or of obliteration of the arachnoid villi that ultimately absorb the CSF (communicating hydrocephalus). Hydrocephalus may be static, in which case no intervention is made, or it may be progressive, requiring the surgical placement of a ventriculoperitoneal shunt.

Clinical Manifestations and Diagnosis

The majority of IVHs occur within the first 3 days of life, and most are asymptomatic. The neonate with severe IVH may develop anemia, pallor, hypotension, focal neurologic signs, seizures, an acute increase in ventilatory assistance needs, apnea, metabolic acidosis, and/or bradycardia.

US through the anterior fontanelle is the method of choice to diagnose, grade, and monitor IVH. All premature infants with birth weights less than 1,500 g should have a diagnostic US performed within the first week of life.

Treatment

The risk of IVH is minimized by preventing premature delivery, if possible, or through the use of appropriate neonatal resuscitation measures to minimize hypoxemia. The goal in acute management of IVH is to maintain adequate cerebral perfusion while controlling intracerebral pressure. IVH is followed by serial US evaluations, because ventriculomegaly occurs before there is an increase in head circumference. Progressive posthemorrhagic hydrocephalus is treated by placement of a ventriculoperitoneal shunt.

HYPOXIC ISCHEMIC ENCEPHALOPATHY

Pathogenesis

Hypoxic ischemic encephalopathy (HIE) occurs with an incidence of approximately 6 per 1,000 full-term infants. HIE is a significant cause of neonatal morbidity and mortality, with long-term neurologic sequelae. It is a consequence of an ischemia-reperfusion injury related to a number of prenatal or perinatal events. Maternal risk factors include hypotension, hypothyroidism, and infertility treatment. Intrapartum events commonly include cord prolapse, placental abruption, breech extraction, or difficult forceps delivery. Postnatal events such as sepsis, severe respiratory failure, or congenital heart disease are far less common causes.

Clinical Manifestations

HIE is the most common cause of neonatal seizures. Most commonly, an infant presents at birth with severe perinatal depression or asphyxia requiring full resuscitation in the delivery room. Significant metabolic and respiratory acidosis is often present, and the infant may have poor respiratory effort. The infant may have depressed mental status for several hours secondary to depressed of cortical activity. Up to 50% of these infants have seizures within the first 6 to 12 hours of birth. Normal infant reflexes such as the Moro or grasp are often absent, and severely affected newborns do not have a gag reflex. This period is often followed by a time of improved alertness; however, infants with significant brain injury frequently regress to a depressed level of consciousness with signs of brainstem dysfunction. Hypotonia, apnea, fixed and dilated pupils, poor suck and swallow, and proximal weakness are all signs of substantial injury. Metabolic disturbances including hypoglycemia, hypocalcemia, hyponatremia, and acidosis are common. A diffusion-weighted MRI obtained within 48 to 72 hours of the injury may demonstrate the extent of injury and in severe cases may help delineate a poor prognosis. EEG may document seizures or a burst suppression pattern indicative of global injury. However, the best predictor of outcome remains the neurologic exam at 1 week of life. If an infant has a normal exam and is able to take full oral feeds, the chances for a full recovery are excellent.

Treatment

Although no treatment is available for established brain injury, preliminary studies of head cooling after acute perinatal depression show promise in reducing the severity of neurologic sequelae. Further studies are needed before this approach is universally recommended.

NEONATAL SEIZURES

The causes of neonatal seizures are delineated in Table 13-9.

TABLE 13-9 Causes of Neonatal Seizures

Metabolic	Hypoglycemia
	Electrolyte abnormalities
	Hypocalcemia
	Hypomagnesemia
	Hyponatremia
	Inborn errors of metabolism
	Organic acidemias
	Error of amino acid metabolism
	Urea cycle defects
	Pyridoxine deficiency
Toxic	Maternal drug ingestion
	Neonatal drug withdrawal
	Hyperbilirubinemia
Hemorrhagic	Intraventricular hemorrhage
	Subdural or subarachnoid hemorrhage
Infectious	Bacterial meningitis
	Viral encephalitis
Asphyxia	Hypoxic ischemic encephalopathy
Genetic/dysmorphic syndromes	Cerebral dysgenesis
	Chromosomal abnormalities
	Phakomatoses (tuberous sclerosis)

Seizures noted in the delivery room may be caused by direct injection of local anesthetic into the fetal scalp, severe anoxia, or congenital brain malformation. Seizures because of hypoxic-ischemic encephalopathy (postasphyxial seizures), a common cause of seizures in the full-term neonate, usually occur 12 to 24 hours after a history of birth asphyxia and are often refractory to conventional doses of anticonvulsant medications. Postasphyxial seizures may also result from metabolic disorders such as hypoglycemia and hypocalcemia. IVH is a common cause of seizures in premature infants and often occurs from the first to third days of life. Seizures with IVH may be associated with a bulging fontanelle, hemorrhagic spinal fluid, anemia, lethargy, and coma. Seizures after the first 5 days of life may be caused by infection or drug withdrawal. Seizures associated with lethargy, acidosis, ketonuria, respiratory alkalosis, and a family history of infantile death may be caused by an inborn error of metabolism.

Clinical Manifestations

A careful prenatal and perinatal history may shed light on the seizure etiology. The diagnostic evaluation of infants with seizures should include a determination of blood levels of glucose, sodium, calcium, magnesium, and ammonia. In the jaundiced neonate, measurement of the bilirubin level is indicated. When infection is suspected, a blood culture and LP are performed. If an inborn error of metabolism is suspected, urine organic acids and serum amino acids may be examined. Further evaluation may include a US or a CT scan of the head. If physical examination or head imaging suggests a congenital infection, appropriate cultures, antibody determinations, and PCR should be done. Continuous bedside video and EEG monitoring provides the best information in defining the type of seizure present. Continuous EEG with pyridoxine infusion helps establish the presence or absence of pyridoxine deficiency. If seizures result from neonatal abstinence syndrome, a controlled narcotic wean is indicated.

Seizures are difficult to differentiate from benign jitters or clonus. In contrast to seizures, jitters and tremors are sensory dependent, elicited by stimuli, and may be interrupted by holding the extremity. Seizure activity is coarse, with fast and slow clonic activity, whereas jitters are characterized by fine, very rapid movement. It is often difficult to identify seizures in the newborn period because the infant, especially the LBW infant, usually does not demonstrate the tonic-clonic major motor activity typical of the older child.

Subtle seizures constitute 50% of seizures in newborns (both term and preterm). Subtle seizure activity may include rhythmic fluctuations in vital signs, apnea, eye deviation, nystagmus, tongue thrusting, eye blinking, staring, and "bicycling" or "swimming" movements. Continuous bedside EEG monitoring can help identify subtle seizures.

Treatment

If possible, the primary cause of the seizure should be identified and treated. Any metabolic disturbances must be corrected. If a toxin (hyperammonemia, hyperbilirubinemia) is isolated as the etiology of the seizure, exchange transfusion may be used to remove it. Meningitis is treated with the appropriate antibiotic agent. In the absence of an identifiable cause, anticonvulsant therapy is used. Agents include phenobarbital, phosphotase (Dilantin), lorazepam (Ativan), and diazepam (Valium). Phenobarbital is standard primary therapy. Fosphenytoin or phenytoin may be used when seizures persist with a phenobarbital level greater than 50 mg/L. The long-term outcome of neonatal seizures is determined by the type and etiology of the seizure.

NEONATAL DISORDERS OF THE ENDOCRINE SYSTEM

HYPOTHYROIDISM

The physical stigmata of congenital hypothyroidism in the newborn are often too subtle for physical diagnosis, so clinicians rely heavily on diagnostic screening. All states currently require newborn screening for hypothyroidism. The sooner treatment is initiated, the better the prognosis for normal intellectual development in the child. In most cases the diagnosis can be made and treatment initiated within 4 weeks.

Clinical Manifestations

Primary hypothyroidism is indicated by a low T_4 level and an elevated thyroid-stimulating hormone (TSH) level. Serum levels should be drawn to confirm abnormal screening results.

A low T_4 level accompanied by a low TSH value may indicate a physiologically normal thyroid status caused by a low concentration of thyroid-binding globulin (TBG). This is frequently observed in premature infants or may be seen on a hereditary basis. Alternatively, a low T_4 and low TSH with a normal TBG level may indicate hypopituitarism or hypothalamic deficiency. Hypothalamic deficiency usually is accompanied by growth hormone or corticotropin deficiency, which may cause acute hypoglycemia. Figure 13-3 delineates an algorithm for the diagnosis of hypothyroidism in the infant.

Treatment

If the screening results indicate primary hypothyroidism, the T_4 and TSH studies should be repeated and therapy started. Serum T_4 is measured after 5 days of therapy, and the thyroxine dosage is adjusted to keep the T_4 level in the upper half of the normal range for age. The TSH concentration may remain elevated for months in some patients despite adequate therapy because of immaturity of the feedback mechanism. If therapy is started within the first month after birth, the prognosis is excellent. The thyroxine dose must be carefully adjusted because too little thyroxine results in persistent hypothyroidism, whereas too much thyroxine may result in advanced bone age and craniosynostosis.

NEONATAL HYPOGLYCEMIA

Full-term neonates frequently have transient asymptomatic hypoglycemia, with blood glucose measurements in the 30s (mg/dL). As a result, published statistical definitions of hypoglycemia generally use a level of less than 40 mg/dL. However, levels of less than 60 mg/dL that persist for more than a few days should prompt consideration of and evaluation for pathologic processes. Various endocrine, congenital, metabolic, and nervous system disorders can result in pathologic hypoglycemia in the neonate (see Table 13-10).

Clinical Manifestations

The onset of hypoglycemia may occur anywhere from a few hours after birth to several days of age. Subtle symptoms such as poor feeding, apathy, lethargy, and hypotonia are most common, but life-threatening manifestations such as seizures, apnea, and cyanosis may also occur.

Inborn errors of metabolism may cause persistent or recurrent hypoglycemia. When the infant is hypoglycemic, serum should be obtained for glucose, insulin, cortisol, growth hormone, lactate, and pyruvate levels. Serum amino acid screening is indicated if no definitive diagnosis is made; the infant need not be hypoglycemic at the time of the sample collection.

Treatment

In asymptomatic infants, oral feedings can be attempted. If oral feedings are not accepted, an intravenous infusion of maintenance dextrose is initiated. In symptomatic infants, an intravenous push of 10% dextrose precedes infusion of intravenous dextrose. The rate is adjusted to keep the blood glucose level between 60 and 120 mg/dL. Rebound hypoglycemia may occur if the dextrose infusion is abruptly decreased. Point of care testing devices are useful for

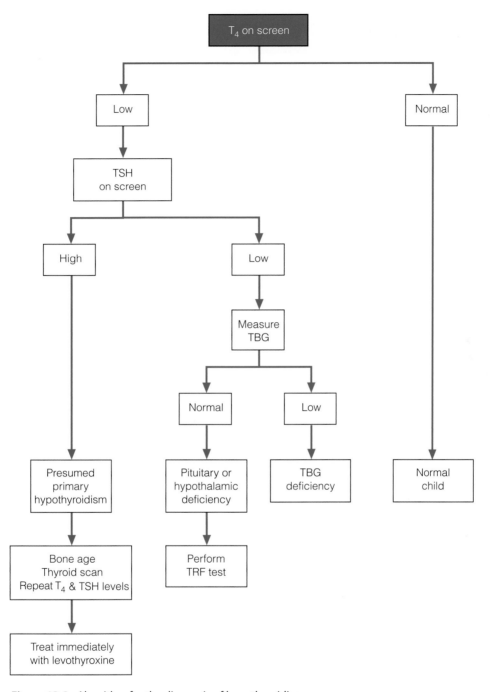

Figure 13-3 • Algorithm for the diagnosis of hypothyroidism.

screening blood sugar; abnormal values should be verified with a true blood sugar. When the infant is stabilized, the dextrose infusion rate is slowly decreased, with careful monitoring of blood glucose. After dextrose infusion is discontinued, the blood glucose level should be monitored for 24 hours.

CONGENITAL ANOMALIES

TRACHEOESOPHAGEAL FISTULA

The lower section of the esophagus develops as an elongation of the superior portion of the primitive

■ **TABLE 13-10** Causes of Neonatal Hypoglycemia

With hyperinsulinism	Transient hyperinsulinism
	Infants of diabetic mothers
	Infants with Rh hemolytic disease
	Protracted hyperinsulinism
	Functional hyperinsulinism
	Beckwith-Wiedemann syndrome
	Islet cell adenomas
Without hyperinsulinism	Transient hypoglycemia
	Intrauterine growth retardation
	Birth asphyxia
	Polycythemia
	Cardiac disease
	CNS disease
	Sepsis
	Maternal use of propranolol, oral hypoglycemic agents, or narcotic addiction
	Protracted hypoglycemia
	Neonatal hypopituitarism
	Defects in carbohydrate and/or amino acid metabolism

foregut endoderm. When there is abnormal anastomosis of superior and inferior portions of the esophagus, esophageal atresia results. Of neonates with esophageal atresia, 85% have tracheoesophageal fistula (TEF). Figure 13-4 shows the five types of tracheoesophageal atresias. Esophageal atresia with distal TEF accounts for 85% of the cases of TEF. Forty percent of patients with TEF have other congenital defects. For example, VACTERL syndrome describes the association of vertebral, anal, cardiac, tracheal, esophageal, renal, and limb anomalies.

Clinical Manifestations

Neonates with TEF have excessive oral secretions, inability to feed, gagging, and respiratory distress. Polyhydramnios often is noted on fetal US. Lateral and anteroposterior chest radiographs of the thoraco-cervical region and abdomen with a Replogle tube in

the proximal esophagus reveal a blind pouch with air in the GI tract. In esophageal atresia without TEF, gas is absent from the GI tract, whereas in TEF without esophageal atresia (H type), infants may have nonspecific symptoms for several months, including chronic cough with feeding and recurrent pneumonia.

Treatment

The usual corrective procedure is division and closure of the TEF and end-to-end anastomosis of the proximal and distal esophagus. If the distance between esophageal segments is too long for primary anastomosis, delayed anastomosis follows stretching of the upper segment. Strictures at the anastomosis site require periodic dilation.

DUODENAL ATRESIA

Duodenal obstruction may be complete (atresia) or partial (stenosis) because of a web, band, or annular pancreas. Duodenal atresia results from a failure of the lumen to recanalize during the eighth to tenth weeks of gestation. Seventy percent of the cases of duodenal atresia are associated with other malformations, including cardiac anomalies and GI defects such as annular pancreas, malrotation of the intestines, and imperforate anus. Twenty-five percent of infants with duodenal atresia are premature. Duodenal atresia is often associated with trisomy 21.

Clinical Manifestations

With complete obstruction, in utero polyhydramnios may be present. After birth, bilious emesis begins within a few hours after the first feeding. Abdominal radiographs usually show gastric and duodenal gaseous distention proximal to the atretic site. This finding is known as the **double bubble** sign. The presence of gas in the distal bowel suggests partial obstruction.

Treatment

Treatment is surgical. Mortality is related to prematurity and other associated anomalies.

CONGENITAL DIAPHRAGMATIC HERNIA

Congenital diaphragmatic hernia results from a defect in the (usually left) posterolateral diaphragm

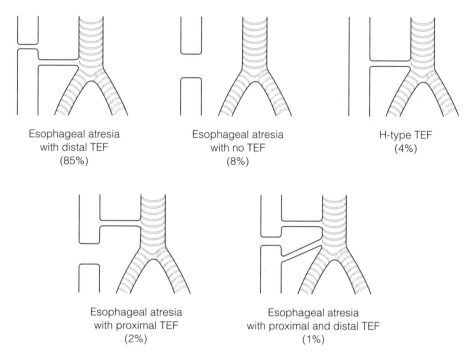

Figure 13-4 • Types of tracheoesophageal fistulas with relative frequencies.

that allows abdominal contents to enter the thorax and compromise lung development. This defect is commonly referred to as a **Bochdalek hernia**. The combination of pulmonary hypoplasia and pulmonary arteriolar hypertension makes this congenital defect lethal in many cases.

Clinical Manifestations

Early symptoms include respiratory distress with decreased breath sounds on the affected side, shifted heart sounds to the opposite side, and a scaphoid abdomen. Diagnosis is sometimes made via fetal US. After birth, the defect is obvious on a simple chest radiograph.

Treatment

Because of pulmonary hypoplasia and pulmonary hypertension, the patient must be intubated and ventilated. Management focuses on gentle ventilation: provision of positive pressure ventilation sufficient to achieve stable acid-base balance without overdistention of the remaining lung parenchyma. Sometimes conventional ventilation is not sufficient to provide adequate oxygen delivery and carbon dioxide excretion; in such cases, high-frequency ventilation or ECMO may be needed to manage the child's pulmonary

hypertension. Treatment of pulmonary hypertension typically precedes surgical correction of the diaphragmatic defect. A Replogle tube is placed to minimize GI distention that would further diminish effective lung volume.

OMPHALOCELE

Omphalocele results when the abdominal viscera herniate through the umbilical and supraumbilical portions of the abdominal wall into a sac covered by peritoneum and amniotic membrane. The defect results from arrested folding of the embryonic disc. Large defects may contain the entire GI tract and the liver and spleen. The sac covering the defect is thin and may rupture in utero or during delivery. The incidence of omphalocele is 1 in 6,000 births.

Clinical Manifestations

Polyhydramnios is noted in utero, and 10% of infants with omphaloceles are born prematurely. Diagnosis is often made by prenatal US. Thirty-five percent of afflicted infants have other GI defects, and 20% have congenital heart defects. Ten percent of children with omphalocele have Beckwith-Wiedemann syndrome (exophthalmos, macroglossia, gigantism, hyperinsulinemia, and hypoglycemia).

Treatment

Cesarean section may prevent rupture of the sac. Small defects are closed primarily, whereas larger defects often require a staged repair that involves covering the sac with prosthetic material.

Definitive treatment requires surgery. In infants with an intact sac, repair can be postponed as long as the sac remains intact. Emergent surgical intervention is required to cover the intestine if the sac is ruptured.

GASTROSCHISIS

Gastroschisis, by definition, contains no sac; the intestine is herniated through the abdominal wall lateral to the umbilicus. The eviscerated uncovered mass is adherent, edematous, dark in color, and covered by a gelatinous matrix of greenish material. The pathogenesis of this abdominal wall defect is not clear.

Clinical Manifestations

Polyhydramnios is noted in utero. Sixty percent of these infants are born prematurely, and 15% have associated jejunoileal stenoses or atresias.

Treatment

Gastroschisis is a surgical emergency; single-stage primary closure is possible in only 10% of infants. In most affected infants a Silastic silo is placed over the exposed bowel allowing for gradual reduction into the abdomen over a period of several days.

CLEFT LIP AND CLEFT PALATE

Epidemiology

Cleft lip (with or without cleft palate) occurs in 1 in 1,000 births and is more common in boys. Multiple genetic and environmental factors play a role in the etiology of the cleft lip. The recurrence risk in siblings is 3% to 4%. The risk for a child with a mother with cleft lip is 14%. Cleft palate occurs in 1 in 2,500 births. Genetic factors are also important in cleft palate, and the recurrence risk is the same as that for cleft lip. Cleft palates are common in patients with chromosomal abnormalities.

Clinical Manifestations

Malformations associated with cleft lip include hypertelorism, hand defects, and cardiac anomalies. In general, feeding difficulties are not seen in isolated cleft lip.

Treatment

Most cleft lips are repaired shortly after birth or once the infant demonstrates steady weight gain. Cleft palate repair is usually undertaken at 9 to 12 months of age. In the newborn period, respiratory and feeding problems may occur. Repositioning the tongue and feeding the infant on his or her side should resolve respiratory difficulties. Most patients do well with a long soft nipple. Complications after cleft palate repair include speech difficulties, dental disturbances, and recurrent otitis media. Although two thirds of children demonstrate acceptable speech, it may have a nasal quality or a muffled tone.

NEURAL TUBE DEFECTS

Neural tube defects are discussed in detail in Chapter 15.

NEONATAL DERMATOLOGIC PROBLEMS

ERYTHEMA TOXICUM NEONATORUM

The rash of erythema toxicum consists of evanescent papules, vesicles, and pustules on an erythematous base that usually occur on the trunk (but sometimes appear on the face and extremities). Rash onset usually occurs 24 to 72 hours after birth but may be seen earlier. Gram stain of vesicular contents reveals sheets of eosinophils. The lesions resolve over 3 to 5 days without therapy. Fifty percent of full-term babies have erythema toxicum. This figure decreases as the gestational age decreases. The rash may be a host response to microbial colonization of hair follicles after birth.

MILIA

Milia are characterized by pearly white or pale yellow epidermal cysts found on the nose, chin, and forehead. The benign lesions exfoliate and disappear within the first few weeks of life. No treatment is necessary.

SEBORRHEIC DERMATITIS

Seborrhea is characterized by erythematous, dry, scaling, crusty lesions. It occurs in areas rich in sebaceous glands (face, scalp, perineum, and postauricular and intertriginous areas). Affected areas are sharply demarcated from uninvolved skin. Seborrhea appears between 2 and 10 weeks and is commonly called "cradle cap" when it appears on the scalp. For severe cradle cap, baby oil is applied to the scalp for 15 minutes, followed by washing with a dandruff shampoo. For seborrhea of the diaper area, 1% hydrocortisone cream can be used. If candidal superinfection occurs, nystatin ointment is recommended.

MONGOLIAN SPOTS

Mongolian spots are transient dark blue-black pigmented macules usually seen over the lower back and buttocks in 90% of African American, Indian, and Asian infants. The spots result from infiltration of melanocytes deep within the dermis and are never elevated or palpable. The hyperpigmented areas fade as the child ages. They present no known long-term problems but may occasionally be mistaken for bruises inflicted by abusive trauma.

DRUG ABUSE

FETAL ALCOHOL SYNDROME

Alcohol is the most common teratogen to which fetuses are exposed. Maternal alcohol ingestion results in a spectrum of effects in the offspring, ranging from mild reduction in cerebral function to classic fetal alcohol syndrome. The amount of alcohol consumed by the mother appears to correlate with the degree to which the fetus is affected. Fetal alcohol syndrome occurs in 1 in 1,000 newborns. The syndrome affects 40% of the offspring of women who consume more than four to six drinks per day while pregnant.

Clinical Manifestations

Features of fetal alcohol syndrome include microcephaly and mental retardation, intrauterine growth retardation, facial dysmorphisms, and renal and cardiac defects. Facial anomalies include midfacial hypoplasia, micrognathia, a flattened philtrum, short palpebral fissures, and a thin vermillion border.

Treatment

Treatment is aimed at minimizing morbidity and mortality from renal and cardiac defects and assisting the child with mental retardation with activities of daily living.

COCAINE

Cocaine causes maternal hypertension and placental vasoconstriction with diminished uterine blood flow and fetal hypoxia. These effects are associated with increased rates of spontaneous abortion, placental abruption, fetal distress, meconium staining, preterm birth, intrauterine growth retardation, and low Apgar scores at birth.

Clinical Manifestations

Maternal cocaine use is associated with an increased incidence of congenital anomalies, intracranial hemorrhage, and NEC. Congenital anomalies include cardiac defects, skull abnormalities, and genitourinary malformations. Cocaine-exposed infants have demonstrated abnormalities in respiratory control and have an increased risk of SIDS. Long-term defects include attention and concentration deficits and an increased incidence of learning disabilities.

Infants may undergo withdrawal, characterized by irritability, increased tremulousness, lability, inability to be consoled, and poor feeding after birth.

Treatment

During the perinatal period, therapy is supportive. Sedative medications may be helpful, but frequently soothing nonpharmacologic interventions are adequate. At school age, many of these children have special learning needs.

HEROIN AND METHADONE

Heroin and methadone are the two narcotics to which fetuses are most commonly exposed. Approximately 10,000 heroin-dependent babies are born in the United States each year, and 5,000 narcotic-addicted pregnant women are in methadone treatment programs. Methadone maintenance is prescribed for pregnant women to decrease the stress that unreliable heroin dosing and uncontrolled withdrawal in utero place on the fetus. However, infants born to mothers participating in methadone maintenance programs may still display symptoms of neonatal abstinence syndrome.

Clinical Manifestations

Opiate abuse is not associated with congenital anomalies, but maternal use causes intrauterine growth retardation, an increased risk of SIDS, and infant narcotic withdrawal syndrome. It is unclear whether the abnormalities of fetal growth seen with narcotic abuse are caused by the direct effect of the drug or to other environmental factors, such as poor maternal nutrition.

Narcotic abstinence withdrawal syndrome, which generally occurs within the first 4 days of life, is characterized by irritability, poor sleeping, a high-pitched cry, diarrhea, sweating, sneezing, seizures, poor feeding, and poor weight gain. The risk of neonatal withdrawal is higher with methadone (75%) than with heroin (50%). Methadone withdrawal tends to be later in onset and more protracted, sometimes lasting as long as 1 month. Symptoms appear soon after birth, improve, and then may recur at 2 to 4 weeks.

Treatment

The treatment for narcotic withdrawal syndrome attempts to minimize irritability, emesis, and diarrhea and to maximize sleep between feedings. Symptomatic care includes holding, rocking, and swaddling the infant and providing the neonate with frequent small feedings of a hypercaloric formula.

Infants of narcotic-abusing mothers should never be given naloxone in the delivery room because it may precipitate seizures. Narcotic withdrawal symptoms unresponsive to nonmedicinal care can be mitigated by a controlled wean of methadone, morphine, phenobarbital, or benzodiazepines.

 KEY POINTS

- A cephalohematoma is a traumatic subperiosteal hemorrhage that does not cross suture lines. A caput succedaneum is a diffuse, edematous, and often dark swelling of the soft tissue of the scalp that extends across the midline and/or suture lines.

- It is useful to divide infants who are small for gestational age into two categories: symmetric (early onset) and asymmetric (late onset or "head sparing"). Intrauterine growth retardation may result from fetal, placental, or maternal causes. Infants who are small for gestational age have a higher risk of intrauterine fetal death.

- Neonates at risk for being large for gestational age are those of diabetic mothers; postmature infants; and neonates with erythroblastosis fetalis or Beckwith-Wiedemann syndrome. Most infants who are large for gestational age are constitutionally large, from large parents or a family with a predilection for large infants.

- Neonatal herpes simplex virus infection is caused by HSV-2 or HSV-1. Neonatal HSV manifests itself in three discrete constellations of symptoms: disseminated infection involving the liver and other organs (often including the CNS), localized CNS disease, or SEM disease. Antiviral therapy with acyclovir is indicated for all forms of neonatal herpes infections because even initially localized disease may disseminate with devastating effects.

- Eighty percent of pediatric AIDS cases result from maternal vertical transmission. Maternal treatment dramatically reduces the risk of transmission to the infant.

- Neonatal sepsis is generally divided into early-onset, late-onset, and nosocomial sepsis.

- Respiratory distress syndrome is the most common cause of respiratory failure in newborn infants, occurs in premature infants and results from deficiency of surfactant. Therapy with artificial surfactant improves RDS dramatically and has significantly decreased the rate of neonatal mortality in premature infants.

- Meconium aspiration syndrome results from aspiration of meconium that has passed from the fetus into the amniotic fluid. The resulting hypoxia and acidosis increase pulmonary vascular resistance and cause right-to-left shunting of blood across the patent foramen ovale or the ductus arteriosus or both.

- PPHN is seen when there is failure of the pulmonary vasculature resistance to fall with postnatal lung expansion and oxygenation. It occurs in term and post-term infants who have experienced acute or chronic hypoxia in utero. The therapies used to treat PPHN include supplemental oxygen, hyperventilation, administration of sodium bicarbonate, pulmonary vasodilators, and support of systemic blood pressure.

- Hyperbilirubinemia may be conjugated or unconjugated. Conjugated hyperbilirubinemia is always pathologic, whereas unconjugated hyperbilirubinemia may or may not be pathologic. The two most common causes of unconjugated hyperbilirubinemia are physiologic jaundice and hemolytic disease.

- Necrotizing enterocolitis refers to a process of acute intestinal necrosis seen in premature infants. Infants with medical NEC present with feeding intolerance, abdominal distention, occult blood in the stool, and dilated bowel loops and pneumatosis intestinalis. Free peritoneal air is evidence of perforation and an indication for surgical intervention.

- Intraventricular hemorrhage is seen almost exclusively in preterm infants and results from bleeding of the germinal matrix. Infants with grade III IVH and grade IV IVH are more likely to develop motor and intellectual disabilities.

- Congenital diaphragmatic hernia results from a defect in the left posterolateral diaphragm that allows abdominal contents to enter the thorax and compromise lung development. The combination of pulmonary hypoplasia and pulmonary arteriolar hypertension makes this congenital defect lethal in some cases.

- Gastroschisis, by definition, contains no sac; the intestine is herniated through the abdominal wall lateral to the umbilicus. Omphalocele results when the abdominal viscera herniate through the umbilical and supraumbilical portions of the abdominal wall into a sac covered by peritoneum and amniotic membrane.

- Alcohol is the most common teratogen to which fetuses are exposed. Features of fetal alcohol syndrome include microcephaly and mental retardation, intrauterine growth retardation, facial dysmorphisms, and renal and cardiac defects.

Chapter 14

Nephrology and Urology

Prasad Devarajan • Shumyle Alam • Curtis Sheldon • Katie S. Fine

The kidneys are the primary regulator of body fluid. They excrete waste products of metabolism, such as urea and creatinine, and preserve the ionic equilibrium by conserving or excreting electrolytes. In addition, the kidneys contribute to the maintenance of osmolarity and pH, synthesis of erythropoietin, and the production of vitamin D. The central role of the kidneys in growth and development places the infant and child at risk when faced with anatomic or physiologic stressors to the kidneys. Infants, in particular, are susceptible to renal challenges. Their kidneys are less effective in filtering plasma, regulating electrolytes, and concentrating urine.

Although the kidneys and urinary tract are separate systems, they are interrelated; irregularities in one system may affect the other. Abnormalities may be anatomic, infectious, cellular, inflammatory, functional, hormonal, or maturational.

RENAL DYSPLASIA AND CYSTIC DISEASES

In **renal agenesis**, one or both kidneys fail to form. Bilateral renal agenesis results in Potter syndrome; affected infants are stillborn or die shortly after birth due to associated pulmonary hypoplasia. Unilateral agenesis is usually an isolated defect but may be associated with other abnormalities.

In **multicystic dysplastic kidney**, the most common renal cystic disease of childhood, the organ consists of numerous noncommunicating, fluid-filled cysts. Affected kidneys are nonfunctional, but the condition is virtually always unilateral. Multicystic kidney is the second most common cause of renal masses in the newborn (exceeded only by hydronephrosis resulting from ureteropelvic junction obstruction). The diagnosis is confirmed by US. Most cases undergo spontaneous involution. Nephrectomy is recommended when the kidney changes in size or appearance (increased risk of Wilms tumor) or when the patient is hypertensive or experiencing pain.

Polycystic kidney disease is an inherited disorder that occurs in two forms: the autosomal recessive type (ARPKD) and the autosomal dominant type (ADPKD). In the former, the kidneys appear enlarged but maintain their symmetric, reniform shape. The renal collecting tubules are dilated, producing small cysts. Unaffected segments are interspersed, but in general the kidneys function poorly. The condition is usually discovered during evaluation of a palpable renal mass in an infant. Similar dilation is found in the hepatic bile ducts, with varying degrees of periportal fibrosis. Life expectancy is appreciably shortened; severely affected infants may die within weeks. The autosomal dominant form of polycystic kidney disease usually is detected in adulthood but may be diagnosed earlier on prenatal US or through workup for a positive family history. The cysts can be quite large and distort the normal shape of the kidney. Hypertension and renal insufficiency develop over time. Transplant is a viable option.

URETEROPELVIC JUNCTION OBSTRUCTION

Ureteropelvic junction obstruction (UPJO) is the most common cause of **hydronephrosis** in childhood. Possible etiologies of *primary* UPJO include intrinsic narrowing at the junction of the renal pelvis and ureter or angulation of the ureter from a crossing renal vessel. *Secondary* UPJO can result from scarring at the ureteropelvic junction, angulation secondary to massive ureteral dilation, or stones. The obstruction leads to elevated intrapelvic pressure, dilation of the renal pelvis and calyces, urinary stasis, and possible loss of the renal parenchyma. Between 10% and 40% of UPJO cases are bilateral.

CLINICAL MANIFESTATIONS

Hydronephrosis due to UPJO is commonly detected on prenatal US. A palpable abdominal mass is the most common presentation in the newborn. Older children may present with abdominal or flank pain, cyclical vomiting, and hematuria in addition to a mass. The renal US confirms the presence of a hydronephrotic kidney; a subsequent diuretic nuclear renogram can further characterize the severity of the obstruction and the relative function of the kidneys.

Treatment

Surgical correction is indicated when a proven obstruction progresses, results in deterioration of function, or causes symptoms. The most common approach to correction of the UPJ in children is laparoscopic or open pyeloplasty, which reestablishes transport of urine from the pelvis to the ureter.

VESICOURETERAL REFLUX

Vesicoureteral reflux (VUR) results when the length of the tunnel of the intravesical submucosal ureter is insufficient to prevent retrograde flow. The condition may be bilateral or unilateral.

CLINICAL MANIFESTATIONS

The most frequent presentation is recurrent urinary tract infections (UTIs), though it is important to realize the VUR in itself does not cause infection. Retrograde flow of infected urine can result in pyelonephritis. Like UPJO, VUR can cause fetal hydronephrosis, but it is a much less frequent etiology.

DIAGNOSTIC EVALUATION

A voiding cystourethrogram (VCUG) detects abnormalities at ureteral insertion sites and permits classification of the grade of reflux based on the extent of retrograde flow and associated dilatation of the ureter and pelvis (Fig. 14-1). It is the initial study of choice when VUR is suspected due to the ability to obtain superior anatomic detail. Radionuclide cystography exposes patients to a lower radiation dose and is useful for following reflux. Low grades of reflux may resolve spontaneously. Higher grades are associated with large, tortuous ureters; marked distortion of the renal pelvis and calyces; and low spontaneous resolution rates. The associated recurrent UTIs and pyelonephritis can lead to progressive renal injury and scarring.

TREATMENT

Antibiotic prophylaxis is the first-line treatment for VUR. Amoxicillin is preferred in infants ≤3 months of age. Older patients can be treated with trimethoprim-sulfamethoxazole or nitrofurantoin. There is current controversy in the literature regarding the need for antibiotic prophylaxis in patients with low-grade VUR; however antibiotic prophylaxis is still recommended for all children with VUR, especially infants and small children. Ureteral reimplantation is indicated when the grade of reflux worsens, multiple antibiotic sensitivities or allergies develop, there is evidence of diminishment of renal function, the patient has recurrent UTIs or pyelonephritis, or noncompliance is an issue. Surgery involves lengthening the intravesicular segment of the tunnel through which the ureter enters the bladder. An alternative to open surgery is injection with bulking agents such as Deflux™ to recreate the tunnel mechanism.

POSTERIOR URETHRAL VALVES

Occurring only in males, posterior urethral valves (PUV) consist of obstructing leaflets within the posterior urethra which result in partial-to-complete bladder outlet obstruction. The increased pressure causes urethral dilation, bladder neck hypertrophy, and bladder trabeculation. VUR occurs with increased frequency and may lead to renal dysplasia. Posterior urethral valves are the most common cause of **end-stage renal disease** in the male child.

CLINICAL MANIFESTATIONS

The disorder may be suspected by detecting hydronephrosis and bladder distention on prenatal US

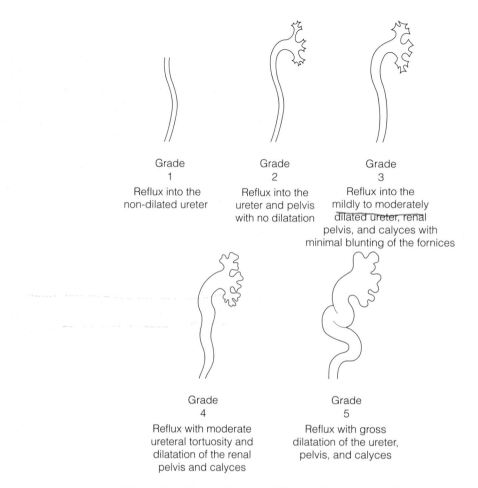

Grade
1
Reflux into the
non-dilated ureter

Grade
2
Reflux into the
ureter and pelvis
with no dilatation

Grade
3
Reflux into the
mildly to moderately
dilated ureter, renal
pelvis, and calyces with
minimal blunting of the fornices

Grade
4
Reflux with moderate
ureteral tortuosity and
dilatation of the renal
pelvis and calyces

Grade
5
Reflux with gross
dilatation of the ureter,
pelvis, and calyces

Figure 14-1 • International classification of vesicoureteral reflux.

or by palpating a distended bladder or renal mass during the newborn examination. In older infants, parents may note a weak or dribbling urinary stream or unexplained daytime wetting. Occasionally, the condition is diagnosed in boys during radiologic evaluation following a UTI. Posterior urethral valves are clearly visualized on a radiographic VCUG.

TREATMENT

First-line treatment involves ablation of the obstructing valve leaflets and, if VUR is present, antibiotic prophylaxis. Sometimes intermittent catheterization or temporary diversion with a vesicostomy is necessary. When VUR is secondary to PUV, rates of resolution are roughly equal for all grades with adequate bladder management; early surgical correction of the reflux is discouraged, as the bladder pathophysiology can change over time and early surgery has a high failure rate. Prognosis is related to the degree of renal and bladder impairment at the time of PUV ablation.

HYPOSPADIAS

Hypospadias, the most common congenital anomaly of the penis, occurs in 1 per 250 male newborns. Incomplete development of the distal urethra leads to positioning of the urethral meatus along the ventral shaft of the penis toward the perineum. The ventral foreskin is usually deficient. Hypospadias may be associated with a curvature of the penis known as chordee. **Circumcision is contraindicated** because surgical repair may require the preputial tissue. The aims of therapy are to extend the urethral meatus to the tip of the glans penis, create a straight erection, and produce the appearance of a normal circumcised phallus. Prognosis is excellent for distal hypospadias; proximal hypospadias may require a staged surgical approach in order to achieve an acceptable cosmetic and functional result. The association of a hypospadias and any degree of testicular cryptorchidism should prompt an ambiguous genitalia workup.

CRYPTORCHIDISM

Cryptorchidism is defined as testes that have not fully descended into the scrotum and, unlike retractile testes, cannot be manipulated into the scrotum with gentle pressure. Isolated cryptorchidism is one of the most common congenital anomalies discovered at birth, occurring in roughly 3% of term male newborns. As a group, preterm infants have a higher incidence of undescended testes, although this may be related more to low birth weight than gestational age. Testes that remain outside the scrotum may develop impaired sperm and hormone production; both the undescended and the contralateral descended testes are at increased risk for malignancy. Bilateral cryptorchidism usually results in oligospermia and infertility.

CLINICAL MANIFESTATIONS

One or both testes may be positioned in the abdomen or anywhere along the inguinal canal. Most are palpable on examination. Ninety percent of patients also have inguinal hernias.

TREATMENT

By 12 months of age, .99% of males have bilateral descended testicles. Spontaneous descent after age 3 months is unlikely. Surgical repair (orchiopexy) takes place at 6 to 12 months of age and has a high success rate (99%). Orchiopexy does not appear to alter the incidence of malignant degeneration (2% to 3%), but it does render the testis accessible for regular self-examination.

TESTICULAR TORSION

Torsion is a **surgical emergency**, requiring prompt recognition and correction to prevent loss of the testicle. Most patients with testicular torsion lack the posterior attachment to the tunica vaginalis that keeps the testis from rotating around the spermatic cord. This creates a mobile testis and results in a **bell-clapper deformity** (the ability of the untethered testis to twist on its stalk).

CLINICAL MANIFESTATIONS

Testicular torsion is a clinical diagnosis. The hallmark of presentation is the acute onset of unilateral scrotal pain typically sufficient to wake the child from sleep. Nausea and vomiting are common. Right-sided torsion sometimes is confused with appendicitis, necessitating examination of the external genitalia in males with abdominal pain. In torsion, the scrotum often appears swollen and erythematous. The testis is exquisitely tender and the cremasteric reflex is usually absent. **Epididymitis**, which is more common during adolescence, presents with a similar clinical picture. Epididymitis may be infectious or secondary to torsion of a testicular or epididymal **appendix**. A Doppler US is helpful in differentiating between epididymitis and testicular torsion but may delay appropriate treatment. The presence of the "blue dot" sign (on the upper aspect of the scrotum) and a normal cremasteric reflex suggest torsion of the appendix testes, though US with Doppler flow is recommended to rule out testicular torsion.

TREATMENT

Early surgical detorsion is critical and should ideally take place within 6 hours of the onset of pain. If the testis is manually detorsed in the ER, US conformation and surgical exploration should be performed during the same admission. Necrotic testes must be removed. The contralateral testis is fixed to the fibrous layer of the posterior scrotal envelope during surgery to prevent subsequent torsion. Torsion of a testicular or epididymal appendix resolves spontaneously; nonetheless, epididymitis due to torsion is often treated with antibiotics.

HYDROCELES AND VARICOCELES

Hydroceles are fluid-filled sacs in the scrotal cavity consisting of remnants of the processus vaginalis. They are often diagnosed in the newborn period or early childhood. Hydroceles communicate with the peritoneal cavity through a patent processus and are at risk for incarceration. These **communicating** hydroceles and hernias should be repaired as soon as possible to prevent the development of an incarcerated hernia. Most noncommunicating or simple hydroceles involute by 12 months of age.

A **varicocele** is defined as dilation of the testicular veins and enlargement of the pampiniform plexus. Varicoceles become detectable in boys during adolescence, occur more commonly on the left, and are usually nontender. They are generally not visible when the patient is supine, but become evident upon standing when the veins distend and produce the characteristic "bag of worms" within the scrotum. Indications for surgical repair include pain, progressive enlargement, and discordant testicular growth. Unrepaired varicoceles may place the patient at an increased risk for infertility.

URINARY TRACT INFECTIONS

PATHOGENESIS

Bacterial UTIs are a frequent cause of pediatric morbidity. Infection may be limited to the bladder (**cystitis**) or may also involve the kidney (**pyelonephritis**). Children with pyelonephritis can sustain damage to the infected area of the renal parenchyma, resulting in localized scarring and decreased function.

In febrile infants, the urinary tract is the most common site of bacterial infection. The source is almost always hematogenous seeding of the kidneys, which results in the high rate of renal scarring observed in this group of patients. In older children, UTIs more often result from ascent of exterior fecal flora into the urinary tract. Common pathogens include *Escherichia coli* (80%) and *Proteus* and *Klebsiella* species.

EPIDEMIOLOGY

After the first year of life (equal incidence), girls have almost a 10-fold risk over boys. Although uncircumcised male infants are more prone to UTIs in the first year of life, this susceptibility alone is not a sufficient indication for universal routine circumcision.

RISK FACTORS

The most significant risk factor is the presence of an anatomic or physiologic urinary tract abnormality that predisposes to stasis of urine. Examples include bladder outlet obstruction, reflux, and dysfunctional voiding.

DIFFERENTIAL DIAGNOSIS

The differential diagnosis includes external genital irritation, meatal stenosis in the circumcised male,

vaginitis, vaginal foreign body, sexual abuse, and pinworm infestation. Adenovirus can cause a self-limited hemorrhagic cystitis that does not respond to antibiotics but may be mistaken for a UTI. Lower lobe pneumonia often presents with fever, chills, and flank pain. In the adolescent, the possibility of a sexually transmitted disease must be entertained. Posterior urethralgia is a benign, self-limiting inflammation of the posterior urethra in boys which may mimic a UTI.

CLINICAL MANIFESTATIONS

In older children, the signs and symptoms of cystitis are similar to those in adults and include low-grade fever, frequency, urgency, dysuria, incontinence, abdominal pain, and hematuria. In contrast, pyelonephritis presents with high fever, chills, nausea, vomiting, and flank pain. Older children are more likely to have an isolated infection of the bladder; upper tract involvement is suggested by elevation of the peripheral white blood count, erythrocyte sedimentation rate, and C-reactive protein. Unexplained high fevers in younger children should prompt at minimum a clean-catch or catheterized urine sample.

Infants warrant special attention because fever may be the only manifestation of a UTI in this age group, and a UTI can be the first clinical suggestion of an obstructive anomaly or vesicoureteral reflux. Ideally, the urine should be examined in all febrile patients younger than 1 to 2 years.

DIAGNOSTIC EVALUATION

Although pyuria, hematuria, and bacteriuria on urinalysis suggest a UTI, a positive urine culture is the gold standard for diagnosis. The absence of white and/or red blood cells in the urine does not rule out a UTI; for instance, pyuria is often absent in febrile infants with pyelonephritis. Urine may be obtained by suprapubic tap (in neonates), sterile catheterization of the bladder, or clean catch (listed in order of increasing likelihood of contamination). Bagged specimens are inadequate for evaluation of UTIs. All febrile infants (and older patients with suspected UTIs) should receive a urine culture (results in 24 to 48 hours) and dipstick urinalysis. Patients with positive dipstick results for leukocyte esterase (with or without positive nitrites) should be treated for a presumed UTI until culture results are available. Susceptibility testing is performed on any singular bacteria isolated to ensure appropriate antibiotic treatment.

The workup of initial UTIs in children is controversial and depends on the patient's age, severity of infection, and response to treatment. Figure 14-2 provides a suggested diagnostic algorithm for children with UTIs. Current American Academy of Pediatrics guidelines recommend that all children younger than 24 months undergo renal US to rule out hydronephrosis or structural lesions that predispose to infection. Those with hydronephrosis on US and those with normal US who do not respond to appropriate antibiotic therapy within 48 hours should also receive a VCUG. In prompt responders with normal US, the VCUG is optional. Other experts argue that all children younger than a certain age (6 to 12 months) should receive a VCUG regardless of response to treatment. It is likely that further studies will result in more evidence-based recommendations.

In cases of suspected pyelonephritis, a nuclear imaging study such as a DMSA is helpful to document areas of injury and possible scar formation.

TREATMENT

Children with suspected cystitis may be treated with an appropriate oral antibiotic such as amoxicillin, ampicillin, nitrofurantoin, or trimethoprim-sulfamethoxazole. If the culture is negative, antibiotics may be discontinued. A positive urine culture should prompt a 5- to 7-day course with an appropriate oral antibiotic (based on sensitivity results).

Nontoxic-appearing children with suspected pyelonephritis should be treated with an oral cephalosporin or intravenous ampicillin plus gentamicin or a cephalosporin until culture results are available. Patients who are toxic-appearing, unable to tolerate oral medications, or younger than 6 months must be admitted to the hospital for 10 to 14 days of intravenous antibiotics and observation. Patients older than 6 months may be discharged on a culture-specific oral antibiotic to finish the course of therapy provided their clinical picture improves. Large defects on DMSA scan suggestive of severe pyelonephritis may benefit from a full course of intravenous antibiotics.

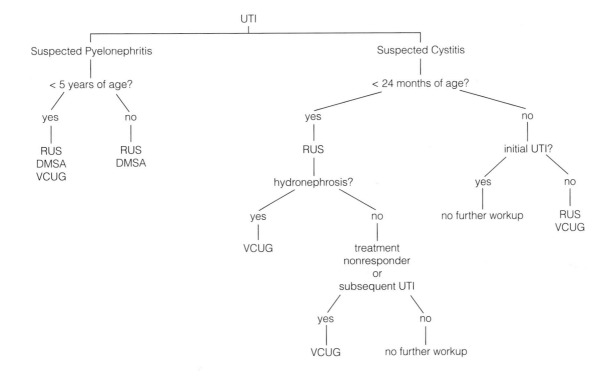

RUS, renal ultrasound; DMSA, technetium-99 dimercaptosuccinic acid renal scan; VCUG, voiding cystourethrogram

Figure 14-2 • Suggested diagnostic algorithm for pediatric urinary tract infection.

The prognosis for patients with isolated cystitis is excellent; morbidity increases with recurrent infection. Most UTI-related complications are the result of pyelonephritis, including perinephric abscesses, renal scarring, and renal failure.

NEPHROTIC SYNDROME

Nephrotic syndrome is a glomerular disorder characterized by proteinuria, hypoalbuminemia, hyperlipidemia, and edema.

EPIDEMIOLOGY

In children, nephrotic syndrome may be idiopathic (90%) or secondary (Table 14-1). **Minimal change disease** (MCD) is by far the most common cause of primary nephrotic syndrome in the pediatric population (more than 80% of all cases). Most patients present between 2 and 6 years of age, and boys outnumber girls. **Focal segmental glomerulosclerosis** (FSGS), **membranoproliferative glomerulonephropathy** (MPGN), and **membranous nephropathy** (MN) account for most of the remainder of idiopathic cases of nephrotic syndrome in children. These forms are typically detected in the older age groups.

CLINICAL MANIFESTATIONS

Patients with early nephrotic syndrome appear quite well. Periorbital edema is commonly the first abnormality noted. This is followed by lower-extremity edema, weight gain, generalized edema, and ascites. Anorexia and diarrhea are variably present.

DIFFERENTIAL DIAGNOSIS

Edema may be renal, hepatic, nutritional, or cardiac in origin. Other conditions associated with proteinuria include exercise, trauma, UTI, dehydration, and acute tubular necrosis; however, none of these causes the degree of protein loss seen in nephrotic syndrome. Of note, glomerular filtration rate (GFR) and blood pressure are less likely to be affected in nephrotic syndrome than in the nephritic syndromes (Table 14-2).

DIAGNOSTIC EVALUATION

The hallmark of nephrotic syndrome is **marked proteinuria**. Nephrotic-range proteinuria is usually defined as proteinuria exceeding $1,000$ mg/m^2 per day, or a spot (random) urinary protein-to-creatinine ratio exceeding 2 mg/mg. The proteinuria in childhood nephrotic syndrome is relatively selective, consisting primarily of albumin, with resultant hypoalbuminemia (<2.5 g/dL). Hyperlipidemia, with elevated serum cholesterol and triglyceride concentrations, is a

---

■ TABLE 14-1 Causes of Childhood Nephrotic Syndrome

Primary

- Minimal change nephrotic syndrome (MCNS)
- Focal segmental glomerulosclerosis (FSGS)
- Membranoproliferative glomerulonephritis (MPGN)
- Membranous nephropathy (MN)

Secondary

- Infections (hepatitis B, hepatitis C, HIV, malaria, syphilis)
- Systemic diseases (SLE, Henoch-Schonlein purpura, diabetes mellitus)
- Allergies (bee stings, food allergens)
- Drugs (nonsteroidal anti-inflammatory drugs, heroin)
- Malignancies (lymphoma, leukemia)
- Genetic (Finnish-type congenital nephrotic syndrome, Denys-Drash syndrome)

■ TABLE 14-2 Diseases That Present with the Nephritic Syndrome

Acute poststreptococcal glomerulonephritis (APGN)
Henoch-Schönlein purpura
IgA nephropathy
Hemolytic-uremic syndrome
Systemic lupus erythematosus (SLE)
Alport syndrome
Membranoproliferative glomerulonephritis (MPGN)
Shunt nephritis

consistent feature of nephrotic syndrome. It is usually transient, resulting primarily from increased hepatic lipoprotein synthesis in response to low plasma oncotic pressure.

Renal biopsy is indicated for patients outside the typical age range for MCD, those with renal insufficiency, and those who do not respond to steroids. Gross sections in MCD show few if any abnormalities; the only consistent finding is effacement of epithelial cell foot processes demonstrated by electron microscopy. Focal segmental glomerulosclerosis is characterized by focal sections of distorted glomeruli, with mesangial hypertrophy, segmental capillary loop fibrosis, and varying degrees of tubular atrophy. Increased mesangial cellularity and glomerular basement membrane thickening are found in diffuse membranoproliferative glomerulonephritis. Membranous nephropathy is characterized by diffuse thickening of the capillary walls due to deposit formation.

TREATMENT

If the clinical presentation is consistent with uncomplicated primary nephrotic syndrome, strict dietary salt restriction and oral steroid therapy are appropriate. If symptoms do not resolve within 8 to 12 weeks or if the patient experiences frequent or severe relapses, renal biopsy is indicated to confirm the diagnosis and identify the histologic subtype.

Steroids result in prompt remission in most cases of MCD. Nephrotic syndrome that does not respond to oral steroids may require treatment with immune suppressants such as cyclophosphamide. Intravenous albumin (followed by a diuretic) can be used as a temporary measure to induce diuresis in the presence of incapacitating anasarca or edema-related respiratory compromise.

Bacterial infections, particularly **spontaneous bacterial peritonitis**, are the most frequent complications of nephrotic syndrome and usually occur while the patient is on immunosuppressant therapy. Other serious complications include thromboembolic events, hypertension, persistent hyperlipidemia, and steroid toxicity.

The prognosis of MCD is excellent; although up to 80% of patients relapse at least once, very few develop any long-standing renal insufficiency. Unfortunately, patients with focal segmental glomerulosclerosis and diffuse membranoproliferative glomerulonephritis do not respond well to steroid therapy, and end-stage renal disease is common. Both diseases may recur following renal transplantation.

GLOMERULONEPHRITIS

The term **glomerulonephritis** implies inflammation within the glomerulus. Antigen-antibody complexes are formed or deposited in the subepithelial or subendothelial areas; immune mediators follow, resulting in inflammatory injury. The term **nephritic syndrome** is characterized by **hematuria** (overt or microscopic) with red cell casts, edema, hypertension, and azotemia. The major glomerulonephritic syndromes of childhood are listed in Table 14-2; distinguishing characteristics are discussed in the following sections.

ACUTE GLOMERULONEPHRITIDES

Acute poststreptococcal glomerulonephritis (APGN), the most common glomerulonephritis in childhood, occurs sporadically in older children and is twice as common in males. Streptococcal infections involving either the throat or the skin (impetigo) precede the clinical syndrome by 1 to 3 weeks. Treating the streptococcal infection does not prevent APGN. Elevated antistreptolysin-O or anti-DNAse B titers suggest recent streptococcal infection. The C3 component of the complement pathway is low. Although biopsies are not usually performed, the renal histology reveals mesangial and capillary cell proliferation, inflammatory cell infiltration, and granular "humps" of IgG and C3 below the glomerular basement membrane.

Henoch-Schönlein purpura (HSP), a systemic vasculitis characterized by a purpuric rash, crampy abdominal pain, and arthritis, can present with a glomerulonephritis-type syndrome that may be difficult to distinguish from IgA nephropathy. The C3 levels remain normal. Two percent of children with HSP develop long-term renal impairment.

Rapidly progressive glomerulonephritis is the description given to a number of glomerulopathies that, for unknown reasons, deteriorate over a few weeks or months to renal failure, uremia, encephalopathy, and even death. All forms demonstrate generalized crescent formation in the glomeruli, thought to represent cellular destruction by macrophages with subsequent necrosis and fibrin deposition. Fortunately, rapidly progressive glomerulonephritis is rare in children.

CHRONIC GLOMERULONEPHRITIDES

IgA nephropathy, once thought to be a benign condition, is now known to slowly progress to renal failure in 25% of cases. The C3 levels are normal. Renal biopsy confirms the diagnosis, demonstrating mesangial deposits of IgA in the glomeruli. Glomerulonephritis associated with systemic lupus erythematosus is discussed in Chapter 11.

INHERITED GLOMERULONEPHRITIDES

Alport syndrome, or hereditary nephritis, is caused by mutations in the gene encoding type IV collagen that result in an abnormal glomerular basement membrane. Inheritance is X-linked, although defective genes encoding other glomerular basement membrane components can cause similar disease. The diagnosis is usually confirmed through renal biopsy, which reveals a characteristic splitting of the basement membranes. Because type IV collagen is an important component of the cochlea, Alport syndrome is associated with sensorineural hearing loss.

Benign familial hematuria, or thin membrane disease, is a common cause of asymptomatic microscopic and occasionally gross hematuria. Renal function is normal, and biopsy, although unnecessary, reveals diffuse thinning of the glomerular basement membrane on electron microscopy. Because transmission is autosomal dominant, asymptomatic microscopic hematuria is usually found in other family members.

CLINICAL MANIFESTATIONS

The initial presentation of glomerulonephritis includes hematuria, azotemia, oliguria, malaise, abdominal pain, edema, and **hypertension**. Red cell casts are invariably present; in fact, the urine is often described as tea colored by parents. Proteinuria occurs as well but is usually much less prominent than in nephrotic syndrome. The GFR is compromised, leading to salt and water retention and circulatory overload. Azotemia is marked by increasing serum BUN and creatinine levels. Sodium and potassium regulation may be temporarily disrupted. Important laboratory studies include UA, urine culture, hemoglobin and platelet counts, coagulation studies, serum electrolytes, BUN and creatinine, streptococcal antibody titers, and complement levels. A low level of complement C3 which

returns to normal in 6 to 8 weeks is typical of APGN, whereas a persistently decreased level of C3 (and C4) is highly suggestive of SLE or MPGN.

DIFFERENTIAL DIAGNOSIS

The differential diagnosis of hematuria, the most prominent manifestation of glomerulonephritis, includes other renal conditions (infection, trauma, malignancy, stones, cystic disease) and hematologic disorders. Vaginal bleeding produces false-positive results if the specimen is collected incorrectly. Both hemoglobin and myoglobin test positive for blood on urine dipstick; however, there are no red blood cells on microscopic urine examination in the presence of myoglobinuria.

TREATMENT

Positive streptococcal cultures are treated with appropriate antibiotic therapy. Hypertension, when present, can be severe, requiring vasodilators, diuretics, and fluid restriction. Steroids may improve the outcome of rapidly progressive glomerulonephritis.

Although the clinical manifestations of APGN may take a few months to resolve, the overall prognosis for return to normal function is excellent. Patients with other types of glomerulonephritis fare less well. Virtually all males and 20% of females with Alport syndrome progress to end-stage renal disease by middle adulthood. The course of rapidly progressive glomerulonephritis is particularly devastating, with most patients becoming dependent on dialysis within a few years. Many chronic glomerulonephritic syndromes progress to renal failure and may eventually recur in the transplanted kidney.

RENAL TUBULAR ACIDOSIS

All forms of renal tubular acidosis (RTA) are characterized by normal anion gap **hyperchloremic metabolic acidosis**, resulting from insufficient renal transport of bicarbonate or acids. The nephron tubules are the site of reabsorption and secretion. Most bicarbonate filtered from the plasma is reabsorbed in the proximal tubule, along with amino acids, glucose, sodium, potassium, calcium, phosphate, and water. In the distal tubule, the remainder of the bicarbonate is reabsorbed and hydrogen ions are secreted into the tubular lumen. Defects in either transport site compromise the kidney's ability to maintain pH homeostasis.

DIFFERENTIAL DIAGNOSIS

In **proximal RTA** (type 2), the proximal tubule fails to reabsorb bicarbonate from the ultrafiltrate. Distal RTA may result from either deficient hydrogen secretion into the filtrate (type 1) or impaired ammonia production in the face of hyperkalemia from hypoaldosteronism or pseudohypoaldosteronism (type 4). Distal RTA type 4 is the most common RTA in both children and adults. Most types of RTA can be hereditary or sporadic, acute or chronic, occurring alone or as part of a disease complex. For example, most patients exhibit proximal RTA type 2 in conjunction with **Fanconi syndrome**, a generalized disorder of proximal tubule transport resulting in excessive urinary losses of bicarbonate, amino acids, small proteins, glucose, electrolytes, and water.

CLINICAL MANIFESTATIONS

Patients who manifest proximal RTA type 2 as part of Fanconi syndrome present with failure to thrive; associated signs and symptoms include chronic acidosis, hypokalemia, vomiting, anorexia, polydipsia and polyuria, volume contraction, and impaired vitamin D metabolism (rickets).

Distal RTA type 1 also presents with metabolic acidosis and failure to thrive. Hypokalemia, hypercalciuria, and kidney stones are common. In contrast, the acidosis in distal RTA type 4 occurs in the setting of hyperkalemia in conjunction with primary or secondary hypoaldosteronism or end-organ resistance.

DIAGNOSTIC EVALUATION

Any patient with hyperchloremic metabolic acidosis of unclear etiology warrants further workup to rule out RTA (Fig. 14-3).

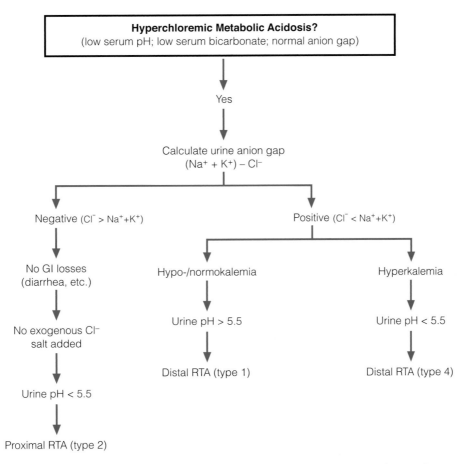

Figure 14-3 • Suggested diagnostic algorithm for hyperchloremic metabolic acidosis of unknown etiology.

TREATMENT

Treatment consists of providing children with sufficient amounts of an **alkalinizing agent** (bicarbonate or citrate) to correct the acidosis completely and restore normal growth. Thiazide diuretics may be administered in proximal RTA to increase proximal tubular reabsorption of bicarbonate. Hypokalemia is treated concurrently when the alkali is coupled with potassium as a salt. Hyperkalemia is usually more difficult to correct; furosemide is prescribed unless the defect results in salt wasting. If RTA is associated with an underlying condition, the primary disorder must be treated.

NEPHROGENIC DIABETES INSIPIDUS

PATHOGENESIS

Diabetes insipidus (DI) involves a disorder in renal concentrating ability. Patients produce large amounts of very dilute urine regardless of hydration status. DI may be central or nephrogenic in origin. In central DI, the production or release of antidiuretic hormone is insufficient (see Chapter 6). Nephrogenic DI arises from end-organ resistance to arginine vasopressin (antidiuretic hormone), either from a receptor defect or from medications or other processes that interfere with aquaporin-2–mediated transport of water at the renal cortical tubules.

EPIDEMIOLOGY

Nephrogenic DI may be congenital or acquired and usually presents within the first several years of life. Acquired nephrogenic DI has been associated with polycystic kidney disease, pyelonephritis, lithium toxicity, and sickle cell disease.

CLINICAL MANIFESTATIONS

All patients present with polyuria and compensatory polydipsia. Other features may include intermittent fever, irritability, vomiting, and growth retardation. Most affected children also have a history of recurrent hypernatremic dehydration. Developmental delay may occur as a result of frequent hypernatremic seizures. Some patients manifest no symptoms until they are stressed with illness. Others remain completely unable to keep themselves in fluid balance without continual therapy.

DIFFERENTIAL DIAGNOSIS

Differentiating central DI from nephrogenic DI is not possible based on symptomatology alone, although the former more commonly follows head trauma or meningitis. Other conditions that may present in a similar manner include diabetes mellitus, RTA, and compulsive water drinking, which is seen in a significant minority of patients with schizophrenia.

DIAGNOSTIC EVALUATION

Patients with nephrogenic DI are unable to concentrate their urine. Despite significant dehydration, their urine specific gravity and osmolarity measurements remain inappropriately low. Figure 14-4 outlines the suggested evaluation of a patient with suspected nephrogenic DI. Perinatal testing to detect arginine vasopressin receptor gene (*AVPR2*) mutations is now available.

TREATMENT

Acute treatment consists of rehydrating the child, replacing ongoing urinary losses, and correcting electrolyte abnormalities. A low-sodium diet (<0.7 mEq/kg/day) should be coupled with thiazide diuret-

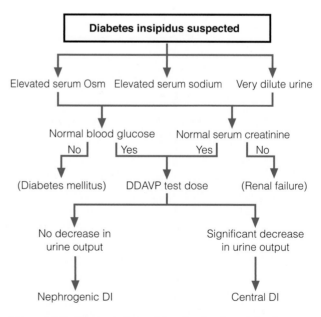

Figure 14-4 • Suggested algorithm for the diagnosis of nephrogenic diabetes insipidus.

ics to decrease urinary sodium reabsorption. The addition of indomethacin may have an additive effect on thiazide diuretics in reducing water excretion.

Children with nephrogenic DI are at risk for poor growth. The disease is life-long but carries a good prognosis, provided that episodes of hypernatremic dehydration are minimized.

HYPERTENSION

Blood pressure rises as a child grows, reaching adult values during adolescence. Hypertension in the pediatric population is defined as blood pressure **greater than 95th percentile for age**, **gender**, **and height** measured on three separate occasions about 1 week apart.

DIFFERENTIAL DIAGNOSIS

Essential (primary) hypertension is the most common form in adults. Children are more likely to man-

ifest **secondary hypertension**, usually related to renal disease. However, because of the increase in childhood obesity and poor diet, the rate of essential hypertension in children is increasing. Endocrine, vascular, and neurologic conditions may also be associated with increased blood pressure (Table 14-3).

CLINICAL MANIFESTATIONS

History

Stable or slowly progressive hypertension is unlikely to cause symptoms. Family history is often positive for hypertension, stroke, or premature heart attack. Patients with secondary hypertension often come to medical attention for complaints related to their underlying disease (e.g., growth failure, edema). Past medical history, state of health, recent medications, and review of systems for urinary tract symptoms provide pertinent information.

■ **TABLE 14-3** Differential Diagnosis of Pediatric Hypertension	
Factitious	*Endocrine*
• Anxiety ("white coat" hypertension)	• Congenital adrenal hyperplasia
• Inappropriate cuff size	• Cushing syndrome
Primary (essential) hypertension	• Hyper- or hypothyroidism
	• Pheochromocytoma
Renal	• Hyperaldosteronism
• Glomerulonephritis	• Hypercalcemia
• Pyelonephritis	
• Cystic disease	*Vascular*
• Obstructive uropathy	• Renal artery stenosis
• Renal trauma	• Coarctation of the aorta
• Renal tumor	• Renal artery thrombosis
• Renal failure	• Renal vein thrombosis
	• Arteriovenous fistula
Neurologic	• Vasculitis
• Pain	*Other*
• Increased intracranial pressure	• Chronic upper airway obstruction
• Brain injury	• Acute intermittent porphyria
• Malignant hyperthermia	
Drugs and Toxins	
• Oral contraceptives	
• Corticosteroids	
• Calcineurin inhibitors	
• Cocaine and other street drugs	

Severe hypertension or hypertension that has developed over a short period of time can cause headache, dizziness, and vision changes. **Hypertensive encephalopathy** is characterized by vomiting, ataxia, mental status changes, and seizures.

Physical Examination

The most important part of the examination is obtaining an accurate blood pressure reading. The air bladder portion of the cuff should encircle the patient's arm and be wide enough to cover 75% of the upper limb. A cuff that is too small will give a falsely elevated reading. At least once, the blood pressure should be taken in all four extremities to exclude aortic coarctation. Particular attention should be given to the heart sounds and peripheral pulses. Poor growth, flank pain, a retroperitoneal mass, large bladder, or abdominal bruit suggests a renal or renal vascular etiology. Obesity contributes to hypertension in a genetically predisposed patient.

DIAGNOSTIC EVALUATION

The initial laboratory evaluation should include a CBC, serum electrolytes, BUN, creatinine, renin level, and UA. Doppler US of the kidneys permits assessment of anatomy as well as renal vasculature. Chest radiograph, electrocardiogram, and echocardiogram evaluate heart size and function, whether cardiac deficits are the cause or the effect of the hypertension.

TREATMENT

The best treatment for essential hypertension is **preventive healthcare**. High-salt diet, sedentary lifestyle, cigarette use, alcohol abuse, drug abuse, high serum cholesterol levels, and obesity compound the disorder and increase the morbidity and mortality. Secondary hypertension responds to treatment of the underlying disorder when possible.

Pharmacologic therapy is indicated in patients with persistent or refractory hypertension. Diuretics, β-blockers, and calcium channel blockers are used in younger children; angiotensin receptor blockers are second-line treatment in this age group but are effective first-line agents in adolescents and adults because of fewer side effects.

In patients with severe hypertension, rapid decreases in blood pressure compromise organ perfusion. Hypertensive crisis is treated with sublingual nifedipine, intravenous nicardipine, intravenous ni-

troprusside, or labetalol. Hydralazine is also effective, especially in neonates. Close monitoring is essential to prevent a rapid drop in blood pressure.

Stroke, heart attack, and renal disease are the most devastating complications of hypertension. Prognosis depends on the underlying disorder and degree of control.

ACUTE RENAL FAILURE

Renal failure is a potentially life-threatening condition with increasing incidence in children. **Acute renal failure** (ARF) consists of an abrupt reduction in renal function, occurring over hours to days, with retention of nitrogenous waste products such as BUN and creatinine (azotemia). Recently, the term **acute kidney injury** (AKI) has been proposed to reflect a complex disorder that occurs in a wide variety of settings with clinical manifestations ranging from a minimal elevation in serum creatinine to anuric renal failure.

DIFFERENTIAL DIAGNOSIS

The mechanisms of ARF include prerenal, intrinsic, or postrenal failure (Table 14-4). **Prerenal** failure is

■ **TABLE 14-4** Causes of Acute Renal Failure
Prerenal
• Hypovolemia (dehydration, shock, hemorrhage, nephrotic syndrome)
• Hypotension (decreased cardiac output, shock, sepsis)
• Peripheral vasodilatation (anaphylaxis, shock, sepsis)
• Renal vasoconstriction (sepsis, NSAIDs, ACE inhibitors, hepatorenal syndrome)
Intrinsic
• Acute tubular necrosis (prolonged prerenal failure, nephrotoxins)
• Acute glomerulonephritis (poststreptococcal, membranoproliferative, crescentic)
• Acute interstitial nephritis (idiopathic, antibiotics)
• Renal vascular disease (hemolytic-uremic syndrome, vasculitis)
Postrenal
• Congenital (posterior urethral valves, ureteropelvic junction obstruction)
• Acquired (stones, clots, neurogenic bladder)
ACE, angiotensin converting enzyme; NSAID, nonsteroidal anti-inflammatory drugs

the functional response of a structurally normal kidney to hypoperfusion. This is the most common form, accounting for about 55% of ARF, with hypovolemia as the most common underlying mechanism. The decreasing GFR produces oliguria (urine output <400 mL/m^2/day) or anuria. Most patients completely recover from prerenal failure unless it is unrecognized or inappropriately treated.

By contrast, **intrinsic** renal failure results from a structural abnormality in the kidney itself, and accounts for about 40% of ARF cases. The most common underlying mechanism is acute tubular necrosis (ATN), and the terms *intrinsic ARF* and *ATN* are frequently used interchangeably. ATN is a poorly understood condition in which damaged tubules become obstructed with cellular debris. ATN may result from prolonged prerenal failure, sepsis, and the use of nephrotoxic medications (such as aminoglycosides, vancomycin, and radio-contrast media). Intrinsic renal failure can also occur in patients with glomerulonephritis, interstitial nephritis, and renal vasculitis. While hemolytic-uremic syndrome used to be the most common cause of intrinsic ARF a decade ago, the epidemiology of ARF has shifted in recent years, with ATN and sepsis accounting for the majority of cases today. Intrarenal conditions can present with oliguria or anuria, although the urine output may also be normal, especially when nephrotoxins are the cause (nonoliguric renal failure). While patients can recover from intrinsic renal failure, a significant number progress to chronic renal insufficiency.

In **postrenal** failure, obstructive lesions at or below the collecting ducts produce increased intrarenal pressure and result in a rapidly declining GFR and hydronephrosis. The lesions may be congenital or acquired, structural or functional. Patients with complete obstruction are anuric. Partial obstructions may present with normal or increased urine output.

CLINICAL MANIFESTATIONS

A history of recent dehydration, shock, cardiac surgery, treatment with nephrotoxic medications, streptococcal infection, or posterior urethral valves may help clarify the etiology. Growth failure, bony abnormalities, anemia, deafness, and previous renal conditions suggest acute deterioration superimposed on chronic renal failure. Depending on the etiology, the physical examination may reveal dehydration, cardiovascular stability, abdominal tenderness, and abdominal or suprapubic masses. Edema, oliguria, and hypertension are usually evident. Findings of congestive heart failure (hepatomegaly, diffuse crackles on lung examination) require immediate intervention.

DIAGNOSTIC EVALUATION

ARF is characterized by hyperkalemia, azotemia, and metabolic acidosis. A progressive increase in BUN and creatinine levels signals diminishing renal function. Anemia is variably present. Urinalysis for hematuria, proteinuria, leukocytes, and casts also provides useful information. RBC casts are typical of acute glomerulonephritis, WBC casts are seen in interstitial nephritis or pyelonephritis, and pigmented coarsely granular casts indicate ATN. Urine and plasma urea nitrogen, creatinine, osmolarity, and sodium can be used to differentiate between prerenal and intrinsic failure (Table 14-5).

Renal US is the single best noninvasive radiographic test for determining the site of obstruction in postrenal failure, as well as kidney size and shape and renal blood flow. It is also a very useful modality to differentiate between acute and chronic renal failure, since kidneys are normal or enlarged in ARF and usually shrunken in chronic renal failure. Renal

---

■ TABLE 14-5 Typical Findings in Prerenal and Intrinsic ARF

Diagnostic Index	Prerenal	Intrinsic Renal
Urinalysis	Few if any abnormalities	Hematuria, proteinuria, casts
Urine specific gravity	>1.020	<1.020
Urine osmolality (mOsm/kg H$_2$O)	>500	<350
Urine/plasma creatinine	>40	<20
Serum BUN/creatinine	>20	<15
Fractional excretion of sodium (FeNa)	<1	>2

FeNa (%) = ([U/P]Na)/([U/P]Cr) × 100

nuclear scans can delineate renal perfusion and functional differences. A voiding cystourethrogram and CT may also be helpful. Renal biopsy is indicated when the diagnosis remains unclear or the extent of involvement is unknown.

Major complications of ARF may be metabolic (hyperkalemia, hyponatremia, hypocalcemia, metabolic acidosis with high anion gap), cardiovascular (hypertension, pulmonary edema, arrythmias), gastrointestinal (gastritis, bleeding), neurologic (somnolence, seizures, coma), hematologic (anemia, bleeding), and/or infectious (increased susceptibility to infections).

TREATMENT

Treatment depends on the etiology. Prerenal failure usually responds to prompt and vigorous correction of the renal hypoperfusion. Once intrinsic ARF is established, treatment is largely supportive, consisting of appropriate fluid management (careful replacement of insensible water loss and ongoing losses), correction of electrolyte abnormalities, and dialysis (for fluid overload, hyperkalemia, or acidosis that is unresponsive to medical therapies). The underlying abnormality must be corrected to achieve optimal resolution and to prevent recurrence. Medications that undergo renal clearance require dosing adjustments in ARF to avoid toxicity or further worsening of the ARF. The prognosis of ARF depends on the underlying etiology, length of impairment, and severity of functional disturbance.

CHRONIC RENAL FAILURE

Chronic renal failure (CRF) implies that renal function has dropped below 30% of normal; function at 10% or less defines **end-stage renal disease**. The most common cause of CRF in the pediatric population is obstructive uropathy, followed by renal dysplasia, glomerulonephropathies (particularly focal segmental glomerulosclerosis), and hereditary renal conditions.

CLINICAL MANIFESTATIONS

Growth failure frequently prompts evaluation for renal disease in the outpatient setting. Subjective complaints range from none to polyuria, episodic unexplained dehydration, salt craving, anorexia, nausea, malaise, lethargy, and decreased exercise tolerance. Hypertension and pallor are noted on examination. Long-standing CRF produces rickets.

DIAGNOSTIC EVALUATION

Patients with CRF demonstrate many of the same laboratory abnormalities seen in ARF, including azotemia, acidosis, sodium imbalance, and hyperkalemia. Anemia is usually more pronounced in CRF than ARF. Chronic hyperphosphatemia leads to secondary hyperparathyroidism, presenting as renal osteodystrophy which may be evident on skeletal radiographs.

TREATMENT

Treatment for CRF includes nutritional, pharmacologic, and dialysis therapy. Close monitoring of clinical and laboratory status is required. Protein restriction is controversial, since it prevents worsening azotemia but can also adversely affect growth and development. Sodium intake should be restricted to control hypertension. Calcium carbonate and activated vitamin D treat renal osteodystrophy. Iron and recombinant erythropoietin improve the anemia. Complete catch-up growth is unlikely even when optimal caloric intake and normalization of metabolic parameters occur.

Children with less than 10% of normal renal function (a creatinine greater than 10 mg-dL) require either dialysis or renal transplant. **Peritoneal dialysis**, which can be performed at home, is the standard for children requiring long-term dialysis. Peritonitis, the most frequent complication of peritoneal dialysis, is usually caused by gram-positive organisms and can usually be treated in the outpatient setting. Hemodialysis, performed at specialized pediatric dialysis centers, provides close to 10% of normal renal function but is time consuming. Hemodialysis-associated mortality is low. Complications of hemodialysis include **disequilibrium syndrome**, which occurs when the serum urea nitrogen level drops too rapidly, resulting in cerebral edema. Signs and symptoms of disequilibrium syndrome include headache, nausea, vomiting, abdominal pain, muscle cramps, seizures, and coma. Other complications related to hemodialysis include bleeding, thrombosis, and infection.

Renal transplantation is the ultimate therapy for all children with end-stage renal disease, and there are few absolute contraindications. The donated kidney may come from a living related or deceased donor; living related donor transplants have better host and graft survival rates.

Children with CRF require complex and time-consuming treatment and, as a consequence, they often experience a decrease in their quality of life and are predisposed to developmental and social delays.

ENURESIS

Successful bladder control is typically achieved between 24 and 36 months of age, although many developmentally normal children take significantly longer. Enuresis is the involuntary loss of urine in a child older than 5 years. It may be nocturnal or daytime, primary or secondary. **Primary** enuretics are patients who have never successfully maintained a dry period, whereas **secondary** enuretics are usually dry for several months before regular wetting recurs.

CLINICAL MANIFESTATIONS

A careful history and physical examination may suggest secondary causes for enuresis such as a UTI, developmental delay, obstruction, emotional strain, or inappropriate parental toilet training expectations.

Primary nocturnal enuresis is thought to be caused by delayed maturational control or inadequate levels of antidiuretic hormone secretion during sleep.

TREATMENT

Behavior modification programs are moderately effective. The most popular method of treatment is a nighttime audio alarm that sounds as soon as the child starts to urinate, eventually conditioning controlled bladder emptying before enuresis. Intranasal desmopressin acetate (generic name for DDAVP; analogous to endogenous vasopressin) acts to concentrate the urine. If given in the evening, less urine is produced overnight, decreasing the likelihood of wetting. Given the potential for central nervous system side effects, DDAVP is limited to situational use in this population (e.g., in conjunction with a sleepover or during overnight camp). With all therapies, the cure rate is 15% per year after 5 years of age; children who remain enuretic past 8 years of age have a 10% risk of never resolving their symptoms.

 KEY POINTS

- In older children, urinary tract infections (UTIs) result from contamination of the urinary tract with exterior fecal flora. Hematogenous seeding is more probable in infants, particularly those younger than 2 months. *Escherichia coli* is the most common pathogen in bacterial UTIs. The most significant risk factor for recurrent UTIs is the presence of a urinary tract abnormality that causes urinary stasis, obstruction, reflux, or dysfunctional voiding.

- Nephrotic syndrome is characterized by proteinuria, hypoalbuminemia, hyperlipidemia, and edema. Minimal change disease is the most common type of pediatric idiopathic nephrotic syndrome.

- Glomerulonephritic syndromes are inflammatory and characterized by hematuria, azotemia, oliguria, edema, and hypertension.

- Alport syndrome is associated with painless hematuria and sensorineural hearing loss, and progresses to renal failure in males by middle adulthood.

- The overall prognosis of acute poststreptococcal glomerulonephritis is excellent, with normalization of C3 levels in 6 to 8 weeks and resolution of clinical manifestations in 90% of cases.

- All classifications of renal tubular acidosis (RTA) are characterized by hyperchloremic metabolic acidosis

with a normal plasma anion gap. The most common type in children is distal RTA type 4 with hyperkalemia (from hypoaldosteronism or pseudohypoaldosteronism).

- Diabetes insipidus (DI) is a disorder of urine concentration and can be central or nephrogenic. Clinical manifestations include polyuria, polydipsia, and growth retardation. Therapy for nephrogenic DI includes a low-sodium diet, thiazide diuretics, and indomethacin.

- Blood pressure norms are related to age, gender, and height. Three blood pressure readings on separate occasions that are greater than the 95th percentile for age, height, and gender constitute hypertension. Rapid drops in blood pressure, even if maintained in the normal range, may compromise cerebral perfusion in a patient with a history of sustained high blood pressure.

- The causes of ARF include prerenal (55%), intrarenal (40%), or postrenal (5%). Laboratory findings include increasing levels of BUN and creatinine, hyperkalemia, and metabolic acidosis.

- Children with growth failure should be screened for renal disease.

Mary Sutton • *Katie S. Fine*

NEURAL TUBE DEFECTS

Failure of neural tube closure during the 3rd and 4th weeks of gestation results in a group of related disorders termed **neural tube defects**. Maternal malnutrition, drug exposure (e.g., valproic acid and carbamazepine), maternal hyperthermia, congenital infections, radiation, and genetic factors are all associated with an increased risk of neural tube defects. There is a 3% to 4% risk of a second affected child being born to parents who already have one child with a neural tube defect. Because failure of closure results in persistent leakage of **alpha-fetoprotein** into the amniotic fluid, the maternal serum alpha-fetoprotein level at 16 to 18 weeks' gestation is an excellent screening tool for identifying high-risk pregnancies. The incidence of neural tube defects is decreased in infants whose mothers receive at least 400 micrograms per day of **folic acid** supplementation prior to conception and during the early weeks of pregnancy. The overall incidence of neural tube defects is declining worldwide due to improved maternal nutrition and widespread prenatal diagnosis with subsequent elective termination of the pregnancy.

CLINICAL MANIFESTATIONS

Abnormalities may occur anywhere along the central nervous system (CNS); the higher the lesion, the more devastating the sequelae. Neonates with **anencephaly** are born with large skull defects and virtually no cortex. Brainstem function is marginally intact. Many are stillborn; others die within days of birth. **Encephaloceles** are protrusions of cranial contents through a bony skull defect, usually in the occipital region. Affected patients manifest severe mental retardation, seizures, and motor deficits. Hydrocephalus is a frequent complication.

Spina bifida includes a variety of conditions characterized by neural tube defects in the spinal region associated with incomplete fusion of the vertebral arches. **Myelomeningocele** are protruding sacs of neural and meningeal tissues, whereas **meningoceles** contain meninges only. Both are most common in the lumbosacral region. Bowel and bladder sphincter dysfunction is the rule, and sensorimotor loss exists below the lesion. In **spina bifida occulta**, the bony vertebral lesion occurs without herniation of any spinal contents. Birthmarks, dimples, subcutaneous masses, or hairy tufts at the base of the back suggest an underlying defect. Although the infant may initially appear neurologically intact, the caudal end of the cord is affixed or tethered to the distal spine. As the vertebral column grows throughout childhood, the tethered distal spinal cord develops traction injury, resulting in gait disturbance, sphincter dysfunction, foot deformities, and increasing motor deficits. Spina bifida defects have a high incidence of infectious complications, cortical malformations, and **Chiari type II malformation** (dysgenesis and downward displacement of the lower brainstem and cerebellum that often results in hydrocephalus and stridor, apnea, and dysphagia).

TREATMENT

Cesarean section delivery prior to the onset of labor results in an improved anatomic level of motor function. Early closure of repairable back lesions and prophylactic antibiotics until closure decreases the risk of infection. The majority of infants with myelomeningocele develop hydrocephalus within the first month of life. Early ventriculoperitoneal (VP) shunt placement, even for mild hydrocephalus, appears to improve intellectual outcome. Infants with severe cyanotic episodes, apnea, stridor, and dysphagia from Chiari type II malformations benefit from early cervical decompression. Early attention to urodynamics, anticholinergic medication, and clean intermittent catheterization result in urinary continence for the majority of patients and reduce the risk of urinary tract complications, the major cause of death after the first year of life. Surgical release of tethered spinal cord can prevent deterioration of motor and sphincter dysfunction and may partially reverse acquired deficits. Fetal surgery is under investigation as a means of repairing some defects in an attempt to preserve motor and sensory function.

HYDROCEPHALUS

PATHOGENESIS

Hydrocephalus is the pathologic enlargement of the ventricles that occurs when cerebral spinal fluid (CSF) production outpaces absorption, usually secondary to outflow obstruction. In **noncommunicating** hydrocephalus, the block exists somewhere within the ventricular system, and the ventricles proximal to the obstruction are selectively enlarged. Noncommunicating hydrocephalus is most commonly caused by narrowing at the cerebral aqueduct or malformations/enlargements of the posterior fossa. Causes include congenital malformations such as Chiari type II malformations, aqueductal stenosis, arachnoid cyst, and Dandy-Walker malformation; intrauterine infection; and intraventricular hemorrhage. Acquired noncommunicating hydrocephalus in older children is most often due to posterior fossa neoplasms and aqueductal stenosis or gliosis.

In contrast, all ventricles are proportionately enlarged in **communicating** hydrocephalus, which occurs when CSF absorption at the arachnoid villi is impaired secondary to meningitis, subarachnoid hemorrhage, or leukemia. Rarely, communicating hydrocephalus is due to excessive CSF production from a choroid plexus papilloma.

CLINICAL MANIFESTATIONS

History and Physical Examination

The clinical manifestations of hydrocephalus depend on the rate of onset and whether the fontanelles are still open. An inappropriate increase in head circumference or bulging anterior fontanelle may be the only indication in infants; poor feeding, irritability, lethargy, downward deviation of the eyes (the "setting sun" sign), spasticity in the legs, apnea, and bradycardia often provide additional clues that the infant has increased intracranial pressure. In older patients with acute courses, the signs are relatively clear and include morning headache that improves after upright positioning or vomiting, irritability and/or lethargy, and papilledema and diplopia (CN VI palsy). Spasticity, clonus, and hyperreflexia most prominent in the legs are additional neurologic signs of hydrocephalus. The **Cushing triad**, consisting of hypertension, bradycardia, and slow irregular respirations, is a late and ominous sign of increased intracranial pressure implying imminent risk of brain herniation.

DIFFERENTIAL DIAGNOSIS

Conditions that lead to increased intracranial pressure without hydrocephalus include acute intraventricular hemorrhage, diffuse brain edema (secondary to traumatic brain injury, hypoxic-ischemic encephalopathy, large ischemic stroke or encephalitis), cerebral venous sinus thrombosis, abscesses, and many tumors, all of which are easily differentiated by computed tomography (CT) or magnetic resonance imaging (MRI).

DIAGNOSTIC EVALUATION

The CT scan is an important adjunct in the evaluation of hydrocephalus. Anatomic malformations, ventricular size, and source of obstruction are clearly delineated. A head ultrasound (US) may be sufficient in the young infant. In children who have a VP shunt, rapid sequence MRI can assess ventricular size without exposing the child to cumulative excessive radiation over time. If a lumbar puncture (LP) is indicated, it **should not** be attempted in the presence of asymmetric or obstructive causes of increased intracranial pressure due to the risk of herniation of the brain across the tentorium or through the foramen magnum.

TREATMENT

Patients with hydrocephalus are at risk for developmental delay, visual impairment, motor disturbances and, in severe cases of obstructive hydrocephalus, death. If the underlying etiology cannot be corrected, surgical diversion with a VP shunt decreases intracranial pressure and relieves the symptoms. An endoscopic **third ventriculostomy** is a surgical alternative to VP shunt when CSF obstruction occurs at or distal to the cerebral aqueduct. A third ventriculostomy (the surgical creation of an opening at the floor of the third ventricle) may occasionally close due to gliosis, but this intervention avoids the risks of mechanical failure or infection present with the VP shunt. Acetazolamide decreases CSF production and may be effective in the short term if the hydrocephalus is transient and mild.

Indwelling shunts can be complicated by mechanical failure of the device, problems due to over-shunting or under-shunting, and infection. *Staphylococcus epidermidis* is the most frequently isolated pathogen. The management of shunt infections is currently a matter of debate. Systemic and intraventricular antibiotics are always administered. Some centers remove the shunt and replace it when the infection is resolved; others replace the shunt immediately, and still others treat the shunt in place. The programmable valve is a technological advance in VP shunts that permits external adjustment to optimize ventricular pressure.

CEREBRAL PALSY

Cerebral palsy (CP) is a nonprogressive disorder of movement and posture that results from a static lesion of the developing brain before, during, or after birth. Approximately one-third of cases develop after full-term birth following an apparently normal gestation. Modern case series have identified a single or mixed etiology for the motor disability in at least 80% of cases of CP. In Shevell's 2003 consecutive case series of children with CP, the top five etiologic entities were periventricular leukomalacia, intrapartum asphyxia, cerebral dysgenesis, intracranial hemorrhage, and vascular infarction. Transient neonatal depression is not predictive of an eventual diagnosis of CP. Excluding extremely premature or low-birth-weight infants, over 90% of infants with Apgar scores of 0 to 3 at 5 minutes do not develop CP. Infants with intrapartum hypoxia-ischemia who have normal neurologic examinations by 1 week of age have a good likelihood of normal outcome. Prenatal factors such as intrauterine infection, prematurity, placental hemorrhage, and multiple gestations raise the risk of CP. Acquired postnatal causes of CP include stroke, trauma, kernicterus from severe hyperbilirubinemia, and infections of the central nervous system.

CLINICAL MANIFESTATIONS

CP is classified by the pattern of motor impairments and by characteristics of muscle tone. The most common form is **spastic** CP, which is the consequence of injury to the pyramidal motor tracts in the brain. Spastic hypertonia is the velocity-dependent increased resistance of a muscle in response to passive stretching. The disorder is further classified by which limbs are involved (Table 15-1). Patients with CP are generally hypotonic through the first few months of life, only later developing the characteristic spasticity. In infancy, the presence of an extensor plantar response and delay in appearance and then disappearance of primitive reflexes (such as the Moro or the asymmetric tonic neck reflex) can be early indicators of CP. It is usually very difficult to make the diagnosis until a patient is failing to meet motor developmental milestones or the spasticity becomes apparent on exam. Maximal treatment of spasticity and aggressive physical and occupational therapy and bracing help maintain and maximize the child's function during growth and development.

Extrapyramidal CP is a rare but important disorder that results from damage to the basal ganglia, which is involved in the regulation of muscle tone and coordination. Affected patients exhibit involuntary choreoathetoid movements and postural ataxia, in addition to hypotonic quadriparesis or spastic diplegia.

■ **TABLE 15-1** Topographic Classification of Spastic (Pyramidal) Cerebral Palsy
Diplegia—bilateral leg spasticity and weakness much greater than arm spasticity and weakness. Often observed in preterm infants with periventricular leukomalacia (PVL)
Quadriplegia—all limbs severely involved. Often related to PVL, asphyxia, cerebral dysgenesis, or hemorrhage
Hemiplegia—one side involved, upper extremity more than lower. Usually due to a unilateral cortical lesion such as dysgenesis or stroke

Kernicterus used to be a major cause of extrapyramidal CP. Now that improved management of hyperbilirubinemia has decreased the incidence of kernicterus, most patients with extrapyramidal CP have an identifiable brain insult (e.g., severe acute perinatal asphyxia, placental infarction, maternal toxemia). Cerebral dysgenesis, including malformations of the cerebellum and brainstem, can cause **ataxic** CP with hypotonia, truncal ataxia, and titubation (bobbing of the head and/or trunk).

The American Academy of Neurology and the Practice Committee of the Child Neurology Society published a practice parameter addressing the diagnostic assessment of the child with cerebral palsy in 2004. The practice parameter suggests that the history and physical examination should be reviewed to exclude a progressive or degenerative brain disorder. The child should be screened for associated conditions including developmental delay, visual or hearing impairments, speech and language delays, and feeding and swallowing dysfunction. An electroencephalograph (EEG) should be obtained if there is a history of possible seizures. Neuroimaging, preferably MRI, is employed to look for an anatomic etiology for the CP. If cerebral malformation is present, a genetic or metabolic evaluation should be considered. Evaluation for a hypercoagulable state is suggested if a stroke is identified.

DIFFERENTIAL DIAGNOSIS

Although CP is nonprogressive, periods of rapid growth may transiently increase spasticity and contribute to contractures, which can make the child appear to have a progressive disorder. Metabolic and genetic evaluation should be considered if the child has deterioration or episodic decompensation, no etiology can be determined, or if there is a family history of childhood neurologic disorder. Progressive or degenerative disorders that can be misdiagnosed as CP include metachromatic leukodystrophy, Friedreich ataxia, ataxia-telangiectasia, and certain metabolic and mitochondrial disorders associated with spasticity.

TREATMENT

A multidisciplinary team approach, including a general pediatrician, physical and occupational therapists, nutritionist, speech-language therapist, and social support services, results in optimal function. Many systemic medicines have been tried to reduce spasticity with variable success. However, significant improvements in motor function have been achieved with botulinum toxin injections along with stretching and/or serial casting to treat joint deformities. Intrathecal baclofen pumps can improve spasticity with fewer central side effects, but the pumps can fail or get infected. Selective dorsal nerve rhizotomy is used in selected cases to decrease spasticity. Many children ultimately require orthopedic surgery to correct deformities and release contractures.

About one-third of children with CP are otherwise cognitively normal; the remaining have varying degrees of cognitive disability ranging from learning disabilities to severe mental retardation. Up to 50% of patients with CP develop epilepsy. Hearing and visual impairments should be monitored and corrected if possible. If a child with CP is nonverbal or language impaired, it is important to rule out hearing impairment and provide for alternate modes of communication including sign language, communication boards, and/or augmentative communication devices.

SEIZURES AND EPILEPSY

PATHOGENESIS

A **seizure** is a transient clinical event that results from abnormal and excessive electrical activity of populations of cerebral neurons. The abnormal electrical activity disrupts brain function, leading to **positive signs** (motor, sensory, psychic) and/or **negative signs** (loss of awareness, loss of motor tone) depending on the cortical localization of the seizure. **Epilepsy** is diagnosed when a patient has had two or more unprovoked seizures. In contrast, "provoked" or acute symptomatic seizures occur in the context of an acute brain insult (trauma, intoxication, intracranial infection) and are not classified as epilepsy unless they become recurrent following resolution of the acute illness. Some children develop epilepsy due to cortical malformations or have specific age-related epilepsy syndromes. For 60% to 80% of children with epilepsy, no apparent cause can be determined.

Neonatal seizures are discussed in Chapter 13.

FEBRILE SEIZURES

Febrile seizures are typically brief, generalized seizures with fever which occur in up to 5% of otherwise healthy children ages 6 months to 6 years. Febrile seizures, even when recurrent, are not considered epilepsy. Febrile seizures are divided into simple febrile seizures and complex febrile seizures. **Simple febrile seizures** are generalized, brief, and single (do not recur within 24 hours). **Complex febrile seizures** are focal, prolonged (greater than 10 or 15 minutes), or repetitive (recur within 24 hours). By definition, the diagnosis of febrile seizure excludes children with intracranial infection or prior history of nonfebrile seizure. Most febrile seizures occur in the first 24 hours of an illness, in children less than 3 years old and with fevers of 39°C or higher.

One-third of all children with febrile seizures will have a recurrence. Risk factors for recurrent febrile seizure include: (a) first febrile seizure before age 1 year; (b) family history of febrile seizures; and (c) low-grade fever/short duration of fever at the time of the seizure. Children with three or more risk factors have a 60% recurrence rate. A long febrile seizure does not increase the risk of recurrence, but it does increase the risk that a recurrent febrile seizure will be prolonged. In general, treatment of children with febrile seizures with a daily anticonvulsant is not recommended. Education about seizure first aid, seizure precautions, and an emergency plan in case of recurrent seizure is important for children with febrile seizures. Repetitive seizures and seizures lasting more than 5 minutes can be treated with rectal diazepam. The child should be transported to the emergency department by ambulance if the seizure continues more than 5 minutes after rectal diazepam. Febrile status epilepticus should be treated aggressively to prevent morbidity and mortality.

The American Academy of Pediatrics has practice parameters that address the **evaluation of first simple febrile seizure** in neurologically healthy children between 6 months and 5 years. The diagnosis of febrile seizure is based on a thorough history. It is important to differentiate nonseizure events (such as rigors in a febrile child, breathholding spells, or syncope) from febrile seizure. In the history and physical examination, it is vital to look for evidence that the child may have meningitis or encephalitis causing the seizure and to consider that affected children less than 18 months old may not have meningismus. It is also important to ask about possible ingestions of drugs or toxins and history suggestive of metabolic disorder or derangement from unusual intake or fluid/electrolyte losses. Seizures are the presenting sign in about 15 percent of children with meningitis, and in about one-third of these children, meningeal signs and symptoms may be absent. The guideline recommends that LP should be strongly considered after first simple febrile seizure in a child less than 12 months and that LP should be considered in the child between 12 and 18 months also because signs of meningismus may be subtle. LP should also be considered for children older than 18 months if they have meningeal signs and in children who have been pretreated with antibiotics. Blood glucose, serum electrolyte, calcium, phosphorus, magnesium, and CBC should not be routinely performed but can be sent under particular circumstances, such as checking serum glucose if the child has a prolonged period of postictal obtundation. EEG and neuroimaging are not recommended in the evaluation of simple febrile seizures.

Children with febrile seizures have an increased risk of developing epilepsy. Between 2% and 7% of all children with febrile seizures develop epilepsy if followed to age 25 years. Three major risk factors increase the risk of later epilepsy: (a) complex febrile seizures, (b) preexisting neurodevelopmental abnormality, and (c) epilepsy in first-degree relatives. Children with all three risk factors have an almost 50% chance of subsequently developing epilepsy. Additional risk factors for developing epilepsy in children with febrile seizures include history of first febrile seizure under age 1 year, short duration of fever prior to the seizure, and number of febrile seizures.

It is important to note that over 90% of children who have febrile seizures do not develop epilepsy. Overall, the morbidity and mortality associated with febrile seizures is extremely low. Two large prospective studies showed no differences in cognition between children with a history of febrile seizures and children without any febrile seizure.

EPILEPSY

Approximately 5% of all children have a provoked or unprovoked seizure by the age of 20 years. By early adulthood, the cumulative incidence of epilepsy is between 1% and 2%. In children who are observed off of anticonvulsants, the risk for recurrence after a single unprovoked seizure is 40% to 50%. Risk factors for seizure recurrence following a first unprovoked seizure in childhood include: (a) prior history of abnormal brain/development, (b) abnormal EEG, (c) prior febrile seizures, (d) transient focal weakness (Todd paresis), or (e) seizure arising out of sleep. Healthy normally developing children whose initial seizure occurs while awake have the best prognosis for remaining seizure free.

In general, the child is observed off of daily anticonvulsants and with an emergency treatment plan after a first unprovoked seizure. The recurrence risk is 80% after a second unprovoked seizure; at that point most children are started on a daily anticonvulsant.

About 50% of children with epilepsy outgrow their seizures, particularly those with age-related epilepsy syndromes such as benign rolandic epilepsy or childhood absence epilepsy. Some adolescents develop epilepsy due to an age-related epilepsy syndrome (juvenile myoclonic epilepsy) or traumatic brain injury. The probable etiology and prognosis of a seizure vary with the child's age, family history of epilepsy, history of preexisting neurodevelopmental disability, identified epilepsy syndrome, and the acute symptomatic cause for the seizure.

Clinical Manifestations

History and Physical Examination

It is vital to take a thorough history of what occurred before, during, and after an event to determine whether the event was an epileptic seizure or a nonepileptic paroxysmal event such as reflux, syncope, or a night terror. The context of the child's age, past medical and family histories, and any prior unusual spells are important in the differentiation of a seizure from a nonseizure event.

The diagnosis of a seizure is based primarily on the historical account of the episode. The history should include questions about what the child was doing and feeling prior to and during the event, how the event evolved over time, how long the event lasted, and how the child behaved following the event. It is important to ask if any abnormal spells have occurred previously and whether the child had any recent illness, injury, ingestion, or prior abnormalities of development, vision, strength, coordination, sensation, or growth. The child's past history and family history provide supplemental supporting information for the diagnosis. At the end of a thorough history, the physician should be able to differentiate an epileptic seizure from a nonseizure paroxysmal event (such as syncope or daydreaming). Occasionally, the available history is not sufficient to make the determination of seizure vs. nonseizure. In that case, the family should be taught seizure first aid and what to observe if the event recurs.

The physical examination should be comprehensive including vital signs, growth parameters, and presence of neurocutaneous lesions, dysmorphic features, retinal abnormalities, signs of infection, cardiac abnormality, or trauma. A full neurological examination assesses mental status, cranial nerve function (including vision), and evidence of any focal abnormalities of tone or strength, sensation, coordination, deep tendon reflexes, or gait.

Diagnostic Evaluation

EEG studies can provide supplementary information to support a diagnosis of epilepsy. An abnormal EEG permits classification of the epilepsy as **focal** (localization-related) or **generalized** and may suggest a specific epilepsy syndrome (such as 3-Hz spike-and-wave pattern typically seen in children with absence epilepsy). The EEG result should be evaluated in light of the child's history. A child with epilepsy can have a normal EEG. Similarly, a child who has had a nonseizure paroxysmal event may have an abnormal EEG, which should not be used to misdiagnose the event as epilepsy. A practice guideline established by the American Academy of Neurology, the Child Neurology Society, and the American Epilepsy Society recommends routine EEG as a standard part of the diagnostic evaluation in a child following a first nonfebrile seizure.

If imaging is performed, MRI of the brain is the preferred modality. MRI shows an abnormality such as cortical dysgenesis in about 20% of cases of new-onset seizure. Emergent neuroimaging may be necessary in a child who is not returning to baseline within hours, in the child with a postictal focal deficit, or the patient with signs or symptoms of increased intracranial pressure. Brain MRI may not be necessary if the clinical history and EEG are consistent with certain epilepsy syndromes (such as childhood absence epilepsy). In general, brain MRI should be performed in any child who has a history of a partial-onset seizure, abnormal neurologic exam, or abnormal developmental history. LP should be considered in any child with persistently altered mental status or meningeal signs and in young infants less than 6 months of age. If increased intracranial pressure is suspected or if the child has focal neurologic signs, an imaging study of the head should precede the LP. Toxicology screening is warranted if there is a question of ingestion of drugs or toxins. Other laboratory tests should be ordered on an individual basis if the child has vomiting, diarrhea, dehydration, or failure to return to baseline alertness.

CLASSIFICATION OF EPILEPTIC SEIZURES AND EPILEPSY SYNDROMES

Table 15-2 delineates the International Classification of Epileptic Seizures.

Partial seizures are those in which the first clinical and electrographic changes start in a system of neurons in one hemisphere. The signs and symptoms of a partial seizure are specific to the area of the brain involved in the seizure and may be motor, sensory, autonomic, or higher cortical psychic symptoms. Partial seizures are further categorized by whether or not consciousness is impaired during the seizure. During **simple partial seizures**, consciousness is fully maintained, and the seizure involves a small focal area of the brain. During **complex partial seizures**, consciousness is altered, the individual is not fully aware or responsive, and a larger portion of the brain, potentially portions of both hemispheres, is involved in the seizure.

- **Motor** seizures may manifest as focal twitching (Jacksonian march if the twitching travels distal to proximal up one extremity or one side of the body);

involuntary movement (turning of the eyes, head and/or trunk); or vocalization or arrest of speech.
- **Sensory** seizures can include tingling, numbness, an unpleasant odor or taste, vertigo, flashing lights, or auditory symptoms.
- **Autonomic** seizures may include an epigastric "rising" sensation, vomiting, sweating, pupillary changes, or piloerection ("goosebumps").
- Simple partial seizures may include **higher cortical psychic symptoms** including feelings of familiarity ("déjà-vu"), sudden intense feelings of fear or sadness, dysphasia, distortions of time, and formed hallucinations.

During complex partial seizures, the child may have repetitive semipurposeful movements (automatisms) including picking at the clothes, oral-buccal movements (chewing, swallowing), or more complex motor movements such as kicking, flailing of the arms, running, jumping, or spinning. During complex partial seizures arising from the frontal lobe, the child may have bilateral motor movements and seem combative if physically restrained. Both simple and complex partial seizures can evolve into secondarily generalized seizures.

Generalized seizures are those in which the clinical and electrographic changes at seizure onset are bilateral and widespread in both hemispheres. Consciousness is impaired. Seizures may be nonconvulsive (such as absence seizures) or convulsive with bilateral tonic, clonic, or myoclonic movements. In a **generalized tonic-clonic** seizure (GTC), the tonic phase consists of sustained flexor or extensor contraction followed by the clonic phase (rhythmic, symmetric, generalized contractions of the face and extremities). Often, the patient exhales and remains in exhalation during the tonic phase of a GTC, with breathing commencing in a grunting or irregular fashion during the clonic phase. Seizures may also be solely tonic or solely clonic. Bowel or bladder incontinence may occur. The child may bite the side of the tongue or buccal mucosa, and can be injured falling to the floor without any protective reflexes. An **aura** or warning prior to the onset of the GTC implies partial-onset seizure with rapid secondary generalization. Similarly, a postictal transient hemiparesis (Todd paralysis) implies a partial onset to the seizure. The **postictal** phase is characterized by unresponsiveness and flaccid muscle tone. The child should have a gradually improving level of consciousness over the following 10 to 30 minutes.

Absence seizures begin between ages 4 and 9 years and consist of brief episodes of staring associated with

■ **TABLE 15-2** International Classification of Epileptic Seizures (ILAE, 1981)
Partial seizures
Simple partial (intact consciousness)
Motor
Sensory
Autonomic
Psychic
Complex partial (impaired consciousness)
Partial seizures with secondary generalization
Generalized seizures
Absence (typical, atypical)
Tonic
Clonic
Tonic-clonic
Myoclonic
Atonic
Infantile spasms

altered consciousness. The typical duration is 5 to 10 seconds. Often, the staring is accompanied by subtle clonic activity in the face or arms or simple automatisms (such as eye blinking, chewing, or perseverative motor activity). Absence seizures start and stop abruptly and have no postictal phase. Although brief, absence seizures can occur in clusters many times a day and interfere with learning and socialization. In a typical absence seizure, the EEG shows abrupt onset and offset of 3-per-second generalized symmetric spike-and-slow wave complexes. In a child with untreated absence epilepsy, 3 to 5 minutes of hyperventilation will often precipitate a typical absence seizure.

Atonic seizures consist of abrupt, total loss of postural tone in the neck ("head drop") or the entire body ("drop seizure") which can cause injury to the child. **Myoclonic seizures** are quick lightning-like jerks similar to those experienced by normal subjects while in light sleep.

Every child with epilepsy should be clinically evaluated to determine if he or she has one of the recognized **childhood epilepsy syndromes**. The International League Against Epilepsy syndrome classification is based on age of onset, seizure types involved, and EEG appearance. An epilepsy syndrome diagnosis provides important prognostic, therapeutic, and at times genetic information.

Differential Diagnosis

Neonates can have unusual movements and automatisms that are not epileptic. Also, encephalopathic neonates can have subclinical seizures that can only be detected with continuous EEG monitoring. Continuous EEG monitoring can be a useful tool to guide therapy in neonates with encephalopathy or ongoing potential seizures (Table 15-3).

In children, **syncope** is often misdiagnosed as a seizure. Common characteristics of syncope are the proper setting (prolonged standing or kneeling, just stood up, dehydration, sudden pain, or seeing blood); pallor; lightheadedness; visual changes ("vision coning down to black"); and muffled hearing. The loss of consciousness is brief, particularly if the child remains lying down; transient stiffening or clonic movements at the end of syncope (convulsive syncope) reflects transient decreased blood flow in the brain and is not an epileptic seizure. Following common vasovagal syncope, a child should have little if any confusion/mental status change. Clues suggestive of potentially life-threatening cardiac syncope include syncope

during exercise, a family history of deafness, or a family history of sudden death in children or young people.

Young children can have pallid or cyanotic **breath-holding spells** characterized by a sudden pain or upset, followed by a cry, color change, and the child holding his or her breath in exhalation. Some children then lose consciousness briefly and may have stiffening or transient clonic movements. If the history is typical for breathholding spells, the only potential evaluation beyond thorough history and examination should be possible EKG to rule out cardiac syncope.

Essential tremor, spasmus nutans, tics, and myoclonus are various movement disorders that may mimic seizures. **Essential tremor** begins in infancy or childhood and may involve the chin, head, neck, and hands; it usually does not interfere with normal functions. **Spasmus nutans** presents in infancy and includes head nodding and tilting and rapid, small-amplitude nystagmus without alteration of consciousness. A child with spasmus nutans should have MRI to rule out an optic pathway tumor. **Myoclonic movements** are sudden, involuntary jerk-like motions similar to startle responses.

Tourette complex consists of motor and vocal tics (sudden, involuntary behaviors that are repetitive) that persist almost daily for more than a year. Common comorbid conditions include obsessive-compulsive tendencies and attention-deficit/hyperactivity disorder. Children can also have less frequent tics of one type or the other. If tics become disruptive and interfere with functioning, they can be treated with behavioral therapy or medications (including botulinum toxin) with variable success.

Other conditions that may be confused with seizures include benign paroxysmal vertigo, temper tantrums, and night terrors. **Pseudoseizures** should be suspected in the patient with implausible findings (e.g., alert and responsive during generalized tonic-clonic movements).

Treatment

Effective treatment of epilepsy combines education and medication. Both the child and the parents should become knowledgeable about acute seizure care and local emergency medical services.

With medication, approximately 50% to 70% of patients become seizure free. Another 10% to 30% have significant reductions in seizure frequency and/or intensity. There has been a dramatic increase

■ TABLE 15-3 Characteristics of Childhood Epilepsy Syndromes

Name of Syndrome	Age of Onset	Types of Seizures	EEG	Remission	Treatment
Juvenile myoclonic epilepsy	10 to 18 years	GTC on awakening, myoclonic seizures on awakening, absence seizures	Rapid, generalized spike waves and poly-spike and wave, may have photosensitivity	Not typical; usually life-long	Valproic acid, levetiracetam, topiramate
Childhood absence epilepsy	5 to 10 years	Absence seizures, occasionally GTC	Ictal EEG: 3 Hz spike and wave, sudden onset and offset	80% remit at puberty, some to develop JME	Ethosuximide, valproic acid, lamotrigine
Juvenile absence epilepsy	7 to 16 years	Absence seizures, GTC, occasional myoclonus	Ictal EEG : 3.5 to 4 Hz spike and wave	Somewhat less likely to remit than childhood absence, may develop JME	Valproic acid, lamotrigine, topiramate
Benign epilepsy of childhood with centrotemporal spikes (BECTS, benign rolandic epilepsy)	5 to 10 years	Simple partial hemifacial motor/ sensory seizures arousing the child from sleep, GTC in sleep	EEG: high-voltage centrotemporal spikes, activated during sleep and tend to spread or shift from side to side	Usually remits by age 15 or 16 years	Seizures typically nocturnal, may elect to observe off of anticonvulsants or treat with carbamazepine or oxcarbazepine
Infantile spasms	2 to 7 months	Clusters of flexor or extensor spasms	Interictal EEG: hypsarrhythmia Ictal EEG: electrodecremental response	Spasms may resolve, many children evolve into Lennox-Gastaut	ACTH, valproic acid, vigabatrin (in children with tuberous sclerosis)
Lennox-Gastaut syndrome	1 to 8 years	Multiple seizure types: tonic, atonic, atypical absence, myoclonic, GTC	Interictal EEG: diffuse slow (1.5 to 2 Hz) spike wave discharges	Intractable epilepsy, resistant to treatment with anticonvulsants; does not tend to remit	Felbamate, lamotrigine, topiramate, valproic acid, zonisamide, benzodiazepines; patient may need more than one anticonvulsant

ACTH, adrenocorticotropic hormone; EEG, electroencephalogram; GTC, generalized tonic-clonic seizures; JME, juvenile myoclonic epilepsy.

in the number of medications available for the management of seizures. The newer medications have a better toxicity profile. Table 15-4 lists their names, indications, and side effects. Conventional anticonvulsants require careful monitoring of serum levels; most new drugs do not require routine monitoring.

Identifying seizure type and epilepsy syndrome helps predict which anticonvulsants may be beneficial.

There is a paucity of class I and class II randomized clinical trials to determine evidence-based recommendations for treatment, particularly for children with generalized seizures. For children with partial-onset

TABLE 15-4 Indications and Side Effects of Anticonvulsants

Medication	Indications	Side Effects/Toxicity
Conventional drugs		
Carbamazepine (Tegretol)	Partial, tonic-clonic	Diplopia, nausea and vomiting, ataxia, leukopenia, thrombocytopenia
Ethosuximide (Zarontin)	Absence	Rash, anorexia, leukopenia, aplastic anemia
Phenobarbital (Luminal)	Tonic-clonic, partial	Hyperactivity, sedation, nystagmus, ataxia
Phenytoin (Dilantin)	Tonic-clonic, partial	Rash, nystagmus, ataxia, drug-induced lupus, gingival hyperplasia, anemia, leukopenia, polyneuropathy
Valproic acid (Depakote)	Tonic-clonic, absence, partial	Hepatotoxicity, nausea and vomiting, abdominal pain, weight gain, anemia, leukopenia, thrombocytopenia
Newer drugs		
Gabapentin (Neurontin)	Partial	Somnolence, dizziness, ataxia, fatigue
Lamotrigine (Lamictal)	Tonic-clonic, partial, absence, and Lennox-Gastaut	Dizziness, ataxia, blurred or double vision, nausea, vomiting, rash (including Stevens-Johnson syndrome)
Oxcarbazepine (Trileptal)	Partial, tonic-clonic	Somnolence, hyponatremia, rash
Topiramate (Topamax)	Tonic-clonic, partial, Lennox-Gastaut, infantile spasms	Somnolence, fatigue, confusion, headache, ataxia, weight loss
Zonisamide (Zonegran)	Partial, generalized, infantile spasms, myoclonic seizures	Somnolence, ataxia, confusion, irritability, renal stones

epilepsy, oxcarbazepine should be considered for initial monotherapy based on current efficacy evidence. Considering all factors, including cost, carbamazepine, valproic acid, topiramate, and phenytoin are other reasonable choices to treat partial-onset seizures. In terms of generalized epilepsy, valproic acid and ethosuximide have equal efficacy for treatment of childhood absence epilepsy; lamotrigine is more effective than placebo but has not been compared head-to-head with the other medications. For other generalized epilepsies, valproic acid, levetiracetam, topiramate, and lamotrigine are reasonable choices.

In most patients, it is reasonable to consider weaning off of anticonvulsant medication after the child has been seizure free for 2 years. In patients with particular epilepsy syndromes such as JME, the seizures are usually life-long, so anticonvulsants are generally not withdrawn. Recommendations to start and stop anticonvulsants must be tailored to the individual patient, with decisions made by the physician together with the patient and family.

For patients with poor seizure control on medication (approximately 10%), additional interventions are available. By monitoring a patient's seizures with con-

tinuous EEG leads, a focus may be discovered that can be removed surgically. The risks and benefits of such a procedure need to be explored carefully with the patient and family. Another option is the ketogenic diet. Inducing ketosis through a high-fat, very low-carbohydrate diet may control symptoms in some children. The vagal nerve stimulator, approved by the Food and Drug Administration in 1997, has proven quite beneficial in some patients. About 50% of children with epilepsy experience remission, after which the medication can be tapered. Unfortunately, remission is less likely to occur for children who have seizure disorders as a result of congenital or acquired brain damage.

EMERGENCY MANAGEMENT OF STATUS EPILEPTICUS

Status epilepticus is defined as a prolonged episode of seizure activity (>30 minutes) or an extended period of recurrent seizures between which the patient does not return to consciousness. **Status epilepticus is a medical emergency**, leading to hypoxia, brain damage, and death. For treatment purposes, any convulsive seizure lasting more than 5 minutes should be addressed with emergency medication. For out of hospital use, rectal diazepam (Diastat) and midazolam (IV form squirted next to the buccal mucosa or sprayed intranasally) are effective and safe in the setting of prolonged seizures. Airway, breathing, and circulation should be evaluated and addressed as necessary. Intravenous or rectal short-acting benzodiazepines (lorazepam or diazepam) often stop the seizure. For a prolonged seizure not responsive to initial treatment, fosphenytoin, midazolam, or phenobarbital loading doses are administered to break the seizure as well as to prevent recurrence. Patients in refractory status may require induction of anesthesia in the intensive care unit with pentobarbital or propofol and continuous EEG monitoring to adjust and evaluate ongoing management. Prognosis after status epilepticus is related to the underlying etiology for the prolonged seizure. If a child has preexisting epilepsy, anticonvulsant levels are drawn. The child who is febrile and toxic-appearing or has new repetitive seizures and altered mental status warrants an evaluation for CNS infection (including LP). A head CT should be obtained prior to LP in a child with focal seizures, postictal focal deficits, or any signs or symptoms of increased intracranial pressure. Targeted or comprehensive toxicology screening is undertaken if there is any concern about ingestion. Historic features consistent with metabolic disorder (unexplained encephalopathy, deterioration during illness, unusual odors) or unexplained acidosis or coma should trigger metabolic evaluation including glucose, ketones, acylcarnitine profile, serum and urine amino acids, urine organic acids, serum ammonia, and serum lactate and pyruvate.

HEAD TRAUMA

Acute head trauma is the most common cause of pediatric death and disability in the developed world. Head injuries in children most often result from motor vehicle accidents, bicycle mishaps, falls, or child abuse. Males are twice as likely as females to sustain significant head trauma. Recovery from a head injury depends on the severity of the initial injury and factors contributing to secondary neuronal injury such as hypotension and hypoxia. Severe injury is often associated with behavioral changes, motor impairment, and memory problems. Approximately 10% of children hospitalized for a traumatic brain injury have a seizure, and 35% of these patients will subsequently develop a seizure disorder.

A **concussion** is defined as a brief alteration or loss of consciousness following relatively mild head trauma. Brain injury is undetectable, and the neurologic examination returns to normal within hours. In contrast, **cerebral contusions** represent a direct injury to the brain itself. Diffuse **axonal injury** results from shearing forces on the white matter of the brain that occur with rapid deceleration of the head. It is frequently followed by brain edema, further disruption of blood flow, inflammation, and ischemia.

Brain hemorrhages that occur secondary to trauma are typically epidural or subdural (Table 15-5;

■ TABLE 15-5 Differentiating Acute Subdural and Epidural Bleeds		
	Subdural	**Epidural**
Location	Between the dura and arachnoid layers	Between the skull and the dura
Symmetry	Usually bilateral	Usually unilateral
Etiology	Rupture of bridging cortical veins or subdural veins	Rupture of middle meningeal artery or vein
Typical injury	Direct trauma or shaking	Direct trauma in the temporal area
Consciousness	Intact but altered	Impaired-lucid-impaired
Common associated findings	Seizures, retinal hemorrhages	Ipsilateral pupillary dilatation, papilledema, contralateral hemiparesis
Appearance on CT with contrast	Crescentic	Biconcave
Prognosis	High morbidity; low mortality	High mortality; low morbidity
Complications	Herniation	Skull fracture; uncal herniation

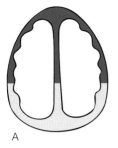
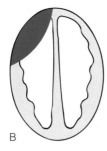

Figure 15-1 • **(A)** Subdural hemorrhage. **(B)** Epidural hematoma.

TABLE 15-6 Glasgow Coma Scale		
Activity (Child/Adult)	**Score**	**Activity (Infant)**
Eye opening		
Spontaneous	4	Spontaneous
To speech	3	To speech
To pain	2	To pain
None	1	None
Verbal		
Oriented	5	Coos, babbles
Confused	4	Irritable
Inappropriate words	3	Cries to pain
Nonspecific sounds	2	Moans to pain
None	1	None
Motor		
Follows commands	6	Normal, spontaneous movements
Localizes pain	5	Withdraws to touch
Withdraws to pain	4	Withdraws to pain
Abnormal flexion	2	Abnormal flexion
Abnormal extension	2	Abnormal extension
None	1	None

Fig. 15-1). Some severe brain injuries may also result in subarachnoid injury and bleeding into the CSF.

CLINICAL MANIFESTATIONS

History

Severe brain injury may occur in the absence of external signs of trauma. The source of injury should be described by the child and caretaker separately whenever possible; a history that is not consistent with a given injury is suggestive of child abuse. Reports of vomiting, severe headache, and mental status changes strongly suggest increased intracranial pressure. Confusion, loss of consciousness, amnesia, seizures, and visual impairment may also be present after significant injury.

Physical Examination

Patients with head injuries should receive a primary survey as soon as possible (see Chapter 1). Moderate to severe injury may result in altered breathing and the need for respiratory support. The Glasgow Coma Scale score (GCS; Table 15-6) provides a rapid, widely used, easily reproducible method of quantifying neurologic function and helps guide initial therapy. When brain injury is mild, the GCS usually remains greater than 12; patients with GCS <8 following head trauma are at risk for severe morbidity and death and generally require immediate intervention.

Bradycardia, hypertension, and slow, irregular respirations form the **Cushing triad**, the hallmark of increased intracranial pressure. Palpation of the head may reveal step-off (depressed) skull fractures or a bulging fontanelle. **Basilar skull fractures** are characterized by periorbital (raccoon eyes) or postauricular (Battle's sign) bruising, hemotympanum, or CSF rhinorrhea or otorrhea. Cranial nerve function, especially pupil size and reactivity, may help localize the injury. Papilledema may be evident on visualization of the fundus. Sensory and motor function is difficult to assess in the patient with impaired mental status, who may respond minimally even to noxious stimuli. Deep tendon and pathologic reflexes should be assessed in all patients. Serial neurologic examinations track evolving lesions and response to interventions.

DIAGNOSTIC EVALUATION

Cervical spine films are indicated for any patient with significant head trauma to rule out cervical injury. A **head CT** is typically recommended for patients with persistently altered mental status/levels of consciousness; a history of loss of consciousness lasting >1 minute; amnesia for the event; recurrent vomiting; severe, persistent headache; focal signs on neurologic examination; signs and symptoms of increased intracranial pressure; evidence of an underlying skull fracture; or a history of significant injury. In patients who have sustained mild trauma, have a normal examination, and have a history of a brief alteration or loss of consciousness with subsequent return to normal mental status, the decision regarding imaging is made by the examining physician. A CT is of little or no benefit in children with mild injury and no loss of consciousness.

TREATMENT

Specific treatment depends on the severity of the injury. Patients with suspected head or neck injury should be positioned on a back board with appropriate cervical spine immobilization in the field. Those with severe injury and GCS <8 generally require intubation. Hypotension is uncommon in isolated head trauma, but associated injuries may lead to shock (hypovolemic shock from hemorrhage; neurogenic shock from spinal cord injury; cardiogenic shock from myocardial contusion). The goal of supportive therapy is to optimize the **cerebral perfusion pressure**, which is the difference between the mean arterial pressure and the intracranial pressure. **Cerebral edema** is the most significant complication in the acute period. Normal oxygenation, normoglycemia, hyperosmolality, and elevation of the head of the bed are recommended to minimize intracranial hypertension and secondary brain injury. Mild hyperventilation, which reduces cerebral blood flow, is used to decrease intracranial pressure during the initial phase of therapy. Patients with evidence of impending herniation should be vigorously hyperventilated and given an osmotic agent such as mannitol and/or furosemide to decrease intracranial pressure acutely. Patients with evidence of significant cerebral edema require intracranial pressure monitoring with a subdural bolt or intraventricular catheter.

Patients with moderate injury and/or a declining GCS should be admitted to the hospital for further observation, serial neurologic examinations, and intervention as needed. Children with mild trauma should be observed in the hospital or at home with a reliable, competent caregiver for at least 24 hours. Any evidence of persistent headache, confusion, irritability, behavior changes, or visual disturbances should prompt further medical attention and workup.

Information regarding specific parameters for "return to play" for head injury that results from sports participation is provided by the Centers for Disease Control and Prevention at http://www.cdc.gov/ConcussionInYouthSports/.

ISCHEMIC/HEMORRHAGIC STROKES

Stroke consists of the sudden onset of focal neurologic impairment caused by an interruption of cerebral blood flow, which may be transient or permanent. In children, stroke is rare and is usually precipitated by one of the following:

- Cardiac disease (congenital heart disease, endocarditis)
- Vascular disease (arteriovenous malformation, aneurysm)
- Hematologic disorders (sickle cell disease and diseases that predispose to the formation of thrombi or bleeding)
- Metabolic disease (most commonly homocystinuria)

Most strokes in children occur in the cerebral hemispheres, presenting with hemiparesis, visual field defects, and/or aphasia. Brainstem and cerebellar strokes are less common. The neurologic manifestations correlate with the location of the ischemia. Magnetic resonance angiography (MRA) can evaluate vessels and reveal areas of ischemia. Additional laboratory tests that may prove helpful include coagulation studies, CBC and cultures, connective tissue/vasculitis profiles (ESR, C3, C4, ANA), and workups to rule out lipid and metabolic abnormalities. Low-molecular-weight heparin is useful in some conditions to dissolve thromboses and prevent recurrences. Large clots may require surgical evacuation.

An arteriovenous malformation (AVM) is an abnormal collection of arteries and veins. Occasionally, a cranial bruit is present on physical examination. More commonly, however, AVMs present in a previously asymptomatic individual with the sudden or insidious onset of headache, vomiting, nuchal rigidity, progressive hemiparesis, diplopia, ataxia, and focal or generalized seizures. Arteriography permits determination of the site of the abnormality and feeding vessels. Surgical removal, embolization, or radiotherapy is necessary to prevent recurrent stroke or hemorrhage.

Thrombosis can occur at both arterial and venous sites. Conditions that predispose to thrombosis include sickle cell hemoglobinopathy, coagulation disorders, congenital heart disease, cardiac procedures, arrhythmias, endocarditis, trauma to the area of the internal carotid artery, bacterial meningitis, and infections leading to cavernous sinus thrombosis.

HEADACHES

PATHOGENESIS

Headaches are a common complaint in the pediatric population. It is important to determine early in the evaluation whether the headaches are **primary** (benign headaches not associated with underlying neuropathology; includes tension, migraine headaches) or **secondary** (pathologic, with the pain typically generated secondary to increased intracranial pressure).

Benign tension headaches are often associated with psychological stress or fatigue. They are typically described as generalized, constant, and band-like in distribution. Most respond to over-the-counter analgesics, removal of the inciting stressor, and rest. Affected patients who take analgesics more than three to four times per week are at risk for the development of chronic, **analgesic overuse headaches**. Frequent tension-type headaches can also be associated with clinical depression.

Migraine headaches are hypothesized to result from sudden progressive depolarization of a hyperexcitable cerebral cortex ("spreading cortical depression"). They are characterized by recurrent attacks of severe, throbbing, typically frontal or frontotemporal pain which lasts for several hours. Photophobia, nausea, and vomiting may also be present. In about one-third of patients, the headaches are preceded by an aura, which is usually visual (e.g., scotomas). Symptoms resolve with sleep. Migraines are classified as **complicated** when they are accompanied and/or followed by transient neurologic deficits such as weakness/paralysis, sensory loss, difficulty speaking, or alterations in vision or mental status. Patients who suffer from migraine headaches remain asymptomatic and have normal neurologic examinations between episodes of pain. Migraine sufferers virtually always have a family history of migraine headaches.

CLINICAL MANIFESTATIONS

History

Patients should be asked about the history (acute vs. chronic), onset, progression, severity, location, duration, and timing of the headaches. Response to medication and alleviating/exacerbating factors are important factors. Any weakness, visual disturbances, or abnormal sensations should be reported. Questions about stress levels, recent life changes, and precipitating factors (foods, menstruation, exercise) may assist in the diagnosis. Asking the patient or caregiver to keep a headache diary can identify possible triggers, including fatigue, sleep deprivation, fasting, caffeine, menstruation, and stress.

Headaches that wake the patient from sleep are suspicious for increased intracranial pressure. These headaches are usually made worse by lying flat or increasing venous pressure by bending, sneezing, or straining. Nausea and vomiting are not uncommon, particularly on wakening, and are concerning in the patient who has no associated complaints of abdominal pain or diarrhea. Pathologic headaches usually increase in both severity and frequency over time. There may be associated personality changes, gait disturbances, and vision abnormalities. Headaches accompanied by worsening focal neurologic deficits warrant emergent evaluation for an intracranial source.

Physical Examination

The physical examination includes assessment of growth parameters, vital signs (including blood pressure), and structures of the head (sinuses, teeth). The funduscopic examination permits detection of **papilledema** (swelling of the optic disc) in cases of increased intracranial pressure; CN VI palsy may also be present. Vision acuity should be documented. Carotid bruits, which may be detected in patients with AVMs, should be ruled out. A full neurologic examination is of paramount importance and includes cranial nerve function, strength, sensation, deep tendon reflexes, gait, balance, and mental status.

DIAGNOSTIC EVALUATION

Neither CT nor MRI of the head is indicated in the patient with nonprogressive recurring headaches and a normal neurologic examination. **Neuroimaging is indicated in the setting of any of the following**: recent onset of severe, debilitating headaches; headaches which are increasing in severity and/or frequency; headaches in the setting of seizures or a history of neurodevelopmental impairment; and headaches accompanied by neurologic signs (i.e., papilledema, strabismus, unilateral weakness or sensory loss, dysarthria, ataxia, or changes in mental status, affect, behavior, or arousability). Such signs typically manifest within 6 months of the onset of headaches in patients with underlying neuropathology. Although structural lesions large enough to result in symptomatic increased intracranial pressure are almost always visible on head CT, the MRI provides additional detail which may be beneficial in patients with abnormal CT scans or suspected posterior fossa lesions.

DIFFERENTIAL DIAGNOSIS

Pseudotumor cerebri is a benign but important cause of headaches that typically occurs in overweight adolescent females or in association with thyroid disease or use of certain medications. It is thought to be caused by impaired CSF resorption. Although the examination is positive for papilledema, the increased intracranial pressure is accompanied by a normal CT. Sequential LPs, which demonstrate increased opening pressure, usually alleviate the headaches. Acetazolamide and furosemide may be helpful in more protracted cases. Pseudotumor cerebri is self-limited and typically resolves without complication.

TREATMENT

Tension headaches respond to nonprescription analgesics and rest. Stress management techniques and biofeedback training may also be beneficial. Daily prophylaxis should be considered in headache patients requiring medication more than two to three times a week. Referral to a mental health professional prior to the initiation of prophylactic treatment for chronic headaches may be beneficial in patients with suspected social or emotional stressors.

Treatment of migraine headaches begins with reassurance that the headache is not due to underlying neuropathology. Nonpharmacologic interventions (e.g., biofeedback, cognitive therapy) are often very beneficial for controlling migraine headaches. Patients should be instructed to eat regular meals and avoid fatigue and sleep deprivation. Over-the-counter medications (acetaminophen, ibuprofen) work well as abortive medications in younger patients; intranasal or oral **sumatriptan** is reserved for children ≥12 years of age with headaches which are severe or unresponsive to over-the-counter medications. Subcutaneous sumatriptan is inappropriate for children. Prophylaxis should be considered if abortive medication is necessary more than three to six times a month; anticonvulsants, antidepressants, and beta-blockers have been prescribed with variable success.

ENCEPHALOPATHY

To function normally, the brain needs adequate blood flow, oxygen, energy substrates, removal of metabolic waste, and appropriate electrolyte balance. Disruption of any of these will lead to generalized cerebral dysfunction with alteration in mental status and/or level of consciousness, termed **encephalopathy**.

CLINICAL MANIFESTATIONS

The differential diagnosis of pediatric encephalopathy, or deterioration in mental status due to generalized cerebral dysfunction, is extensive (Table 15-7). Fortunately, the age of the patient, past medical history, history of present illness, and physical examination often suggest the etiology. Encephalopathy secondary to a systemic process such as electrolyte imbalance, infection, or liver failure is characterized by fluctuating mental status and nonlocalizing neurologic manifestations (myoclonus, tremors, temperature instability). In contrast, levels of consciousness are abnormal but fairly stable when encephalopathy results from structural lesions in the brain (tumor, abscess, hemorrhage), and focal neurologic signs are more common. Recent or concurrent febrile illness is consistent with infectious encephalitis. Focal findings (hemiparesis, ataxia, cranial nerve defects) on examination and seizures are more common with **herpes simplex (HSV) encephalitis** than other viral etiologies. **Reye syndrome**, a rare mitochondrial disorder characterized by acute-onset encephalopathy and degenerative liver disease, may follow a viral illness, especially when aspirin has been administered. Signs and symptoms include severe vomiting, delirium, stupor, hypoglycemia, and elevated transaminase and ammonia levels. **Metabolic disorders** typically present with recurrent episodes of mental status changes that clear when the acute process is corrected. A careful history may suggest environmental exposures or drug use. Particular areas of interest on examination include vital signs, liver size, pupil and funduscopic assessment, and neurologic findings (cranial nerves, reflexes, strength, sensation, and cerebellar function).

DIAGNOSTIC EVALUATION

Electrolyte abnormalities, uremia, hypoglycemia, acidemia, and hyperammonemia can be ruled out with simple blood tests. The WBC count is elevated in the presence of infection. Urine and blood should

TABLE 15-7 Causes of Encephalopathy in Children

Infection	Metabolic disorders
• Infection of the central nervous system is by far the most common cause of acute encephalopathy in children.	• aminoacidopathies
	• organic acidopathies
• Infections which may present with altered level of consciousness include meningitis, encephalitis, postinfectious encephalomyelitis, brain abscess, and subdural empyema.	• disorders of carbohydrate metabolism
	• disorders of fatty acid oxidation
	Mitochondrial disorders
	• Reye syndrome
• Sepsis can produce generalized cerebral depression in the absence of central nervous system involvement.	**Disorders of the liver**
	• hepatic encephalopathy
• Infection with *Shigella* species occasionally presents with isolated encephalopathy.	**Renal Disease**
	• hypertensive encephalopathy
Trauma/Abuse	• kidney failure/uremia
Central nervous system disorders	**Pulmonary disease**
• increased intracranial pressure/hydrocephalus/shunt malfunction; seizures, postictal phase	• acute, chronic hypoxia
	Cardiovascular disease
• neoplastic infiltration or brain tumor	• cardiovascular failure/shock/compromised perfusion
• arteriovenous malformation, embolism, stroke	**Endocrinopathy**
Ingestions (see Chapter 2)	• hypoglycemia
Electrolyte imbalances	• diabetic ketoacidosis
• hyponatremia	• adrenal insufficiency
• hypernatremia	• Hashimoto encephalopathy
• hypocalcemia	**Gastrointestinal disorders**
• hypercalcemia	• intussusception
• hypomagnesemia	

be sent for toxicology screening. An emergent head CT scan is indicated in patients with evidence of increased intracranial pressure or focal neurologic signs. A LP is appropriate when meningitis or encephalitis is suspected and increased intracranial pressure has been ruled out. HSV encephalitis is characterized by focal mediotemporal spikes superimposed on a diffuse slow wave pattern on EEG and temporal lobe abnormalities on CT and MRI.

TREATMENT

Specific identification of the underlying disorder is critical to resolving the encephalopathy and preserving brain function. Treatment depends on the cause and whether increased intracranial pressure is present. Patients with severe disease require intubation and close intracranial pressure monitoring in an ICU. Antibiotics are added in cases of bacterial infection; high-dose IV acyclovir is recommended for patients with HSV. Metabolic disorders are discussed in Chapter 9. Ingestions are discussed in Chapter 2.

WEAKNESS

Abnormalities leading to weakness or paralysis, or both, may occur at any level of the neuromotor axis, from the motor cortex and pyramidal tracts to the anterior horn cell, peripheral nerve, neuromuscular junction, and muscle.

DIFFERENTIAL DIAGNOSIS

Guillain-Barré syndrome (GBS) is an acute-onset, progressive, ascending weakness caused by autoimmune-mediated demyelination of peripheral nerves. More than half of cases develop 7 to 21 days after an acute respiratory or gastrointestinal viral illness. Sensory and autonomic impairments are often present but not prominent. Initial symptoms include numbness of the distal extremities followed by progressive (usually) ascending weakness. Deep tendon reflexes wane and disappear. Severity varies from mild weakness to progressive involvement of the trunk and cranial nerves. Respiratory muscle involvement may necessitate mechanical ventilation. A significantly increased CSF protein level is consistent with GBS. Motor nerve conduction studies may be helpful, particularly early in disease. Symptoms may progress for up to 4 weeks, with resolution typically beginning approximately 4 weeks thereafter. Recovery is usually complete in children, although the rare patient experiences permanent lingering disability. Intravenous immune globulin shortens the duration and severity of the illness.

Tick paralysis resembles GBS, although ocular palsies and pupillary abnormalities are more commonly seen. Certain ticks in the Appalachian and Rocky Mountains are capable of producing a neurotoxin that blocks acetylcholine release. The patient recovers completely when the tick is removed from the skin.

Myasthenia gravis (MG) is a chronic autoimmune disorder of the neuromuscular junction. Autoantibodies bind to the postsynaptic acetylcholine receptor and block its activity. The rate of receptor breakdown also increases, so fewer receptors are present. The principal symptoms are easy fatigability and weakness that is exacerbated by sustained activity and improves with rest. Juvenile MG typically presents in late childhood or adolescence; the onset may be rapid or insidious, and symptoms wax and wane over time. Almost half of patients experience ocular muscle involvement, resulting in ptosis and/or diplopia. Bulbar weakness leads to dysarthria and difficulty swallowing. Administration of an intravenous anticholinesterase (edrophonium chloride) results in a transient increase in muscle strength by blocking the breakdown of acetylcholine in the synaptic cleft. Repetitive electrical nerve stimulation studies demonstrate a significant fall in response strength over several rapid-fire trials. Acetylcholine receptor antibodies are measurable in the serum. MG may go into complete or partial remission after several years; however, most patients continue to experience periodic exacerbations throughout adulthood. Anticholinesterase therapy (neostigmine or pyridostigmine bromide) may relieve all or most of the symptoms in patients with mild involvement. Corticosteroids and other immune suppressants help curb the autoimmune response. Thymectomy results in significant improvement in many patients with MG, presumably because the thymus is thought to sensitize the lymphocytes producing the offending antibodies.

Duchenne-type muscular dystrophy (DMD), an X-linked recessive disease of muscle tissue, is the classic myopathy. Serum creatinine kinase levels are drastically elevated, even at birth. The disease presents in early childhood with motor delay. Weakness is greatest in the proximal muscle groups, so the patient must rise from sitting on the floor in two steps: first leaning on the hypertrophied calves, and then pushing the trunk up with the arms (Gower's sign). Eventually, ambulation is lost, the muscles atrophy, and contractures develop. Cardiac and cognitive abnormalities are often present as well. Treatment is mostly supportive; corticosteroids slow but do not stop the progressive muscle destruction. Most children become wheelchair bound early in the second decade, with death in adolescence or early adulthood from respiratory failure or cardiomyopathy.

Spinal muscle atrophy (SMA) is an inherited disorder involving degeneration of the anterior horn cells and cranial nerve motor nuclei. The most severe form, SMA type I (Werdnig-Hoffmann disease), becomes evident in early infancy with generalized hypotonia and weakness. SMA type 2 presents between 6 and 12 months of age and is usually less severe. Cognitive abilities remain unaffected in both forms of the illness. No specific therapy is available; death occurs from repeated aspiration or lung infections. Both SMA and DMD are suggested by characteristic changes on EMG and muscle biopsy and confirmed by specific gene tests.

Tumors that compress the spinal cord result in weakness and paralysis below the lesion and constitute a surgical emergency. Cervical spinal cord injuries produce sudden-onset paresthesias and paralysis. Environmental toxin exposure may induce acquired neuropathies or myopathies. For example, infants in certain endemic areas (or those fed honey) may be exposed to spores of Clostridium botulinum and develop progressive paralysis from the elaborated toxin, which irreversibly blocks release of acetylcholine at the motor endplate.

TREATMENT

Diagnostic workup is tailored by findings on history and physical examination. Patients with asymmetric weakness or signs of increased intracranial pressure should undergo neuroimaging to rule out mass effect and hydrocephalus. Findings localized to a particular level of the spinal cord warrant evaluation for cord compression or injury. An LP is helpful when infection is suspected. Supportive treatment may be required at some point; more definitive treatment, if available, is disease specific.

NEURODEGENERATIVE DISORDERS

Neural tissue degeneration can occur at any level of the nervous system, from the brain cell bodies to the peripheral nerves. Many of the diseases are inherited; most are progressive and debilitating. Neurodegenerative disorders may be divided into gray matter disorders, white matter disorders, and systemic disorders.

Gray matter disorders, which include Tay-Sachs, Gaucher, and Niemann-Pick diseases, result from lipid buildup in neuronal cell bodies. Hypotonia, mental retardation, seizures, retinal degeneration, and ataxia are common.

White matter disorders (leukodystrophies) are inherited progressive degenerative diseases resulting from abnormally formed myelin, impaired conduction, and rapid myelin breakdown. They present in younger patients with spasticity and developmental milestone loss; older children and adolescents experience visual disturbances (optic atrophy), changes in personality, and dropping school grades. **Adrenoleukodystrophy**, so named because of its frequent association with adrenal insufficiency, is characterized by areas of demyelination coupled with an intense perivascular inflammatory reaction. Psychomotor retardation progresses to spasticity, extensor posturing, and death by early adulthood.

System diseases are categorized according to the particular neural pathway affected. **Rett syndrome** is an X-linked but usually sporadic disorder of cerebral atrophy. Affected males succumb in utero. Females initially show normal development; however, after 1 year of age, microcephaly and developmental milestone regression occur. Repetitive hand wringing is the most characteristic behavior; other manifestations include seizures, ataxia, mental retardation, and autistic behavior. Life expectancy is appreciably shortened.

ATAXIA

Ataxia is the inability to coordinate purposeful movement and control balance. Conditions that affect the cerebellum, connected sensory/motor pathways, or the inner ear are likely to cause ataxia in children.

The most common causes in the pediatric population are infectious labyrinthitis, acute cerebellar ataxia, and drug ingestion (e.g., phenytoin, carbamazepine, sedatives, hypnotics, phencyclidine). Metabolic derangements, hydrocephalus, head trauma, and cerebellar hemorrhages may also cause ataxia.

DIFFERENTIAL DIAGNOSIS

Viral infection of the labyrinthine structures can cause acute ataxia which is often associated with horizontal nystagmus. The incoordination resulting from **acute cerebellar ataxia** may be relatively minor; alternatively, the child may be unable to walk or stand. The condition is most common between the ages of 2 and 7 years and often follows a viral illness. The patient appears otherwise well, with no changes in level of consciousness or mental status. Headache and nuchal rigidity are absent, and the CSF is sterile. The prognosis of acute cerebellar ataxia which involves only the trunk, limbs, and mild nystagmus is quite good, with return of normal coordination within a few weeks. Cases associated with opsoclonus or tremors of the head and neck may require treatment with systemic corticosteroids or intravenous immunoglobulin and can result in permanent neurologic impairment.

Ataxia that is slowly progressive is more likely to be caused by a brain tumor or a degenerative spinocerebellar disease such as ataxia-telangiectasia or Friedreich ataxia. **Ataxia-telangiectasia** is an autosomal recessive neurodegenerative disorder that presents in toddlers and progresses to wheelchair dependence. The ataxia is associated with extensive telangiectasias and immunodeficiency. The genetic defect is located on chromosome 11.

Friedreich ataxia presents later in childhood with progressive ataxia, weakness, and muscle wasting. Skeletal deformities invariably follow. Most patients die of cardiomyopathy-related heart disease before 30 years of age. Inheritance is autosomal recessive, linked to a defect on chromosome 9.

CLINICAL MANIFESTATIONS

History and Physical Examination

The history should include questions concerning disease onset (acute vs. chronic) and progression (slow vs. rapid). Associated symptoms may include fever, headache, vomiting, vertigo, photophobia, and altered mental status. Recent precipitating events (seizures, infections, head trauma) and exposures (medications, heavy metals, solvents, gases) should be documented. Some ataxias have a genetic basis, so the family history may be positive for neurologic illnesses.

The examination includes evaluation of truncal balance, mental status, gait, deep tendon reflexes, and muscle tone and strength. An abnormal gait may be caused by weakness (reduced reflexes and muscle strength) rather than imbalance. The examiner should note the presence of any nystagmus and/or signs of increased intracranial pressure (bradycardia, hypertension, papilledema, meningismus). If the child is old enough and cooperative, tests such as heel-to-knee, finger-to-nose, and rapid alternating movement help evaluate cerebellar function. The Romberg test evaluates function of the peripheral nerves and posterior columns. With the patient standing balanced with feet together and eyes open, the Romberg sign is present (abnormal) if the child cannot maintain balance when he or she closes the eyes.

DIAGNOSTIC EVALUATION

Toxicology screens should be considered in ambulatory patients or patients with suspected abuse. Neuroimaging permits assessment for cerebellar masses (tumor, abscess, hemorrhage). CT of the head should always precede lumbar puncture in patients with ataxia unless deep tendon reflexes (DTRs) are absent on examination; intracranial processes do not interfere with DTRs. A brain MRI may be preferable in some cases given the superior detail of the posterior fossa with this study. LP permits analysis for abnormalities noted in meningitis, acute disseminated encephalomyelitis, and Guillain-Barré syndrome. Chronic or recurrent ataxia warrants metabolic and genetic workup.

PHAKOMATOSES

Phakomatoses are neurocutaneous diseases characterized by lesions in the nervous system, skin, and eyes. Three autosomal dominant conditions are described: neurofibromatosis, tuberous sclerosis, and von Hippel-Lindau disease. Sturge-Weber disease, a purely sporadic disorder, is traditionally included as well.

NEUROFIBROMATOSIS

Neurofibromatosis types 1 (von Recklinghausen disease) and 2 (bilateral acoustic neuromas) are the most

■ **TABLE 15-8** Diagnosis of Neurofibromatosis Type 1
Two of the following must be present:
1. Six or more café-au-lait spots, >5 mm in size in children and >15 mm in adolescents or adults
2. Axillary or inguinal freckling
3. Two or more Lisch nodules (hamartomas) in the iris
4. Two or more neurofibromas or one plexiform neurofibroma
5. A distinctive osseous lesion, such as sphenoid dysplasia
6. Optic gliomas
7. Affected first-degree relative diagnosed based on the preceding criteria

common variants in children. **Neurofibromatosis type 1** is a clinical diagnosis based in part on the presence of six or more café-au-lait spots of a specific size (Table 15-8). A large gene on chromosome 17 coding for neurofibromin has a high spontaneous mutation rate. Patients with neurofibromatosis type 1 are at increased risk for optic pathway gliomas and other low-grade gliomas in the central nervous system. They typically require evaluation and treatment for the associated seizures, learning disorders, renovascular hypertension, and scoliosis. Routine vision screening is critical. Neurofibromas that cause impairment may be surgically removed; however, most will recur.

Bilateral acoustic neuromas are the hallmark of **neurofibromatosis type 2**. Complications include hearing loss and vestibular disorientation. Brain MRI demonstrates bilateral eighth cranial nerve masses. Neurofibromas, meningiomas, schwannomas, and astrocytomas are also associated with type 2 neurofibromatosis. Cataracts and retinal hamartomas are not uncommon. Surgical debulking is appropriate when hearing impairment becomes pronounced. Cochlear implants have restored hearing in some patients. The genetic abnormality occurs on chromosome 22.

TUBEROUS SCLEROSIS

Tuberous sclerosis, like neurofibromatosis, is a progressive autosomal dominant neurocutaneous disorder, although sporadic cases are more common than inherited ones. Two separate genes have been identified for tuberous sclerosis (chromosome sites 9q34 and 16p13). The normal genetic product is tuberin, a protein thought to suppress the development of tumors.

Disease severity varies greatly from patient to patient. Typical skin lesions include **ash-leaf spots** (flat, hypopigmented macules), **shagreen patches** (areas of abnormal skin thickening), sebaceous adenomas, and ungual fibromas. Ash-leaf spots are the earliest manifestation and are best detected under Wood lamp examination. Neuroimaging demonstrates the distinctive periventricular knob-like areas of localized swelling, or tubers. Subependymal nodules and giant cell astrocytomas may also be present. Mental retardation and seizures (including infantile spasms) are common. Tumors also have a predilection for the kidney, heart (particularly cardiac rhabdomyomas), and retina. Treatment consists of antiepileptic therapy and surgical removal of related tumors when indicated.

VON HIPPEL-LINDAU DISEASE

Von Hippel-Lindau disease is characterized by retinal angiomas (abnormal masses of thin-walled capillaries), cerebellar hemangioblastomas, and associated neoplasms, including renal cell carcinoma and pheochromocytoma. Ocular lesions respond to laser therapy; no specific treatment exists for the CNS growths. The genetic abnormality occurs on chromosome 3p25 and exhibits variable penetrance. Von Hippel-Lindau disease generally does not present until adolescence or beyond.

STURGE-WEBER SYNDROME

Sturge-Weber syndrome (leptomeningeal angiomatosis) is a disorder of neurologic deterioration associated with a port-wine stain (nevus flammeus) over the area innervated by the first division of the trigeminal nerve. Affected children manifest progressive mental retardation, seizures, hemiparesis, and visual impairment; approximately a third develops glaucoma. *Tunable (pulsed) dye laser therapy* fades the port-wine stain but does not address the underlying neurologic dysfunction. Lesions should be treated early in life to optimize cosmetic outcome. Optimal control of seizures may limit subsequent developmental delay. About 10% of children with a unilateral port wine stain over the dermatome innervated by CNV_1 will

be affected with Sturge-Weber syndrome; this percentage is higher if the lesion is bilateral.

SKULL ABNORMALITIES

Microcephaly describes a head circumference that is greater than 2 standard deviations below mean head size for age. It often results from genetic abnormalities (e.g., trisomy 21, Prader-Willi syndrome) or congenital insults (maternal drug ingestions, congenital infections, or insufficient placental blood flow). Affected children often demonstrate both cognitive and motor delay; associated seizure disorders are not uncommon.

Macrocephaly, in contrast, refers to a head circumference greater than 2 standard deviations above the mean. Macrocephaly may be familial; however, cranioskeletal dysplasias, storage diseases, and hydrocephalus should be explored as possible causes, particularly if the growth rate crosses percentile lines over time.

Positional plagiocephaly is the benign flattening of the back of the head often seen in infants placed to sleep exclusively on their backs. A variant results when an infant preferentially lies with the head turned toward one side; flattening of the parieto-occipital area is accompanied by prominence of the forehead on the same side. Most cases require no intervention beyond counseling the parents to encourage the child to lie with the head tilted to the opposite side (by moving a mobile or colorful object to that side). If there is a cosmetic concern, a soft plastic helmet fitted by a plastic surgeon may be successful in gently molding the back of the head into a more acceptable shape when instituted prior to 9 months of age.

Craniosynostosis is the premature fusion of one or more cranial sutures. It may be idiopathic or occur as part of a syndrome. Bony growth continues along the open suture lines, resulting in an abnormally shaped head. If early obliteration of the sagittal suture occurs (most common), the child has a long head and a narrow face (scaphocephaly). In contrast, premature closure of the coronal sutures results in a very wide face with a short, almost box-like, skull. The need for and timing of surgical intervention, which consists of reopening the sutures and retarding their subsequent fusion, is controversial. Most defects are repaired before 2 years of age for cosmetic reasons. Craniosynostosis with associated hydrocephalus, subnormal brain growth, and development issues was addressed earlier.

KEY POINTS

- An elevated maternal serum alpha-fetoprotein level at 16 to 18 weeks of gestation is an excellent screen for neural tube defects. The incidence of neural tube defects is decreased in infants whose mothers receive folic acid supplementation prior to conception and in the early weeks of pregnancy.

- Clinical manifestations of hydrocephalus include inappropriately large head circumference, bulging fontanelle, and poor feeding (in infants); irritability and/or lethargy; morning headaches and vomiting; papilledema and diplopia; and hyperreflexia of the lower limbs. A lumbar puncture (LP) is contraindicated if herniation of the brain is a concern.

- Cerebral palsy (CP) is a nonprogressive disorder of movement and posture resulting from a fixed lesion of the brain. If a child with CP exhibits progressive deterioration, an alternate diagnosis should be sought.

- Febrile seizures are typically brief, generalized seizures with fever which occur in up to 5% of otherwise healthy children ages 6 months to 6 years. About a third of children with a history of febrile seizure will have recurrent febrile seizures. Febrile seizures, even when recurrent, are not considered epilepsy. Children with a history of febrile seizure are at greater risk than their peers for the development of epilepsy later in life.

- The context of the child's age, past medical and family histories, and any prior unusual spells are important in the differentiation of a seizure from a non-seizure event. The diagnosis of a seizure is based primarily on the historical account of the episode.

- Subdural and epidural hemorrhages are more common than intraparenchymal bleeding when head injury is related to trauma. Clinical manifestations of basilar skull fractures include raccoon eyes, Battle's sign, hemotympanum, and CSF rhinorrhea or otorrhea.

- When evaluating a patient with headaches, it is important to determine whether the headaches are primary (tension or migraine headaches) or secondary (pathologic) in etiology. Clinical manifestations that should prompt consideration of pathologic headaches include symptom focality; frontal or occipital location; debilitating episodes of pain; increasing frequency and/or severity; headaches and vomiting upon awakening; and neurologic signs.

- Abnormalities leading to weakness or paralysis, or both, may occur at any level of the neuromotor axis, from the motor cortex and pyramidal tracts to the anterior horn cell, peripheral nerve, neuromuscular junction, and muscle. Guillain-Barré syndrome is an acute-onset, progressive, ascending weakness caused by autoimmune-mediated demyelination of peripheral nerves. Myasthenia gravis is a chronic autoimmune disorder of the neuromuscular junction. Duchenne-type muscular dystrophy is an X-linked recessive disease involving direct destruction of muscle tissue.

- The most common causes of acute ataxia in the pediatric population are infectious labyrinthitis, acute cerebellar ataxia, and toxic ingestion.

- Positional plagiocephaly is the benign flattening of the back of the head often seen in infants placed to sleep exclusively on their backs. Most cases require no intervention beyond counseling the parents to encourage the child to lie with the head tilted to the opposite side (by moving a mobile or colorful object to that side).

16 Nutrition

Katie S. Fine

Good nutrition is essential for optimal physical growth and intellectual development. A healthy diet protects against disease, provides reserve in times of stress, and contains adequate amounts of protein, carbohydrates, fats, vitamins, and minerals. Children with vegan diets (ingesting no animal products) are at risk for vitamin B_{12} deficiency and, if exposed to inadequate sunlight, vitamin D deficiency as well. Iron supplementation/fortification should be considered for both vegan and lacto-ovo vegetarians. Infant feeding intolerance, failure to thrive, iron-deficiency anemia (Chapter 10), and obesity are the most common pediatric conditions associated with malnutrition in the developed world.

In order to assess a child's nutritional status and growth, pediatricians follow the patient's **growth chart**. Growth charts represent cross-sectional data from the National Center for Health Statistics. The patient's weight, height, and **body mass index** (BMI; weight in kilograms divided by height in meters squared) are recorded as points on the chart at each health maintenance visit. Separate growth charts are generated for preterm infants and children with certain genetic disorders, including Down syndrome and Turner syndrome.

INFANT FEEDING ISSUES

Infant feeding addresses the physical and emotional needs of both mother and child. Babies double in weight by age 4 to 5 months, and typically triple their birth weight by their first birthday. Height reaches twice birth length by age 3 to 4 years. Although breastfeeding is almost always preferable, many commercially prepared iron-fortified formulas provide appropriate calories and nutrients. Preterm infants require specifically balanced formula or breast milk with added fortifier. Newborns feed on demand, usually every 1 to 2 hours. Neonates typically lose up to 10% of their birth weight over the first several days; formula-fed babies regain that weight by the second week of life, whereas breastfed babies may take about a week longer. Healthy infants automatically regulate intake to meet caloric demand for basic metabolism and growth.

All infant formulas contain the recommended amounts of vitamins and minerals. Iron-fortified cereals should be added to the infant diet between 4 and 6 months of age. After 6 months of age, other baby foods may be started, including fruits and vegetables. When introducing new foods, only one novel product should be introduced at a time to evaluate for potential adverse reactions. Whole-fat cow milk may be introduced at age 12 months and should continue until age 24 months, when skim milk should be substituted. Infants and children sent to bed with a bottle containing anything but water are at risk for **milk-bottle teeth caries**.

BREASTFEEDING

The American Academy of Pediatrics recommends **exclusive breastfeeding** during the first 6 months of life and continuation of breastfeeding during the second 6 months for optimal infant nutrition. Studies have shown that breastfed infants have a lower incidence of infections, including otitis media, pneumonia, sepsis, and meningitis. Human milk contains bacterial and viral antibodies (secretory IgA) and macrophages. **Lactoferrin** is a protein found in breast milk that increases the availability of iron and has an inhibitory effect on the growth of *Escherichia coli*.

Breastfed infants are less likely to experience feeding difficulties associated with allergy (eczema) or intolerance (colic).

Breastfed infants should receive oral **vitamin D supplementation** beginning in the weeks after birth to prevent **rickets**, a condition in which developing bone fails to mineralize due to inadequate 1,25-dihydroxycholecalciferol. Rickets in breastfed infants becomes clinically and chemically evident in late infancy (Table 16-1). Rickets due solely to vitamin D deficiency begins to respond to supplementation within weeks. According to the American Academy of Pediatrics, breastfed infants may require fluoride supplementation if the concentration of the mineral in their main water source is extremely low.

In developed countries, mothers with human immunodeficiency virus (HIV) infection or untreated active tuberculosis and those who are using illegal drugs should not breastfeed. Other contraindications include infants with galactosemia and certain maternal medications (antithyroid agents, lithium, isoniazid, and most chemotherapy drugs).

INFANT FEEDING INTOLERANCE

Feeding intolerance may lead to food aversion and failure to thrive; the most significant cause is cow milk protein intolerance or allergy.

Clinical Manifestations

History and Physical Examination

Feeding intolerance may present with any number of clinical manifestations. **Malabsorption** is characterized by poor growth and chronic, nonbloody diarrhea. **Allergy** may be accompanied by eczema or wheezing. A severe local allergic reaction within the bowel results in **colitis**, indicated by anemia and/or obvious blood in the stools. Other possible nonspecific symptoms include vomiting, irritability, and abdominal distention.

Differential Diagnosis

Infectious gastroenteritis, necrotizing enterocolitis, intussusception, intermittent volvulus, celiac disease, cystic fibrosis, chronic protein malnutrition, aspiration, and eosinophilic enteritis should be considered. The most common condition mistaken for milk protein intolerance is colic, which is generally limited to infants 3 weeks to 3 months of age. **Colic** is a

■ TABLE 16-1 Clinical and Laboratory Manifestations of Rickets

Craniotabes (thinning of the outer skull layer)
Rachitic rosary (enlargement of the costochondral junctions)
Epiphyseal enlargement at the wrists and ankles
Delayed closing of abnormally large fontanelle
Bowlegs
Delayed walking
Normal-to-low serum calcium
Low serum phosphorus
Elevated serum alkaline phosphatase
Low serum 25-hydroxycholecalciferol

syndrome of recurrent irritability that persists for several hours, usually in the late afternoon or evening. During the attacks, the child draws the knees to the abdomen and cries inconsolably. The crying resolves as suddenly and spontaneously as it begins.

Treatment

Exclusive breastfeeding during the first year of life eliminates the problem posed by cow milk protein intolerance, except in severely allergic infants. If there is no evidence of any underlying disease in formula-fed infants with characteristic symptoms, substitution of a protein hydrolysate formula is recommended, because as many as 25% of children with cow milk protein allergy are also intolerant of soy protein.

FAILURE TO THRIVE

Failure to thrive (FTT) is defined here as persistent weight below the third percentile or falling off a previously established growth curve. It is not uncommon for a child to cross a growth percentile curve between 9 and 18 months of age, as growth begins to relate more closely to genetic potential rather than maternal nutrition. However, a growth curve which flattens or crosses one or more growth percentile curves is cause for concern. Risk factors for FTT include low birth weight, low socioeconomic status, physical or mental disability, and caretaker neglect. FTT is often associated with developmental delay, particularly if it occurs during the first year of life when brain growth is maximal.

Differential Diagnosis

FTT may result from inadequate caloric intake, excessive caloric losses, or increased caloric requirements. **Most cases of FTT in developed countries are nonorganic or psychosocial in origin**; that is, there is no coexistent medical disorder. The list of organic diagnoses predisposing to FTT is extensive, and virtually all organ systems are represented (Table 16-2). **Organic FTT virtually never presents** with isolated growth failure; other signs and symptoms are generally evident with a detailed history and physical examination.

Clinical Manifestations

History

The caretaker must be questioned in detail about the child's diet, including how often the child eats,

TABLE 16-2 Differential Diagnosis of Failure to Thrive	
Nonorganic	
Neglect	Inadequate amount fed
Abuse	Incorrect preparation of formula
Cardiac	
Congenital heart malformations	
Gastrointestinal	
Malabsorption	Inflammatory bowel disease
Cow milk protein intolerance/allergy	Celiac disease
Gastroesophageal reflux	Hirschsprung disease
Pyloric stenosis	
Pulmonary	
Cystic fibrosis	Chronic aspiration
Bronchopulmonary dysplasia	Respiratory insufficiency
Infectious	
HIV	Intestinal parasites
Tuberculosis	Urinary tract infection
Chronic gastroenteritis	
Neonatal	
Prematurity	Congenital or perinatal infection
Low birth weight	Congenital syndromes
Endocrine	
Diabetes mellitus	Adrenal insufficiency or excess
Hypothyroidism	Growth hormone deficiency
Neurologic	
Cerebral palsy	Degenerative disorders
Mental retardation	Oral-motor dysfunction
Renal	
Renal tubular acidosis	Chronic renal insufficiency
Other	
Inborn errors of metabolism	Immunodeficiency syndromes
Malignancy	Collagen vascular disease
Cleft palate	

how much is consumed at each feeding, what the child is fed, how the formula is prepared, and who feeds the child. Information regarding diarrhea, fatty stools, irritability, vomiting, food refusal, and polyuria should be documented. Recurrent infections suggest congenital or acquired immunodeficiency. Constitutional growth delay can usually be diagnosed by family history alone. Foreign and domestic travel, source of water, and developmental delay are occasionally overlooked topics. The psychosocial history includes questions concerning the caretaker's expectations of the child, parental and sibling health, financial security, recent major life events, and chronic stressors.

Physical Examination

Weight, height, and head circumference should be recorded on an appropriate growth chart. Relatively recent growth failure is usually limited to weight alone, whereas height and (late) head circumference are also affected in chronic deficiency. Severely deprived children may present with lethargy, edema, scant subcutaneous fat, atrophic muscle tissue, decreased skin turgor, coarsened hair, dermatitis, and distended abdomen.

Observation of caretaker–child interactions and feeding behavior is critical. Children who are listless, minimally responsive to the examiner and/or caretaker, withdrawn, or excessively fearful often have contributing psychosocial issues. Findings suggestive of physical abuse or neglect (see Chapter 2) should be sought and documented.

A complete physical examination, with careful attention for dysmorphism, pallor, bruising, cleft palate, rales or crackles, heart murmurs, and muscle tone may suggest the etiology.

Diagnostic Evaluation

Information obtained from the history and physical examination determines the direction of further diagnostic workup. Any child with FTT should receive a complete blood count, serum electrolytes, blood urea nitrogen and creatinine, protein and albumin measurements, urinalysis, and urine culture. Bone age films may also be helpful in children beyond infancy. Severely malnourished children and patients with suspected nonorganic FTT should be admitted to the hospital. Adequate catch-up growth during hospitalization on a regular diet is virtually diagnostic of psychosocial FTT.

OBESITY

When a pediatric patient's BMI is greater than the 95th percentile for age, that individual is considered **overweight**. A child whose BMI falls between the 85th and 95th percentiles is considered **at risk for overweight**. These percentile cutoffs may be modified as use of BMI in the pediatric population increases. According to the most recent National Health and Nutrition Examination Survey, about 14% of 2- to 5-year-olds and 19% of older children are overweight. A period of adipose cell proliferation occurs from age 2 to 4 years and again during puberty, placing pediatricians in an ideal position to affect their patients' health well into adulthood.

While the root cause is simply caloric intake in excess of expenditure, the presence of certain gene markers results in increased risk. Factors associated with an increased risk of obesity in children include genetic, parental, family, and lifestyle issues (Table 16-3). The social and psychological consequences of being a "fat" child may be particularly damaging to self-esteem at a critical age. Obese patients of normal or above-average height are unlikely to have a predisposing health condition. The workup of the short obese child should include consideration of endocrine disorders (hypothyroidism, Cushing syndrome), genetic syndromes, and hypothalamic tumors.

Metabolic syndrome is the combination of **obesity, hypertension, insulin resistance, and dyslipidemia** (increased triglycerides, decreased HDL levels, and relatively high levels of abnormally dense LDL particles). Rates of type 2 diabetes, cardiovascular disease, and fatty liver disease are increased in patients with metabolic syndrome. Other potential complications

■ **TABLE 16-3** Risk Factors for Obesity in Children
Overweight parent(s)
Large birth weight
Diabetic mother
Low parental education level
Poverty
Overweight child at age 3 years
Increased length of TV viewing
Poor dietary choices
Lower activity levels

of obesity include depression, sleep apnea, gallbladder disease, slipped capital femoral epiphysis, and early-onset puberty in females.

Obesity is treated by altering caloric intake/dietary habits, developing a regular exercise program, and behavioral modification (setting goals and monitoring self-control). Careful attention must be paid to maintaining patients' growth and development while at the same time decreasing their BMI over time. Surgical options and appetite suppressants are currently considered inappropriate for use in the pediatric population.

KEY POINTS

- The American Academy of Pediatrics recommends exclusive breastfeeding during the first 6 months of life, with continued breastfeeding through age 12 months.

- Newborns initially lose weight, but should ultimately gain in weight back to birthweight by the 3rd week of life.

- Cow milk protein intolerance can result in colitis and failure to thrive.

- The sporadic nature and sudden onset of colic usually distinguish this condition from feeding intolerance.

- The healthy formula-fed infant with presumed cow milk protein intolerance should be switched to a protein hydrolysate formula rather than one formulated with soy protein.

- Most cases of failure to thrive in developed countries are due wholly or in large part to neglect.

- Children with BMIs greater than the 95th percentile for age are considered overweight.

- Metabolic syndrome (obesity, insulin resistance, dyslipidemia, and hypertension) increases the risk for development of type 2 diabetes and cardiovascular disease.

17 Oncology

Karen C. Burns • Rajaram Nagarajan • Franklin O. Smith • Bradley S. Marino

There are approximately 12,500 new diagnoses of pediatric cancers in patients under the age of 20 years each year in the United States. Approximately two-thirds occur below the age of 15 years. The most common types of cancers in children under the age of 15 years are leukemia and brain tumors. In the older adolescent group, Hodgkin disease and germ cell tumors predominate (Figs. 17-1 and 17-2).

Common therapeutic modalities for treating childhood cancer include surgery, radiation, chemotherapy, hematopoietic stem cell transplantation, and biologic agents. The most commonly used chemotherapeutic agents are listed in Table 17-1.

Although childhood cancer represents a small number of childhood diseases, it accounts for a substantial number of deaths in children. It is the second most common cause of death under the age of 15 years (11%)—first is accidents (40%). In older adolescents, cancer-related deaths account for 5% of all deaths—fourth behind accidents, suicide, and homicide. Overall, tremendous progress has been made, with cure rates now exceeding 80% overall.

This has lead to increasing numbers of childhood cancer survivors. Issues relating to survivorship are now being appreciated and need to be acknowledged in pediatric and general practices. Primary care physicians need to be aware that long-term complications of cancer therapies exist and that appropriate lifelong follow-up is needed. It is also important that childhood cancer survivors (and their caregivers) are aware of their history of cancer and the therapies given to them, so that they are empowered to be advocates for their own health as they grow older.

The following sections describe the more common cancers in children and adolescents.

LEUKEMIA

The leukemias account for the greatest percentage of cases of childhood malignancies. There are more than 3,000 new cases of leukemia each year in the United States, and approximately 35 to 40 children per million are affected. Figure 17-1 lists types of childhood cancers (0 to 14 years of age) and the fraction of the total childhood malignancies that each accounts for annually.

PATHOGENESIS

Leukemia results from malignant transformation and clonal expansion of hematopoietic cells at an early stage of differentiation that are then unable to undergo further maturation. Leukemias are classified on the basis of leukemic cell morphology into **lymphoblastic leukemias** (lymphoid lineage cell proliferation) and **myeloid leukemias** (granulocyte, monocyte, erythrocyte, or platelet lineage cell proliferation). **Acute leukemias** constitute 97% of all childhood leukemias and are subdivided into acute lymphoblastic leukemia (ALL) and acute myeloid leukemia, also known as acute myelogenous leukemia (AML). If untreated, they are rapidly fatal within weeks to a few months of diagnosis, but with treatment they are potentially curable. **Chronic leukemias** make up only 3% of childhood leukemias, the majority of which are chronic myelogenous leukemia (CML) seen in adolescents. Unlike patients with acute leukemias, CML can be indolent and patients may survive without treatment for months to years. If left untreated, the chronic leukemias may undergo an acute transformation that

Percent Distribution of Childhood Cancers Under the Age of 15 Years

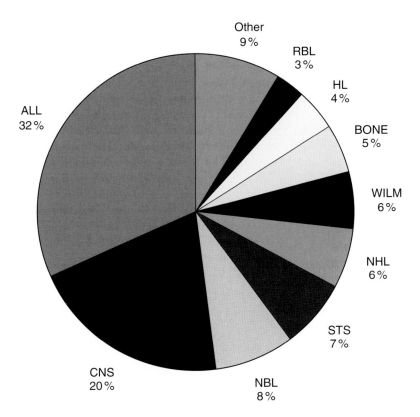

Figure 17-1 • Percent distribution of childhood cancers under the age of 15 years. ALL, acute lymphoblastic leukemia; BONE, osteosarcoma and Ewing sarcoma; CNS, central nervous system tumor; HL, Hodgkin disease; NBL, neuroblastoma; NHL, non-Hodgkin lymphoma; RBL, retinoblastoma; STS, soft tissue sarcoma; WILM, Wilms tumor. (Compiled from Ries L, Smith MA, Gurney JG, et al., eds. *Cancer Incidence and Survival among Children and Adolescents: United States SEER Program 1975–1995.* Bethesda, MD: National Cancer Institute, SEER program. NIH Pub. No. 99-4649; 1999.)

requires immediate therapy to survive. Because CML is so rare in children, a discussion of the chronic leukemias is beyond the scope of this review text. The following discussion focuses on ALL and AML of childhood and adolescence.

CLASSIFICATION

ALL is classified by both morphologic and immunologic methods. **Morphologic classification** is based on the appearance of the lymphoblasts. The L1-type lymphoblast is the most common (85%), followed by the L2 morphology (14%), with L3 lymphoblasts the rarest form. Therapy and outcome are not different for L1 versus L2 lymphoblasts. L3 blasts (or Burkitt or mature B leukemia) are treated more like Burkitt lymphoma with spread to the bone marrow. **Immunologic classification** is based on immunophenotype, which is described by surface antigen expression and flow cytometric analysis. The most frequent childhood ALL immunophenotype, precursor B-cell, accounts for 80% of cases and is associated with a good prognosis in the

majority of cases. Outcomes for T-cell ALL, which is responsible for 19% of childhood ALL, have improved significantly over the past several years and are now comparable to the outcomes of some precursor B-cell ALL. Mature B-cell ALL or Burkitt leukemia, which accounts for 1% of cases, is treated like Burkitt lymphoma with a good outcome.

AML is classified into eight subtypes by morphologic and histochemical information using the French-American-British (FAB) classification system: M0 is undifferentiated stem cell leukemia, M1 is myeloblastic leukemia without differentiation, M2 is myeloblastic leukemia with differentiation, M3 is promyelocytic leukemia, M4 is myelomonocytic leukemia, M5 is monoblastic leukemia, M6 is erythroleukemia, and M7 is megakaryoblastic leukemia. The prognosis for AML is dependent on both subtype and risk factors. Patients with M3 AML, and trisomy 21 patients with M7 AML, have a good prognosis, as do patients with favorable risk factors. Patients with poor risk factors have a poor prognosis. Risk factors will be discussed later in this chapter.

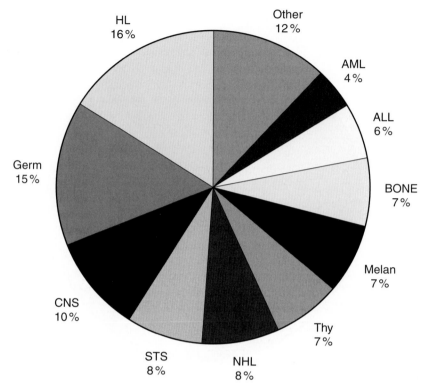

Percent Distribution of Cancer Types for 15 to 19 Year Olds

Figure 17-2 • Percent distribution of cancer types for 15 to 19 year olds. ALL, acute lymphoblastic leukemia; AML, acute myeloid leukemia; BONE, osteosarcoma and Ewing sarcoma; CNS, central nervous system tumor; Germ, germ cell, trophoblastic, and other gonadal tumors; HL, Hodgkin disease; Melan, malignant melanoma; NBL, neuroblastoma; NHL, non-Hodgkin lymphoma; STS, soft tissue sarcoma; Thy, thyroid carcinoma. (Compiled from Ries L, Smith MA, Gurney JG, et al., eds. *Cancer Incidence and Survival among Children and Adolescents: United States SEER Program 1975–1995.* Bethesda, MD: National Cancer Institute, SEER program. NIH Pub. No. 99-4649; 1999.)

EPIDEMIOLOGY AND RISK FACTORS

Table 17-2 compares the epidemiology of ALL and AML. ALL, the most common pediatric neoplasm, accounts for 75% of all cases of childhood acute leukemia. ALL is 1.3 times more common in boys than in girls and more common in white children than in African American children. The incidence of ALL peaks between 2 and 5 years of age. AML accounts for 20% of all cases of childhood acute leukemia. There is no race or gender predilection in patients with AML. The incidence of AML, in contrast to ALL, is increased in adolescence.

Syndromes with an increased risk for leukemia include trisomy 21, Fanconi anemia, Bloom syndrome, ataxia-telangiectasia, X-linked agammaglobulinemia, and severe combined immunodeficiency. Twins have an increased risk of leukemia if one twin develops ALL or AML during the first 5 years of life. Children who have undergone chemotherapy or radiation therapy for a first malignancy have an increased risk of developing a secondary leukemia 1 to 10 years after treatment. Children with congenital bone marrow failure

states, such as Shwachman-Diamond syndrome (exocrine pancreatic insufficiency and neutropenia) and Diamond-Blackfan syndrome (congenital red cell aplasia), have an increased risk of developing AML.

CLINICAL MANIFESTATIONS

History and Physical Examination

Symptoms usually develop days to weeks before diagnosis. Nonspecific constitutional symptoms include lethargy, malaise, and anorexia. Children may complain about bone pain or arthralgias caused by leukemic expansion of the marrow cavity. Progressive bone marrow failure may lead to pallor from anemia and ecchymoses or petechiae from thrombocytopenia. The anemia is normochromic and normocytic. Decreased marrow production of RBCs leads to a low reticulocyte count. The WBC count is low ($<5,000$ per mm^3) in a third of patients, normal (5,000 to 20,000 per mm^3) in a third of patients, and high ($>20,000$ per mm^3) in a third of patients. Many children have hepatosplenomegaly and cervical

TABLE 17-1 Listing of Common Chemotherapeutic Agents and Their Toxicities

Chemotherapy	Mechanism of Action	Acute and Long-Term Toxicity
Alkylating agents		
Cyclophosphamide	Alkylation; cross linking	Hemorrhagic cystitis; SIADH; cardiac toxicity; fertility
Iphosphamide	Alkylation; cross linking	Hemorrhagic cystitis; renal toxicity; ototoxicity; fertility
Cisplatinum	Platination; cross linking	Ototoxicity; renal toxicity; delayed nausea
Antimetabolites		
Methotrexate	Interferes with folate metabolism	Mucositis; Hepatic and renal toxicity; neurotoxicity
Mercaptopurine	Blocks purine synthesis	Mucositis; hepatic toxicity
Thioguanine	Blocks purine synthesis	Mucositis; hepatic toxicity
Cytarabine	Inhibits DNA polymerase	Mucositis; flu-like syndrome; ocular toxicity
Antitumor antibiotic		
Doxorubicin	Intercalation; DNA strand breaks	Mucositis; cardiac toxicity
Plant products		
Vincristine	Mitotic inhibitor; blocks microtubule polymerization	SIADH; neurotoxicity—footdrop, constipation
Etoposide	DNA strand break	Mucositis; infusion reactions; secondary leukemias
Asparaginase	Asparagine depletion	Coagulopathy; pancreatitis; anaphylaxis
Corticosteroids	Receptor-mediated lympholysis	Increased appetite; hypertension; hyperglycemia; myopathy; avascular necrosis; cataracts

Chemotherapy: Brief listing of commonly used chemotherapeutic agents and their toxicities. To a greater or lesser extent the following common toxicities are seen with most chemotherapy: nausea, alopecia, myelosuppression, and immunosuppression. Additionally infertility and second malignancies are a concern following chemotherapy.
Adapted from Pizzo PA, Poplack DG, eds. *Principles and Practice of Pediatric Oncology*, 5th ed. Philadelphia: Lippincott Williams & Wilkins, 2006.

lymphadenopathy at diagnosis. Extramedullary involvement is also seen in the CNS, skin, and testicles. CNS infiltration causes neurologic signs and symptoms, such as headache, emesis, papilledema, and sixth cranial nerve palsy. Patients with AML may develop a soft-tissue tumor called a **chloroma** in the spinal cord or on the skin. Table 17-3 compares the presentations of ALL and AML.

DIFFERENTIAL DIAGNOSIS

The differential diagnosis includes aplastic anemia, idiopathic thrombocytopenic purpura, viral infection (Epstein-Barr virus, parvovirus), metastatic disease secondary to another malignancy, bone marrow suppression secondary to a drug reaction, rheumatologic diseases such as lupus or juvenile rheumatoid arthritis, and viral-induced or familial hemophagocytic syndrome.

DIAGNOSTIC EVALUATION

A complete blood count (CBC) with manual differential and review of the blood smear to look for blast cells should be obtained in any child with suspected leukemia. The peripheral blood can be sent for flow cytometry to determine the type of leukemia. Bone marrow biopsy and aspirate remain the gold standard for diagnosis, even if peripheral blood has been used to type the leukemia. Biopsy and aspirate material are sent for morphology, immunophenotype, and cytogenetics which are critical elements used to risk stratify the leukemia into a treatment group. A comprehensive metabolic panel, LDH, uric acid, calcium,

■ **TABLE 17-2** Epidemiology of Acute Lymphocytic Leukemia and Acute Myelogenous Leukemia

Characteristic	ALL	AML
Incidence	2,500 to 3,000 cases/yr (75%)	350 to 500 cases/yr (15% to 20%)
Peak age	4 yr	Increased in adolescence
Race	White > African American	Equal (APML more common in Hispanic population)
Gender	Male > Female	Equal
Genetics	Trisomy 21, Bloom syndrome, Fanconi anemia, ataxia telangiectasia, Shwachman syndrome, neurofibromatosis, twins, siblings at increased risk	Trisomy 21 (AML much more likely <3 yr), Bloom syndrome, Fanconi anemia, ataxia telangiectasia, Kostmann syndrome, NF-1, Diamond-Blackfan syndrome, Li-Fraumeni syndrome
Noninherited		Aplastic anemia, myelodysplastic syndromes (MDS), PNH
Pathogenesis		
• Environment	Ionizing radiation	Ionizing radiation, benzene, epipodophyllotoxins, alkylating agents (nitrogen mustard, melphalan, cyclophosphamide)
• Viral	Epstein-Barr virus and L3 ALL	None
• Immunodeficiency	Wiskott-Aldrich, congenital hypogammaglobulinemia, ataxia telangiectasia	

APML, acute promyelocytic leukemia; MDS, myelodysplastic syndrome; PNH, paroxysmal nocturnal hemoglobinuria.
From Frank G, Shah SS, Catallozzi M, et al., eds. *The Philadelphia Guide: Inpatient Pediatrics.* Malden, MA: Blackwell; 2005:303.

magnesium, and phosphorus are obtained to define baseline values prior to chemotherapy and possible tumor lysis syndrome. Coagulation studies are sent to exclude disseminated intravascular coagulation (DIC). Blood, urine, and viral cultures are obtained if infection is suspected. A chest radiograph is sent to evaluate for mediastinal mass. If mediastinal mass is suspected, an echocardiogram is needed to look for possible cardiac dysfunction or cardiac effusion. A chest CT is frequently obtained to evaluate airway compression. No sedation should be used in the patient with mediastinal mass until these studies are performed and an anesthesia consultation is acquired. A lumbar puncture (LP) is performed to evaluate for central nervous system (CNS) disease. If the patient has thrombocytopenia or coagulation abnormalities, these must be corrected prior to the LP.

TREATMENT

The treatment strategy for both ALL and AML is to stabilize the patient at diagnosis, put the leukemia in remission, and manage the complications of therapy.

Managing leukemic complications at presentation involves blood product transfusions, empirical treatment of potential infection with IV antibiotics, prevention of the sequelae of hyperviscosity, and correcting metabolic abnormalities and renal insufficiency from tumor lysis syndrome. Neutropenia, defined as an absolute neutrophil count less than 500 per mm^3, predisposes children to serious bacterial and fungal infections. The development of fever in a child with neutropenia warrants careful evaluation for bacteremia or sepsis and empiric, broad-spectrum IV antibiotic therapy.

Acute Lymphocytic Leukemia Therapy

Patients with ALL have a high risk of **tumor lysis syndrome**, a triad of metabolic abnormalities (hyperuricemia, hyperphosphatemia, and hyperkalemia) resulting from spontaneous or treatment-induced tumor cell death, with rapid release of intracellular contents into the circulation that exceeds the excretory capacity of the kidneys. Tumor lysis syndrome is generally seen in tumors with high growth rates such

TABLE 17-3 Comparison of the Clinical Presentation of Acute Lymphocytic Leukemia and Acute Myelogenous Leukemia

Characteristic	ALL	AML
Marrow failure		
• Anemia (g/dL)	Hb <7 (43%)	Hb <9 (50%)
• Thrombocytopenia (per mm^3)	Hb 7 to 11 (45%)	Plt <100,000 (75%)
	Hb >11 (12%)	WBC >100,000 (20%)
• Neutropenia (per mm^3)	Plt <20,000 (20%)	
	Plt 21,000 to 99,000 (47%)	
	Plt >100,000 (25%)	
	WBC <10,000 (53%)	
	WBC 10,000 to 49,000 (30%)	
	WBC >50,000 (17%)	
Fever	60%	30% to 40%
Mediastinal mass	10% (mostly in T-cell)	
CNS involvement	5%	2%
Chloromas		Common in M4, M5 subtype
		Common in periorbital area
Testicular involvement	2% to 5%	Rare
Disseminated intravascular coagulation		Common (esp. in APML)
Bone pain	20%	20%
Hepatosplenomegaly	60% to 65%	50%
Other		Leukemia cutis (10%)
		• Neonates
		• Blueberry muffin spots
		Gingival hypertrophy (15%)

APML, acute promyelocytic leukemia.
From Frank G, Shah SS, Catallozzi M, et al., eds. *The Philadelphia Guide: Inpatient pediatrics.* Malden, MA: Blackwell; 2005:304.

as T-cell ALL or Burkitt lymphoma, and patients with mediastinal mass or high white blood cell (WBC) count, but should be anticipated in all cases of acute leukemia. Rapid release of intracellular contents leads to hyperphosphatemia, hyperkalemia, and hyperuricemia. Hyperkalemia can cause cardiac arrhythmias. Initial IV fluids should never contain potassium. Phosphate, especially at high serum levels, binds to calcium, resulting in precipitation of calcium phosphate in renal tubules, hypocalcemia, and tetany. Purines are processed to uric acid. Hyperuricemia can result in precipitation of uric acid in renal tubules and renal failure. Prevention and management of tumor lysis syndrome includes vigorous hydration, urine alkalinization, uric acid reduction with allopurinol, and potassium and phosphate reduction. The risk for tumor lysis is greatest during the first 3 days of chemotherapy.

Hyperleukocytosis (WBC count >200,000 per mm^3) occurs in 9% to 13% of patients with ALL. Hyperleukocytosis can cause significant vascular stasis. This is often seen in the patient with ALL whose WBC count is greater than 300,000 per mm^3. Symptoms include mental status changes, headache, blurry vision, dizziness, seizure, and dyspnea. Without therapy, hyperleukocytosis may cause hypoxemia and secondary acidosis or stroke from sludging in the lungs and CNS, respectively. The WBC count may be lowered using hyperhydration or leukophoresis. It is recommended that the hemoglobin concentration be kept ≤10 g/dL to minimize viscosity, and that the platelet count be maintained at >20,000/mm³ to minimize the risk of hemorrhage.

Large collections of malignant cells in the mediastinum (mediastinal mass), common in T-cell leukemia, can compress vital structures and cause tracheal compression or superior vena cava syndrome. Superior vena cava syndrome is characterized by distended neck veins; swelling of the face, neck, and upper limbs; cyanosis; and conjunctival injection. The mass and the compressive symptoms it creates usually resolve with chemotherapy and radiation. Patients with severe symptoms may warrant empiric steroid therapy and/or emergent radiation therapy.

The ALL treatment regimen includes induction, consolidation, interim maintenance, delayed intensification, and maintenance therapies. At diagnosis children with ALL undergo **induction therapy**, during which maximum log kill is achieved. If remission is achieved, leukemic blasts in the bone marrow decrease to less than 5% of marrow cells, and the CBC values return to normal. Induction therapy occurs over 28 days with vincristine, steroids, intrathecal methotrexate, and asparaginase. For high-risk patients, daunomycin is added. The disease response is generally re-evaluated every 7 to 14 days. Failure to achieve adequate response by the end of induction requires intensification of therapy. More than 95% of patients with ALL achieve remission after induction therapy. The goals of **consolidation** are to kill additional leukemic cells with further systemic therapy and to prevent leukemic relapse within the CNS by giving intrathecal methotrexate. **Interim maintenance**, which follows induction and consolidation, is less intense and includes vincristine, 6-mercaptopurine, and methotrexate. The delayed intensification course provides another round of intense chemotherapy to induce a deeper remission. **Maintenance therapy** completes the therapeutic course and includes intrathecal methotrexate every 3 months, monthly vincristine and steroid therapy, weekly oral methotrexate, and daily oral 6-mercaptopurine. The objectives of maintenance therapies are to continue the remission achieved in the previous phases and to provide additional cytoreduction to cure the leukemia. Patients with high-risk leukemia receive an additional interim maintenance and delayed intensification course prior to entering maintenance therapy.

Leukemia can recur during or after the completion of maintenance therapy. The earlier the relapse, the worse the prognosis (<36 months from diagnosis), although isolated extramedullary (CNS, testes) relapses have better outcomes than bone marrow relapses. Radiation is utilized for CNS and testicular disease. It is also used for CNS prophylaxis in those patients who take >14 days to enter remission. Discontinuation of chemotherapy occurs when the patient has remained in remission throughout the prescribed course of maintenance therapy. The total length of therapy is approximately 2.5 years for females and 3.5 years for males.

Factors associated with poor prognosis in patients with ALL include age greater than 10 years or less than 1 year at diagnosis, WBC count greater than 50,000 per mm³ at diagnosis, failure to respond to induction therapy, and the presence of the Philadelphia chromosome or hypoploidy in the leukemia cells. Factors associated with a particularly good prognosis include trisomy 4, 10, and 17 in the leukemia cells or a TEL-AML translocation (t[12;22]).

Acute Myeloid Leukemia Therapy

Hyperleukocytosis occurs in 5% to 22% of patients with AML. The most common symptoms for patients with AML-induced hyperleukocytosis include dyspnea and hypoxemia, from pulmonary leukostasis, and mental status change or seizure due to stroke from CNS leukostasis. Patients may require hyperhydration or leukapheresis similar to ALL. In contrast to ALL, patients with AML and hyperleukocytosis are treated at a lower WBC count because AML cells are larger and stickier than the lymphocytes found in ALL. Similar to ALL treatment, a hemoglobin concentration not greater than 10 g/dL is recommended to reduce viscosity, and a platelet count of more than 20,000 is advisable to minimize the risk of CNS hemorrhage.

AML chemotherapy is more intensive than that used for ALL. Induction therapy includes an anthracycline with cytosine arabinoside. Although 70% to 85% of patients with AML achieve remission with induction therapy, many patients relapse within a year. Myelosuppression is severe, and good supportive care is essential. Patients should remain in the hospital for close monitoring for signs of infection until they show signs of bone marrow recovery. If remission can be achieved, patients are assigned a risk group based on chromosome alterations in the leukemic cells. Patients with low-risk disease (inv 16, t[16;16], or t[8;21]) are treated with chemotherapy alone. Patients with high-risk disease (monosomy 5 or 7, or no remission) are treated with bone marrow transplantation from a related or unrelated donor. All other patients are considered intermediate-risk patients. If a matched related donor is available they go on to bone marrow transplant. If no matched related donor is found, they continue with chemotherapy.

Acute promyelocytic leukemia (APML), M3 subtype, has a higher overall survival rate (80%) than the other AML subtypes. Similarly, patients with AML and trisomy 21 also have excellent overall survival. In general, patients who present with a WBC count greater than 100,000/mm^3 at diagnosis have a worse prognosis. Patients with secondary AML/myelodysplastic syndrome have a poor response to therapy.

NON-HODGKIN LYMPHOMA

PATHOGENESIS

Non-Hodgkin lymphomas (NHLs) are a heterogeneous group of diseases characterized by neoplastic proliferation of immature lymphoid cells, which, unlike the malignant lymphoid cells of ALL, accumulate outside the bone marrow. NHLs can be divided into T- and B-cell categories. Histopathologic subtypes in childhood NHL include lymphoblastic (pre-T- or pre-B-cell), Burkitt lymphoma or large B-cell lymphoma (B-cell), and anaplastic large cell lymphoma (T or null cell). Other peripheral T-cell lymphomas are under the category of NHL but very uncommon in children. Burkitt lymphoma is interesting in that the presentation and pathogenesis in equatorial Africa is different than in developed countries. It almost uniformly presents as a rapidly expanding jaw lesion and 95% of these tumors carry EBV genomes in their cells, whereas 15% to 20% of North American tumors are associated with EBV.

EPIDEMIOLOGY

Lymphomas are the third most common malignancy in childhood and account for 10% of childhood cancers. There is a distinct geographic frequency of NHL; in equatorial Africa, NHL accounts for 50% of childhood cancer. In the United States, approximately 60% of pediatric lymphomas are NHLs; the remainder are Hodgkin lymphoma. Lymphoblastic lymphoma accounts for 50% of cases, and Burkitt and anaplastic large cell lymphomas account for approximately 35%

and 15%, respectively. NHL occurs at least three times more frequently in boys than in girls and has a peak incidence between 7 and 11 years of age.

RISK FACTORS

Children with congenital immunodeficiency (e.g., Wiskott-Aldrich syndrome, X-linked lymphoproliferative disease, severe combined immunodeficiency) and acquired immunodeficiency (e.g., AIDS, iatrogenic immunosuppression in organ and bone marrow transplant recipients) have an increased incidence of NHL. Patients with Bloom syndrome and ataxia-telangiectasia also have a higher incidence of NHL than the general pediatric population.

CLINICAL MANIFESTATIONS

T-cell lymphoblastic lymphoma is most often associated with a mediastinal mass (50% to 70%), whereas B-cell lymphoblastic lymphoma often involves bone, isolated lymph nodes, and skin. Superior vena cava syndrome may be associated with the T-cell type secondary to mediastinal mass. Burkitt lymphoma often exhibits extremely rapid growth and can be associated with tumor lysis syndrome even before chemotherapy is started. The sporadic form of Burkitt lymphoma can present as an abdominal tumor associated with nausea, emesis, or intussusception. Other Burkitt locations may include tonsils, bone marrow (20%), and the CNS. The endemic form of Burkitt lymphoma involves the jaw, orbit, and/or maxilla. Anaplastic large cell lymphoma is a slowly progressive disease with fever; weight loss is rare.

DIAGNOSTIC EVALUATION

The evaluation before therapy should include a CBC to look for leukocytosis, thrombocytopenia, and anemia. A comprehensive metabolic panel includes calcium, phosphorus, uric acid, and LDH to evaluate for tumor lysis syndrome. A chest radiograph should be performed to assess for mediastinal mass prior to sedation and biopsy of accessible affected nodes. An echocardiogram and anesthesia consultation is required prior to sedation in the patient with a mediastinal mass. A bone marrow aspiration and biopsy with flow cytometry, cell markers/immunophenotyping, and cytogenetics should be performed to isolate the type of lymphoma. An LP with cytology is performed to evaluate for CNS involvement. A CT scan of the neck, chest, abdomen, and pelvis helps to assess the extent of disease, and a gallium or Positron Emission Tomography (PET) scan is useful for diagnostic purposes and follow-up for residual disease or recurrence.

TREATMENT

Similar to ALL therapy, lymphoblastic non-Hodgkin lymphoma is generally treated with combination chemotherapy. ALL and lymphoblastic non-Hodgkin lymphoma therapy are immunophenotypically similar but with a different distribution of disease (nodal vs. marrow).

Chemotherapy is the mainstay of treatment for Burkitt lymphoma unless the tumor is localized and complete surgical resection is possible. Therapy is quite intense and given over a short period of time (4 to 6 months) using drugs including cyclophosphamide, prednisone, vincristine, methotrexate, cytarabine, doxorubicin, and etoposide. Patients with CNS involvement are known to have a poorer prognosis. Patients with tumor lysis syndrome require extremely careful management with increased fluid intake, alkalinization of the urine, frequent electrolyte observation, and allopurinol. Patients with Burkitt lymphoma are at high risk of developing kidney failure requiring dialysis from their tumor lysis syndrome.

Anaplastic large cell lymphoma is treated with combination chemotherapy. Children are most commonly treated using B-cell lymphoma protocols.

HODGKIN LYMPHOMA

PATHOGENESIS

The cause of **Hodgkin disease** (HD) is unknown, and a number of studies investigating potential etiologies have shown that age, ethnicity, socioeconomic status, and geographic distribution suggest both environmental and genetic components and a multifactorial etiology. Patients who develop HD have an increased incidence of immune dysregulation. There is increased risk in siblings, twins, and an association with EBV, although the EBV genome is not universally found in tumor tissue. Additionally, there is an increased risk of HD in patients with ataxia-telangiectasia and Wiskott-Aldrich and Bloom syndromes. Histopathologic subtypes in childhood HD include nodular sclerosing (40% to 55%),

lymphocyte predominant (10% to 15%), mixed cellularity (30%), and lymphocyte depleted (5%).

EPIDEMIOLOGY

Hodgkin disease accounts for 5% of all cases of childhood cancer prior to 15 years of age and 9% prior to 20 years of age. Epidemiologic studies have identified three distinct forms of HD: a childhood form (younger than 14 years); a young adult form (15 to 34 years of age); and an older adult form (55 to 74 years of age). Its incidence has a bimodal distribution with peaks occurring at 15 to 30 years of age and after the age of 50. It rarely occurs in children younger than 10 years. There is a 3:1 male predominance in the childhood form of HD.

CLINICAL MANIFESTATIONS

History and Physical Examination

The most common presentation is painless, rubbery, cervical lymphadenopathy in 80% of patients. Two-thirds of patients also have mediastinal lymphadenopathy, and this presentation is more common in adolescent patients. Systemic symptoms ("B" symptoms) are present in 20% to 30% of patients and include unexplained fever, drenching night sweats, and unintentional weight loss of more than 10% over the preceding 6 months. Other common presenting symptoms include anorexia, fatigue, and extreme pruritus.

DIFFERENTIAL DIAGNOSIS

The differential diagnosis for HD includes other diseases that can result in lymphadenopathy with or without systemic symptoms. Reactive or inflammatory nodes as a result of bacterial lymphadenitis, infectious mononucleosis, tuberculosis, atypical mycobacterial infection, cat-scratch disease, HIV infection, histoplasmosis, and toxoplasmosis should be considered. Other primary or metastatic malignant processes resulting in cervical adenopathy or a mediastinal mass include leukemia, NHL, head/neck rhabdomyosarcoma, and germ cell tumors.

DIAGNOSTIC EVALUATION

Evaluation for HD should include a detailed history and physical examination with attention to the signs and symptoms that require a more urgent evaluation including cough, dyspnea, orthopnea, chest pain, bleeding, bruising, jaundice, or pallor. The physical examination should include a careful evaluation of all lymph node groups including the tonsils. Lymphadenopathy in the upper anterior and posterior cervical chains tends to be more commonly associated with childhood infections, whereas nodes in the supraclavicular area are consistent with malignancy. Lymph nodes that are >1 cm, matted, and nontender are of greatest concern. Enlargement of the liver or spleen is consistent with more advanced disease.

Evaluating a child for HD necessitates imaging and should begin with a chest radiograph prior to any biopsy or procedure to determine whether or not there is clinically significant mediastinal involvement. The presence and size of a mediastinal mass and whether there is airway compromise or cardiac compression influence the way in which the biopsy is performed and the type of anesthesia required. Patients with a mediastinal mass should have pulmonary function testing and an echocardiogram before undergoing general anesthesia. Node biopsy is required to make the diagnosis, preferably excisional lymph node biopsy. The hallmark of diagnosis is the identification of Reed-Sternberg cells in tumor tissue.

Recommended basic tests include a CBC, erythrocyte sedimentation rate (ESR), soluble IL-2, C-reactive protein (CRP), chemistry panel including liver function tests (LFTs), direct antibody testing (DAT) if there is evidence of jaundice or anemia, and ferritin. Eosinophilia is seen in 15% to 30% of patients, and anemia is seen either secondary to advanced disease or hemolysis. Global immune defects are common at diagnosis of HD, and anergy is seen in 25% of patients. This immune dysregulation seen at diagnosis predisposes patients to opportunistic infections during their treatment. Imaging studies include a CT scan of the neck, chest, abdomen, and pelvis. PET is quite useful and has a role in diagnosis and in following for residual or recurrent disease. The gallium scan was previously used but has fallen out of favor with the emergence of PET scanning. Although uncommon, evidence of cytopenias should prompt bone marrow aspirate and biopsy, which is routinely performed in patients with extensive disease and "B" symptoms. Bone scan is only recommended for patients with bone pain.

TREATMENT

Treatment depends on the histologic subtype of disease, staging, and response to therapy (Table 17-4).

Most pediatric protocols involve multiagent chemotherapy given in a risk-adapted and response-based manner. Involved field radiation therapy is used for patients with bulky disease or with residual tumor after initial chemotherapy. Vincristine, prednisone, cyclophosphamide, and procarbazine were used commonly in the past, although newer chemotherapy combinations are being used in patients with low- or intermediate-risk disease, given the certain infertility for males with the use of cyclophosphamide and procarbazine together. Prognosis varies from 70% to 90% depending on the

■ TABLE 17-4 Staging for Hodgkin Lymphoma	
Stage	**Definition**
I	Involvement of single lymph node region or single extralymphatic site
II	Involvement of two or more lymph node regions on the same side of diaphragm or localized involvement of an extralymphatic site and one or more lymph node regions on the same side of the diaphragm
III	Involvement of lymph node regions on both sides of the diaphragm with involvement of the spleen or localized involvement of an extralymphatic site
IV	Disseminated involvement of one or more extralymphatic organs with or without lymph node involvement
"B" symptoms	Fever higher than 38°C for 3 consecutive days
	Drenching night sweats
	Unexplained weight loss >10% during the prior 6 months
	Those without B symptoms have stage [number] A disease.

extent of disease and response to therapy. Recurrent disease is often responsive to therapy but extremely difficult to cure. As in adults, lymphocyte predominance has the most favorable prognosis. There are many late effects secondary to therapy including secondary malignant neoplasms (breast, thyroid, sarcomas); cardiac toxicity (anthracyclines and radiation therapy [XRT]); pulmonary (bleomycin); hypothyroidism (XRT); infertility (alkylating agents as above, pelvic radiation); and musculoskeletal/growth (XRT). Current upfront therapies are now being modified to reduce the occurrence of late effects while maintaining high cure rates.

CENTRAL NERVOUS SYSTEM TUMORS

CNS tumors are the most common solid tumors in children and are second to leukemia in overall incidence of malignant diseases. In contrast to adults, in whom supratentorial brain tumors are more common, brain tumors in children are predominantly infratentorial, involving the cerebellum and brainstem. Table 17-5 denotes the location, clinical manifestations, and prognosis of CNS tumors in children. Childhood brain tumors are differentiated further from those in adults in that they are usually low-grade astrocytomas or malignant neoplasms such as medulloblastomas, whereas most CNS tumors in adults are malignant astrocytomas or metastases from non-CNS cancers.

CLINICAL MANIFESTATIONS

The presenting signs and symptoms of CNS tumors depend on the age of the child and location of the tumor (Table 17-5). Any CNS tumor may cause increased intracranial pressure (ICP) by obstructing CSF flow. Symptoms of increased ICP include early morning headaches, vomiting, and lethargy. The headache is usually present upon awakening, improves with standing, and worsens with coughing or straining. It is intermittent but recurs with increasing frequency and intensity. Obstructive hydrocephalus may produce macrocephaly if it occurs before the sutures have fused. Strabismus with diplopia can result from a sixth nerve palsy induced by ICP. Papilledema may be detected on funduscopic examination. The Cushing triad (hypertension, bradycardia, and irregular respirations) is a late finding.

Children with **infratentorial tumors** often present with deficits of balance or brainstem function (truncal ataxia, problems with coordination and gait, cranial nerve dysfunction). Because it can result from increased ICP, a sixth nerve palsy is not considered a localizing focal neurologic deficit, whereas other cranial nerve deficits, by definition, localize the lesion to the brainstem. Head tilt, as a compensation for loss of binocular vision, is noted with focal deficits of cranial nerves III, IV, or VI, which cause extraocular muscle weakness. Nystagmus is usually caused by cerebellovestibular pathway lesions, but it may also be seen with a marked visual deficit (peripheral or cortical blindness).

Children with **supratentorial tumors** commonly present either with signs of increased ICP or seizures. Although most seizures are generalized, less dramatic episodes with incomplete loss of consciousness (complex partial seizures) and transient focal events without loss of consciousness (partial seizures) are also seen. Personality changes, poor school performance, and change in hand preference suggest a cortical lesion. Endocrine abnormalities are noted with pituitary and hypothalamic tumors. Babinski reflex, hyperreflexia, spasticity, and loss of dexterity occur with either brainstem or cortical tumors.

DIFFERENTIAL DIAGNOSIS

The differential diagnosis includes arteriovenous malformation, aneurysm, brain abscess, parasitic infestation, herpes simplex encephalitis, granulomatous disease (tuberculosis, cryptococcal, sarcoid), intracranial hemorrhage, pseudotumor cerebri, primary cerebral lymphoma, vasculitis, and, rarely, metastatic tumors.

DIAGNOSTIC EVALUATION

CT and MRI are the procedures of choice for diagnosing and localizing tumors and other intracranial masses. A head CT can be performed much faster than a head MRI, and is safer in an unstable patient. A CT is useful as an initial screen and to assess for hydrocephalus, hemorrhage, or calcification. MRI is the gold standard for localization of brain tumors to assist with surgical planning. Brain MRI is especially helpful in diagnosing tumors of the posterior fossa and spinal cord. Examination of CSF cytology is essential to determine the presence of metastasis in medulloblastoma and germ cell tumors.

■ **TABLE 17-5** Location and Manifestations of Primary CNS Tumors

Tumor	Age at Onset (yr)	Manifestations*	5-Year Survival (%)	Comments
Infratentorial				
Cerebellar astrocytoma	5 to 8	Ataxia; nystagmus; head tilt; intention tremor	90	20% of all primary CNS tumors
Medulloblastoma	3 to 5	Obstructive hydrocephalus; ataxia; CSF metastasis	50	Acute onset of symptoms; 20% of all primary CNS tumors
Ependymoma	2 to 6	Obstructive hydrocephalus; rarely seeds spinal fluid	50	25% to 40% supratentorial
Brainstem glioma (intrinsic pontine glioma)	5 to 8	Progressive cranial nerve dysfunction; gait disturbance; pyramidal tract and cerebellar signs	<10	Worst prognosis of all childhood CNS tumors
Supratentorial				
Cerebral astrocytoma	5 to 10	Seizures; headache; motor weakness; personality changes	10 to 50	Survival for high-grade glioma is poor
Craniopharyngioma	7 to 12	Bitemporal hemianopsia; endocrine abnormalities; postoperative diabetes insipidus common	70 to 90	Calcification above sella turcica; postoperative diabetes insipidus common
Optic glioma	<2	Poor visual acuity; exophthalmos; nystagmus; optic atrophy; strabismus	50 to 90	Neurofibromatosis in NF-1 in 70% of patients
Germ cell tumor (pineal or pituitary)	—	Paralysis of upward gaze (Parinaud syndrome); lid retraction (Collier sign); precocious puberty; may seed spinal fluid	75	Germ cell line: may secrete BhCG or alpha-feto protein

*All CNS tumors may cause increased intracranial pressure.
CNS, central nervous system; CSF, cerebrospinal fluid; hCG, human chorionic gonadotropin.

TREATMENT

Treatment of CNS tumors is complex and is best managed by a multidisciplinary approach. Table 17-6 outlines the general principles of treatment of primary CNS tumors.

NEUROBLASTOMA

PATHOGENESIS

Neuroblastoma is a childhood embryonal malignancy of the postganglionic sympathetic nervous system. Neuroblastoma can be located in the abdomen, thoracic cavity, or head and neck. Abdominal tumors account for 70% of tumors, a third of which arise from the retroperitoneal sympathetic ganglia and two-thirds from the adrenal medulla itself. Thoracic masses, accounting for 20% of the tumors, tend to arise from paraspinal ganglia in the posterior mediastinum. Neuroblastoma of the neck occurs in 5% of cases and often involves the cervical sympathetic ganglion.

EPIDEMIOLOGY

Neuroblastoma and other sympathetic nervous system tumors account for approximately 8% of all childhood cancers under the age of 15 years. The prevalence is approximately 1 case per 7,000 live births, and there are approximately 600 new cases of neuroblastoma per year. It is also the most common solid tumor outside the CNS under the age of 15 years. The median age at diagnosis is between 17 and 22 months; more than 50% of children are diagnosed before 2 years of age, 90% are diagnosed before 5 years of age, and 97% are diagnosed by 10 years of age. There is a slight male predominance. Neuroblastoma accounts for 15% of the pediatric cancer-related deaths in the United States each year.

RISK FACTORS

The etiology is unknown in most cases, and no causal environmental factor has been isolated. No prenatal or postnatal exposure to drugs, chemicals, viruses, electromagnetic fields, or radiation has been associated strongly or consistently with an increased incidence of neuroblastoma. A family history of the disease can be found in 1% to 2% of cases. Neuroblastoma has been reported in patients with Hirschsprung disease, congenital central hypoventilation syndrome (Ondine curse), pheochromocytoma, and/or neurofibromatosis type 1, suggesting the existence of a global disorder of neural crest–derived cells.

CLINICAL MANIFESTATIONS

The clinical manifestations are extremely variable because of the widespread distribution of neural crest tissue and the length of the sympathetic chain. Additionally the biologic behavior is very diverse, from self-resolving asymptomatic disease to widely metastatic disease requiring substantial treatment.

■ **TABLE 17-6** Approach to Treatment of Childhood CNS Tumors	
Treatment	**Goals**
Surgery	Establish diagnosis
	Debulk and/or resect tumor
	Treat increased ICP (ventricular shunt, if required)
Radiation	Control residual disease
	Control tumor dissemination
	Cure
Chemotherapy	Adjuvant therapy for malignant tumors
	Minimize radiation exposure
	Delay and/or obviate need for radiation
Newer approaches	Immunotherapy to scavenge for minimal residual disease
	Antiangiogenic therapy to suppress abnormal tumor blood vessel development
	Molecularly targeted therapy to suppress abnormal growth factor pathways

CNS, central nervous system; ICP, intracranial pressure.
Adapted from Pizzo PA, Poplack DG, eds. *Principles and Practice of Pediatric Oncology*, 3rd ed. Philadelphia: Lippincott-Raven, 1997.

History and Physical Examination

Abdominal tumors are hard, smooth, nontender abdominal masses that are most often palpated in the flank and displace the kidney anterolaterally and inferiorly. Abdominal pain and systemic hypertension occur if the mass compresses the renal vasculature. Respiratory distress is the primary symptom seen in thoracic neuroblastoma tumors. Sometimes the thoracic variant is asymptomatic, and the tumor is discovered as an incidental finding on chest radiograph obtained for an unrelated reason. Neuroblastoma of the neck presents as a palpable tumor causing Horner syndrome (ipsilateral ptosis, miosis, and anhidrosis) and heterochromia of the iris on the affected side. Sometimes thoracic or abdominal tumors invade the epidural space posteriorly in a dumbbell fashion, compromising the spinal cord and resulting in back pain and symptoms of cord compression.

The signs and symptoms vary according to location of primary disease and degree of dissemination. Metastatic extension occurs in lymphatic and hematogenous patterns. Nonspecific symptoms of metastatic disease include weight loss and fever. Specific metastatic sequelae include bone marrow failure, resulting in pancytopenia; cortical bone pain, causing a limp (Hutchinson syndrome); liver infiltration, resulting in hepatomegaly (Pepper syndrome); periorbital infiltration, resulting in proptosis and periorbital ecchymoses (raccoon eyes); distant lymph node enlargement; and skin infiltration, causing palpable nontender subcutaneous bluish nodules in infants with **International Neuroblastoma Staging System** (INSS) stage IVS tumors. See Table 17-7. Paraneoplastic effects, such as watery diarrhea in patients with differentiated tumors that secrete vasoactive intestinal peptide and opsoclonus-myoclonus (chaotic eye movements, myoclonic jerking, and truncal ataxia), have been noted.

DIFFERENTIAL DIAGNOSIS

The differential diagnosis of abdominal neuroblastoma includes benign lesions such as adrenal hemorrhage, hydronephrosis, polycystic kidney disease, and splenomegaly and malignant tumors such as renal cell carcinoma, Wilms tumor, hepatoblastoma, leukemia, lymphoma, and retroperitoneal rhabdomyosarcoma and others.

DIAGNOSTIC EVALUATION

Once a mass is confirmed by CT of chest, abdomen, and pelvis, the diagnosis of neuroblastoma can be made by pathologic identification of tumor tissue, or by the unequivocal presence of tumor cells on bone marrow aspirate combined with elevated urinary catecholamines (vanillylmandelic acid and homovanillic acid). Tissue biopsy for histology, DNA ploidy, and myc myelocytomatosis viral-related oncogene, neuroblastoma derived (MYCN) analysis is helpful with prognosis. Measurement of urinary catecholamines, which are breakdown products of epinephrine and norepinephrine, is also useful for following response to therapy and for detecting recurrence. Additional imaging required for staging includes bone marrow biopsies, bone scan, metaiodobenzylguanidine (MIBG) scintigraphy, and at times PET scanning. Although not done frequently, an intravenous pyelogram can help differentiate a kidney (Wilms tumor) from neuroblastoma.

■ **TABLE 17-7** Staging for Neuroblastoma. International Neuroblastoma Staging System (INSS)	
Stage	**Definition**
I	Localized tumor with complete gross excision
II	Localized tumor with incomplete gross excision; ipsilateral lymph node sampling (LNS) negative for tumor (IIA), or ipsilateral nodes positive for tumor (IIB)
III	Tumor extends beyond the midline, with or without regional lymph node involvement, or localized unilateral tumor with contralateral regional lymph node involvement
IV	Dissemination of tumor to distant lymph nodes, bone, bone marrow, liver, and/or other organs (except as defined in stage IVS)
IVS	Age younger than 1 year with dissemination of tumor to liver, skin, or bone marrow without bone involvement and with a primary tumor that would otherwise be stage I or II

TREATMENT

Treatment often involves a multimodal approach and can involve surgery and chemotherapy and at times radiotherapy and/or biologic therapies. In general, after surgical resection of the primary tumor and any lymph nodes or selected metastases, surgical and radiologic data are gathered to stage the tumor based on the **INSS**.

Several biological variables have prognostic values and are used in addition to INSS staging for patients with neuroblastoma. These include age at diagnosis, stage as per INSS criteria, Shimada histopathology, DNA index of the tumor, and MYCN gene amplification. Depending on stage and biological features, treatment can range from observation or surgery alone to multimodal therapy with chemotherapy, stem cell transplantation, radiation, and biotherapy.

Chemotherapy varies in duration and intensity depending on the stage and biologic features, whereas postsurgical radiation is used to treat residual local disease and selected metastatic foci. Chemotherapy regimens usually include vincristine, cyclophosphamide, doxorubicin (Adriamycin), and cisplatin.

Infants younger than 1 year have the best prognosis. Stages I, II, and IVS have a good prognosis, whereas stages III and IV have a poor prognosis and may require aggressive treatment with bone marrow transplantation. Serum markers associated with a poor prognosis include elevated neuron-specific enolase, ferritin, and lactic dehydrogenase. Certain genetic features, such as N-myc oncogene amplification within the tumor cells, are associated with a poor prognosis. Respective 5-year survival rate for low-, intermediate-, and high-risk groups are as follows: low-risk disease (stages I and II): 90% to 95% event-free survival; intermediate-risk disease (stage III, MYCN single-copy): 85% to 90% event-free survival; high-risk disease (stage IV): 35% event-free survival. Stage IVS tumors represent unique biology that has spontaneous regression or only requires very minimal chemotherapy.

WILMS TUMOR

PATHOGENESIS

Wilms tumor is the most common renal tumor in children. It results from neoplastic proliferation of embryonal renal cells of the metanephros. The most often cited genetic anomalies in Wilms tumor involve chromosomal loci 11p13 (WT1) and 11p15 (WT2).

EPIDEMIOLOGY

Renal tumors account for 6% of all childhood cancers under the age of 15 years. The majority are unilateral with only 7% being bilateral. It is predominantly diagnosed in the first 5 years of life.

RISK FACTORS

Associated anomalies include sporadic aniridia, hemihypertrophy, cryptorchidism, hypospadias, and other genitourinary anomalies. Associated syndromes include Beckwith-Wiedemann (hemihypertrophy, macroglossia, omphalocele, and genitourinary abnormalities); Denys Drash; Wilms tumor, aniridia, genitourinary abnormalities, and mental retardation (WAGR) and Perlman syndrome (unusual facies, islet cell hypertrophy, macrosomia, hamartomas).

CLINICAL MANIFESTATIONS

History and Physical Examination

Most children (85%) are diagnosed after incidental detection of an asymptomatic abdominal mass by the child's parents while bathing or dressing the child or by the pediatrician during a routine physical examination. Abdominal pain or fever may develop after hemorrhage into the tumor. Other associated findings include microscopic or gross hematuria (33%) and hypertension (25%). Hypertension occurs as a result of either renin secretion by tumor cells or compression of the renal vasculature by the tumor. Additionally, varicocele can be present on physical examination if there is spermatic vein cord compression of the tumor. Von Willebrand disease is present in 8% of patients. It is important to evaluate the patient for associated anomalies and syndromes associated with Wilms tumor.

DIFFERENTIAL DIAGNOSIS

The differential diagnosis of Wilms tumor includes benign lesions such as hydronephrosis, polycystic kidney disease, and splenomegaly, as well as malignant tumors such as renal cell carcinoma, neuroblastoma, lymphoma, retroperitoneal rhabdomyosarcoma, and ovarian tumors.

DIAGNOSTIC EVALUATION

Radiologic studies include abdominal ultrasound to establish the presence of an intrarenal mass, assess the renal vasculature, and examine the contralateral kidney. An abdominal CT scan assesses the degree of local extension and involvement of the inferior vena cava. A CT scan of the abdomen is routinely performed to detect hematogenous metastases, which are present at diagnosis in 10% to 15% of patients. The most common patterns of spread include the renal capsule, extension through adjacent vessels (inferior vena cava), regional nodes, lung, and liver. The lung is the most common site of metastatic spread. Chest radiograph continues to be the radiographic standard for evaluation of pulmonary metastases, although the use of chest CT is controversial. Bone scan and MRI of the head are only indicated for clear cell sarcoma or rhabdoid tumor of the kidney. These are not Wilms tumor variants, but other types of renal tumors.

TREATMENT

Treatment involves surgical removal of the kidney if it can be safely done; otherwise a biopsy only is performed. Surgery also involves thorough abdominal exploration including the contralateral kidney to provide accurate assessment of tumor spread for staging. Chemotherapy and/or radiation are then prescribed depending on the staging and pathology of the resected kidney. Table 17-8 notes chemotherapeutic and radiation guidelines.

If tumor histology demonstrates anaplasia, clear cell sarcoma of the kidney, or rhabdoid tumor, the treatment can differ from that just described. Favorable prognostic factors include small tumor size, patient older than 2 years, favorable histology, and no lymph node metastases or capsular/vascular invasion. The 4-year overall survival of patients with stages II through IV favorable histology disease is approximately 90%.

BONE TUMORS

Primary malignant bone tumors account for 5% of childhood cancers. Two forms predominate: Ewing sarcoma and osteosarcoma.

EWING SARCOMA

Pathogenesis

Ewing sarcoma is an undifferentiated sarcoma that arises primarily in bone. The clonal nature of the

■ TABLE 17-8 Chemotherapeutic and Radiation Guidelines

Chemotherapy for favorable histology tumors	
Stage I	Tumor limited to kidney and completely excised. Dactinomycin/vincristine × 6 mo.
Stage II	Regional tumor extension, but completely resected. Dactinomycin/vincristine × 6 mo.
Stage III	Residual tumor present, but confined to the abdomen. Dactinomycin/vincristine × 6 mo. XRT as below.
Stage IV	Metastatic disease. As stage III.
Stage V	Bilateral disease. Special considerations depending on extent of disease in each kidney.
Radiation	
Stage III	XRT to tumor bed and extends across vertebral column to avoid scoliosis.
Stage III as a result of peritoneal spill	Whole abdominal XRT.
Stage IV	XRT to primary disease site (only if stage II and to lung, liver, or other metastases).

disease is revealed by the consistent translocation from chromosome 11 to chromosome 22 in affected cells. Ewing sarcoma is thought to arise from a pluripotent neural crest cell of the parasympathetic nervous system. Other tumors with the same or similar translocations occurring outside of bone are known as peripheral primitive neuroectodermal tumors, and they are also members of the Ewing family of soft-tissue tumors.

Epidemiology

Ewing sarcoma is seen primarily in adolescents and is 1.5 times more common in males than females. It is an extremely rare occurrence in African Americans. Like osteosarcoma, it is more likely to occur in adolescents than in young children.

Clinical Manifestations

Pain and localized swelling at the site of the primary tumor are the most common presenting complaints. Unlike osteosarcoma, in which the long bones are predominantly involved, flat and long bones are equally represented. The most commonly involved sites are the femur (20%), pelvis (20%), fibula (12%), and humerus and tibia (10%). Other sites include ribs, clavicle, and scapulae. In the long bones, Ewing sarcoma often begins midshaft, rather than at the ends as in osteosarcoma. Systemic manifestations are more common in children with metastases and include fever, weight loss, and fatigue.

Differential Diagnosis

The differential diagnosis for Ewing sarcoma includes osteomyelitis, eosinophilic granuloma (Langerhans cell histiocytosis), and osteosarcoma. Metastasis to the bone by neuroblastoma or rhabdomyosarcoma should be considered in younger children with a solitary bone lesion.

Diagnostic Evaluation

Radiographs characteristically reveal a lytic bone lesion with calcified periosteal elevation (onion skin) and/or a soft-tissue mass. Bone scans are needed to assess for other metastatic sites. Bone marrow biopsies are needed to evaluate bone marrow involvement. Biopsy confirms the diagnosis. Leukocytosis and an elevated ESR are often seen.

Treatment

Treatment involves both global (chemotherapy) and local control (radiation therapy or surgery). Chemotherapy is critical to both reduce the size of the primary tumor and treat metastases, even if overt metastases are not seen, because almost all patients with Ewing sarcoma have microscopic metastatic disease at the time of diagnosis. Specific agents include vincristine, doxorubicin, cyclophosphamide, etoposide, and ifosfamide. If the tumor affects an expendable bone (proximal fibula, rib, or clavicle), complete surgical excision may be warranted.

The prognosis is excellent for patients with distal extremity nonmetastatic tumors; the 5-year survival rate is greater than 66% in patients without metastatic disease. Children with metastatic disease at diagnosis have less favorable outcomes.

OSTEOGENIC SARCOMA

Pathogenesis

Osteosarcoma, also called osteogenic sarcoma, is a malignant tumor of the bone-producing mesenchymal stem cells. Osteosarcoma arises in either the medullary cavity or the periosteum. The primary tumor is usually located at the metaphyseal portion of bones that are associated with maximum growth velocity, which include the distal femur, proximal tibia, and proximal humerus.

Epidemiology

Osteosarcoma is seen mainly in adolescence, with a male-to-female ratio of 2:1. Peak incidence occurs during the maximum growth velocity period.

Clinical Manifestations

Similar to Ewing sarcoma, pain and localized swelling are the most common presenting complaints, but in contrast to Ewing sarcoma, systemic manifestations are rare. Because these tumors occur most frequently in adolescents, initial complaints may be attributed to trauma. The most common tumor sites are the long bones of the body including the distal femur (40%), proximal tibia (20%), and proximal humerus (10%). Metastases are present at diagnosis in 20% of cases, the majority of which are in the lungs. Gait disturbance and pathologic fractures also may be present.

Differential Diagnosis

The differential diagnoses for osteosarcoma are similar to Ewing sarcoma, and include Ewing sarcoma, benign bone tumors, and chronic osteomyelitis.

Diagnostic Evaluation

A lytic bone lesion with periosteal reaction is characteristic on radiograph. The periosteal inflammation has the appearance of a radial sunburst that results as the tumor breaks through the cortex and new bone spicules are produced. A CT scan of the chest is essential to detect pulmonary metastases, which appear as calcified nodules. Additionally, a bone scan is needed to assess for other metastatic bony disease. The ESR and CBC are generally normal, and the serum alkaline phosphatase level may be elevated at diagnosis.

Treatment

At diagnosis, 20% of patients have clinically detectable metastatic disease, and most of the remaining patients have microscopic metastatic disease. Management of the primary tumor is surgical, either with amputation or limb-sparing surgery. Unlike Ewing sarcoma, osteosarcoma is relatively resistant to radiation therapy. The addition of both neoadjuvant (before surgery) and adjuvant (after surgery) chemotherapy has raised the survival rate substantially; before chemotherapy, survival from osteosarcoma was 20% with amputation alone. Currently, with aggressive chemotherapy, long-term relapse-free survival is greater than 70%. Specific chemotherapeutic agents include cisplatin, doxorubicin, and methotrexate. Aggressive treatment of metastatic disease is indicated because some patients can be cured with high-dose chemotherapy and surgical resection of all metastases.

RETINOBLASTOMA

Pathogenesis

Retinoblastoma (Color Plate 26) is the most common intraocular malignancy in children and is considered a malignant tumor of the embryonic neural retina. The majority of retinoblastoma is sporadic (60%), but the remaining hereditary forms are transmitted as an autosomal trait with high but incomplete penetrance. The genetic mutation associated with retinoblastoma is located at chromosome 13q14 at the RB1 locus.

Epidemiology

Retinoblastoma accounts for approximately 3% of childhood cancers. It occurs in 1 in 18,000 live births in the United States with approximately 300 new cases per year. Two-thirds of cases occur before the age of 2 years, and 95% before the age of 5 years. Virtually all bilateral disease (both eyes involved with retinoblastoma) is hereditary and accounts for 25% of cases and presents in the first 2 years of life. Sixty percent of cases are nonhereditary and unilateral (one eye) and the remaining 15% are hereditary and unilateral.

Differential Diagnosis

The differential is rather limited and includes congenital cataract, medulloepithelioma, *Toxocara canis*

endophthalmitis, persistent hyperplastic primary vitreous, and Coats disease. It is important that an ophthalmologist with experience in retinoblastoma is involved in the care.

Diagnostic Evaluation

Retinoblastoma is one tumor where routine well-child checks and physical examinations can help detect a cancer and possibly detect it early. The presence of leukocoria (absence of a red reflex) is a finding often seen with retinoblastoma, and its presence can serve as a red flag for further workup. Additionally, a parent or guardian may be the first to notice an abnormality in the child's eye (in photographs) and/or vision; such reports should not go unheeded.

The most important aspect of evaluation is the ophthalmologic examination, which should be performed by an experienced ophthalmologist. Both eyes need careful evaluation to determine the extent of the tumor and depending on these findings, further workup is needed. It may include an MRI of the orbits and head to grossly assess involvement of the optic nerve and determine if there is involvement of the pineal or parasellar sites (if involved it is called trilateral retinoblastoma). At times, a bone scan and/or bone marrow biopsies are obtained if there is a high suspicion of systemic retinoblastoma involvement (high-risk features such as optic nerve involvement, choroidal invasion or extraorbital spread, etc.).

Treatment

Treatment for retinoblastoma varies and can include enucleation, chemotherapy, local therapies (laser, cryotherapy), radioplaques, and external beam radiation. Chemotherapy can be used to help shrink the tumors so that local therapies can be more effective. Treatment is dependent on the extent of disease as graded by the Reese-Ellsworth classification. At times, upfront enucleation of the involved eye (if unilateral) is needed if the local therapies (laser or cryotherapy), with or without systemic chemotherapy, are unlikely to cure the eye. Enucleation is also performed in the setting of bilateral disease if one eye is more involved than the other and cannot be salvaged to preserve vision. Subsequent therapy is then based on the pathology of the enucleated eye and whether the remaining eye is involved. It is important that a team approach involving the ophthalmologist, oncologist, and radiation oncologist is used.

Of note, a child born to a parent with bilateral retinoblastoma or to a parent with unilateral retinoblastoma with a known genetic mutation should be screened by an ophthalmologist for retinoblastoma at birth and at regular intervals until the child is 4 to 5 years old.

SOFT TISSUE SARCOMAS

PATHOGENESIS

Soft tissue sarcomas (STS) are a very diverse group of tumors. As there are different tumors that develop in different age groups, there are different types of soft tissue sarcomas that tend to develop depending on the age. In general, STS are divided into either rhabdomyosarcomas (slightly less than half) or nonrhabdomyosarcoma sarcomas. Rhabdomyosarcomas have been associated with certain familial syndromes, including neurofibromatosis and Li-Fraumeni syndrome. Nonrhabdomyosarcoma sarcomas are very heterogeneous and their pathogenesis and presentation are dependent on the histology. For example, malignant peripheral nerve sheath tumors are associated with neurofibromatosis type I, while some tumors such as malignant fibrous histiocytoma or leiomyosarcoma are seen in fields of radiation for a prior tumor.

EPIDEMIOLOGY

STS make up 7% to 8% of tumors in children and adolescents, which represent approximately 850 to 900 cases diagnosed each year in the United States. The most common STS in children under the age of 10 years is rhabdomyosarcoma, while in those over the age of 10 years it is fibrosarcoma and other tumor types. Rhabdomyosarcoma has two major subtypes, embryonal (53%) and alveolar (21%). The nonrhabdomyosarcomas encompass a number of different histologies such as fibrosarcoma, malignant fibrous histiocytoma, synovial sarcoma, and malignant peripheral nerve sheath tumor.

Of note, many of the STS have associated chromosomal abnormalities. Rhabdomyosarcoma has been associated with the t(2;13) and t(1;13) translocations. Synovial sarcoma is associated with t(X;18) translocation.

DIFFERENTIAL DIAGNOSIS

The differential diagnosis is quite variable depending on the site of the primary tumor; therefore, STS may present as a variety of benign and malignant conditions depending on the site. Approximately 35% of rhabdomyosarcoma occurs in the head and neck, 22% in genitourinary sites, and almost 20% in the extremities. The most common sites for nonrhabdomyosarcoma sarcomas are the extremities, trunk/abdomen, and the head and neck.

DIAGNOSTIC EVALUATION

Radiologic evaluation includes appropriate imaging of the primary site of the tumor and may include a CT or MRI scan of the site to assess the extent of disease and involvement of nearby structures. Additional imaging for metastatic disease includes CT of the chest and a bone scan. Further workup involving bone marrow biopsies is dependent on the STS diagnosis and is required for rhabdomyosarcoma. For rhabdomyosarcoma, 25% of newly diagnosed cases have distant metastases with lung being the most frequent site. Other sites include regional lymph nodes, bone, and bone marrow.

TREATMENT

Treatment is quite variable depending on the diagnosis and the staging of the tumor. For rhabdomyosarcoma, treatment can utilize all three treatment modalities, surgery, radiation, and chemotherapy. Complete surgical removal, if possible, is key with radiation for residual bulk disease or microscopic tumor. Chemotherapy is used in virtually all cases to help with the reduction of tumor size and eradication of metastasis. The duration and aggressiveness of the chemotherapy are dependent on multiple factors including surgical resection, histology, age at presentation, site of disease, and the presence of metastases.

For nonrhabdomyosarcomas, treatment is dependent on the histology, size of tumor, natural history of the tumor, and the presence of metastatic disease. Again, surgery, radiation, and chemotherapy all play important parts in the treatment.

KEY POINTS

- The leukemias account for the greatest percentage of cases of childhood malignancies. Leukemias are classified on the basis of leukemia cell morphology into lymphoblastic leukemias or nonlymphoblastic (myeloblastic) leukemias. ALL is the most common pediatric neoplasm and accounts for about 85% of all childhood acute leukemias.

- NHLs are a heterogeneous group of diseases characterized by neoplastic proliferation of immature lymphoid cells, which, unlike the malignant lymphoid cells of ALL, accumulate outside the bone marrow.

- Hodgkin lymphoma accounts for 40% of the lymphoma cases in the pediatric population.

- The overall prognosis for HD is better than NHL. Late effects of treatment are very common.

- CNS tumors are the most common solid tumors in children and second to leukemia in overall incidence of malignant diseases.

- In contrast to brain tumors in adults, in whom supratentorial tumors are more common, brain tumors in children are predominantly infratentorial (posterior fossa), involving the cerebellum, midbrain, and brainstem.

- Neuroblastoma may occur in the abdomen, thoracic cavity, or head and neck; 70% of children present with abdominal tumors.

- Neuroblastoma has a variable presentation and biological behavior, ranging from spontaneous regression to aggressive dissemination requiring bone marrow transplantion.

- Staging for Wilms tumor is done after exploratory laparotomy, and the therapy involves surgery, chemotherapy, and sometimes radiation.

- Ewing sarcoma is an undifferentiated sarcoma that arises primarily in bone and affects young children and adolescents. Pain and localized swelling are the most common presenting complaints of Ewing sarcoma, and the most common sites for Ewing sarcoma are the femur and the bones of the pelvis.

- Osteogenic sarcoma is a malignant tumor of the bone-producing cells of the mesenchyma, and arises most often during maximum growth velocity in the distal femur, proximal tibia, or proximal humerus.

- Similar to Ewing sarcoma, pain and localized swelling are the most common presenting complaints in osteogenic sarcoma, but in contrast to Ewing sarcoma, systemic manifestations are rare.

- Treatment of Ewing sarcoma and osteosarcoma may involve chemotherapy and surgery.

- Well-child checks are important to screen for leukocoria to assess for retinoblastoma.

- The most common soft tissue sarcoma is rhabdomyosarcoma, and the most common site of rhabdomyosarcoma is the head and neck.

18 Ophthalmology

Constance West • Katie S. Fine • Bradley S. Marino

VISION SCREENING

Vision screening in children is critical because the young eye is part of a dynamic system that may be quickly damaged by visual deprivation. The development of normal vision requires the production of *clear retinal images* and *proper eye alignment*. Table 18-1 lists the American Academy of Ophthalmology's recommendations for vision screening and referral. Children older than 8 years can be screened according to adult guidelines. Patients with a history of prematurity, intrauterine infection, CNS disease, or family history of ocular disease are at higher risk for eye pathology and require more extensive follow-up by a pediatric ophthalmologist.

STRABISMUS

Strabismus, or misalignment of the eyes, occurs in approximately 4% of children. When strabismus occurs in a child younger than 4 to 6 years, the child's brain may begin to "suppress" the image from the deviating eye, resulting in amblyopia. Amblyopia is found in the majority of patients with esotropia, and sometimes with exotropia or vertical deviations. Certain neurologic diseases are associated with an especially high incidence of strabismus, including cerebral palsy, Down syndrome, hydrocephalus, and brain tumors. Unilateral visual deprivation (e.g., ptosis) may also be associated with or lead to strabismus.

CLINICAL MANIFESTATIONS

The deviating eye of a patient with strabismus may turn inward (esotropia), outward (exotropia), upward,

or downward. Diagnosis is made using the corneal light reflex and cover tests. (Note: With one eye covered, the patient fixes vision on an object. When the obscured eye is quickly uncovered, no eye movement should be detectable. The test is repeated on the other side. If eye drift is noted when either eye is uncovered, this is considered a positive cover test.)

TREATMENT

The most important consequences of untreated strabismus, aside from the cosmetic deformity, are **amblyopia** (discussed later in the chapter) and reduced stereopsis (depth perception). Treatment is aimed at eliminating or preventing amblyopia, realigning the eyes, and addressing any underlying/predisposing condition (if present). Some causes of strabismus respond to corrective lenses, occlusion, and/or atropine penalization, but usually surgery is needed as well. **Early medical and surgical intervention results in an improved chance for establishing normal acuity and alignment.**

AMBLYOPIA

Amblyopia, literally meaning "dull sight," describes the development of reduced vision in an otherwise normal eye. The condition occurs in 2% to 5% of the general population. Children are most susceptible between birth and 7 years of age. The earlier amblyopia develops, the more severe the visual defect. Strabismic amblyopia (about one-third of cases) is caused by suppression of retinal images from a misaligned eye. Anisometropic amblyopia (unequal refractive errors in the two eyes) causes a blurred retinal

TABLE 18-1 Pediatric Vision Screening Recommendations of the American Academy of Ophthalmology		
Age	**Examination**	**Referral**
Newborn	Corneal light reflex test	Abnormal red reflexes
	Red reflexes	Any other ocular abnormality
By age 6 mo	Fixation to light or small toys	Aversion to occlusion
	Monocular occlusion	Strabismus
	Corneal light reflex test	Nystagmus
	Cover/uncover test	Abnormal red reflexes
	Red reflexes	Any other ocular abnormality
Age 3 to 4 yr	Visual acuity	Visual acuity less than 20/40 in either eye and/or no more than one-line difference between the two eyes on vision testing
	Corneal light reflex test	
	Fundus examination	Strabismus
		Any other ocular abnormality
Age 5 or older	Visual acuity	Visual acuity of 20/40 or less in one or both eyes
	Corneal light reflex test	Strabismus
	Cover/uncover test	Any other ocular abnormality
	Fundus examination	

From Communication of the American Academy of Ophthalmology, San Francisco, 2001.

image in one eye and is responsible for amblyopia about a third of the time. The remaining cases are mixed mechanism, and associated with both strabismus and anisometropia. Visual deprivation amblyopia due to opacities of the visual axis (e.g., corneal opacity, cataracts) is the least common cause of amblyopia. Other risk factors include premature birth and a family history of amblyopia or strabismus.

CLINICAL MANIFESTATIONS

Subnormal vision is the only sign of amblyopia. Untreated amblyopia leads to permanent vision loss and diminished stereopsis.

TREATMENT

The first step in treating amblyopia involves correcting any refractive errors with glasses. Visual opacities such as cataracts, if present, should be removed. Proper alignment must be restored. Finally, **occlusion** of the better-seeing eye forces visual development of the affected eye and the visual centers in the brain corresponding with that eye. Early intervention is crucial to promote normal vision; **beyond 8 years of age, treatment is usually unlikely to be successful.**

LEUKOCORIA

Leukocoria (white pupil or absence of the red reflex) in an infant or child may be caused by a number of entities, ranging from isolated ocular abnormalities to life-threatening systemic disease. All cases of leukocoria require prompt ophthalmologic referral.

DIFFERENTIAL DIAGNOSIS

Retinoblastoma, the most common intraocular malignancy of childhood, is a life-threatening cause of leukocoria. The disease occurs in approximately 1 in 20,000 live births, resulting in 300 new cases in the United States each year. The associated genetic defect is found on the q14 band of chromosome 13. Untreated retinoblastoma leads to death from brain and visceral metastasis in almost all cases.

Cataracts (opacities of the crystalline lens) occur in 1 of every 250 newborns, thus making cataracts the most common cause of leukocoria. They may be congenital or acquired and may be unilateral or bilateral. Cataracts are often genetically determined but may result from metabolic diseases or intrauterine infections.

Retinopathy of prematurity (ROP) is a retinal vascular disease of premature infants that can also lead to leukocoria. Risk factors include birth weight less than 1,250 g, gestational age less than 32 weeks, mechanical ventilation, and need for supplemental oxygen.

Other causes of leukocoria include congenital glaucoma and ocular toxocariasis (a parasitic infection most frequently acquired in infancy or young childhood).

CLINICAL MANIFESTATIONS

Leukocoria is detectable by routine screening of the **red reflex** in all neonates. Infants at high risk for retinoblastoma (positive family history in a first- or second-degree relative) or the development of ROP should be examined by an experienced ophthalmologist.

TREATMENT

Successful therapy combines treatment of the underlying condition with attention to associated amblyopia. Treatment of retinoblastoma may include **enucleation** (removal of the eye), chemotherapy, radiation therapy, and/or cryotherapy. Small or localized tumors may not require enucleation. Prognosis is directly related to the size of the tumor at diagnosis, and cure rates approach 90%. If retinoblastoma is not bilateral at presentation, the patient should be closely followed because 20% will develop another tumor in the previously unaffected eye.

Unilateral or bilateral congenital cataracts may be surgically removed. The visual prognosis for children requiring cataract extraction is not as good as that seen in adults because amblyopia or associated ocular abnormalities may limit the ultimate level of visual acuity. Congenital cataracts that are not removed by 2 to 3 months of age result in significant, usually irreversible, amblyopia.

Most cases of ROP regress spontaneously; however, laser ablation of the retina or cryotherapy performed at an intermediate stage of ROP reduces progression to retinal detachment and scarring. Infants with treated or regressed ROP remain at risk for the development of amblyopia, strabismus, myopia, and visual impairment. Some premature infants with periventricular leukomalacia develop central visual loss and may have difficulty with special orientation and other complex visual tasks.

NASOLACRIMAL DUCT OBSTRUCTION

Congenital nasolacrimal duct obstruction (dacryostenosis), a common cause of overflow tearing, occurs in about a quarter of neonates. Obstruction is usually caused by failure of the distal membranous end of the nasolacrimal duct to open.

CLINICAL MANIFESTATIONS

Chronic tearing in the absence of conjunctival injection is the hallmark of nasolacrimal duct obstruction. The presence of mucopurulent discharge and tenderness over the medial aspect of the lower lid suggests superimposed infection of the nasolacrimal sac (dacryocystitis). Less common causes of excess tearing in infancy include chronic irritation from allergens and infantile glaucoma.

Congenital nasolacrimal duct obstruction causes tearing with some mattering on the lashes, while infantile glaucoma is associated with corneal clouding, photophobia, and limbal conjunctival injection. Buphthalmos (increased corneal diameter accompanying infantile glaucoma) is a later finding in infantile glaucoma; evaluation by an ophthalmologist is warranted if there is any concern about infantile glaucoma.

TREATMENT

Treatment varies according to the severity of symptoms. The obstruction resolves spontaneously by 1 year of age in 96% of infants. Referral to an ophthalmologist is indicated if symptoms persist. **Probing** of the nasolacrimal duct system is performed at 12 to 15 months of age unless severe symptoms warrant earlier intervention. Superimposed dacryocystitis should be treated with warm compresses, nasolacrimal massage, and systemic antibiotics (i.e., a first-generation cephalosporin) in select cases.

OPHTHALMIA NEONATORUM

Ophthalmia neonatorum refers to conjunctivitis occurring within the first month of life. Any ocular discharge in the neonate requires evaluation because tears are usually absent in the first few weeks of life.

DIFFERENTIAL DIAGNOSIS

Common causes of ophthalmia neonatorum include chemical irritation, *Chlamydia trachomatis*, and *Neisseria gonorrhoeae*. Chemical conjunctivitis can be caused by birth trauma or by antibiotic prophylaxis given at birth to prevent gonococcal infection. Less common infectious causes, including herpes simplex virus (HSV), *Staphylococcus aureus*, *Haemophilus influenzae*, and *Pseudomonas aeruginosa*, typically manifest after the first week of life. Nasolacrimal duct obstruction should be considered in older neonates with persistent conjunctival discharge.

CLINICAL MANIFESTATIONS

Infants usually present with eyelid edema, conjunctival hyperemia, and ocular discharge. Age at onset and clinical features may suggest the diagnosis, but appropriate laboratory evaluation is required (Table 18-2).

TREATMENT AND PREVENTION

Infants with suspected gonococcal, HSV, or *P. aeruginosa* conjunctivitis should be referred to an ophthalmologist. Infants with conjunctivitis related to other causes require referral if signs worsen or symptoms persist after 3 days of treatment. Parents and their sexual partners should be treated for *Chlamydia* and gonococcal infections in the usual manner.

The incidence of neonatal conjunctivitis has decreased dramatically since the introduction of ocular prophylaxis with silver nitrate. **Erythromycin**, effective against both *C. trachomatis* and *N. gonorrhoeae*, currently is preferred.

INFECTIOUS CONJUNCTIVITIS

After the newborn period, infectious conjunctivitis (**pink eye**) is very common in childhood and may be bacterial or viral in origin. The infection causes inflammation in the conjunctiva, which overlies the sclera. Adenovirus in particular is a frequent cause of viral conjunctivitis.

■ TABLE 18-2 Distinguishing Features of Ophthalmia Neonatorum

Features	Chemical	*N. gonorrhoeae*	*C. trachomatis*
Age at onset	24 hours	2 to 4 days	4 to 10 days
Clinical features	Bilateral	Bilateral	Unilateral or bilateral
	Serous discharge	Purulent discharge	Mucopurulent discharge
	Conjunctival hyperemia	Marked eyelid edema	Conjunctival hyperemia
		Chemosis	
Complications	Self-limited	Sepsis	Corneal scarring
		Meningitis	Pneumonia
		Arthritis	
		Corneal ulceration	
		Blindness	
Diagnosis	Exclude serious causes	Conjunctival culture on chocolate or Thayer-Martin agar	Conjunctival *Chlamydia* culture
			Direct immunofluorescent antibody test
Treatment	None	Topical erythromycin; intravenous cefotaxime; treat parents	Oral plus topical erythromycin; treat parents

DIFFERENTIAL DIAGNOSIS

Inflammation of the conjunctiva may be precipitated by exposure to allergens, toxins, chemicals, or irritants. Some systemic diseases may also have "red eyes" as part of the presentation.

Corneal abrasions may present with a red, painful, tearing eye that is sensitive to light. Examination of the eye with a blue-filtered light following instillation of **fluorescein** reveals the denuded area. Corneal abrasions are treated with eye patching (to decrease pain and promote healing) and topical antibiotics. Most heal within 24 hours.

CLINICAL MANIFESTATIONS

Table 18-3 compares and contrasts the clinical manifestations of viral, bacterial, and allergic conjunctivitis.

TREATMENT

In practice, most cases of infectious conjunctivitis are treated with a trial of antibiotic drops or ointment for 5 to 7 days. Choices include polymyxin-bacitracin, trimethoprim-polymyxin B, sodium sulfacetamide, gentamicin, or ofloxacin. Refractory cases require culture results to guide therapy. Although both viral and most bacterial conjunctivitis are usually self-limited diseases, antibiotics limit infectivity and decrease disease duration by approximately 2 days. (Notable exceptions include *Neisseria gonorrhoeae* conjunctivitis, which must be treated with parenteral ceftriaxone, and *Haemophilus influenzae* conjunctivitis that occurs in conjunction with same-sided otitis media, which must be treated with appropriate oral agents.)

Antibiotic drops that contain steroids (to decrease inflammation) must **not** be given if HSV-1 is thought to be the cause of the infection because there is an increased risk of more severe disease and visual impairment.

HORDEOLUM AND CHALAZION (STYES)

A **hordeolum** is an acute infection of the meibomian glands (internal hordeoolum), or the sebaceous glands surrounding the eyelash follicle (external hordeolum). *Staphylococcus aureus* is the usual culprit. Localized tender swelling progresses to a point, which ruptures to the outside. Treatment involves warm compresses; the value of ophthalmic antibiotics is questionable. Occasionally, incision and drainage or systemic antibiotics may be indicated if an acute cellulitis develops.

Chalazions are areas of sterile lipogranulomatous reaction within the meibomian glands in the tarsal plate that may progressively enlarge. The affected area is typically firm but nontender. Excision may be required for cosmetic purposes or if the area becomes irritated and produces a mass effect. The condition may be chronic and recurrent; good lid hygiene can reduce the risk of recurrence.

PERIORBITAL CELLULITIS

Periorbital (preseptal) cellulitis is caused by bacterial infection of the eyelids and surrounding skin anterior to the orbital septum, a fibrous band that separates the subcutaneous lid from the orbit itself.

■ **TABLE 18-3** Comparison of Viral, Bacterial, and Allergic Conjunctivitis			
Symptom	**Viral**	**Bacterial**	**Allergic**
Pain	Mild	Mild to moderate	None
Discharge	Clear	Mucopurulent	Clear
	Mild to copious	Mild to copious	Mild to moderate
	Prone to crusting	Definite crusting	No crusting
Itching	Usually absent	Absent	Present
Injection	Diffuse	Diffuse	Diffuse
Vision	Normal	Normal	Normal
Possible etiologies	Adenovirus, ECHO virus, coxsackievirus	*Haemophilus influenzae, Streptococcus pneumoniae, Neisseria gonorrhoeae*	Seasonal pollen or other allergen exposure

PATHOGENESIS

Bacteria gain access to the area around the eye through breaks in the skin (*Staphylococcus aureus*, group A *streptococcus*), hematogenous dissemination (*Streptococcus pneumoniae, Haemophilus influenzae*), insect bites, or via extension from infected sinuses or other upper respiratory structures (*S. pneumoniae, H. influenzae, Moraxella catarrhalis*). Both the Hib vaccine and the pneumococcal conjugate vaccine have contributed to a measurable decline in the incidence of periorbital infections.

DIFFERENTIAL DIAGNOSIS

Orbital cellulitis, in which the infection extends posterior to the orbital septum, is an emergency. Severe pain with eye movement, proptosis, vision changes, and decreased ocular mobility accompany this disease. A CT scan should be considered to confirm the diagnosis, identify any coinfected structures (e.g., sinuses), and delineate extension. Associated orbital abscesses sometimes require surgical drainage. Empirical parenteral antibiotic therapy should provide coverage against *S. aureus, S. pyogenes, S. pneumoniae, H. influenzae, M. catarrhalis,* and anaerobic bacteria found in the upper respiratory tract. Suggested regimens include cefuroxime (with clindamycin added if anaerobic infection is suspected) or ampicillin/sulbactam. Periorbital edema and erythema that accompany orbital cellulitis may be slow to resolve. When the patient appears recovered, he or she may be released with oral antibiotics to complete a 3-week course. Brain abscesses, meningitis, and cavernous sinus thrombosis are infrequent but serious complications of orbital cellulitis.

Other causes of a swollen eyelid include trauma, edema, allergies, and tumor.

CLINICAL MANIFESTATIONS

In periorbital cellulitis, the skin around the eye is indurated, warm, and tender, although there is no true eye pain. Fever is variably present in cases of localized skin trauma. In the young child with hematogenous seeding or extension as the source, the fever is generally quite high, with rapid progression of the swelling. The physical examination may reveal sinus tenderness, sore throat, or a point of entry on the skin. It is important to mark the area of induration to assist in documenting subsequent resolution (or lack thereof). Any child with signs or symptoms consistent with meningitis (Chapter 12) should receive a lumbar puncture.

TREATMENT

Intravenous antibiotics should begin as soon as possible and continued until resolution of induration. For periorbital cellulitis that follows a break in the skin, a penicillinase-resistant penicillin or a first-generation cephalosporin is appropriate. Vancomycin may be required depending on local resistance patterns. Cefuroxime is the antibiotic of choice in other cases; occasionally, a third-generation cephalosporin is used to prevent extension to the meninges in the young child. The patient may be released with oral antibiotics to complete a 10-day course when symptoms abate.

 KEY POINTS

- Screening for strabismus by means of cover testing should be included in every pediatric health maintenance examination. Early recognition and treatment offer the best chance for avoiding permanent visual abnormalities.
- Amblyopia represents a common and potentially reversible cause of vision loss in children. Strabismus is the most common cause of amblyopia in children. Successful treatment depends on early recognition and referral for occlusion therapy and elimination of predisposing conditions.

- The most common cause of leukocoria is a congenital cataract. All cases of leukocoria require prompt ophthalmologic referral.
- All infants at high risk for retinopathy of prematurity should be seen by an ophthalmologist before discharge from the nursery.
- Retinoblastoma should be diagnosed early and treated aggressively to secure a favorable outcome.
- Nasolacrimal duct obstruction is a common cause of tearing in infants and neonates and typically resolves spontaneously. Referral is indicated if symptoms per-

KEY POINTS *(continued)*

- sist beyond 9 to 12 months of age and for infants with recurrent dacryocystitis.

- Conjunctivitis in the neonate may represent chemical irritation or acquired infection. *Chlamydia trachomatis* and *Neisseria gonorrhoeae* are the most common infectious agents.

- Conjunctivitis in the older child can be caused by infectious agents (bacteria, viruses) as well as systemic disease, irritants, and allergen exposure.

- Corneal abrasions may be diagnosed by examining the surface of an eye that has been exposed to fluorescein drops under a blue-filter light.

- Orbital cellulitis, characterized by (a combination of) eye pain, decreased mobility, vision changes, and proptosis, is a true emergency. Surgical drainage of associated abscesses may be required. Periorbital cellulitis may originate from a break in the skin, hematogenous spread, or by extension of respiratory or sinus bacteria.

Orthopedics

Eric J. Wall • *Katie S. Fine*

Pediatricians and family practitioners benefit from a basic knowledge of orthopedics, because musculoskeletal complaints comprise a significant percentage of office visits in this population. The timely diagnosis and management of congenital, developmental, traumatic, and infectious bone and joint conditions in children can minimize potential deformities and loss of function.

DEVELOPMENTAL DYSPLASIA OF THE HIP

PATHOGENESIS

Developmental hip dysplasia (DDH) refers to an abnormal relationship between the hip ball and socket, which occurs in about 1 in 1,000 births. This most commonly comes about during delivery, but can occasionally develop in utero or during childhood. If dislocation persists, the acetabulum will not develop into a cup-like shape, and the head of the femur is forced further out of the socket. Once the ball is repositioned in the socket of an infant, the socket usually regains its cup-like shape.

EPIDEMIOLOGY

DDH is much more likely in the newborn with breech presentation or a positive family history of DDH. Risk is slightly increased in females and first-born children. There is also an association with other anomalies, including clubfoot, congenital torticollis, metatarsus adductus, and infantile scoliosis.

CLINICAL MANIFESTATIONS

Early diagnosis of hip dislocation usually results in a better outcome; therefore, careful examination of the newborn is critical. Gluteal fold asymmetry may accompany hip dislocation in the newborn; however, up to 71% of normal infants have gluteal fold asymmetry, resulting in very low specificity for this sign. The **Barlow and Ortolani provocative tests** are most helpful. With the infant's hip and knee each flexed to 90 degrees, the examiner places the fingertips on the greater trochanter, with the thumb webspace over the knee and the thumb on the inner thigh. Gentle pressure is applied to the flexed and adducted hip in a posterior direction during the Barlow maneuver, and a positive result occurs when there is a palpable clunk as the hip dislocates in a posterior-superior direction. This test can be immediately followed by the Ortolani maneuver (hip abduction with a resulting clunk as the head relocates into the joint) (Fig. 19-1). DDH can evolve over time, so children should be screened at regular intervals until they are ambulatory. In examining a somewhat older infant in which the dislocation becomes relatively fixed, a **Galeazzi sign** and limited hip abduction should be sought. By holding the ankles with the knees bent and hips flexed, the examiner looks for any foreshortening of the (affected) limb. Older patients may also present with limited hip abduction, a limp, and apparent shortening of the involved extremity.

Because most of the hip and pelvis are not ossified at birth, radiographs are not helpful until 4 to 6 months of age. Ultrasound is more accurate for the detection of DDH from birth to about 4 months,

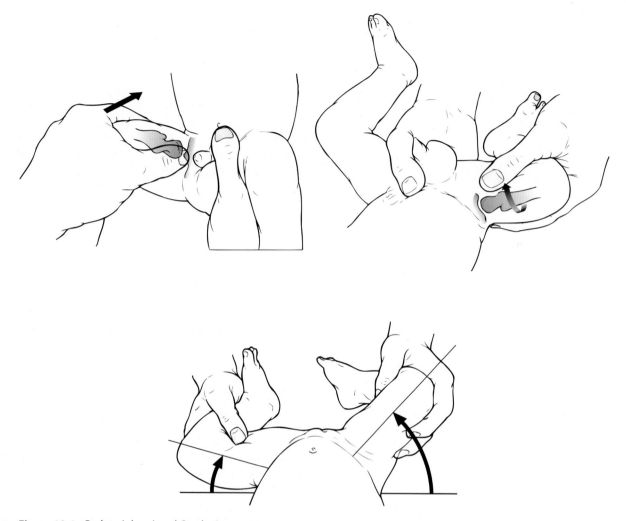

Figure 19-1 • Barlow (*above*) and Ortolani maneuvers.

but screening is best delayed until 6 weeks of age, when the rate of false positive examinations decreases. Routine ultrasound screening of all infants is not recommended but should be considered for babies with a family history of DDH and for those born in the breech position.

TREATMENT

When an abnormal clunk, limited hip abduction, or limb asymmetry is noted at the newborn examination (or thereafter), the patient should be referred for orthopedic consultation. Most dislocatable hips stabilize without intervention within the first 2 weeks of life. If treatment is indicated in children younger than 6 months, a Pavlik harness (which keeps the hip abducted and flexed) is the best initial treatment. Body

casting is used in older patients. Cases that do not respond to conservative measures require surgical reduction or hip reconstruction.

FOOT DEFORMITIES

Flexible foot deformities, such as flexible flatfoot, rarely predispose children to difficulty walking, poor shoe fit, and/or pain. Almost any deformity of the foot that can be molded by the examiner's hands to an anatomically correct position requires minimal intervention.

Metatarsus adductus (isolated in-toeing of the forefoot) is a common, relatively benign condition caused by intrauterine positioning. As opposed to clubfoot, ankle joint range of motion is unrestricted. Mild metatarsus adductus is flexible; the examiner can temporarily straighten the forefoot to the anatomically correct position. In cases of severe metatarsus adductus, the foot is inflexible. Severe cases are treated with serial bracing or casting starting at age 6 to 12 months. Surgery is rarely indicated.

Talipes equinovarus, or clubfoot, is a more rare and debilitating deformity that consists of medial rotation of the tibia, fixed plantar flexion at the ankle, inversion of the heel, and forefoot adduction (metatarsus adductus). Dorsiflexion at the ankle is restricted in patients with clubfoot. Without treatment, the foot becomes progressively more deformed, and calluses or ulcerations can develop when the child is old enough to limp. Early intervention is essential for subsequent normal function and development. Initial treatment consists of serial casting; patients with unsatisfactory improvement require surgical repair, preferably before the age of anticipated ambulation. Associated congenital malformations are relatively common.

LIMP

Limp is probably the most common musculoskeletal complaint prompting medical evaluation in children. Pain, weakness, decreased range of motion, and leg-length discrepancy all can disrupt the normal gait.

DIFFERENTIAL DIAGNOSIS

The list of conditions that can present with limp is extensive (Table 19-1). **Trauma** is the most common cause of limp at any age.

The patient's age affects the differential diagnosis. Infection, inflammation, and paralytic syndromes are common etiologies in children from 1 to 3 years of age. From 3 to 10 years of age, Legg-Calvé-Perthes disease, toxic synovitis, and juvenile idiopathic arthritis become more common. Slipped capital femoral epiphysis is a consideration in pubertal patients.

Legg-Calvé-Perthes disease is defined as avascular necrosis (ischemic compromise) of the femoral head. The etiology is unknown. Eventually (over approximately 2 to 5 years), the ischemic bone is resorbed and reossification occurs. Legg-Calvé-Perthes disease occurs more often in males and younger children (4 to 8 years of age). A painless or mildly painful limp that develops insidiously is the most common presenting complaint. The pain is often referred to the knee or thigh, clouding the diagnostic picture. Range of motion is limited upon abduction, flexion, and

■ **TABLE 19-1** Differential Diagnosis of Limp by Disease Category
Trauma or overuse
Fracture
Soft-tissue injury
Infectious
Septic arthritis
Osteomyelitis
Lyme arthritis
Discitis
Inflammatory
Transient synovitis
Rheumatic disease
Reactive arthritis
Developmental/Acquired
Developmental dysplasia of the hip
Avascular necrosis
Slipped capital femoral epiphysis
Neurologic
Muscular dystrophy
Peripheral neuropathy
Neoplasia
Bone tumors
Leukemia
Spinal cord tumors
Metabolic
Rickets
Hematologic
Sickle cell disease
Hemophilia
Other
Appendicitis
Pelvic inflammatory disease
Testicular torsion

internal rotation. Initial radiographic studies may appear normal; subsequent films demonstrate epiphyseal radiolucency (Fig. 19-2). A bone scan may be helpful to detect early impairment in the blood supply and fragmentation and flattening of the femoral head. Treatment involves containing the softened femoral head within the acetabulum, preserving its

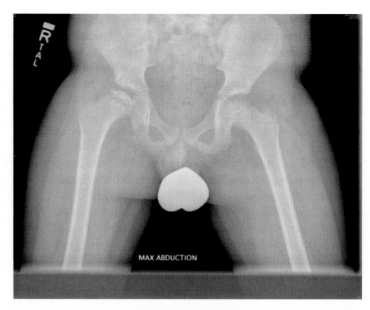

Figure 19-2 • Legg-Calvé-Perthes disease of left hip. Nine-year-old male with stiffness in right hip who presented with complaint of limp. Radiograph shows 50% collapse with sclerosis of the right femoral head as compared to his normal opposite (left) hip. (Courtesy of Cincinnati Children's Hospital Medical Center, Department of Pediatric Orthopaedics.)

spherical contour, and maintaining normal range of motion. Younger children with minimal involvement and full range of motion may be observed. Bracing, casting, or surgery is necessary in older patients with significant changes in the femoral head. The amount and area of ischemic damage affects the prognosis. Subluxation of the femoral head out of the hip socket is the most serious acute complication; long-term disability is related to healing of the femoral head in a misshapen pattern (nonspherical), and the subsequent development of arthritis in the fifth decade of life for 50% of patients.

Slipped capital femoral epiphysis (SCFE) is the gradual or acute separation of the proximal femoral growth plate, with the femur head slipping off the femoral neck and rotating into an inferior/posterior position. The cause is unknown but may be hormonal (most common during puberty) in origin or related to excessive weight bearing (more common in overweight individuals). It occurs slightly more often in males. Antecedent trauma is not a contributing factor. Although usually asymmetric at presentation, 25% of cases eventually progress to bilateral involvement. The typical patient presents with a limp and pain, which may be centered in the hip or groin but often is referred to the knee. Limited internal rotation at the hip and limb shortening are present on examination. Radiographs with the child's hips in the **frog-leg lateral position** are the study of choice for noting epiphyseal displacement (Fig. 19-3). Radiographs may show physeal plate

widening, decreased epiphyseal height and a Klein line (line drawn along the femoral neck) that does not intersect the lateral epiphysis. The primary goal of treatment is prevention of further misalignment. Pin fixation is effective in the acute setting. Chronic cases generally require osteotomy. Long-term complications include avascular necrosis and late degenerative changes similar to those seen with osteoarthritis.

CLINICAL MANIFESTATIONS

History

The history should include questions about the onset, timing, and evolution of the limp. Pain may be severe (fracture, infection), constant, associated with activity (injury), acute, or chronic. The absence of pain suggests weakness or instability. Swelling and stiffness are common in rheumatologic disease. Toxic synovitis may follow a recent viral illness. Any history of bowel or bladder incontinence suggests spinal cord compression.

Physical Examination

Watching the child walk is particularly important because certain gaits are associated with specific disorders. Each joint should be examined for range of motion, swelling, warmth, erythema, and tenderness. Fractures produce point tenderness and

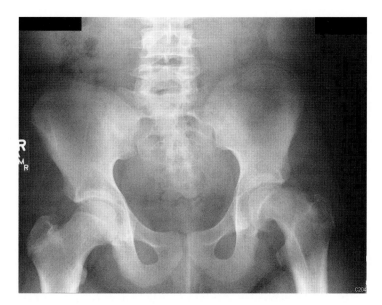

Figure 19-3 • Radiograph of a slipped capital femoral epiphysis. Fourteen-year-old adolescent male with complaint of pain and limp in right thigh. Radiograph shows about 30% medial slippage of the femoral head off the femoral neck on the left as compared to his normal right hip.
(Courtesy of Cincinnati Children's Hospital Medical Center, Department of Pediatric Orthopaedics.)

occasionally angulation. Neurologic evaluation includes deep tendon reflexes, strength, and sensation. Extremities are assessed for adequate perfusion and deformities. Muscle atrophy and fasciculation may be present in neuromuscular disease.

DIAGNOSTIC EVALUATION

All patients with significant limp should have a physical examination to localize the area of tenderness or stiffness, followed by plain radiographs of any area with positive findings. A blood test with elevation of the sedimentation rate (ESR), C-reactive protein (CRP), and/or white blood cell (WBC) count can suggest infection, inflammatory arthritis, or occasionally malignancy. A bone scan is an excellent advanced imaging study for poorly localized limp or pain, demonstrating areas of increased bone turnover consistent with infection, fracture, or bone marrow malignant invasion. Ultrasound (US), magnetic resonance imaging (MRI), and computed tomography (CT) scans are most helpful when symptoms localize to a specific bone or joint. US is useful for evaluating for the presence of joint effusion, especially when a septic joint is considered. MRI permits detailed localized evaluation of joints, bones, cartilage, and soft tissues. The presence of an abscess and/or necrotic bone detected via gadolinium-enhanced MRI may require surgical debridement and drainage. Patients with weakness should have electrolytes, calcium, serum creatinine kinase (CPK), and urine myoglobin studies performed; electromyography and nerve conduction studies may also be helpful. If the weakness is progressive and limited to the lower extremities, spinal cord compression must be ruled out with imaging studies (i.e., MRI).

OSGOOD-SCHLATTER DISEASE

Osgood-Schlatter disease involves swelling, pain, and tenderness over the tibial tuberosity. It is caused by repetitive stress to the distal insertion of the patellar tendon attachment to the proximal tibia. Osgood-Schlatter disease typically occurs between 10 and 15 years of age, during the adolescent growth spurt. Pain is worsened with kneeling, running, jumping, or squatting but is always relieved by rest. Radiographs reveal irregularities of the tubercle ossification center and soft tissue swelling. Most cases are mild and treated with activity modification and stretching exercises. Severe cases may require casting for up to 6 weeks. Long-term morbidity is quite low; the disorder almost always resolves when skeletal maturity is reached.

IDIOPATHIC SCOLIOSIS

Idiopathic scoliosis is spinal curvature detected in otherwise healthy children with normal bones, muscles, and vertebral discs. The cause is unknown, but heredity definitely plays a role. **Scoliosis**, or lateral curvature with rotation, is more common than kyphosis (roundback).

EPIDEMIOLOGY

Five percent of children display some degree of spinal deformity. Routine screening is critical for detection. Severe scoliosis requiring bracing or surgery is about eight times more common in females than males. Progression of the curve is most rapid during the adolescent growth spurt.

HISTORY AND PHYSICAL EXAMINATION

Idiopathic scoliosis is usually not associated with back pain or fatigue; such symptoms warrant further investigation. The physical examination consists of two parts. First, the child is examined from the rear while standing up. Shoulder girdle and iliac crest areas are noted for asymmetry and unequal height. Then, the Adam forward bending test is performed. The child bends forward from the waist with the arms hanging freely. The examiner should examine the patient's back for a rib cage or low back prominence on one side of the spine versus the other. This asymmetry of the back can be measured with a scoliometer, and patients with a reading of 7 degrees or more should obtain a standing scoliosis x-ray.

DIFFERENTIAL DIAGNOSIS

Occasionally, scoliosis may be caused by neuromuscular abnormalities or congenital deformities. **Kyphosis** is an abnormally large posterior rounding of the spine. Kyphosis is often related to poor posture and may be treated with physical therapy or observation. Inflexible kyphosis may be associated with wedge-shaped vertebral bodies (**Scheuermann disease**) and may require bracing or corrective surgery.

Treatment

Most scoliosis is minor and requires only observation during the growing years to make sure it does not progress into a treatable range. Bracing is usually recommended to limit progression for curves over 25 to 30 degrees in growing children; it does not reduce the curve. Curves over 45 to 50 degrees often require surgical treatment due to the risk of late progression in adulthood. Only curves over 90 to 100 degrees cause significant cardiopulmonary compromise in children or adults with idiopathic scoliosis.

ACHONDROPLASIA

Achondroplasia is a disorder of cartilage calcification and remodeling. Inheritance is autosomal dominant. The physical appearance is strikingly characteristic: these patients are very short with proportionally large heads. Long bones tend to be wide, short, and curved, and digits are short and stubby. Kyphoscoliosis and lumbar lordosis may be quite pronounced. Heterozygotes have fairly normal intelligence, sexual function, and life expectancy. Homozygotes fare less well, given their increased susceptibility to pulmonary complications and an abnormally small foramen magnum that predisposes to **brainstem compression**.

COMMON FRACTURES IN CHILDREN

Children's bones are more flexible than adults and can bend, bow, or partially break. Incomplete "buckle" and greenstick fractures are more common than displaced fractures due to this flexibility and the presence of a thicker periosteum wrapped around the bones. Because ligaments and tendons are relatively stronger in children than bones and growth plates, fractures are much more common than sprains prior to adolescence. It is usually safest to assume that any posttraumatic severe bone or joint pain is secondary to a fracture rather than a sprain, even if the radiographs are normal. The hallmark of a fracture is severe **point tenderness** over a bone. Fractures through the growth plate require particular care because they may result in crooked or shortened limbs.

DIFFERENTIAL DIAGNOSIS

Fractures can disrupt the growth plate, which is the weakest portion of the child's skeletal system. **Epiphyseal fractures** are categorized according to the Salter-Harris classification (Fig. 19-4). Bowing or bending without any visible fracture after trauma typifies a **bow fracture**. Tenderness over a growth plate is often a nondisplaced fracture. **Stress fractures** due to repetitive forces in athletes are frequently invisible on initial films. **Pathologic fractures** result when underlying disease weakens the bone, as may occur in osteogenesis imperfecta, malignancies, long-term steroid use, infection,

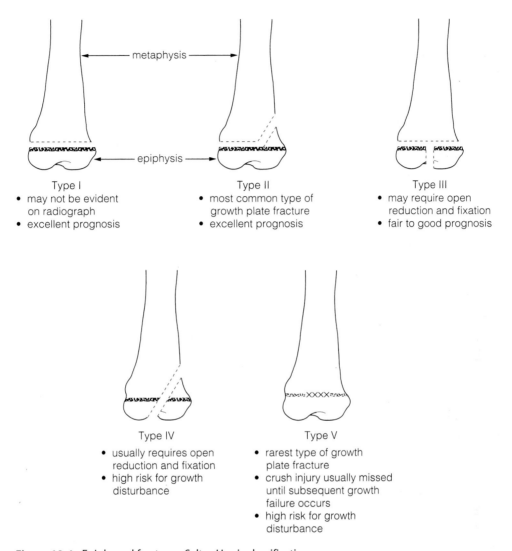

Figure 19-4 • Epiphyseal fractures: Salter-Harris classification.

endocrine disorders, and some inborn errors of metabolism.

DIAGNOSTIC EVALUATION

Radiographs should include AP and lateral views of the involved bone as well as the joints immediately adjacent to the injury. Salter-Harris types I and V may not be appreciated on these views; oblique views or serial radiographs may be necessary to confirm the diagnosis. It is important to remember that at least 5% of fractures are not visible on the initial radiographs, only becoming apparent 2 to 3 weeks later on follow-up films. Children with severe limb pain after trauma should be splinted even if initial studies are normal due to the likelihood of an occult fracture.

TREATMENT

Most fractures can be adequately treated with casts or splints. Fractures that are unstable, misaligned, or involve the growth plate typically require manipulation in the emergency department. Open fractures usually need operative washout and debridement to minimize the risk of infection. Femur fractures, elbow fractures, and fractures that penetrate the joint often benefit from surgical fixation with pins, plates, or rods.

OSTEOGENESIS IMPERFECTA

Osteogenesis imperfecta (OI) describes a group of closely related genetic disorders resulting in fragile, brittle bones. The common denominator in all variants is the abnormal synthesis of type I collagen, which normally constitutes approximately 90% of the bone matrix but is also dispersed in the teeth, ligaments, skin, ears, and sclerae. The most severe form is type II, or fetal OI, which results in multiple intrauterine and birth fractures and is uniformly fatal in the perinatal period.

CLINICAL MANIFESTATIONS

Clinical severity depends on the subclass of OI (Table 19-2). Some variants cause death early in life; others present with only moderately increased susceptibility to fractures. Blue sclerae are a characteristic feature in some forms of the disease. Short stature is not uncommon as a result of frequent, recurrent fractures. Fractures associated with OI occasionally raise suspicion for child abuse.

TREATMENT

Treatment involves standard fracture care, pneumatic bracing, and careful avoidance of even minor trauma. Patients with severe disease may benefit from pamidronate therapy, which inhibits osteoclastic resorption.

SUBLUXATION OF THE RADIAL HEAD

Nursemaid's elbow, or radial head subluxation, is a common injury seen in young children. The history is often remarkable for a sudden strong jerking of the child's hand, resulting in rapid extension at the elbow. The child dangles the affected arm close to the body, with the elbow slightly flexed and the forearm pronated. Motion at the elbow is limited and painful. "Radial head subluxation" is a misnomer, and radiographs appear normal. Treatment consists of extending the elbow and supinating the hand, a procedure which is often inadvertently performed by the radiology technician during radiologic assessment of

	TABLE 19-2 Classification of Osteogenesis Imperfecta			
Syndrome	**Mode of Inheritance**	**Orthopedic Manifestations**	**Non-orthopedic Manifestations**	**Life Expectancy**
Type I	Autosomal dominant	Frequent fractures from the neonatal period through adolescence;* severe bone fragility; bow legs; joint laxity; short stature	Blue/gray sclerae; adult-onset sensorineural hearing loss (deafness); abnormal dentition	Generally shortened
Type II	Autosomal recessive	Short, deformed limbs; multiple in utero and neonatal fractures; severe bone fragility	Intrauterine growth retardation; stillbirth; blue/gray sclerae	Days
Type III	Autosomal recessive	Frequent fractures which heal with deformation; severe bone fragility; lower limb deformities; short stature	Normal or mildly blue/gray sclerae	Generally shortened
Type IV	Autosomal dominant	Increased susceptibility to fractures*	Normal sclerae; increased risk for aortic dilatation	Near normal

*Susceptibility to fractures progressively decreases during adolescence; pathologic fractures in adulthood are rare.

the elbow. A second validated method is flexion the patient's arm to 90 degrees and pronation the forearm. A successful reduction is usually accompanied by a click as the entraped annular ligament pops into place. Usually the child begins to move the arm normally within minutes.

OSTEOMYELITIS

PATHOGENESIS

Bone infections require early recognition and aggressive treatment to secure a favorable outcome. Hematogenous seeding is the usual source of origin; trauma seems to increase susceptibility. The femur and tibia account for two-thirds of cases. Infection usually begins in the metaphysis, an area of relative blood stasis and few phagocytes. Fifty percent of neonates with a bone infection have an associated septic joint.

EPIDEMIOLOGY AND RISK FACTORS

Incidence peaks in the neonatal period and again in older children (9 to 11 years of age) when it becomes more common in males. The predominant organism in all age groups is **Staphylococcus aureus** (S. aureus). Group B streptococci and *Escherichia coli* (E. coli) are important pathogens in the neonate. Patients with sickle cell disease are particularly susceptible to *Salmonella* osteomyelitis. *Pseudomonas aeruginosa* can cause foot osteomyelitis or septic arthritis following a puncture wound through sneakers.

CLINICAL MANIFESTATIONS

History and Physical Examination

Infants present with a history of fever and refusal to move the involved limb. Older patients also complain of localized bone pain and often are febrile. The physical examination may reveal soft-tissue swelling, limited range of motion, erythema, and point tenderness. Occasionally, sinus tracts drain purulent fluid onto the skin surface.

DIFFERENTIAL DIAGNOSIS

Traumatic injury and malignant invasion of the bone may present with similar symptoms. Range of motion generally remains intact in patients with osteomyelitis as opposed to those with septic arthritis.

DIAGNOSTIC EVALUATION

The WBC is often within the normal range. Approximately 50% to 60% of peripheral blood cultures are positive. **Aspiration** of the involved bone **before antibiotics are started** is often key to isolation, identification, and sensitivity testing of the causative organism, especially if initial blood cultures are negative. Radiographs are initially normal but demonstrate periosteal elevation or radiolucent necrotic areas at 2 to 3 weeks. Bone scans are positive within 24 to 72 hours of symptom onset. Gadolinium-enhanced MRI can be obtained to evaluate for subperiosteal or intraosseous abscess or necrotic bone, especially in patients who have severe symptoms or who are refractory to IV antibiotic therapy. Serum markers of inflammation are usually elevated; an elevated C-reactive protein value is observed in 98% of cases and returns to normal within 7 days of effective treatment. The ESR is elevated in 90% of cases but requires longer (3 to 4 weeks) to return to normal.

TREATMENT

Treatment consists of intravenous or high-dose oral antibiotics for 4 to 6 weeks. Initially, broad-spectrum antistaphylococcal agents, such as cefazolin, nafcillin or oxacillin, are appropriate. Neonates require coverage for group B streptococci and gram-negative bacilli. Patients with sickle cell disease should initially receive a third-generation cephalosporin for *Salmonella* coverage. When the organism has been recovered and sensitivities are available, therapy may be narrowed. Most patients do not require surgery unless they develop abscesses or necrotic bone (sequestrum).

SEPTIC ARTHRITIS

PATHOGENESIS

Septic arthritis (purulent infection of the joint space) is more common and potentially more debilitating than osteomyelitis. Pathogens are theorized to enter the joint during episodes of bacteremia.

EPIDEMIOLOGY

The incidence is highest in infants and young children. Neonates may be infected with group B streptococcus, E. coli, *Streptococcus pneumoniae* (S. pneumoniae), or S. aureus. In infants older than 6 weeks and young children, the hip is the most commonly affected site.

The knee is more frequently involved in older children. *S. aureus* is the most likely pathogen outside the neonatal period. Other bacteria with a predilection for joints in younger children include *Kingella kingae* and *S. pneumoniae*. In older children, streptococci and gram-negative bacteria are not uncommon. *Neisseria gonorrhoeae* (*N. gonorrhoeae*) must be considered in the sexually active adolescent, especially if multiple joints are involved.

CLINICAL MANIFESTATIONS

History and Physical Examination

Septic arthritis presents as a painful joint, often accompanied by fever, irritability, and refusal to bear weight. On examination, range of motion is clearly limited. The joint is tender and may be visibly swollen.

DIFFERENTIAL DIAGNOSIS

Osteomyelitis and inflammatory arthritis should be considered in the differential diagnosis. In addition, many causes of reactive or postinfectious arthritis may present in a similar manner. **Toxic synovitis** is a frequent cause of hip pain and stiffness in children. It has not been definitively proven to be an infectious condition, although it often follows a viral illness. In contrast to septic arthritis, range of motion is minimally limited, the child is generally afebrile and will usually bear weight, the ESR is less than 40 mm/hr, and the WBC count is typically less than 12,000/μL.

DIAGNOSTIC EVALUATION

The standard of care for septic arthritis involves aspiration of the joint. The synovial fluid typically yields a WBC count in excess of 25,000/μL and a pathologic organism. The exception is *N. gonorrhoeae*, which is difficult to recover; blood, cervical, rectal, and nasopharyngeal cultures may be helpful in the sexually active adolescent with septic arthritis.

TREATMENT

Delay in treatment may result in permanent destructive changes and functional impairment. A septic hip is an orthopedic emergency. Intravenous antibiotic therapy remains the treatment of choice; conversion to oral therapy is appropriate when sensitivities are known and symptoms substantially improve. Ceftriaxone is an appropriate initial choice in the young child; a semisynthetic penicillin or (first- or second-generation) cephalosporin is preferred in older children due to the overwhelming likelihood of *S. aureus* arthritis in this age group. Cefotaxime is a better choice in the neonate. Antibiotic therapy can be specifically targeted to the pathogen when culture results become available.

KEY POINTS

- Developmental dysplasia of the hip (DDH) may be demonstrated on physical examination by performing the Barlow and Ortolani maneuvers (in newborns) and evaluating limb length and hip adduction in infants older than 3 months. DDH must be diagnosed and treated early in life to obtain a favorable outcome.

- Plantar and dorsiflexion are intact in metatarsus adductus; in talipes equinovarus, the hindfoot is fixed in plantar flexion.

- Trauma is the most common cause of limp in all age groups. The typical patient with Legg-Calvé-Perthes disease is a young male who presents with a painless or moderately painful limp and knee pain. The typical SCFE patient is an obese adolescent male who presents with hip or knee pain and no history of trauma.

- Scoliosis is more common in adolescent females than in males. Bracing is usually recommended for curves from 25 to 45 degrees until the growth spurt is complete. Bracing halts curve progression; it does not correct the curvature already there.

- Fractures through a growth plate may result in deformity or leg-length discrepancy.

- Epiphyseal fractures categorized as Slater-Harris type IV or V have the greatest risk for disruption of growth.

- Only approximately half of blood cultures are positive in patients with osteomyelitis, so aspiration of the bone prior to antibiotic administration yields invaluable information. *S. aureus* is the most common pathogen in all age groups. Patients with sickle cell disease are particularly susceptible to *Salmonella* osteomyelitis.

- The most common cause of septic arthritis in infants and children is *S. aureus*. *N. gonorrhoeae* should be considered in the sexually active adolescent with septic arthritis.

- Patients with toxic synovitis have lower ESR and WBC counts than those with septic arthritis, and although the joint is generally tender, they typically do not refuse to bear weight.

Chapter 2

Pulmonology

Robert E. Wood • Carolyn Kercsmar • Katie S. Fine

Respiratory diseases are among the leading causes of death in young children worldwide, and respiratory symptoms are a complaint in the majority of pediatric sick visits. While these symptoms are usually related to acute infection, they may be a consequence of congenital or acquired pulmonary disorders. Respiratory disorders specific to the newborn period (including bronchopulmonary dysplasia) are discussed in Chapter 13.

The primary function of the lungs is the exchange of oxygen and carbon dioxide between the blood and the atmosphere. Many abnormalities can affect this exchange adversely, including airway *obstruction*, *restrictive* lung disease (decreased compliance of the lungs and/or chest wall), ventilation-perfusion mismatch, and abnormal respiratory control. Effective respiration requires proper interaction between the respiratory, cardiovascular, and central nervous systems, with adequate support from the musculoskeletal system as well.

DIAGNOSTIC TECHNIQUES IN PEDIATRIC PULMONOLOGY

A standard **chest radiograph** is a vitally important tool in the evaluation of children with respiratory disorders. **Airway films** provide visualization of the trachea and nasopharyngeal airway. **Computed tomography** (CT) studies yield more detailed information and can be combined with vascular contrast. The images obtained are influenced by body position and stage of inspiration or exhalation.

Pulmonary function testing measures lung volume and rates of airflow, permitting assessment of lung capacity and airway obstruction. Pulmonary function tests (PFTs) are generally performed only in patients old enough to cooperate (older than age 5 to 6 years). The data generated is dependent on patient effort and technique, and training of subjects is necessary before reproducible data are obtained.

In older children, **microscopic examination and culture** of expectorated sputum may yield important information, although the results are often somewhat equivocal due to contamination of the specimen with saliva or upper airway secretions.

Bronchoscopy—the direct visual examination of the airways—is a powerful diagnostic tool for evaluation of airway structure and dynamics, as well as to obtain definitive specimens from the lower airways. Rigid or flexible instruments of appropriate size may be used; in general, flexible instruments are best for evaluation of the lower airways (but not for extraction of aspirated foreign bodies) and airway dynamics; rigid instruments give a more detailed image, but result in some anatomic distortion because the rigid instrument does not follow the anatomic pathway.

UPPER AIRWAY OBSTRUCTIVE DISEASE

The upper airway extends from the nostril to the thoracic inlet. In general, obstruction of the upper airway leads to *inspiratory* obstruction, while obstruction below the thoracic inlet results in *expiratory* obstruction.

UPPER AIRWAY OBSTRUCTION IN THE NEONATE/YOUNG INFANT

Choanal atresia or stenosis (narrowing of the nasal passages) can be life-threatening in newborns, who are obligate nose breathers. Mandibular hypoplasia often results in posterior displacement of the tongue (glossoptosis); some children (typically, with trisomy 21) have large, obstructive tongues. Vocal cord paralysis can be unilateral or bilateral, and congenital or (more frequently) acquired. Laryngeal webs are uncommon congenital lesions that may produce respiratory distress in the delivery room and often disappear following intubation. **Laryngomalacia** due to large, floppy arytenoid cartilages or a floppy epiglottis is the most common cause of congenital stridor, and usually resolves with growth over the first 1 to 3 years of life. Subglottic masses (hemangioma or cyst) may present in the first year of life; in the child with persistent stridor and a cutaneous hemangioma, a subglottic hemangioma should be suspected. Subglottic stenosis is rarely congenital; acquired stenosis should be considered in any child who has been intubated, even transiently. Children presenting in the first year of life with persistent stridor and/or hoarseness most likely have either vocal cord paralysis or laryngeal papillomatosis. Vascular compression of the trachea by an anomalous vessel is a relatively common cause of upper airway obstruction in the first year of life.

Clinical Manifestations

Clinical manifestations of upper airway obstruction include noisy inspiration, increased work of breathing (nasal flaring, use of accessory muscles), and retractions (especially in the suprasternal region of the neck). The character and intensity of the noise depend on the structures involved, the degree of muscle tone, and the rate of flow. In general, obstruction in the subglottic space (i.e., at the vocal cords or arytenoid cartilages) results in a high-pitched, monophonic stridor. Obstruction above the glottis produces a more variable, often fluttering stridor which typically varies considerably with position of the head and neck. Upper airway obstruction is often more pronounced during feeding, especially in neonates.

Diagnostic Evaluation

Diagnostic evaluation of upper airway obstruction involves assessment of the severity of the physiologic disturbance and identification of the etiology of the obstruction. Physiologic studies include **pulse oximetry** which measures oxygen saturation in peripheral blood, and **blood gas analysis,** which measures blood pH and carbon dioxide level. During severe obstruction, oxygen saturation can remain within normal limits despite a significant rise in carbon dioxide levels. Patency of the nasal airway is confirmed by passage of a suction catheter through each nostril or by instillation of radiographic contrast material. Radiographs of the nasopharynx and neck can be helpful, but flexible bronchoscopy is often required to definitively evaluate the anatomy and dynamics of the upper airway.

Treatment

Treatment of upper airway obstruction depends on the nature of the obstruction. Following definitive exclusion of more serious pathology most infants with laryngomalacia or unilateral vocal cord paralysis need only be followed. If the airway obstruction is severe (e.g., hypoxemia, failure to thrive, feeding difficulties), provision of an artificial airway followed by surgical intervention is warranted. In many patients, tracheostomy provides an effective and safe long-term solution until more definitive treatment can be provided.

UPPER AIRWAY OBSTRUCTION IN THE OLDER CHILD

Children beyond the first year of life may have upper airway obstruction as a result of a congenital lesion, but acquired lesions are much more likely. Large adenoids and tonsils often result in inspiratory obstruction, with symptomatic exacerbations during periods of viral respiratory infection. Nasal obstruction can also be caused by a foreign body, polyps, or allergic rhinitis. There are many infectious causes of acute upper airway obstruction, such as acute laryngotracheitis and peritonsillar or retropharyngeal abscess.

OBSTRUCTIVE SLEEP APNEA

Many children have upper airway obstruction only during sleep, as a result of changes in upper airway muscle tone. Most have some degree of anatomic obstruction as well (i.e., large adenoids and/or tonsils). Symptoms of obstructive sleep apnea (OSA) include restless sleep with frequent position changes, snoring that is irregular (especially with pauses and gasps), daytime somnolence, poor growth, behavioral problems, enuresis, and poor academic performance. OSA associated with marked obesity can lead to chronic hypoventilation with attendant complications, termed **Pickwickian syndrome**.

Polysomnography is the diagnostic study of choice, measuring respiratory muscle activity, air flow, oxygenation, sleep stage, and heart rate. This test can define the degree and type of physiologic disturbance, whether central, obstructive, or mixed in nature. Treatment of OSA should be directed toward normalizing airway anatomy through the removal of enlarged tonsils and/or adenoids, if indicated. If initial interventions fail and the degree of disturbance is significant, then continuous positive airway pressure (CPAP) is indicated. Severe, untreated OSA may lead to **congestive heart failure** and even death.

LOWER AIRWAY OBSTRUCTIVE DISEASE

The intrathoracic airways narrow during exhalation; thus, any form of lower airway obstruction will be more apparent during exhalation. **Wheezing** is the sound of air squeezing past an intrathoracic obstruction of virtually any type. While most patients with asthma wheeze, *not all patients who wheeze have asthma*. There are two major lower airway obstructive diseases in childhood: asthma and cystic fibrosis. Primary ciliary dyskinesia, a rarer entity, is also primarily an obstructive disease.

ASTHMA

Asthma is a chronic disease of the airways characterized by *reversible airway obstruction*, inflammation, and bronchial hyper-responsiveness. The diagnosis is based on recurrence of symptoms and symptom responsiveness to bronchodilator and/or anti-inflammatory agents. Bronchospasm, which results from smooth muscle constriction, may occur in response to allergic, environmental, infectious, or emotional stimuli (the trigger). Common precipitants include cigarette smoke, upper respiratory infections, pet dander, dust mites, weather changes, exercise, and seasonal or food allergens. Cellular mediators of inflammation are recruited to the lower airway surfaces, inciting mucous production and further increasing airway hyper-responsiveness. The inflammatory response typically involves both immediate and late-phase components; it is the latter that results in the prolonged nature of an asthma exacerbation.

Asthma **severity** is classified based on the degree of impairment prior to initiation of appropriate therapy (Tables 20-1 and 20-2). Following initiation of treatment, asthma **control** is monitored in two domains: impairment (current symptoms and lung function) and risk (future exacerbations and medication side effects) (Tables 20-3 and 20-4). Additional information regarding the 2007 Expert Panel Report 3 Guidelines for the diagnosis and treatment of asthma can be found at www.nhlibi.nih.gov/guidelines/asthma/index.htm.

Epidemiology

Asthma is the most frequently encountered pulmonary disease in children, and its prevalence is on the rise despite advances in therapy. It is among the most common reasons for hospitalization in pediatric practice. More than 50% of patients present before 6 years of age. Boys are affected more often than girls prior to adolescence; thereafter, the ratio is reversed.

Risk Factors

Risk factors include genetic predisposition (parent[s] with asthma or allergy), atopy, cigarette smoke exposure, living in urban areas in poverty, and African American race. Hospitalization due to infection with respiratory syncytial virus is also associated with the development of asthma; this may represent an underlying increased propensity to wheeze rather than an independent risk factor.

Differential Diagnosis

When a child presents with wheezing and respiratory distress, the differential diagnosis includes intraluminal inflammation or failure to clear secretions (bronchiolitis, gastroesophageal reflux with aspiration, cystic fibrosis, tracheoesophageal fistula, primary ciliary dyskinesia); intraluminal mass effects (foreign body aspiration, tracheal or bronchial tumors or granulation tissue); dynamic airway collapse (tracheobronchomalacia); intrinsic narrowing of the airway (congenital or acquired stenosis); and extrinsic compression (vascular ring, mediastinal lymph nodes or masses). Anaphylaxis and angioneurotic edema may cause wheezing at any age. **Cough-variant asthma**, which is relatively uncommon, produces a chronic cough that may be triggered by exercise or noted primarily at night during sleep; wheezing may or may not be present.

TABLE 20-1 Classifying Asthma Severity and Initiating Therapy in Children (Ages 0 to 11 years)

Components of Severity

| | | Intermittent | | Persistent | | | | | |
| | | | | **Mild** | | **Moderate** | | **Severe** | |
		Ages 0 to 4	Ages 5 to 11	Ages 0 to 4	Ages 5 to 11	Ages 0 to 4	Ages 5 to 11	Ages 0 to 4	Ages 5 to 11
Impairment	Symptoms	≤2 days/week		>2 days a week but not daily		Daily		Throughout the day	
	Nighttime awakenings	0	≤2×/month	1 to 2×/month	3 to 4×/month	3 to 4×/month	>1×/week but not nightly	>1×/week	Often 7×/week
	Short-acting beta$_2$-agonist use for symptom control	≤2 days/week		>2 days a week but not daily		Daily		Several times per day	
	Interference with normal activity	None		Minor limitation		Some limitation		Extremely limited	
	Lung function -FEV$_1$ (predicted) or peak flow (personal best) -FEV$_1$/FEC	N/A	Normal FEV$_1$ between exacerbations >80% >85%	N/A	>80% >80%	N/A	60% to 80% 75% to 80%	N/A	<50% <75%
Risk	Exacerbations requiring oral systemic corticosteroids (consider severity and interval since last exacerbation)	0 to 1/year (see notes)	≥2 exacerbations in 6 months requiring oral systemic corticosteroids, or ≥4 wheezing episodes/1 year lasting >1 day AND risk factors for persistent asthma	≥2/year (see notes) Relative annual risk may be related to FEV$_1$					

Recommended Step for Initiating Therapy (See "Stepwise Approach for Managing Asthma" for treatment steps.) The stepwise approach is meant to assist, not replace, the clinical decision making required to meet individual patient needs	Step 1 (for both age groups)	Step 2 (for both age groups)	Step 3 and consider short course of oral systemic corticosteroids	Step 3: medium-dose ICS option and consider short course of oral systemic coricosteroids	Step 3 and consider short course of oral systemic corticosteroids	Step 3: medium-dose ICS option OR step 4 and consider short course of oral systemic corticosteroids

In 2 to 6 weeks, depending on severity, evaluate level of asthma control that is achieved.

Children 0 to 4 years old: If no clear benefit is observed in 4 to 6 weeks, stop treatment and consider alternative diagnoses or adjusting therapy.

Children 5 to 11 years old: Adjust therapy accordingly.

Level of severity is determined by both impairment and risk. Assess impairment domain by caregiver's recall of previous 2 to 4 weeks. Assign severity to the most severe category in which any feature occurs. Frequency and severity of exacerbations may fluctuate over time for patients in any severity category. At present, there are inadequate data to correspond frequencies of exacerbations with different levels of asthma severity. In general, more frequent and severe exacerbations (e.g., requiring urgent, unscheduled care, hospitalization, or ICU admission) indicate greater underlying disease severity. For treatment purposes, patients with ≥2 exacerbations described above may be considered the same as patients who have persistent asthma, even in the absence of impairment levels consistent with persistent asthma.
FEV₁, forced expiratory volume in 1 second; FVC, forced vital capacity; ICS, inhaled corticosteroids; ICU, intensive care unit; N/A, not applicable.
Adapted from 2007 Expert Panel Report 3 Guidelines for the Diagnosis and Treatment of Asthma. Available online at http://www.nhlbi.nih.gov/guidelines/asthma/index.htm.

■ TABLE 20-2 Classifying Asthma Severity and Initiating Treatment (Ages ≥12 years)

Components of Severity		Classification of Asthma Severity ≥12 Years of age			
				Persistent	
		Intermittent	Mild	Moderate	Severe
Impairment Normal FEV_1/FVC: 8 to 19 yr 85% 20 to 39 yr 80% 40 to 59 yr 75% 60 to 80 yr 70%	Symptoms	≤2 days/week	>2 days/week but not daily	Daily	Throughout the day
	Nighttime awakenings	≤2×/month	3 to 4×/month	>1×/week but not nightly	Often 7×/week
	Short-acting beta$_2$-agonist use for symptom control (not prevention of EIB)	≤2 days/week	>2 days/week but not daily, and not more than 1× on any day	Daily	Several times per day
	Interference with normal activity	None	Minor limitation	Some limitation	Extremely limited
	Lung function	- Normal FEV_1 between exacerbations - FEV_1 >80% predicted - FEV_1/FVC normal	- FEV_1 >80% predicted - FEV_1/FVC normal	- FEV_1 >60% but <80% predicted - FEV_1/FVC reduced 5%	- FEV_1 <60% predicted - FEV_1/FVC reduced >5%
Risk	Exacerbations requiring oral systemic corticosteroids	0 to 1 year (see note)	≥2/year (see note)		
		Consider severity and interval since last exacerbation. Frequency and severity may fluctuate over time for patients in any severity category. Relative annual risk of exacerbations may be related to FEV_1.			
Recommended Step for Initiating Treatment (See "Stepwise Approach for Managing Asthma" for treatment steps.)		Step 1	Step 2	Step 3 and consider short course of oral systemic corticosteroids	Step 4 or 5 and consider short course of oral systemic corticosteroids
		In 2 to 6 weeks, evaluate level of asthma control that is achieved and adjust therapy accordingly.			

The stepwise approach is meant to assist, not replace, the clinical decision making required to meet individual patient needs.

Level of severity is determined by assessment of both impairment and risk. Assess impairment domain by patients/caregivers 2 to 4 weeks and spirometry. Assign severity to the most severe category in which any feature occurs.

At present, there are inadequate data to correspond frequencies of exacerbations with different levels of asthma severity. In general, more frequent and intense exacerbations (e.g., requiring urgent, unscheduled care, hospitalization, or ICU admission) indicate greater underlying disease severity. For treatment purposes, patients had ≥2 exacerbations requiring oral systemic corticosteroids in the past year may be considered the same as patients who have persistent asthma, even in the absence of impairment levels consistent with persistent asthma.

EIB, exercise-induced bronchospasm; FEV_1, forced expiratory volume in 1 second; FVC, forced vital capacity; ICU, intensive care unit.

Adapted from 2007 Expert Panel Report 3 Guidelines for the Diagnosis and Treatment of Asthma. Available online at http://www.nhlibi.nih.gov/guidelines/asthma/index.htm.

TABLE 20-3 Assessing Asthma Control and Adjusting Therapy in Children (Ages 0 to 11)

Components of Control		Assessing Asthma Control and Adjusting Therapy in Children					
		Well Controlled		**Not Well Controlled**		**Very Poorly Controlled**	
		Ages 0 to 4	Ages 5 to 11	Ages 0 to 4	Ages 5 to 11	Ages 0 to 4	Ages 5 to 11
Impairment	Symptoms	≤2 days/week but not more than once on each day		>2 days/week or multiple times on ≤2 days/week		Throughout the day	
	Nighttime awakenings	≤1×/month		>1×/month	≥2×/month	>1×/week	≥2×/week
	Interference with normal activity	None		Some limitation		Extremely limited	
	Short-acting beta₂-agonist use for symptom control (not prevention of EIB)	≤2 days/week		>2 days/week		Several times per day	
	Lung function - FEV₁ (predicted) or peak flow personal best - FEV₁/FVC	N/A	>80% >80%	N/A	60% to 80% 75% to 80%	N/A	<60% <75%
Risk	Exacerbations requiring oral systemic corticosteroids	0 to 1×/year		2 to 3×/year	≥2×/year	>3×/year	≥2×/year
	Reduction in lung growth	N/A	Requires long-term follow-up	N/A		N/A	
	Treatment-related adverse effects	Medication side effects can vary in intensity from none to very troublesome and worrisome. The level of intensity does not correlate to specific levels of control but should be considered in the overall assessment of risk.					
Step for Initiating Therapy (See "Stepwise Approach for Managing Asthma" for treatment steps.)		- Maintain current step - Regular follow-up every 1 to 6 months		Step up 1 step	Step up at least 1 step	- Consider short course of oral systemic corticosteroids	
The stepwise approach is meant to assist, not replace, the clinical decision making required to meet individual patient needs		- Consider step down if well controlled for at least 3 months				- Step up 1 to 2 steps	
				- Before step up: Review adherence to medication, inhaler technique, and environmental control. If alternative treatment was used, discontinue it and use preferred treatment for that step.			

continues

TABLE 20-3 Assessing Asthma Control and Adjusting Therapy in Children (Ages 0 to 11) *(continued)*

Components of Control	Assessing Asthma Control and Adjusting Therapy in Children					
	Well Controlled		**Not Well Controlled**		**Very Poorly Controlled**	
	Ages 0 to 4	Ages 5 to 11	Ages 0 to 4	Ages 5 to 11	Ages 0 to 4	Ages 5 to 11
			- Reevaluate the level of asthma control in 2 to 6 weeks to achieve control; every 1 to 6 months to maintain control - Control 0 to 4 years old: If no clear benefit is observed in 4 to 6 weeks, consider alternative diagnoses or adjusting therapy. - Children 5 to 11 years old: Adjust therapy accordingly. - For side effects, consider alternative treatment options.			

The level of control is based on the most severe impairment or risk category. Assess impairment domain by patient's or caregiver's recall of previous 2 to 4 weeks. Symptom assessment for longer periods should reflect a global assessment, such as whether the patient's asthma is better or worse since the last visit.

At present, there are inadequate data to correspond frequencies of exacerbations with different levels of asthma control. In general, more frequent and intense exacerbations (e.g., requiring urgent, unscheduled care, hospitalization, or ICU admission) indicate poorer disease control.

EIB, exercise-induced bronchospasm; FEV_1, forced expiratory volume in 1 second; FVC, forced vital capacity; ICU, intensive care unit; N/A, not applicable.

Adapted from 2007 Expert Panel Report 3 Guidelines for the Diagnosis and Treatment of Asthma. Available online at http://www.nhlibi.nih.gov/guidelines/asthma/index.htm.

Clinical Manifestations

The presentations of asthma are varied. The history may be positive for wheezing with viral respiratory infections. Other possible signs and symptoms include prolonged respiratory infections, decreased exercise tolerance, and persistent day or nighttime coughing. Children with acute exacerbations present in respiratory distress with dyspnea, wheezing, subcostal retractions, nasal flaring, tracheal tugging, and a prolonged expiratory phase resulting from obstruction of airflow. Cyanosis is uncommon. The absence of wheezing with poorly heard breath sounds is an ominous sign, indicating severe airway obstruction with very limited air movement. Mental status changes suggest significant hypercarbia and/or significant hypoxemia with impending respiratory failure.

Diagnostic Evaluation

In children older than 6 years, PFTs can help delineate disease severity at baseline and during exacerbations. Patients with *persistent asthma* should undergo PFTs at least once a year in order to monitor control and adjust therapy. Baseline chest radiographs typically show mild hyperinflation and/or increased bronchial markings. Peak flow (PF) monitoring may

be useful for patients with moderate to severe asthma or those who poorly perceive their symptoms. PF meters are small, portable, and easy to use. They measure how fast a patient can forcibly expire air after a maximal inhalation; decreased readings indicate obstruction to airflow. PF readings may begin to fall hours or even days before symptoms become evident. Reductions to 50% to 80% of predicted values indicate mild to moderate disease exacerbation; readings less than 30% of predicted values are associated with severe obstruction. Unfortunately, peak flow meters are heavily dependent on technique and thus variably reliable.

During acute exacerbations, the chest radiograph demonstrates significant hyperinflation and occasionally focal or subsegmental atelectasis (Fig. 20-1). CO_2 retention can occur with fatigue and may be quite dramatic; hypoxemia is usually less pronounced.

Treatment

With appropriate therapy and good compliance, most patients with persistent asthma can remain symptom-free with few exacerbations. The most effective treatment involves removal of inciting agents (triggers) from the patient's environment and

■ TABLE 20-4 Assessing Asthma Control and Adjusting Therapy (Ages ≥12 years)

Components of Control		Classification of Asthma Control (≥12 years of age)		
		Well Controlled	**Not Well Controlled**	**Very Poorly Controlled**
Impairment	Symptoms	≤2 days/week	>2 days/week	Throughout the day
	Nighttime awakenings	≤2×/month	1 to 3×/week	≥4×/week
	Interference with normal activity	None	Some limitation	Extremely limited
	Short-acting beta$_2$-agonist use for symptom control (not prevention of EIB)	≤2 days/week	>2 days/week	Several times per day
	FEV$_1$ or peak flow	>80% predicted/personal best	60% to 80% predicted/personal best	<60% predicted/personal best
	Validated questionnaires ATAQ ACQ ACT	0 ≤0.75* ≥20	1 to 2 ≥1.5 16 to 19	3 to 4 N/A ≤15
Risk	Exacerbations requiring oral systemic corticosteroids	0 to 1/year	≥2/year (see note)	
		Consider severity and interval since last exacerbation		
	Progressive loss of lung function	Evaluation requires long-term follow-up care.		
	Treatment-related adverse effects	Medication side effects can vary in intensity from none to very troublesome. The level of intensity does not correlate to specific levels of control but should be considered in the overall assessment of risk.		
Recommended Action for Treatment (See "Stepwise Approach for Managing Asthma" for treatment steps.)		- Maintain current step - Regular follow-up at every 1 to 6 months to maintain control - Consider step down if well controlled for at least 3 months	- Step up to 1 step - Reevaluate in 2 to 6 weeks - For side effects, consider alternative treatment options	- Consider short course of oral systemic corticosteroids - Step up 1 to 2 steps - Reevaluate in 2 weeks - For side effects, consider alternative treatment options

*ACQ values of 0.76 to 1.4 are indeterminate regarding well-controlled asthma.

The stepwise approach is meant to assist, not replace, the clinical decision making required to meet individual patient needs.

The level of control is based on the most severe impairment or risk category. Assess impairment domain by patient's recall of previous 2 to 4 weeks by spirometry/or peak flow measures. Symptom assessment for longer periods should reflect a global assessment, such as inquiring whether the patient's asthma is better or worse since the last visit.

At present, there are inadequate data to correspond frequencies of exacerbations with different levels of asthma control. In general, more frequent and intense exacerbations (e.g., requiring urgent, unscheduled care, hospitalization, or ICU admission) indicate poorer disease control. For treatment purposes, patients who had ≥2 exacerbations requiring oral systemic corticosteroids in the past year may be considered the same as patients who have not-well-controlled asthma, even in the absence of impairment levels consistent with not-well-controlled asthma.

ATAQ, Asthma Therapy Assessment Questionnaire©; ACQ, Asthma Control Questionnaire©; ACT, Asthma Control Test™; Difference: 1.0 for the ATAQ; 0.5 for the ACQ; not determined for the ACT.

Before step up in therapy:

Review adherence to medication, inhaler technique, environmental control, and comorbid conditions.

If an alternative treatment option was used in a step, discontinue and use the preferred treatment for that step.

Adapted from 2007 Expert Panel Report 3 Guidelines for the Diagnosis and Treatment of Asthma. Available online at http://www.nhlibi.nih.gov/guidelines/asthma/index.htm.

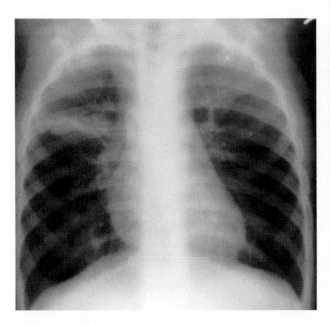
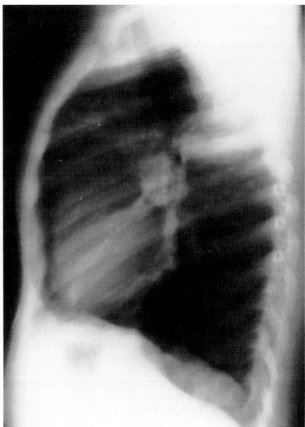

Figure 20-1 • Chest radiograph of a 3-year-old patient obtained during an asthma exacerbation test demonstrates severe hyperinflation, increased anteroposterior diameter of the chest, a depressed diaphragm, and several areas of atelectasis.

appropriate use of maintenance anti-inflammatory medication. Cigarette smoke should be strictly avoided. Limiting dust mite, mold, and pet exposure is beneficial to patients with an allergic component to their asthma. The National Institutes of Health has issued guidelines for the pharmacologic management of asthma based on disease severity and control (Tables 20-5 and 20-6).

The mainstays of medical maintenance therapy include **inhaled corticosteroids** (ICSs), β-2-adrenergic agonists, and **leukotriene receptor antagonists** (LTRAs). **β-2-agonists** such as albuterol reduce smooth muscle constriction and can be administered via nebulization or metered-dose inhalation. Levalbuterol (single isomer R-albuterol) offers a theoretical advantage of better efficacy at lower dosage; however, research has yet to confirm this benefit. Longer-acting preparations (salbutamol, formoterol) may be used in patients who fail to achieve good control with ICS therapy alone. In adolescents, the additive effect of the

β-2-agonists may allow for reduction of ICS dosing. Long-acting β-agonists are not appropriate for monotherapy. Short-acting β-2-agonists are effective in preventing exercise-induced asthma if used 5 to 20 minutes before vigorous activity. The abuse of inhaled bronchodilators may result in some tolerance to their therapeutic effects.

Inhaled corticosteroid therapy is the most effective treatment for chronic asthma and results in excellent control in the vast majority of patients. Topically active ICSs typically have very low systemic bioavailability and result in few systemic adverse effects. Options include beclomethasone, budesonide, flunisolide, fluticasone, mometasone, and triamcinolone. Although early studies with beclomethasone, a first-generation inhaled corticosteroid, suggested small but measurable decreases in short-term linear growth, significant growth suppression in children using daily inhaled corticosteroids have largely been put to rest; in long-term studies using budesonide and fluticasone at low doses,

■ TABLE 20-5 Stepwise Approach for Managing Asthma Long Term in Children (Ages 0 to 11 Years)

	Step 1	Step 2	Step 3	Step 4	Step 5	Step 6
Children 0 to 4 years of age	*Intermittent Asthma*	*Persistent Asthma: Daily Medication**				
Preferred	SABA PRN	Low-dose ICS	Medium-dose ICS	Medium-dose ICS + LABA or Montelukast	High-dose ICS + LABA or Montelukast	High-dose ICS + oral corticosteroids ICS + LABA or Montelukast
Alternative		Cromolyn or Montelukast				
	Each Step: Patient Education and Environmental Control					
Quick-Relief medication	- SABA as needed for symptoms. Intensity of treatment depends on severity of symptoms. - With viral respiratory symptoms: SABA q 4 to 6 hours up to 24 hours (longer with physician consult). Consider short course of oral systemic corticosteroids if exacerbation is severe or patient has history of previous severe exacerbations. Caution: Frequent use of SABA may indicate the need to step up treatment.					
Children 5 to 11 years of age	*Intermittent Asthma*	*Persistent Asthma: Daily Medication**				
Preferred	SABA PRN	Low-dose ICS	Lose-dose ICS + LABA, LTRA, or theophylline or medium-dose ICS	Medium-dose ICS + LABA	High-dose ICS + LABA	High-dose ICS + LABA + oral corticosteroids
Alternative		Cromotyn, LTRA, nedocromil, or theophylline		Medium-dose ICS + LTRA or theophylline	High-dose ICS + LTRA or theophylline	High-dose ICS + LTRA or theophylline + oral corticosteroids
	Each Step: Patient Education, Environmental Control, and Management of Comorbidities Step 2 to 4: Consider subcutaneous allergen immunotherapy for patients who have persistent, allergic asthma					
Quick-relief medication	- SABA as needed for symptoms. Intensity of treatment depends on severity of symptoms: up to 3 treatments at 20-minute intervals as needed. Short course of oral systemic corticosteroids may be needed. Caution: Increasing use of SABA or use >2 days a week for symptom relief (not prevention of EIB) generally indicated inadequate control and the need to step up treatment.					

* Consult with asthma specialist if step 3 care or higher is required. Consider consultation at step 2.

Children 0 to 4 Years of Age
The stepwise approach is meant to assist, not replace, the clinical decision making required to meet individual patient needs.
If an alternative treatment is used and response is inadequate, discontinue it and use the preferred treatment before stepping up.
If clear benefit is not observed within 4 to 6 weeks, and patient's/family's medication technique and adherence are satisfactory, consider adjusting therapy or an alternative diagnosis.
Studies on children 0 to 4 years of age are limited. Most recommendations in this age group are based on expert opinion and extrapolation from studies in older children.

Children 5 to 11 Years of Age
The stepwise approach is meant to assist, not replace, the clinical decision making required to meet individual patient needs.
If an alternative treatment is used and response is inadequate, discontinue it and use the preferred treatment before stepping up.
Theophylline is a less desirable alternative due to the need to monitor serum concentration levels.
Rationale for recommendations in this age group is available at the NIH website.
Alphabetical listing is used when more than one treatment option is listed within either preferred or alternative therapy.
ICS, inhaled corticosteroid; LABA, inhaled long-acting beta$_2$-agonist; LTRA, leukotriene receptor antagonist; oral corticosteroids, oral systemic corticosteroids; SABA, inhaled short-acting beta$_2$-agonist.
Adapted from 2007 Expert Panel Report 3 Guidelines for the Diagnosis and Treatment of Asthma. Available online at http://www.nhlbi.nih.gov/guidelines/asthma/index.htm.

■ **TABLE 20-6** Stepwise Approach for Managing Asthma (Ages ≥12 years)

Intermittent Asthma	Persistent Asthma: Daily Medication					Step up if
	Consult with asthma specialist if step 4 care or higher is required. Consider consultation at step 3					needed (first, check adherence, environmental control, and comorbid conditions). Assess control. Step down if possible (and asthma is well controlled at least 3 months).
Step 1 Preferred: SABA PRN	Step 2 Preferred: Low-dose ICS Alternative: Cromolyn, LTRA, nedocromil, or theophylline	Step 3 Preferred: Low-dose ICS + LABA or Medium-dose ICS Alternative: Low-dose ICS + either LTRA, theophylline, or zileuton	Step 4 Preferred: Medium-dose ICS + LABA Alternative: Medium-dose ICS + either LTRA, theophylline, or zileuton	Step 5 Preferred: High-dose ICS+LABA and Consider Omalizumab for patients who have allergies	Step 6 Preferred: High-dose ICS + LABA + oral corticosteroid and consider Omalizumab for patients who have allergies	

Each step: Patient education, environmental control, and management of comorbidities.
Step 2 to 4: Consider subcutaneous allergen immunotherapy for patients who have allergic asthma (see notes).

The stepwise approach is meant to assist, not replace, the clinical decision making required to meet individual patient needs.
If alternative treatment is used and response is inadequate, discontinue it and use the preferred treatment before stepping up.
Zileuton is a less desirable alternative due to limited studies as adjunctive therapy and the need to monitor liver function. Theophylline requires monitoring of serum concentration levels.
In step 6, before oral corticosteroids are introduced, a trial of high-dose ICS + LABA + either LTRA, theophylline, or zileuton may be considered, although this approach has not been studied in clinical trials.
Rationale for recommendations for preferred therapies in this age group is available at the NIH website. http://www.nhlbi.nih.gov/guidelines/archives/epr-2_upd/asthmafullrpt_archive.pdf
Alphabetical order is used when more than one treatment option is listed within either preferred or alternative therapy.
ICS, inhaled corticosteroid; LABA, long-acting beta₂-agonist; LTRA, leukotriene receptor antagonist; oral corticosteroids, oral systemic corticosteroids; SABA, inhaled short-acting beta₂-agonist.
Adapted from 2007 Expert Panel Report 3 Guidelines for the Diagnosis and Treatment of Asthma. Available online at http://www.nhlibi.nih.gov/guidelines/asthma/index.htm.

linear growth velocity declined initially but then rebounded, and subjects obtained expected adult height. Short courses of oral steroids (3 to 7 days) are used for acute exacerbations; long-term use is reserved for severe, persistent, poorly controlled asthma.

LTRAs (montelukast, zafirlukast) are oral medications also recommended for the initial treatment of mild persistent asthma; they may be used as add-on medications to an ICS. They are most effective in younger patients and those with a shorter duration of asthma. LTRAs also provide some protection from exercise-induced symptoms. Cromolyn sodium, a mast cell stabilizer, is currently used infrequently since it is less effective than inhaled steroids.

The use of theophylline, once a commonly prescribed oral bronchodilator, has fallen out of favor as a first-line treatment option. Although it has some anti-inflammatory properties, theophylline may be poorly tolerated, has significant interactions with multiple other medications, and requires frequent drug-level monitoring. It is presently reserved for use as an add-on therapy in patients who do not respond to conventional medications, and is sometimes used in the intensive care setting as adjunctive treatment for severe exacerbations. Patients (>12 yr old) with severe allergic asthma that remains poorly controlled with use of inhaled corticosteroids, leukotriene receptor antagonists, and long-acting β-agonists may benefit from treatment with omalizumab, an injectable monoclonal antibody directed against IgE. This treatment is expensive and must be given every 2 to 4 weeks.

Mild to moderate exacerbations are managed by the addition of short-acting inhaled bronchodilators to maintenance regimens. Additional steps may include quadrupling the dosage of inhaled steroids for 7 to 10 days or initiating a 5-day pulse of oral steroids. Moderate to severe exacerbations usually require an emergency department visit, and in some cases, hospitalization.

Children who present to the emergency department in an acute asthma attack are initially assessed for airway patency, work of breathing, and ability to adequately oxygenate. Pulse oximetry is a simple, rapid screen for hypoxemia. Patients in severe respiratory distress require blood gas measurements to assess for increasing $PaCO_2$, a sign of impending respiratory failure. A normal $PaCO_2$ in the face of tachypnea and fatigue is an equally ominous sign because the $PaCO_2$ should be well below 40 mm Hg in the patient with a rapid respiratory rate. Nebulized bronchodilators are administered frequently (every 20 minutes or continuously) for severe episodes. Delivery of inhaled β-agonists using a metered dose inhaler (MDI) with a valved holding chamber is equally effective as using a nebulizer. Ipratropium, an anticholinergic agent, may provide additive relief of symptoms in those patients with the most severe obstruction, as measured by PEF or spirometry. The drug is usually given simultaneously with albuterol. Subcutaneous epinephrine or terbutaline can rapidly decrease airway obstruction in severely affected patients who may be too fatigued or uncooperative to use inhaled albuterol. Corticosteroids, administered orally or intravenously, are indicated for treatment of acute exacerbations that fail to improve significantly after the first albuterol treatment in the emergency department. The effect of systemic corticosteroids takes at least 4 hours to begin to appear. Children who do not respond with significant resolution of symptoms after several hours (i.e., children in status asthmaticus) and those who require ongoing oxygen therapy should be hospitalized for continued treatment and close observation.

Despite advances in therapy, some patients still die from asthma. However, the mortality rate for asthma in children is relatively low in developed countries and has stabilized in the past several years. Factors that increase the risk of death include noncompliance, poor recognition of symptoms, delay in treatment, history of intubation, African American race, and steroid dependence.

CYSTIC FIBROSIS

Pathogenesis

Cystic fibrosis (CF) is an inherited multisystem disease characterized by disordered exocrine gland function. The product of the **cystic fibrosis transmembrane regulator (CFTR) gene** is a cell membrane protein that functions as a cAMP-activated chloride channel on the apical surface of epithelial cells in the respiratory tract, pancreas, sweat and salivary glands, intestines, and reproductive system. This channel is nonfunctional in patients with CF, so chloride remains sequestered inside the cell. Sodium and water are drawn into the cell to maintain ionic and osmotic balance, resulting in relative dehydration at the apical surface of the cell. This in turn results in abnormally viscid secretions and impairment of mucociliary clearance in the respiratory tract. Other abnormalities resulting from the inactivity of this chloride channel include impaired binding of *Pseudomonas* in the lungs and a decrease in nitrous oxide production, leading to exaggerated inflammation and diminished bacterial killing.

Epidemiology

CF is acquired through autosomal recessive inheritance, with a disease frequency of 1 in 3,500 Caucasian births (much lower in other races). More than 1,000 distinct gene mutations on chromosome 7 have been described; 70% of known mutant alleles involve a single nucleotide deletion (the ΔF508 mutation). The average life expectancy is currently in the mid- to late 30s in developed countries and has increased dramatically in the past 4 decades.

Clinical Manifestations

History and Physical Examination

Table 20-7 lists the most common presenting signs and symptoms of CF. All levels of the respiratory tract may be affected, including the nasal passages, sinuses, and lower airways. **Nasal polyps** in any pediatric patient should prompt further testing for CF. Opacification of the sinuses and sinusitis are extremely common. Mucus stasis and ineffective clearance lead to bacterial colonization and frequent pneumonias. Typical early childhood pathogens include *Staphylococcus aureus* and *Haemophilus influenzae*. This is generally followed by colonization with *Pseudomonas aeruginosa* in late childhood and early adolescence; more than 90% of patients eventually acquire *P. aeruginosa*, and it is rarely eradicated. Colonization with *Burkholderia cepacia* is particularly ominous and may be associated with accelerated pulmonary deterioration and early death.

Gastrointestinal manifestations include pancreatic insufficiency, bowel obstruction and rectal prolapse, diabetes, and hepatic cirrhosis. Loss of pancreatic enzyme secretion leads to decreased fat absorption; parents may notice that the child's stools are large, bulky, and foul smelling. Later, stool becomes extremely dense, sometimes leading to distal intestinal obstruction. **Failure to thrive** is the most common

TABLE 20-7 Clinical Manifestations of Cystic Fibrosis

Chronic Sinopulmonary Disease

Persistent colonization/infection with pathogens typical of CF lung disease, including

  Staphylococcus aureus

  Pseudomonas aeruginosa (mucoid and nonmucoid)

  Nontypeable *Haemophilus influenzae*

  Burkholderia cepacia complex

  Stenotrophomonas maltophilia

Endobronchial Disease Manifested by

Cough and sputum production

Wheezing and air trapping

Radiographic abnormalities

Evidence of obstruction on PFTs

Digital clubbing

Chronic sinus disease

  Nasal polyps

  Radiographic changes

Intestinal Abnormalities

Meconium ileus

Exocrine pancreatic insufficiency

Distal intestinal obstruction

Rectal prolapse

Recurrent pancreatitis

Chronic hepatobiliary disease manifested by clinical and/or laboratory evidence of

  Focal biliary cirrhosis

  Multilobular cirrhosis

Failure to thrive (protein-calorie malnutrition)

Hypoproteinemia-edema

Fat-soluble vitamin deficiencies

Genitourinary Abnormalities

Obstructive azoospermia in males

Reduced fertility in females

Metabolic Abnormalities

Salt-loss syndromes

Acute salt depletion

Chronic metabolic alkalosis

---

manifestation of CF in infants and children. In the neonate, **meconium ileus** is virtually pathognomonic for CF.

Diagnostic Evaluation

The classic diagnostic findings in CF are related to the elevated sweat chloride concentration, pancreatic insufficiency, and chronic pulmonary disease. Recurrent lower airway infection results in bronchiectasis, fibrosis, parenchymal loss, and the characteristic bleb formation found on chest radiographs (Fig. 20-2). Pulmonary function tests demonstrate mostly obstructive and (later) some restrictive changes. The **sweat chloride test** is the initial diagnostic study of choice. A level greater than 60 mEq/L is generally considered abnormal, but both false positives and false negatives occur, and occasionally a borderline test is hard to interpret. Sweat testing, though simple in concept, is difficult in practice, and should only be performed in specialized centers with experience and expertise. Genetic and prenatal testing are now available; the finding of two mutations at the CFTR site, known to produce disease, is considered diagnostic of CF. Some mutations produce less CFTR dysfunction;

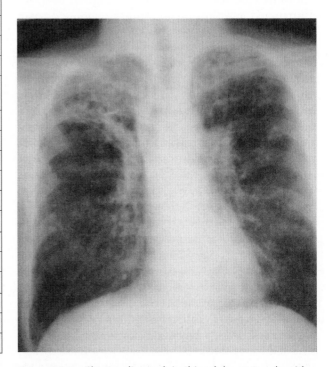

Figure 20-2 • Chest radiograph in this adolescent male with cystic fibrosis demonstrates marked chronic disease and bleb formation.

if at least 10% of normal CFTR activity is present, the individual may remain symptom free.

Treatment

The most fundamental aspect of CF therapy is the maintenance of effective airway clearance. Chest physical therapy, vigorous exercise, and frequent coughing are helpful in mobilizing secretions. Bronchodilators relax smooth muscle walls and increase mucociliary clearance. Antibiotics decrease the production of bacterial toxins, reduce inflammation, and curb tissue destruction. Recombinant human deoxyribonuclease, administered via nebulization, breaks down thick DNA complexes present in mucus as a result of cell destruction and bacterial colonization. Alternate months of regular inhaled tobramycin may be indicated for patients infected with *Pseudomonas*. More recently, azithromycin has been added as a possible immune modifier.

Acute disease exacerbations may be triggered by viral or bacterial infections and are treated by more aggressive chest physical therapy and antibiotics, which may be taken orally or inhaled if the exacerbation is mild and the organisms are not resistant. Frequently, however, bacterial infections must be treated with an aminoglycoside (e.g., tobramycin) and a semisynthetic penicillin or cephalosporin, depending on organism sensitivities. Research aimed at the specific gene mutation is currently under way. Patients often improve in clinical status during hospital admission for reasons that are not entirely clear but may in part involve improved adherence to prescribed therapy and reduced exposure to allergens and other irritants.

Near-normal growth can often be achieved with pancreatic enzyme replacement, fat-soluble vitamin supplements, and high-calorie, high-protein diets. Nasogastric or gastrostomy tube feedings may be instituted if oral intake is inadequate. Maintenance of height and weight above the 25th percentile for age has a better long-term prognosis. Many patients develop relative insulin deficiency and may benefit from insulin therapy.

Prognosis continues to improve with aggressive treatment of pulmonary exacerbations and optimal nutritional support. Respiratory complications remain the major contributors to morbidity and mortality in CF.

Hemoptysis is an alarming development that may occur in patients with severe bronchiectasis. Frequent coughing and inflammation lead to erosion of the walls of bronchial arteries in areas of bronchiectasis, and expectorated sputum becomes streaked with blood. Frank blood loss of more than 500 mL in 24 hours (or more than 300 mL/day for 3 days) is considered an emergency, often requiring bronchial arterial embolization.

Spontaneous pneumothorax is another potentially life-threatening complication of CF. It is usually manifest by the sudden onset of severe chest pain and difficulty breathing. Placement of a chest tube results in rapid re-expansion, but approximately half of pneumothoraces recur unless pleurodesis is performed. Pleurodesis is generally avoided if possible because lung transplantation becomes more difficult following this procedure.

Progressive airway obstruction and hypoxia in advanced disease can lead to **chronic pulmonary hypertension** and **cor pulmonale**. For CF patients with a predicted life expectancy limited to 1 to 2 years, lung transplantation is a potentially viable option. Survival postlung transplantation is on the order of 50% at 5 years.

PRIMARY CILIARY DYSKINESIA

Primary ciliary dyskinesia (PCD) is a group of recessive disorders of ciliary structure/function in which mucociliary clearance is markedly impaired because of ciliary dysfunction. Failure to clear secretions leads to bronchial obstruction, sinusitis, chronic otitis media, and recurrent respiratory infections. Symptoms may be similar to those of CF or asthma. The diagnosis is made by demonstration of abnormal ciliary beat under light microscopy or characteristic ultrastructural changes in samples of ciliated cells obtained from scrapings of the nasal or bronchial epithelium. Treatment is similar to that of the pulmonary component of CF, although patients with PCD do not have the same propensity to infection with *P. aeruginosa*. Most patients with PCD develop bronchiectasis by the end of the second or third decade of life.

RESTRICTIVE LUNG DISEASES

Restrictive lung diseases result from decreased compliance of the chest wall or of the lung itself. They cause a decrease in most measurements of lung volume, including functional residual capacity, tidal volume, and vital capacity. Restrictive lung disease is much less common in the pediatric population than obstructive pulmonary disorders.

Pectus excavatum refers to a depression in the sternum, and **pectus carinatum** refers to an outward deformity. Severe congenital forms of these malformations may result in restrictive lung disease as a result of mechanical interference with normal respiration, but typically these deformities are more cosmetic than functional. Severe scoliosis will usually have a greater effect, with restriction as well as airway compression. Marked obesity, in addition to being a risk for upper airway obstructive disease, may also be a cause of restrictive lung disease. **Neuromuscular disease** may result in restrictive lung disease as a consequence of insufficient respiratory muscle strength (Guillain-Barré syndrome, muscular dystrophy, spinal muscular atrophy).

Any lesion that occupies intrathoracic space, if large enough, will interfere with normal pulmonary expansion. Pleural effusion, pericardial effusion, chylothorax, hemothorax, pneumothorax, chest wall tumors, mediastinal masses, congenital lobar emphysema, cystic adenomatous malformations, diaphragmatic hernias, and pulmonary sequestrations may all compete with normal lung for thoracic space, resulting in restrictive pulmonary compromise.

Interstitial lung disease refers to disorders in which there is disease in the tissues of the lung outside the airways and alveoli. This usually results in decreased compliance and therefore, restrictive physiology. A number of rare diseases can lead to interstitial changes, including chronic interstitial lung disease, desquamative interstitial pneumonitis, and sarcoidosis. **Pulmonary hemosiderosis** involves an abnormal accumulation of hemosiderin in the lungs as a result of diffuse alveolar hemorrhage. It may be idiopathic or the result of problems which produce repeated bleeding into the lung. Diagnosis is based on the presence of hemosiderin-laden macrophages (siderophages) in bronchial washings or gastric aspirates; a specific cause of the bleeding should be sought. Recurrent aspiration can also cause intersti-

---

■ TABLE 20-8 Apnea of Infancy: Apparent Life-Threatening Events

Cause	Helpful Diagnostic Tests
Infectious	
Sepsis	CBC/Blood culture
Meningitis	LP
Pneumonia	Chest radiograph
Bronchiolitis (RSV)	RSV antigen test in season
Pertussis	PCR or fluorescent antibody staining
Neurologic	
Seizures	EEG
Central apnea	Polysomnography
Intraventricular hemorrhage	Cranial US
Respiratory	
Airway obstruction	Airway radiographs or bronchoscopy
Aspiration	Swallowing study
Cardiac	
Arrhythmias	ECG
Gastrointestinal	
Gastroesophageal reflux	Barium swallow or pH/impedance probe
Other	
Metabolic disorders	Tests for inborn errors of metabolism
Electrolyte disorders	Electrolyte panel/blood glucose
Abuse	Skeletal survey/fundoscopic exam

tial disease, as can acute chest syndrome in sickle cell disease (see Chapter 10).

Symptoms of restrictive lung disease typically reflect decreased pulmonary compliance, which may not become clinically apparent until the process is relatively advanced. Exercise intolerance, tachypnea, and eventually dyspnea at rest are common. Space-occupying lesions may or may not be detected by chest auscultation (noting decreased breath sounds over the affected area) and may be seen on chest radiographs or even an echocardiogram. The chronic nature of many restrictive lesions can put patients at risk for developing prolonged respiratory insufficiency. Pulmonary hypertension may develop; an accentuated pulmonic component of the second heart sound may be heard, but echocardiography is usually the diagnostic method of choice. Clubbing of fingers and toes may be noted. Clinical manifestations of pulmonary hemosiderosis may include hemoptysis/hematemesis and a microcytic hypochromic anemia with elevated reticulocyte counts. Many patients with hemosiderosis are mistakenly diagnosed clinically to have recurrent pneumonia.

APNEA OF INFANCY

Apnea is defined as the cessation of breathing for longer than 20 seconds or pauses of any duration associated with color changes (cyanosis, pallor), hypoto-

nia, decreased responsiveness, or bradycardia. It may be central (neurally mediated), obstructive, or mixed. Apnea is not a diagnosis but a potentially dangerous sign requiring aggressive evaluation to define the underlying cause. In contrast to apnea of prematurity, apnea of infancy occurs in full-term infants. Table 20-8 lists some of the more common potential causes.

Apnea of infancy may come to medical attention after an **apparent life-threatening event** (ALTE). ALTEs are very frightening to the caretaker; the infant either stops breathing or is found apneic and may be cyanotic or pale, hypotonic, difficult to rouse, or choking and gagging. The observer often believes that the child would have died without intervention (vigorous stimulation, cardiopulmonary resuscitation).

The goal of the diagnostic workup is to identify or rule out any treatable, life-threatening causes. Table 20-8 lists potential tests to be considered depending on the results of the history and physical examination. In approximately half the cases of apnea of infancy, no predisposing condition is ever found.

Management involves treating the underlying disorder. When no treatable cause can be found, the infant may be placed on a home monitor that senses chest movement (breathing) and heart rate and sounds an alarm when the child becomes apneic or bradycardic. Apnea of infancy does not raise an infant's risk of dying of sudden infant death syndrome (SIDS), which may be why **home monitors have never been proven to decrease the likelihood of SIDS**.

KEY POINTS

- Infants with bilateral choanal atresia often present with life-threatening respiratory distress in the delivery room, although oxygenation improves when the infant is crying.

- Severe obstructive sleep apnea can result in cor pulmonale which may be fatal.

- The three main components of asthma are reversible airway obstruction, increased airway responsiveness, and inflammation. Disease severity is classified before the onset of treatment as intermittent, mild persistent, moderate persistent, and severe persistent.

- Inhaled bronchodilators are the treatment of choice in an acute asthma exacerbation. Inhaled corticosteroids are the treatment of choice for symptom control and avoidance of exacerbations for patients with persistent asthma.

- The disappearance of wheezing with increased respiratory distress signals increased obstruction rather than improvement.

- Cystic fibrosis (CF) is a disorder of exocrine gland function, affecting the lungs, sinuses, pancreas, sweat and salivary glands, intestines, and reproductive system. Failure to thrive is the most common presentation of CF in children. Meconium ileus in the neonate is virtually pathognomonic for CF.

- A diagnosis of CF is made by an elevated sweat chloride level in the presence of pulmonary disease/pancreatic insufficiency or by a genotype with two abnormal CFTR alleles.

- Apnea of infancy does not increase the risk of sudden infant death, and the use of home apnea monitors does not reduce the risk of SIDS.

Adolescent Medicine

Katie Fine

Puberty is defined as the process of hormonal and physical changes whereby the body of a child matures into that of an adult, physiologically capable of sexual reproduction. **Adolescence**, on the other hand, encompasses the physical changes of puberty as well as the cognitive, social, and psychological advances that mark the transition from youth to maturity. Some references further subdivide adolescence into an *early* period (middle school, age 10 to 13 years), a *middle* period (high school, age 14 to 17 years), and a *late* period (age 18 to 21 years). Developmental tasks of adolescence include:

- Achievement of independence (testing authority, establishing autonomy)
- Development of a strong self-identity (defining the self, maintaining healthy self-esteem)
- Establishing appropriate peer relationships
- Transition from relatively concrete thinking to more abstract concepts, such as cause/effect, long-term consequences, and complicated moral dilemmas

Although adolescents are less likely than younger children to regularly appear for health maintenance visits, regular contact with a primary care physician is particularly important in this age group. Many of the diseases and injuries that occur in adolescence result from lifestyle choices that increase the risk of morbidity and mortality. Such behaviors include high-risk sexual activity, eating disorders, substance use and abuse, and actions resulting in accidental or intentional injury.

THE ADOLESCENT OFFICE VISIT

Observing the parent–child interaction is informative, and the parent should be encouraged to raise any concerns with the physician. However, it is imperative that *the majority of the interview and exam take place without the parent present*, particularly in the middle and older adolescent. Many teenagers will not be forthright about health-related issues when they believe their parents may find out about their responses. While virtually all states mandate the reporting of suspected abuse, potential harm (violence or suicide), and certain infectious diseases (including some sexually transmitted diseases [STDs]), most also provide for **confidentiality** of information related to sexual activity and substance abuse. Some states allow all adolescents access to medical care without their parents' knowledge; in other states, only emancipated minors are permitted this right. Emergency treatment should never be withheld pending parental notification or approval.

Although studies show that adolescents are willing to discuss high-risk behaviors and preventative care issues with their physicians, most are uncomfortable initiating these conversations themselves. The acronym HEADSS (Table 21-1) is helpful in identifying pertinent areas in the adolescent social history. An indirect, nonjudgmental method of questioning may be more effective in eliciting truthful answers.

Height, weight, and blood pressure should be recorded at every adolescent health maintenance visit (or at least every 2 years). Other recommended procedures include a hearing screen (once during adolescence); a vision screen (every 2 to 3 years); and hemoglobin/hematocrit, serum cholesterol, and urinalysis (at least once during adolescence). Tuberculosis testing is appropriate in individuals at high risk. The recommended examination and laboratory screening for sexually active patients is discussed in the following section. Immunizations recommended during adolescence are listed in Table 12-1.

■ **TABLE 21-1** The Adolescent Psychosocial History: HEADSS*

Home (family members, relationships, and living arrangements)
Education (academic performance/educational goals)
Activities (peer relationships, work and recreational activities)
Drugs (substance use/abuse, including tobacco, alcohol, steroids, inhalants, and illicit drugs)
Sexuality (dating, sexual activity, contraception, sexual orientation)
Suicide (depression, anxiety, other mental health concerns)

*Some experts suggest that a second "E" should be added to remind physicians to screen for behaviors associated with **E**ating disorders, and that a third "S" should be included to prompt questions concerning **S**afety (the potential for abuse or violent behavior [e.g., gang membership, owning a firearm]).

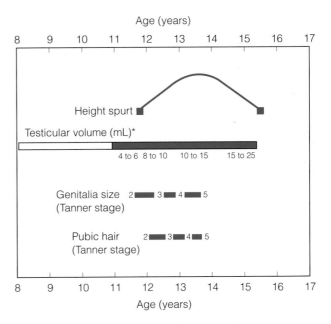

Figure 21-1 • Sequence of pubertal events in the average (American) male.

SEXUAL DEVELOPMENT/ REPRODUCTIVE HEALTH

As mentioned, **puberty** refers to those biologic changes that lead to reproductive capability. The events of puberty occur in a predictable sequence, but the timing of the initiation and the velocity of the changes are highly variable among individuals. The integration of the pubertal changes into the individual's self-identity is crucial to successful progression through adolescence.

In males, the initiation sequence of sexual development is testicular enlargement, followed by pubic hair growth, lengthening of the penis, and achievement of maximal height velocity. This progression is depicted in Figure 21-1.

In females, the order of pubertal events in sexual development is thelarche (breast budding), followed by pubarche, maximal height velocity, and menarche. Figure 21-2 shows these changes.

The **Tanner staging system** is used to determine where an individual is in the pubertal process. Tanner stages for the male genitalia, female breasts, and male and female pubic hair are described in Table 21-2 and illustrated in Figures 21-3 through 21-5. Pubertal abnormalities are addressed in Chapter 6 (Endocrinology).

About two-thirds of high school seniors in the latest Centers for Disease Control and Prevention survey reported that they had engaged in sexual in-

tercourse. Preventative healthcare for sexually active adolescents includes additional examination procedures and laboratory screening. Annual pelvic exams are recommended for all sexually active young women. Screening tests include Pap smear, cervical gonorrhea and chlamydia studies, and a wet mount

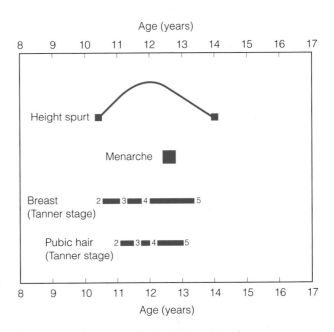

Figure 21-2 • Sequence of pubertal events in the average (American) female.

TABLE 21-2 Secondary Sex Characteristics: Tanner Sexual Maturity Rating (SMR) Scale

Breast development (females)	
Stage I	Preadolescent; elevation of papilla only
Stage II	Breast bud beneath the areola; enlargement of areolar diameter
Stage III	Further enlargement and elevation of breast and areola
Stage IV	Projection of areola to form secondary projection above contour of breast
Stage V	Mature stage; smooth breast contour
Note: Stages IV and V may not be distinct in some patients.	
Genital development (male)	
Stage I	Preadolescent
Stage II	Enlargement of scrotum and testes; skin of scrotum reddens and changes in texture
Stage III	Enlargement of penis, particularly length; further growth of testes and scrotum
Stage IV	Increased size of penis with growth in thickness and development of glans; further enlargement of testes and scrotum and increased darkening of scrotal skin
Stage V	Adult genitalia
Pubic hair (male and female)	
Stage I	Preadolescent (no pubic hair)
Stage II	Sparse growth of longer, slightly pigmented hair, chiefly at base of penis or along labia
Stage III	Increasingly darker, coarser, and more curled hair spreads over junction of pubis
Stage IV	Adult-type pubic hair with no spread to medial surface of thighs
Stage V	Adult in quantity and type with spread to thighs

of vaginal fluids. Adolescent males who are sexually active should have leukocyte esterase testing performed on first-void urine and should be offered urethral or urine-based nucleic acid amplification testing for gonorrhea and chlamydia. Screening for young men who report same-gender sexual contact includes anal and pharyngeal cultures for STDs as well as hepatitis B serology. Patients with evidence of an STD and/or self-report of high-risk behaviors should be offered contraception counseling and testing for syphilis and HIV.

EATING DISORDERS

PATHOGENESIS

The need to be attractive to peers leads to a preoccupation with body image during adolescence. **Anorexia nervosa** is an eating disorder characterized by impaired body image and intense fear of weight gain, culminating in the refusal to maintain at least 85% of normal body weight for age and height. External or internal psychological and/or social stressors superimposed on an inherited vulnerability lead to the development of anorexia.

Binge eating, followed by some compensatory behavior to rid the body of the ingested calories, is the hallmark of **bulimia nervosa**. Patients may purge (induce vomiting or take laxatives) or employ other methods (fasting, intense exercise). Bulimics are usually aware that their behavior is abnormal.

EPIDEMIOLOGY

Estimates of the incidence of anorexia in developed countries range from 1 in 200 to 1 in 2,000 adolescent females. Bulimia is more common, affecting 1% to 2% of Western young women. Up to 10% of patients with eating disorders are male.

RISK FACTORS

Risk factors for eating disorders include positive family history and female gender. Both anorexia and bulimia

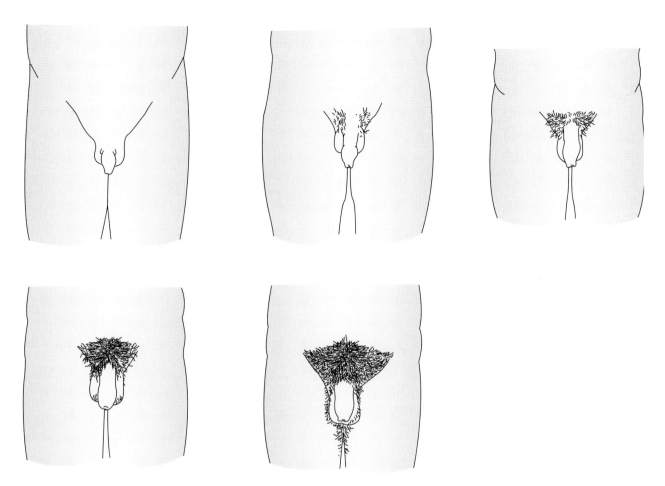

Figure 21-3 • Pictorial representation of Tanner stages of male genital and pubic hair development.

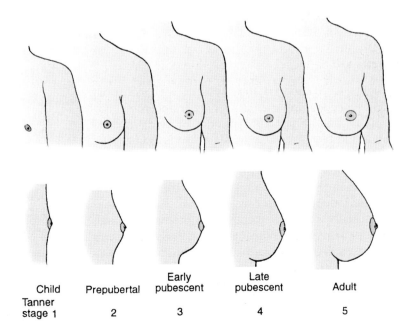

Figure 21-4 • Pictorial representation of Tanner stages of female breast development.

| Child Tanner stage 1 | Prepubertal 2 | Early pubescent 3 | Late pubescent 4 | Adult 5 |

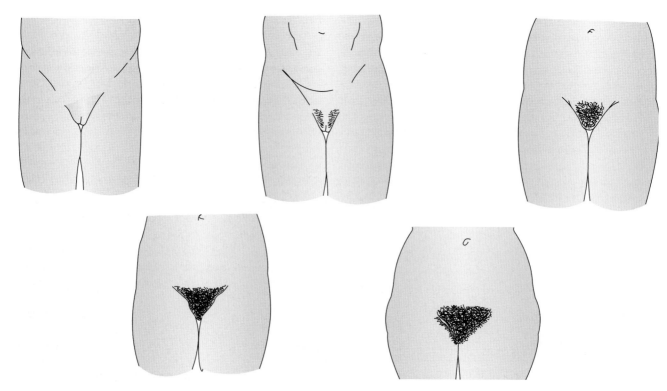

Figure 21-5 • Pictorial representation of Tanner stages of female pubic hair development.

are more common in Caucasians. Personality risk factors associated with anorexia nervosa include intense preoccupation with appearance, low self-esteem, and obsessive traits.

CLINICAL MANIFESTATIONS

History

Patients with anorexia may present with constipation, syncope, upper or lower gastrointestinal discomfort, and/or periodic episodes of cold, mottled hands and feet. *Secondary amenorrhea* is a diagnostic criterion for anorexia nervosa. If the chief complaint is weight loss, this invariably comes from the parents rather than the adolescent; patients with anorexia do not view their behavior as abnormal. Bulimia does not usually produce specific symptoms, although these patients are significantly more likely than their peers to suffer from major depression. Patients may be brought to the physician because they have been caught purging or because their behavior has been reported by someone else.

Physical Exam

Adolescents who suffer from anorexia are severely underweight (usually with a body mass index <17) and may appear cachectic. Vital signs often reveal hypothermia, bradycardia, and orthostatic hypotension. The skin may be dry, yellowish, and hyperkeratotic. Thinning of scalp hair, increased lanugo hair, cool extremities, and nail pitting are additional signs. Thirty to 40% of patients will have a cardiac murmur consistent with mitral valve prolapse.

Patients with bulimia may be of normal weight or slightly overweight. Frequent self-induced vomiting (if present) results in calluses on the backs of the knuckles, eroded tooth enamel, and parotid gland enlargement.

DIFFERENTIAL DIAGNOSIS

Adolescents who participate in certain athletic activities (ballet, wrestling, gymnastics, cheerleading) in which weight gain is thought to negatively impact performance may manifest some of the behaviors associated with eating disorders such as purging and severe calorie restriction. However, most of these elite athletes have a normal body image.

The marked weight loss seen with anorexia may cause the clinician to consider malignancy, inflammatory bowel disease or malabsorption syndromes, and other chronic diseases (infections, endocrine disorders). The differential diagnosis for vomiting (bulimia) is discussed in Chapter 8.

DIAGNOSTIC EVALUATION

Anorexia and bulimia are both clinical diagnoses. Laboratory studies are used to assess the need for specific medical intervention rather than to confirm the disease. Table 21-3 lists diagnostic tests that are used to rule out or quantify certain conditions associated with anorexia and bulimia.

TREATMENT

The treatment for eating disorders is multifactorial and includes nutritional support, behavioral and psychotherapy, and correction of any medical complications resulting from the severe weight loss or purging. Indications for hospitalization/inpatient therapy are noted in Table 21-4. Research is ongoing as to whether psychotropic medicines (particularly selective serotonin reuptake inhibitors) are useful in the treatment of these diseases. Full recovery can take up to several years and is more common in adolescents with bulimia. The publish mortality rate for adolescents with anorexia ranges as high as 4%.

SUBSTANCE USE AND ABUSE

Drug use is defined as the intentional use of any substance that results in alteration of the physical, psychological, cognitive, or mood state of the individual

■ TABLE 21-3 Suggested Laboratory Tests for Adolescents with Eating Disorders

Study	Suspected Result
All patients	
Complete blood count	Neutropenia; also anemia and thrombocytopenia
Serum electrolytes	Hypokalemia/alkalosis (if purging)
	Hyponatremia (due to manipulation of water intake)
Blood urea nitrogen/creatinine	Increased BUN
Glucose	Normal or low
Calcium/phosphate/magnesium	Normal or low
Electrocardiogram	Bradycardia, T-wave inversions, ST depression (anorexia)
	Prolonged QTc interval (bulimia, if hypokalemic)
Patients with anorexia	
ESR*	Normal or low
Urinalysis	Decreased specific gravity
Liver function tests	Elevated
Cholesterol	Elevated
Serum protein/albumin	Low
TSH/T_4	Normal/normal to low
Bone density scan	Osteopenia (if amenorrheic >6 mo)
Patients with bulimia	
Serum amylase	Elevated if vomiting

*Useful for ruling out other conditions in the differential.
ESR, erythrocyte sedimentation rate; TSH, thyroid stimulating hormone

■ TABLE 21-4 Anorexia and Bulimia: Indications for Hospitalization

Both conditions
Failure to improve with outpatient therapy
Hypokalemia (serum potassium <3.2 mmol/L)
Hypochloremia (serum chloride <88 mmol/L)
Cardiac arrhythmias/prolonged QTc interval/bradycardia
Medical complications requiring inpatient intervention
Anorexia
Unstable vital signs
Severe weight loss
Need for enteral nutrition (food refusal)
Arrested pubertal development

despite the potential for personal harm. Patients become addicted when they begin to use the drug in a compulsive, dependent manner despite significant functional impairment (**drug abuse**). This addiction can result from *physical dependence* (physiological symptoms of withdrawal when the drug is removed) or *psychological dependence*. Adolescents may have poor impulse control and prefer instant gratification, leading to high-risk behavior such as drug experimentation. The various substances that are used and abused by adolescents are listed in Table 21-5.

EPIDEMIOLOGY

Unfortunately, substance use among adolescents is not uncommon. Estimates (based on anonymous self-reports) are that about half of 18-year-olds have tried an illegal drug. One in three has used an illicit drug other than marijuana. At least 30% admit to binge drinking within the previous month. More than 1 in 4 high school students reports daily tobacco use. Almost as many admit to marijuana use within the last 30 days. Marijuana, a "gateway" drug, is the most commonly used illicit drug in the United States.

RISK FACTORS

Risk factors and protective factors related to substance use in adolescents are listed in Table 21-6.

CLINICAL MANIFESTATIONS

The clinical manifestations of acute intoxication with the substances of interest are listed in Table 21-5, along with specific treatments for each drug.

Adolescents should be questioned at every maintenance visit regarding tobacco, alcohol, and substance use.

DIAGNOSTIC EVALUATION

Although drug testing is easily available through most labs, testing an adolescent at the request of the parents without the patient's knowledge is generally discouraged. Attempts should be made to involve the suspected user in the discussion and obtain consent for any recommended diagnostic studies.

MANAGEMENT

Patients suspected of drug/alcohol dependence should be referred to an addiction specialist and may require intensive inpatient or outpatient therapy. Adolescents who use tobacco must be encouraged and supported to quit. If the patient is interested in smoking cessation, nicotine replacement therapy ("the patch," gums, etc.) should be offered. Some adolescents may require more intensive behavioral therapy or bupropion.

VIOLENCE IN THE ADOLESCENT POPULATION

EPIDEMIOLOGY

Traumatic injury is the leading cause of death in the adolescent population (Chapter 2). Homicide and suicide are second and third on this list, respectively. Adolescents may be victims of violence, perpetrators of violence against others, and/or intentionally harmful to themselves.

RISK FACTORS

Individual risk factors for violent behavior include previous arrest for juvenile crime, early exposure to violence (domestic violence and in the media), being a victim of abuse, and drug and alcohol use. While young women are more likely than young men to experience sexual abuse, adolescent males are far more likely to be the victims and perpetrators of violent acts. Other factors associated with an increased likelihood of violent behavior include low socioeconomic status and easy access to guns.

The strongest risk factor associated with attempted suicide is a **prior attempt**. Other factors that increase the likelihood of attempted suicide include an existing psychiatric disorder (depression, etc.), substance abuse, a history of being abused, a family history of a major affective disorder and/or suicide, and a recent life stressor. *Adolescents who live in a home with a firearm have a 10-fold greater risk of suicide than their peers.*

CLINICAL MANIFESTATIONS

Physicians and other healthcare personnel who interact regularly with adolescents are in a position to question them about whether they feel safe and whether they have witnessed or been the victims of aggression. Asking how patients deal with anger, if they have ever been in a fight, and whether there

■ **TABLE 21-5** Clinical Manifestations and Managements of Drug Intoxication in Adolescents

Substance	Symptoms of Acute Use	Signs of Acute Use	Specific Treatment
Alcohol	Decreased inhibition, impaired coordination, poor judgment; progressing to slurred speech, ataxia, confusion, coma, and respiratory depression	Nausea/vomiting, flushed skin, sluggish pupils, decreased reflexes, hypoglycemia	Respiratory support; gastric lavage/charcoal; thiamine, glucose administration as indicated
Marijuana	Euphoria, relaxation, impaired cognition; progressing to mood instability and hallucinations	Drowsiness, slowed reaction times, tachycardia, orthostatic hypotension, injected conjunctiva, dry mouth	Benzodiazepines if severe agitation present
MDMA (Ecstasy)	Sense of happiness, enhanced well-being; progressing to agitation, confusion, shock	Hyperthermia, hypertension, tachycardia, tachypnea, dilated pupils, agitation, hyponatremia	Activated charcoal; benzodiazepines for agitation/hypertension; fluid and electrolyte management; cooling blanket if needed
Cocaine/amphetamines	Elation, increased alertness, insomnia, anxiety; progressing to delirium, chest pain, psychosis, seizures, coma	Delirium, hyperthermia, tachycardia, hypertension, dilated pupils, hyperreflexia, tremor	Benzodiazepines/ haloperidol; cooling blanket if needed; treatment of hypertension, arrhythmias as indicated*
Phencyclidine (PCP)	Euphoria or anxiety, impaired cognition, ataxia, hallucinations; progressing to psychosis, respiratory depression, coma, death	Restlessness, labile affect, hyperthermia, tachycardia, hypertension, flushing, nystagmus, small pupils, impaired coordination, seizures	Respiratory support, gastric lavage/charcoal, benzodiazepines/halo- peridol, treatment of hypertension, seizures if indicated
Hallucinogens (including LSD)	Euphoria, increased alertness; progressing to nausea, anxiety, paranoia, hallucinations, seizures, coma	Restlessness, labile affect, hyperthermia, tachycardia, hypertension, flushing, dilated pupils with injected conjunctiva, hyperreflexia	"Talking down" in a calm environment with minimal stimulation; benzodia- zepines; cooling blanket if hyperthermic; treatment of hypertension, seizures as indicated
Heroin	Euphoria followed by sedation, impaired cognition, nausea/vomiting, stupor, respiratory depression, coma	Altered (depressed) mental status, hypo- thermia, decreased respiratory rate, hypotension; pinpoint, unresponsive pupils	Cardiorespiratory support; gastric lavage, charcoal (if ingested); naloxone
Inhalants	Euphoria, impaired judgment; progressing to hallucinations, psychosis, seizures, coma	Agitation or stupor, slurred speech, nystagmus/ eye watering, rhinorrhea, increased salivation	Cardiorespiratory support if needed

*Lidocaine should not be used to treat arrhythmias in patients with cocaine intoxication because it can precipitate seizures in this population.

■ TABLE 21-6 Risk Factors for Substance Use

Illicit drugs
Genetic predisposition (for addiction)
Use of drugs by family and friends
Easy access to drugs
Low levels of parental involvement and support
Poverty
Academic failure
Alcohol
Genetic predisposition (for alcoholism)
Use and abuse of alcohol by parents, peers
Low levels of parental involvement
Tobacco
Parental smoking and tobacco use
Easy access to cigarettes, other tobacco products
No restrictions on smoking in the home
Protective factors
Stable home environment
Parental supervision
Membership in positive social organizations
Academic achievement
Association with abstinent peers

needed to make the transition to a productive adulthood and limit involvement with the juvenile justice system.

As previously mentioned, doctor-patient confidentiality does not extend to information which suggests the potential for immediate harm. Any patient who attempts suicide, even if the attempt is interpreted as merely a "gesture," should be hospitalized and undergo psychiatric evaluation.

KEY POINTS

- It is recommended that adolescents receive a hearing screen, urinalysis, serum cholesterol, and hemoglobin/hematocrit at least once during adolescence. Height, weight, blood pressure, and vision screening should be completed at least every other year.

- In males, the initiation sequence of sexual development is testicular enlargement, followed by pubic hair growth, penile lengthening, and attainment of maximal height velocity.

- In females, the order of pubertal events in sexual development is thelarche (breast budding), followed by pubic hair growth, attainment of peak height velocity, and menarche.

- Annual pelvic examinations are recommended for all sexually active young women. Adolescent males who are sexually active should be offered testing for gonorrhea and chlamydia.

- Secondary amenorrhea is a diagnostic feature of anorexia nervosa. Mitral valve prolapse is not uncommon.

- Marijuana is the most commonly used illicit drug in the United States.

- Patients who are smokers should be encouraged to quit at each health visit. Those who express interest in doing so should be offered nicotine replacement therapy, behavioral therapy, social support, and (in some cases) bupropion.

- Traumatic injury is the leading cause of death in the adolescent population.

- Adolescents who live in a home with a firearm have a 10-fold greater risk of suicide than their peers.

is a gun in the home may also open avenues of discussion.

All adolescent patients should be subjected to screening questions for depression (sadness, despair, hopelessness) and, if these are positive, suicidal ideation. Those patients who admit to having a plan for suicide are at particular risk.

MANAGEMENT

Encouraging parents to limit exposure to violence in the media should be part of preventive health counseling beginning in the toddler years. Securing mental health services for the affected adolescent (and social services for the family) may provide the support

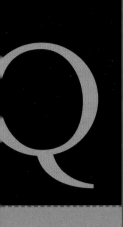
1. A 2-year-old female child presents with VT, severe ventricular dysfunction, hypotension, and metabolic acidosis. The patient is cardioverted into ventricular fibrillation which degenerates into asystole. What is the most appropriate indication for using intravenous epinephrine in this patient?
   a. ventricular ectopy
   b. asystole
   c. severe refractory metabolic acidosis and/or hyperkalemia
   d. bradycardia
   e. supraventricular tachycardia

2. A 16-year-old female patient presents with short stature and no secondary sexual characteristics. What diagnosis must be considered?
   a. Turner syndrome
   b. isolated growth hormone deficiency
   c. Cushing disease
   d. familial short stature
   e. Addison disease

3. Galactosemia, a disorder of carbohydrate metabolism, is inherited in an autosomal recessive fashion. What is the risk of galactosemia in a child whose parents are both carriers for the disorder?
   a. 100%
   b. 75%
   c. 50%
   d. 25%
   e. 0%

4. Which of the following statements is true regarding children with sickle cell disease?
   a. Vaccinations are not required because they receive penicillin prophylaxis.
   b. Gallstones typically develop before the age of 3 years.
   c. Episodes of dactylitis should be treated with antibiotics.
   d. Hydroxyurea maintenance therapy decreases the number and severity of vasoocclusive crises.
   e. Acute chest syndrome requires only supportive care.

5. A mother brings her 5-year-old son to your office in New Mexico for his regular health maintenance visit. A quick review of the patient's chart reveals that he and his family are strict vegans (i.e., they eat no animal products of any kind). Their house is very small, so all the children spend a good deal of time outside. The mother states that her son eats plenty of dark green vegetables and iron-fortified grains. She does not believe in providing supplemental vitamins and minerals. This child is most at risk for nutritional deficiency involving which of the following?
   a. vitamin B_{12}
   b. vitamin B_6
   c. niacin
   d. riboflavin
   e. vitamin D

6. A 6-year-old boy presents with a newly appreciated heart murmur. He is asymptomatic, with normal growth and development and normal exercise tolerance. On examination S1 and S2 are normal; a II/VI low-frequency midsystolic murmur is heard at the left lower sternal border. His pulses are normal. The most likely diagnosis is:
   a. bicuspid aortic valve
   b. Still's murmur
   c. ventricular septal defect
   d. atrial septal defect
   e. coarctation of the aorta

7. You are called to the delivery room for a routine birth. The infant cries when the cord is cut. You examine the child under the warmer and notice that when he stops crying, his chest heaves, and he turns blue. You are unable to pass the NG tube through the nose for suctioning. Which

condition is most likely causing this infant's respiratory distress?
a. choanal atresia or stenosis
b. vocal cord paralysis
c. subglottic stenosis
d. recurrent laryngeal nerve damage
e. laryngeal web

8. A 3-year-old girl is diagnosed with new-onset insulin-dependent diabetes mellitus. Which of the following laboratory findings is consistent with diabetic ketoacidosis?
a. hypoglycemia
b. hypercarbia
c. ketones in urine
d. increased venous blood pH
e. decreased BUN

9. During a male newborn examination, the testes are not palpable in the scrotal sacs. One testis is palpable high in the right inguinal canal and cannot be gently manipulated into the anatomically correct position. The left testis is not palpable but is discovered in the abdomen after consultation with a pediatric urologist and an abdominal ultrasound. In counseling the parents, which one of these statements regarding cryptorchidism is true?
a. More than 99% of males have bilateral descended testes at age 1 year.
b. Impaired sperm production is not a concern if neither testis descends.
c. Malignant degeneration is not a risk factor for testes which do not descend as long as they are placed within the scrotal sac through surgery by 1 year of age.
d. This infant is no more likely than his peers to manifest an inguinal hernia.
e. Microphallus is a common associated condition.

10. A 5-year-old boy presents with a waddling limp and has had a stiff right hip for the last 2 months. He has minimal complaints of pain. The most likely diagnosis is:
a. Legg-Calve-Perthes disease
b. slipped capital femoral epiphysis
c. toddler's fracture
d. septic arthritis
e. juvenile idiopathic arthritis

11. A 17-year-old young girl on oral contraceptive therapy for regulation of her menstrual periods presents with a 1-week history of left leg pain and swelling. Evaluation with a Doppler ultrasound reveals absence of flow in the left femoral and popliteal veins. The clot extends proximally to the left external iliac vein. The most important potential complication that one should be cautious about in this girl is:
a. venous insufficiency
b. limb overgrowth

c. pulmonary embolism
d. edema
e. gangrene

12. A woman with a seizure disorder under medical management wants to conceive a child. Her risk of having a child with a neural tube defect is greatest if her current medical regimen includes which of the following?
a. phenobarbital
b. phenytoin
c. ethosuximide
d. carbamazepine
e. primidone

13. A 2-month-old infant presents to your emergency department with a heart rate of 220 beats/minute, pulses, and adequate perfusion. After giving the infant oxygen, you note abnormal P waves and a narrow QRS (≤ 0.08 sec) on the cardiac monitor. Which of the following is the best course of action?
a. administer IV/IO epinephrine
b. administer IV adenosine by rapid bolus
c. administer IV calcium chloride
d. administer IV atropine by rapid bolus
e. administer IV sodium bicarbonate

14. A 3-month-old infant presents with a history of abnormal movements that his parents think might be seizures. You observe an episode of recurrent rhythmic flexor-extensor spasms that repeat about 30 times before subsiding. The EEG shows hypsarrhythmia, and a Wood lamp exam is positive for several flat, hypopigmented macules scattered over the skin surface. This child's infantile spasms are most likely a result of which of the following underlying disorders?
a. von Recklinghausen disease
b. tuberous sclerosis
c. von Hippel-Lindau disease
d. Sturge-Weber disease
e. bilateral acoustic neurofibromatosis

15. A 21-month-old girl arrives at clinic in May with a vaccination record that indicates that she has received 3 DTaP doses, 3 Hib doses, 3 IPV doses, 3 pneumococcal conjugate vaccine doses, 2 hepatitis A vaccine doses, and 3 hepatitis B vaccine doses. Which of the following should be administered at this visit?
a. DTaP, Hib, IPV, varicella
b. DTaP, Hib, pneumococcal conjugate vaccine, MMR, and varicella
c. DTaP, hepatitis A, IPV, pneumococcal conjugate vaccine
d. DTaP, hepatitis B, MMR, and varicella
e. DTaP, hepatitis A, IPV, MMR, and varicella

16. The mother of a 30-month-old boy is concerned that the child's speech is "garbled." The child uses "ma-ma" and "da-da" appropriately. He uses about 30 other words, but most of them are mispronounced (for instance, "boo" instead of "blue"). The boy's aunt, uncle, and cousins came to visit for a weekend and were unable to understand more than half of what he said. Examination of the ears reveals normal canals with translucent, mobile tympanic membranes, and visible landmarks. Which of the following evaluations for speech delay should be performed first?
    a. receptive language testing
    b. phonetic testing
    c. dysfluency evaluation
    d. tympanogram testing
    e. audiologic (hearing) assessment

17. A 13-year-old girl presents with recurrent abdominal pain over the last 3 months. She has missed a total of 8 days of school. There is no associated fever, weight loss, gastrointestinal bleeding, and the pain does not occur in relation to meals or awaken her from sleep. There is diffuse abdominal tenderness but no other abnormal findings on examination. Which approach is likely to help in the diagnosis and management of her condition?
    a. abdominal CT scan with contrast
    b. upper and lower endoscopy and biopsies
    c. explaining the likely etiology of her symptoms using a biopsychosocial model and symptomatic therapy
    d. a diet history and a diet elimination trial
    e. referral to a psychiatrist

18. A newborn male child has a flat facial profile, upslanted palpebral fissures, epicanthal folds, a small mouth with a protruding tongue, small genitalia, and simian creases on his hands. What of the following chromosomal disorders is most likely in this child?
    a. trisomy 21
    b. trisomy 18
    c. trisomy 13
    d. Klinefelter syndrome
    e. Turner syndrome

19. At a 2-year well-child visit, you collect information that your patient lives in a very old rental home with peeling paint. Both the capillary (screening) and venous blood lead measurements are 50 μg/dL. The patient has a history of constipation but is otherwise asymptomatic. Which of the following courses of action is most appropriate?
    a. Initiate chelation therapy in a lead-free environment within 48 hours.
    b. Redraw the blood lead level in 1 week and test all siblings; treat if ≥50 μg/dL.
    c. Optimize calcium and iron intake and repeat the blood lead level in 1 month; treat if ≥50 μg/dL.

    d. Refer the family to a lead-removal company; repeat the blood lead level 1 month after decontamination of the home, and treat if ≥50 μg/dL.
    e. Refer the case to child protective services for parental neglect.

20. A young couple is in your office for their prenatal visit, and you are discussing infant feeding. The father states that he prefers that the mother breastfeed the baby. The mother is hesitant to commit to breastfeeding because she plans on returning to full-time employment 6 weeks after the child is born. Neither her mother nor her sisters chose to breastfeed. She is concerned that human breast milk may not provide all the nutrients that the child needs, and she believes formula is a more complete nutritional source for infants. She is willing to consider exclusive breastfeeding based on the American Academy of Pediatrics recommendation. If her baby is exclusively breastfed, when should the child begin receiving oral vitamin D supplementation?
    a. never
    b. within the first month of life
    c. age 2 months
    d. age 4 months
    e. age 6 months

21. A 12-year-old female patient presents with fever, night sweats, weight loss, fatigue, anorexia, and painless, rubbery, cervical lymphadenopathy. What is the most common presentation of Hodgkin disease?
    a. fever, night sweats, and/or weight loss of >10% in the preceding 6 months (i.e., "B" symptoms)
    b. mediastinal lymphadenopathy
    c. painless, rubbery, cervical lymphadenopathy
    d. pruritus
    e. extreme fatigue and anorexia

22. Which of the following medication groupings is most appropriate for a patient 12 years old with persistent asthma who has failed to achieve well-controlled asthma while receiving step 2 treatment?
    a. none
    b. a daily low-dose inhaled corticosteroid
    c. a daily medium-dose inhaled corticosteroid and a long-acting inhaled β-2-agonist
    d. a daily low-dose inhaled corticosteroid and a long-acting β-agonist
    e. a daily medium-dose inhaled corticosteroid and nedocromil

23. Crops of papular, vesicular, pustular lesions starting on the trunk and spreading to the extremities, in addition to small, irregular red spots with central gray or bluish-white

specks that appear on the buccal mucosa, is the classic description of which of the following infections?
a. measles
b. erythema infectiosum (fifth disease)
c. roseola infantum
d. zoster (shingles)
e. rubella
f. hand-foot-mouth disease
g. chickenpox

24. A 20-month-old boy who was treated with high-dose amoxicillin (90 mg/kg per day) for acute otitis media 3 weeks ago now presents with acute-onset ear pain, a bulging, erythematous right tympanic membrane, and decreased mobility on pneumatic otoscopy examination. Which of the following is the most appropriate antibiotic choice for this child?
a. azithromycin
b. amoxicillin-clavulanate
c. erythromycin
d. trimethoprim-sulfamethoxazole
e. dicloxacillin

25. Which of the following is considered a risk factor for neonatal respiratory distress syndrome?
a. neonatal sepsis
b. poorly controlled maternal diabetes
c. maternal preeclampsia
d. neural tube defects
e. trisomy 21

26. A mildly febrile 6-year-old patient presents to your office with dysuria and urinary frequency and urgency. She has a history of one prior UTI about 8 months ago. You obtain a dipstick urinalysis and send a urine culture. The dipstick is positive for nitrites and leukocyte esterase. Which of the following is the most appropriate course of action at this time?
a. Await culture results and tailor therapy based on bacterial sensitivities.
b. Begin empiric amoxicillin.
c. Begin empiric amoxicillin and schedule the child for a renal ultrasound within the next 6 weeks.
d. Begin empiric amoxicillin and schedule the child for a renal ultrasound and voiding cystourethrogram within the next 6 weeks.
e. Admit the child to the hospital for IV ampicillin and gentamycin and schedule a DMSA scan.

27. A 3-month-old infant presents with cyanosis and an echocardiogram reveals that the child has tetralogy of Fallot. What four associated lesions describe tetralogy of Fallot?
a. ventricular septal defect, over-riding aorta, pulmonary stenosis, right ventricular hypertrophy

b. ventricular septal defect, atrial septal defect, pulmonary stenosis, right ventricular hypertrophy
c. ventricular septal defect, atrial septal defect, aortic stenosis, right ventricular hypertrophy
d. ventricular septal defect, coarctation of the aorta, aortic stenosis, right ventricular hypertrophy
e. ventricular septal defect, mitral valve prolapse, pulmonary stenosis, left ventricular hypertrophy

28. A 3-year-old boy with a known diagnosis of factor XI deficiency presents to the emergency department with uncontrolled bleeding from a lip laceration following a fall. The most appropriate product that can be used for factor replacement in this child prior to suturing is:
a. cryoprecipitate
b. granulocyte infusions
c. fresh frozen plasma (FFP)
d. platelet transfusion
e. DDAVP

29. At the health maintenance visit for a 12-year-old male, you note that he has entered his pubertal height growth spurt. The patient's mother asks about what changes her son should be expecting in his body over the next several years. As part of your review, you mention that the most typical sequence of pubertal events in males is which of the following?
a. peak height velocity, pubarche, penile enlargement, testicular enlargement
b. peak height velocity, testicular enlargement, penile enlargement, pubarche
c. testicular enlargement, pubarche, penile enlargement, peak height velocity
d. testicular enlargement, peak height velocity, penile enlargement, pubarche
e. pubarche, testicular enlargement, peak height velocity, penile enlargement

30. A 4-year-old child with known asthma presents to the emergency department with a chief complaint of wheezing for the past 8 hours. On examination he is alert and cooperative, mildly tachypneic, has diffuse loud expiratory wheeze, and has a pulse oximetry reading of 89% while breathing room air. He has already taken 3 albuterol aerosols at home in the past hour. He is unchanged after receiving another albuterol inhalation treatment in the emergency department. Appropriate next management would include:
a. supplemental oxygen
b. albuterol inhalation
c. ipratropium bromide inhalation
d. oral corticosteroids
e. all of the above

31. A previously healthy 3-year-old boy presents with a history of fever and diarrhea for the past 2 days. The fever has not responded to ibuprofen, and his urine output has decreased today. On examination, he is alert, has a temperature of 101°F, heart rate of 115 beats per minute, blood pressure of 105/60 mm Hg, and mild diffuse abdominal tenderness. The serum electrolytes are normal, but his BUN is 60 mg/dL and his serum creatinine is 1.8 mg/dL. The complete blood count is normal. Urinalysis shows 1+ protein, small blood, and occasional hyaline casts. The kidney ultrasound is normal. Which of the following statements regarding his acute renal failure is most accurate?
   a. It is due to hemolytic-uremic syndrome.
   b. It is due to pyelonephritis.
   c. It is due to interstitial nephritis.
   d. It is due to the use of ibuprofen in a dehydrated state.
   e. It is due to urinary tract obstruction.

32. A 14-year-old girl presents with several weeks of profound fatigue, intermittent low-grade fevers, a facial rash, and joint pain. The rash recently worsened markedly after sun exposure. On physical examination, she has a malar rash extending over the bridge of the nose, but sparing the nasolabial folds, painless oral ulcers, and painful limitation of movement in her wrists and finger joints. On laboratory testing, her WBC is 3,500/mm^3, Hgb 9.5 g/dL, platelet count 120,000/mm^3. A urinalysis shows 15 to 19 RBC/hpf and an elevated protein of 100 mg/dL. Which of the following tests will most likely be positive?
   a. antinuclear (ANA) antibody
   b. rheumatoid factor (RF)
   c. anti-double-stranded DNA (dsDNA) antibody
   d. anti-Smith (Sm) antibody
   e. anti-Ro (SS-A) antibody

33. A 3-month-old female infant presents to your emergency department unresponsive and with fever, tachypnea, bradycardia, and hypotension. What order should you follow in your initial assessment?
   a. airway, breathing, circulation, disability, exposure
   b. breathing, airway, circulation, disability, exposure
   c. circulation, airway, breathing, exposure, disability
   d. exposure, breathing, airway, circulation, disability
   e. exposure, airway, breathing, circulation, disability

34. A 4-year-old male child presents with abrupt-onset petechiae and ecchymoses. Other than the skin findings, the child appears well and is hemodynamically stable. No splenomegaly is noted. A complete blood count reveals a normal white blood cell count, a normal hematocrit, and a platelet count of 12,000 per mm^3. Large platelets are seen on the peripheral smear. No premature white cell forms are seen on peripheral smear. The parent reports that the child had a viral illness 2 weeks before presentation. Which of the following is the *most* likely diagnosis?
   a. isoimmune thrombocytopenia
   b. leukemia
   c. sepsis
   d. immune thrombocytopenic purpura
   e. hypersplenism

35. A child presents with a reduced number of CD3+ T cells, an increased number of B lymphocytes that are mildly abnormal in function, has a conotruncal heart lesion, hypoplastic thymus, and hypocalcemia. Which of the following chromosomal disorders is most likely in this child?
   a. Zellweger syndrome
   b. microdeletion of 22q11.2
   c. trisomy 13
   d. Gaucher disease
   e. Wilson disease

36. A 4-month-old former 30-week premature infant is seen in late October for well-child care. His mother is concerned about the transfusions that the infant required during her course in the neonatal intensive care unit and wishes to restrict her exposure to blood products. Referral for administration of which of the following would be most appropriate to limit her risk of severe bronchiolitis?
   a. ribavirin
   b. nasal influenza vaccine
   c. injected influenza vaccine
   d. IV RespiGam
   e. IM palivizumab

37. The mother of a 2-month-old infant brings her daughter to your office during the summer for her regular health maintenance visit. The child is cared for by her maternal grandmother 3 days a week while the mother is at work. The infant is exclusively fed a cow milk-based commercial formula when she is with the mother; the grandmother believes that the child should also receive juice diluted with water due to the warm weather. Which of the following represents the most appropriate dietary counseling regarding this infant's diet?
   a. Formula-fed infants at this age require free water supplementation during warm months to maintain optimal hydration.
   b. Formula-fed infants at this age require glucose supplementation during the warm months to maintain optimal caloric intake.
   c. Formula-fed infants do not require any additional vitamin, mineral, caloric, or fluid supplement beyond their formula for the first 6 months of life.

d. Dilution of this infant's formula with water or juice on the days that she is with the maternal grandmother is unnecessary but harmless.

e. This infant should be switched to a soy protein-based formula.

38. No red reflex is seen on funduscopic examination of a newborn. Which of the following is the most likely diagnosis?

a. retinoblastoma

b. leukocoria

c. congenital cataract

d. congenital glaucoma

e. toxocariasis

39. A 5-year-old boy is brought to your office complaining of progressive fatigue, weakness, and nausea over the past few months. He was a model student, but he is now having trouble in school and displaying frequent outbursts, the last of which resulted in his being sent home for hitting another child. Initial lab results show mild hypoglycemia, hyponatremia, and hyperkalemia. The child is diagnosed with adrenal insufficiency and treated appropriately; however, his behavior continues to worsen, and he begins to have difficulty walking and speaking. Which of the following is the most likely etiology of his behavior problems?

a. Tay-Sachs disease

b. Gaucher disease

c. Niemann-Pick disease

d. adrenoleukodystrophy

e. Rett syndrome

40. An 8-year-old girl thought to have attention-deficit disorder (inattentive-type) undergoes EEG testing and is found to have a 3-Hz spike-and-wave pattern. Results of the EEG, coupled with videotaping of episodes of the patient's "inattention," lead to a diagnosis of childhood absence epilepsy. Which of the following is most appropriate for initial treatment of the child's disorder?

a. methylphenidate

b. carbamazepine

c. ACTH

d. ethosuximide

e. phenobarbital

41. A child presents with lymphedema of the hands and feet, a shield-shaped chest, widely spaced hypoplastic nipples, short stature, and multiple pigmented nevi. In addition, she had a coarctation of the aorta that was repaired and has renal disease. Her parents continue to be worried that there is something in addition to her heart condition that is causing failure to thrive. Which of the following chromosomal disorders is most likely in this child?

a. trisomy 21

b. trisomy 18

c. trisomy 13

d. Klinefelter syndrome

e. Turner syndrome

42. A 14-year-old patient familiar to the emergency room staff due to multiple visits in the last 3 months is brought in by her mother for ingestion of an unknown number of acetaminophen tablets. The mother states that she keeps all the medicines in the house locked up because "this is just the sort of thing my daughter would do to me." She saw the girl stuffing something into her bedside drawer while she was passing the girl's room and discovered a bottle marked "acetaminophen, 250 tablets." Only 4 tablets remained in the bottle. The mother did not believe that the daughter took the tablets until she began vomiting about an hour later. The girl refuses to speak in her mother's presence but eventually admits that she took "many tablets" about 4:00 p.m. (3 hours ago). Which of the following is recommended as an antidote for this patient's ingestion?

a. atropine sulfate

b. hemodialysis

c. whole bowel irrigation

d. oral *N*-acetyl cysteine

e. activated charcoal

43. Which of the following scenarios is consistent with abuse rather than accidental injury?

a. a 30-month-old child with a bucket handle fracture

b. a 12-month-old infant with a rib fracture

c. a 6-month-old infant with retinal hemorrhages in the absence of signs of external head trauma

d. abdominal bruises in a 9-month-old infant

e. all of the above

44. A 2-year-old presents with painless rectal bleeding. The hemoglobin is 9 g/dL. Capillary refill remains normal. The best next step to positively identify the cause of bleeding is:

a. colonoscopy

b. transfusion with packed red blood cells

c. meckel diverticulum scan

d. gastric lavage

e. stool culture

45. A 3-week-old male infant presents to the emergency department with 24-hour history of vomiting and poor feeding. He is found to be hypotensive and hypoglycemic. His serum electrolyte values are as follows: Na 121 mmol/L, K 6.9 mmol/L, CO_2 20 mmol/L, chloride 105 mmol/L, BUN 17 mg/dL, creatinine 0.7 mg/dL, glucose 36 mg/dL. He receives 20 mL/kg NS fluid bolus and 2 mL/kg dextrose 25. What other life-saving intervention should this infant receive?

a. IV azithromycin

b. IV bicarbonate

c. IV hydrocortisone

d. IV albumin

e. IV calcium

46. A 7-year-old girl presents with a 3-week history of dozens of asymptomatic red, scaly 5 to 10 mm plaques appearing on the trunk. When the scales are pulled off, they bleed. Her nails are pitted. The most appropriate laboratory test is:

a. a bacterial culture of the red plaques

b. a fungal culture of the red plaques

c. a throat culture

d. a Tzanck smear

e. a complete blood count

47. An 8-year-old patient of yours with attention-deficit/hyperactivity disorder is experiencing unacceptable adverse effects due to his stimulant medication. You have prescribed immediate- and extended-release preparations of two separate agents in the past. You believe that the patient may benefit from switching to a nonstimulant medication. Which of the following medications approved for the treatment of attention-deficit/hyperactivity disorder is classified as a nonstimulant?

a. oral atomoxetine

b. oral lisdexamfetamine

c. oral methylphenidate

d. oral dextroamphetamine

e. oral mixed amphetamine salts

48. A 9-month-old girl presents with a 3-day history of fever to 103°F (39.4°C). This morning, the girl developed a rash. On physical examination, the girl is afebrile and has an erythematous, maculopapular rash over her trunk, arms, and legs. Which of the following is the most likely cause of this patient's illness?

a. human parvovirus B19

b. measles

c. human herpesvirus 6

d. chickenpox

e. group A beta-hemolytic streptococci

49. A 2-year-old child is brought to the emergency department following a brief (<2 minutes) generalized seizure. Initial vitals include a temperature of 102.9°F. Following the history, physical examination, and laboratory studies, you determine that the patient has had a febrile seizure. The parents are appropriately concerned and have a number of questions. You would be correct in telling them which of the following?

a. Children who experience a single febrile seizure have no greater risk of subsequently developing epilepsy than children who have not experienced a febrile seizure.

b. The morbidity and mortality associated with febrile seizures is extremely high.

c. At least half of patients who experience an initial febrile seizure will experience seizures with subsequent episodes of fever.

d. Patients who have experienced a single febrile seizure should be placed on preventative anticonvulsant medication.

e. Febrile seizures are usually associated with intracranial infections.

50. A 3-year-old boy presents with an elbow hemarthrosis after falling on his elbow. There is no history of spontaneous bleeding. There is no history of epistaxis, gingival bleeding, or cutaneous bruising. The child's maternal grandfather had frequent spontaneous bleeding and hemarthroses after trauma on multiple occasions. Laboratory results revealed a prolonged PTT, normal PT, and a platelet count of 150,000 per mm^3. The factor VIII coagulant activity (VIII:c) is low and the factor IX level is normal. What is the most likely diagnosis?

a. idiopathic thrombocytopenic purpura

b. von Willebrand disease

c. vitamin K deficiency

d. hemophilia A

e. liver disease

51. A 10-week-old boy is brought to the emergency department by his mother with a history of failure to thrive and poor feeding. He occasionally vomits small amounts of formula. His birth weight, length, and head circumference were at the 50th percentile; however, his weight has dropped to the 10th percentile and his length to between 25th and 40th percentiles. His vital signs are normal, and the physical exam is otherwise unrevealing. Venous blood gas and electrolyte study results include: pH 7.32, sodium 134 mEq/L, potassium 4.5 mEq/L, chloride 106 mEq/L, and bicarbonate 10 mEq/L. Which of the following diagnoses is the most likely?

a. inborn error of metabolism

b. renal tubular acidosis

c. pyloric stenosis

d. chronic diarrhea

e. cystic fibrosis

52. A 2-year-old girl presents with a swollen left knee, limping, and morning stiffness in the left knee of 3 months' duration. On physical examination, there is a left knee joint effusion, synovial thickening, and limitation of movement. In addition, the left leg is longer than the right and there is atrophy of the quadriceps. The remainder of the review of systems and physical examinations is normal. On laboratory testing, a complete blood count is normal. An antinuclear (ANA) antibody test is positive at

a titer of 1:320. This child is at most risk for which of the following sequelae/complications?

a. glomerulonephritis
b. hemolytic anemia
c. chronic, nongranulomatous anterior uveitis (iridocyclitis)
d. acute anterior uveitis (iridocyclitis)
e. rheumatic heart disease

53. A 9-year-old boy diagnosed with pneumonia 2 days ago presents to the emergency department via ambulance in respiratory distress. His past medical history is noncontributory, and he is at low risk for contracting tuberculosis. He is hypoxic and requires oxygen. A STAT portable chest radiograph reveals a large right-sided pleural effusion, which shifts in the decubitus position. Fluid is obtained via thoracentesis for Gram stain and culture. Which of the following is the most likely pathogen responsible for this boy's pneumonia?

a. *Staphylococcus aureus*
b. Nontypeable *Haemophilus influenzae*
c. *Chlamydophila pneumoniae*
d. *Klebsiella pneumoniae*
e. *Mycoplasma pneumoniae*

54. During a routine annual physical examination, a 9-year-old previously healthy girl has a blood pressure of 140/75 mm Hg in all four extremities. The physical examination is otherwise completely normal, except for obesity. The family history is positive for hypertension in the father and paternal uncle. The blood pressure remains in the 140/70 mm Hg range on two repeat examinations performed 1 week apart, using a cuff that is appropriate for her obesity. The urinalysis, serum electrolytes, and serum creatinine levels are normal. Which of the following is the most appropriate next step in the management of this patient?

a. Reassure the patient that her blood pressure is normal for her size.
b. Advise observation, with repeat blood pressure checks every month.
c. Advise an immediate evaluation by a nephrologist and cardiologist.
d. Advise a regimen of weight reduction and regular exercise.
e. Advice a regimen of diuretic therapy.

55. A parent brings her 12-week-old child to your office because he has a scaly facial rash. The boy was exclusively breastfed for 8 weeks but was switched to commercial cow milk-based formula about a month ago when his mother went back to work. She has been putting lotion on the rash, but it has not helped. The child's birth weight was at the 50th percentile but has now dropped toward the 25th percentile line. The physical examination reveals an eczematous rash over both cheeks. The stool is guaiac-positive but not grossly bloody. Based on the history and physical examination, you suspect that the patient may be allergic to cow milk protein. Which of the following is the best next step in the management of this patient?

a. Recommend that the mother see her obstetrician about medication to help her begin lactating again.
b. Switch the patient from cow milk-based formula to whole cow's milk.
c. Switch the patient from cow milk-based formula to soy formula.
d. Switch the patient from cow milk-based formula to a protein hydrolysate formula.
e. Begin parenteral alimentation to permit total bowel rest.

56. A 16-year-old male is brought to your office by his mother, who insists that you perform a urine drug screen on her son. You begin by interviewing the mother and the young man together, but explain to the parent that you will also be conducting part of the interview and the physical examination without her present in the room. She states that she will only agree to let you speak with him alone if you agree to discuss with her any high-risk behaviors that he admits to engaging in. Concerning patient confidentiality in regard to adolescents, you are required by law to inform the parent of this minor of which of the following?

a. use of marijuana
b. suicidal ideation
c. petty theft
d. consensual sexual relations with another minor of the opposite gender
e. consensual sexual relations with another minor of the same gender

57. You see a 4-year-old child for declining school performance and behavior problems. His mother notes that he is a poor sleeper. He snores loudly and often gasps in his sleep. Sometimes she sleeps with him because she is afraid he will stop breathing. You note a slight fall off the growth curve and very large tonsils. A neck film demonstrates large adenoids as well. The child's insurance company will not pay to have the tonsils and adenoids removed unless you can prove they are causing him significant health problems. Which test is the most likely to give you that information?

a. bronchoscopy
b. overnight pulse oximetry monitoring
c. polysomnography
d. fluoroscopy
e. overnight EEG monitoring

58. An infant who was discharged from the hospital on day 2 of life presents to your office 3 days later for follow-up. The mother did not receive prenatal care. You notice bilateral purulent discharge from the eyes. There is marked eyelid

edema and conjunctival swelling (chemosis). What is the most likely pathologic agent?

a. *Chlamydia trachomatis*
b. *Neisseria gonorrhoeae*
c. group B *Streptococcus*
d. *Toxoplasma gondii*
e. *Treponema pallidum*

59. An unresponsive adolescent patient is brought to the emergency department with suspected ingestion of an unknown substance. EMS received a call from the hotel room where the youth was found, but no one else was there when they arrived. The patient is on 100% inspired oxygen and has required several bouts of positive pressure ventilation in the ambulance. On exam, the patient has a heart rate of 55, blood pressure 85/50, pinpoint pupils, and track lines on his left arm. Along with ongoing cardiovascular and respiratory support, which of the following should be administered to this patient?

a. pralidoxime chloride
b. physostigmine
c. naloxone
d. atropine sulfate
e. desferrioxamine

60. A 15-month-old boy is brought to the emergency department with a fever and difficulty breathing. Right-sided wheezing is noted on the physical examination. The patient does not improve with aerosolized nebulizer treatment. An inspiratory chest radiograph is normal; however, the expiratory film demonstrates right-sided hyperinflation, with mediastinal shift to the left. This patient's respiratory symptoms are most likely due to which of the following?

a. pneumonia
b. foreign body aspiration
c. pneumothorax
d. empyema
e. viral upper respiratory infection

61. You are seeing an 18-month-old boy who is new to your practice. His father is concerned about his child's development in relation to his two older brothers. The boy avoids eye contact and does not respond to efforts to engage him in reciprocal play such as peek-a-boo and patty cake games. He does not generate spontaneous language but can repeat certain words if spoken to him over and over. He spends a lot of time by himself rocking back and forth and becomes very agitated if this activity is interrupted. Which of the following conditions is most consistent with this child's reported behaviors?

a. Down syndrome
b. hearing impairment
c. autism

d. attention-deficit/hyperactivity disorder
e. Asperger syndrome

62. An 8-year-old boy is referred to the emergency department by his pediatrician for a chief complaint of weakness. The weakness has been slowly progressive over the last several weeks. A review of symptoms reveals a history of constipation, polyuria, and polydipsia. The child is on no medications, and past medical history is noncontributory. In the primary physician's office, the patient had a serum potassium measurement of 2.8 mEq/L. A blood pressure measurement in the emergency department is normal for age, height, and gender. Urine electrolyte studies reveal an elevated urine potassium value. Which of the following conditions is the most likely cause of this patient's hypokalemia?

a. excessive sweating
b. renal tubular acidosis
c. anorexia nervosa
d. Cushing syndrome
e. renovascular disease

63. A 2-week-old female infant presents with generalized hypotonia, duodenal atresia and hypothyroidism. What other structural defect is she most likely to have?

a. malrotation
b. endocardial cushion defects
c. cleft palate
d. renal disease
e. sensorineural hearing loss

64. Which of the following conditions are often associated with polyhydramnios?

a. duodenal atresia
b. tracheoesophageal fistula
c. congenital hydrocephalus with myelomeningocele
d. renal agenesis
e. A, B, and C

65. A 3-year-old boy presents with violent episodes of intermittent colicky pain, emesis, and blood per rectum. A tubular mass is palpated in the right lower quadrant. The abdominal radiograph reveals a dearth of air in the right lower quadrant and air-fluid levels consistent with ileus. Which of the following procedures will best assist in diagnosis and treatment?

a. esophagogastroduodenoscopy
b. rectal biopsy
c. air contrast or double contrast enema
d. stool culture
e. colonoscopy

66. An 18-month-old female child presents with blood-streaked stool. The stool is grossly positive on occult

blood testing. Which of the following diagnoses is most likely?

a. anal fissure
b. peptic ulcer disease
c. Mallory-Weiss tear
d. inflammatory bowel disease
e. necrotizing enterocolitis

67. A 4-year-old boy was seen by his pediatrician for fever and abdominal pain. The pain began after a sledding accident the day before his visit in which he fell on his right side. His mother noticed that his abdomen appeared distended today, particularly on the right side. In the pediatrician's office, he is noted to be hypertensive and has gross hematuria. What is the most likely diagnosis?

a. pyelonephritis
b. liver contusion
c. renal contusion
d. Wilms tumor
e. neuroblastoma

68. You are called to evaluate a newborn with an apparent foot deformity. On close examination, you note adduction of the forefoot, inversion of the foot, and plantar flexion at the ankle that is relatively fixed. Which of the following is true of this patient's condition?

a. This clinical picture is most consistent with metatarsus adductus.
b. This deformity will respond to stretching exercises.
c. This deformity will correct spontaneously when the child is able to bear weight.
d. This deformity will require surgical repair.
e. This deformity may be associated with other congenital malformations.

69. A 12-year-old boy with Crohn disease for 2 years is seen with an acute exacerbation. He is complaining of abdominal pain and diarrhea and has right lower quadrant fullness. The most effective approach in this acute setting is which of the following?

a. Perform a colonoscopy for cancer surveillance.
b. Obtain a stool culture and to exclude acute infectious colitis and imaging studies to evaluate for abscess or fistula.
c. Initiate therapy with mercaptopurine or azathioprine.
d. Perform a capsule endoscopy.
e. Start biologic therapy with anti-TNF alpha antibody.

70. A 3-year-old girl periodically experiences swelling around her lips and breaks out in hives when she eats the snacks provided at daycare. Which of the following is the most appropriate for determining whether the child's symptoms are due to food allergies?

a. skin prick testing to foods
b. food-specific IgE levels
c. skin prick testing to foods followed by double-blind placebo-controlled food challenges
d. open-label food challenges
e. endoscopy

71. An 11-year-old girl is referred to your office following an abnormal screen for scoliosis. You diagnose idiopathic scoliosis on exam using Adam's forward bending test. Subsequent radiographs reveal a lateral curvature of 35 degrees. The patient is premenarchal. You refer the patient to an orthopedic surgeon and counsel the parent that the specialist will probably recommend:

a. external bracing
b. follow-up radiographs every 6 months
c. stretching exercises
d. surgical fixation
e. no intervention

72. A child in the emergency department has point tenderness over the proximal tibia and an appropriate history of trauma. The radiograph shows a fracture through the growth plate that extends into the epiphysis and joint space. This type of fracture would be characterized as:

a. Salter-Harris Type I
b. Salter-Harris Type II
c. Salter-Harris Type III
d. Salter-Harris Type IV
e. Salter-Harris Type V

73. A 4-year-old Caucasian boy presents for evaluation of persistent jaundice. The family reports that the boy had neonatal jaundice on the first day of life, and was treated with phototherapy. He has always had mild icterus, but has had increased icterus at times, especially following other mild illnesses, such as ear infections and colds. There is a family history of his father and paternal grandmother having undergone splenectomy. On examination, the boy has mild scleral icterus, and his spleen is palpable about 3 cm below the left costal margin. The laboratory evaluation reveals a total bilirubin of 1.9 mg/dL (unconjugated fraction is 1.5 mg/dL), normal liver transaminases, hemoglobin of 11.2 gm/dL, a normal MCV, and an elevated reticulocyte count of 8%. An osmotic fragility test is performed and demonstrates positive results. What is the most likely diagnosis?

a. iron-deficiency anemia
b. hereditary spherocytosis
c. acute blood loss
d. acute leukemia
e. sickle cell disease

74. An adolescent comes to you with a chief complaint of painless vaginal discharge. You note projection of the breast areola as a secondary mound above the contour of

the breast and pubic hair of adult texture and color with no spread to the medial surface of the thighs. This patient's examination is most consistent with which Tanner stage of development?

a. Stage I
b. Stage II
c. Stage III
d. Stage IV
e. Stage V

75. Which of the following statements about acute myeloid leukemia (AML) is true?

a. The preferred treatment for all types of AML is bone marrow transplant.
b. Chemotherapy used for AML is more intense than that used for ALL.
c. Hyperleukocytosis is not a problem with AML.
d. Patients with Down syndrome and AML have a worse prognosis.
e. Secondary AML has a good response to therapy.

76. A 13-year-old male patient presents with intermittent abdominal pain, diarrhea, weight loss, and growth failure, and is noted on colonoscopy to have inflammatory skip lesions throughout the colon with rectal sparing. Which of the following statements is true?

a. Ulcerative colitis typically is characterized by rectal sparing.
b. Ulcerative colitis typically is characterized by skip lesions.
c. Crohn disease typically is characterized by transmural disease.
d. Ulcerative colitis typically is associated with growth failure.
e. Ulcerative colitis typically is associated with perianal disease.

77. You are moonlighting in the pediatric emergency department when a 10-year-old male arrives by ambulance with lethargy, confusion, dizziness, and a severe headache. His parents and maternal grandmother are in the adult emergency department with less severe but similar symptoms. The emergency medical technicians report that they were called by the police who found the family sleeping in their car with the engine running at their Christmas tree stand. Carbon monoxide poisoning is suspected. Which of the following should be the first step in the evaluation and management of this patient?

a. obtain an EKG
b. draw an arterial blood gas
c. draw a blood carboxyhemoglobin level
d. administer 100% oxygen
e. stabilize the patient for transfer to a hyperbaric oxygen chamber

78. A 5-year-old girl presents to the emergency department with a 12-hour history of fever and respiratory distress. On physical examination, the girl appears toxic, is drooling, and leaning forward with her chin extended. She has a temperature of 104°F (40°C), and a respiratory rate of 32 breaths/min. Which of the following is the most likely diagnosis?

a. epiglottitis
b. croup
c. bacterial pneumonia
d. diphtheria
e. anaphylaxis

79. In response to your question concerning guns in the home during a routine adolescent health maintenance visit, the mother of the patient tells you that her husband, the boy's stepfather, keeps a loaded handgun in the bed table drawer for protection. You would be correct in telling this family that an adolescent who lives in a home with a gun:

a. is less likely than peers who do not live with guns to die from homicide.
b. is less likely than peers who do not live with guns to commit suicide.
c. is mature enough to use good safety precautions, so storing the handgun separately from the ammunition is unnecessary.
d. has a 10-fold greater risk of dying from suicide than peers who do not live in homes with guns.
e. is less likely than peers who do not live with guns to be shot during a domestic dispute.

80. You are seeing a new patient for a health maintenance visit. The child is able to tell you his age and gender and speaks in five to eight word sentences. His grandmother tells you that he is able to pedal a tricycle. He can perform a broad jump when the behavior is modeled and is able to copy a circle. However, he cannot yet balance on one foot or copy a cross. You record that the patient's developmental achievement is consistent with his age. Which of the following most closely correlates with this child's age in years?

a. 2 years
b. 3 years
c. 4 years
d. 5 years
e. 6 years

81. A child weighing 27 kg with a history of vomiting for 36 hours is judged to be 10% dehydrated based on vital signs and physical examination. The serum sodium measurement is 134 mEq/L. An initial 540-mL bolus of normal saline results in stabilization of the heart rate and

improved capillary refill. Which of the following is the most appropriate parenteral fluid choice for the next 8 hours?

a. D_5 0.2 normal saline with 20 mEq/L KCl (added after urination) at 120 mL/hr
b. D_5 0.2 normal saline with 20 mEq/L KCl (added after urination) at 180 mL/hr
c. D_5 0.2 normal saline with 20 mEq/L KCl (added after urination) at 220 mL/hr
d. D 0.45 normal saline with 20 mEq/L KCl (added after urination) at 220 mL/hr
e. D_5 0.45 normal saline with 20 mEq/L KCl (added after urination) at 180 mL/hr

82. An 8-year-old boy presents with growth failure and vague abdominal pain. The abdomen is distended. There is no perianal disease, abdominal mass, or tenderness. The next set of diagnostic tests should include:

a. CBC, CRP, tissue transglutaminase assay
b. CT scan of the abdomen
c. urinalysis, sweat chloride, laparotomy
d. colonoscopy, upper endoscopy
e. stool culture for ova and parasites

83. A 3-year-old boy presents to the pediatrician with fever, pallor, anorexia, joint pain, petechiae, and hepatosplenomegaly. Which of the following is the most likely diagnosis?

a. acute lymphoblastic leukemia
b. acute myelogenous leukemia
c. juvenile chronic myelogenous leukemia
d. aplastic anemia
e. osteosarcoma

84. A 16-year-old girl who is 2 years postmenarche presents with mildly uneven shoulders and a small degree of one-sided rib prominence. Radiographs reveal a 25 degree scoliosis. Which of the following represents the best treatment?

a. posterior spinal fusion
b. intensive physical therapy
c. scoliosis bracing
d. spinal manipulation
e. observation with repeat x-ray in 1 year

85. A 5-year-old boy who returned from a camping trip to his grandparents' farm in Virginia develops a fever of 103°F, a headache, vomiting, and an erythematous, macular rash on his wrists and ankles. On physical examination, he is moderately tachycardic with otherwise stable vital signs and no focal signs of infection. A CBC reveals a normal WBC count and differential and normal hemoglobin. However, the boy's platelet count is 65,000/mm³. Serum electrolytes are normal. Blood cultures and immunofluo-

rescent studies are sent. Which of the following is the most appropriate next course of action?

a. Discharge home on amoxicillin with close follow-up and reliable caregivers.
b. Discharge home on amoxicillin-clavulanic acid with close follow-up and reliable caregivers.
c. Hospitalization for observation pending further test results.
d. Hospitalization for intravenous doxycycline and cefotaxime.
e. Hospitalization for intravenous doxycycline.

86. A 5-year-old boy presents with painful swelling of the hand and feet since the day before. Since earlier today, he has palpable purpura on the lower extremities, and also developed intermittent, colicky midabdominal pain. Prior to these events, he had a cold for 1 week. He did not have fevers, and overall is well appearing. On physical examination, he has normal vital signs. He has palpable purpura on the lower extremities and buttocks. He has scrotal swelling. His hand and feet are puffy, and he has pain with movement of the ankle joints. His abdominal examination is unremarkable. A complete blood count shows normal results with a platelet count of 350,000/mm³. Which of the following laboratory tests is most often abnormal in this disease process?

a. antinuclear antibody (ANA)
b. antineutrophil cytoplasmic antibody (ANCA)
c. complement C3 and C4 levels
d. urinalysis
e. serum creatinine

87. A 12-month-old male infant presents with a hemoglobin of 7.5 and a hematocrit of 22%. The mean corpuscular volume is 65 and the adjusted reticulocyte count is 1.0%. What is the *most* likely cause of anemia in this child?

a. iron-deficiency anemia
b. anemia of chronic disease
c. transient erythrocytopenia of childhood
d. thalassemia syndrome
e. parvovirus B19 aplastic crisis

88. A 12-year-old male adolescent presents with a 1-month history of fever, weight loss, fatigue, and pain and localized swelling of the midproximal femur. Which of the following is the most likely diagnosis?

a. Ewing sarcoma
b. osteosarcoma
c. chronic osteomyelitis
d. benign bone tumor
e. eosinophilic granuloma

89. You are examining a 3-year-old girl at her well-child visit. While she is staring at her stuffed cow in your hands, you quickly cover her right eye with an index card. When the index card is removed seconds later, you notice that the right eye "drifts" back toward the center. This reaction in response to the cover test indicates what abnormal condition?
    a. strabismus
    b. amblyopia
    c. leukocoria
    d. retinoblastoma
    e. nasolacrimal duct obstruction

90. A 14-year-old girl is brought to your office by her mother because she is complaining of "seeing double." The history is significant for headaches that waken the patient from sleep in the morning but are relieved by vomiting. On physical examination, you note that she is unable to abduct either eye. Lower extremity reflexes are slightly exaggerated. Which of the following physical signs is most likely to be present in this patient?
    a. hypotension
    b. papilledema
    c. tachycardia
    d. patency of the anterior fontanelle
    e. erythema migrans

91. A previously healthy 4-year-old girl presents with a history of diarrhea and vomiting for the past 3 days and decreased urine output for the past 12 hours. On examination, she has a heart rate of 120 beats per minute, blood pressure of 105/65 mm Hg, and no edema. The blood tests reveal serum sodium of 128 mEq/L, potassium 5.6 mEq/L, bicarbonate 12 mEq/L, BUN 55 mg/dL, creatinine 1.6 mg/dL. The urine tests reveal a fractional excretion of sodium of 0.1. The kidney ultrasound is normal. Which of the following constitutes the most appropriate immediate management of this child's acute renal failure?
    a. intravenous normal saline bolus to correct the renal hypoperfusion
    b. intravenous bicarbonate to correct the metabolic acidosis
    c. intravenous furosemide to correct the fluid overload
    d. intravenous antibiotics to correct the infectious gastroenteritis
    e. initiation of dialysis to correct the acute renal failure

92. A very tired mother brings her 6-week-old infant to your office because "he screams for hours and hours a day and nothing makes him stop." His parent describes the crying spells as occurring daily and lasting several hours, usually through the late afternoon and early evening. Nothing seems to console the child during these episodes. While he is crying, the infant often pulls his knees to his abdomen as if he is in pain. Other than the crying spells, the child is asymptomatic. He feeds well and moves his bowels regularly. The child's weight, length, and head circumference are normal, and his physical examination is normal. This patient's history and physical examination are most consistent with which of the following conditions?
    a. feeding intolerance
    b. cow milk protein allergy
    c. intussusception
    d. Hirschsprung disease
    e. colic

93. A newborn infant has a slight hip click on hip examination. Which of the following risk factors would most strongly support further evaluation?
    a. female patient
    b. first born
    c. torticollis
    d. metatarsus adductus
    e. breech presentation or family history of developmental dysplasia of the hip

94. A 14-year-old patient in your practice with anorexia nervosa has fallen to 80% of her ideal body weight for height and gender. She has not menstruated in 9 months. She has postural hypotension and a low heart rate. Which of the following murmurs is most likely to be present on this patient's cardiac examination?
    a. a midsystolic click, followed by a murmur
    b. a fixed split S_2
    c. a vibratory holosystolic murmur in both axilla
    d. a third heart sound
    e. a nonspecific ejection murmur at the base of the heart

95. You are offering preventive counseling to the parent of a 12-month-old child at a health maintenance visit. The child weighs 18 lbs. You would be correct in informing the parent that this child should be:
    a. restrained in a rear-facing infant car seat in the back seat of the car until he has reached 20 lbs. in weight
    b. restrained in a forward-facing infant car seat in the back seat of the car since he is now ≥1 year of age
    c. restrained in a rear-facing infant car seat in the front seat of the car until he has reached 20 lbs. in weight
    d. restrained in a forward-facing infant car seat in the front seat of the car since he is now ≥1 year of age
    e. restrained in a forward-facing booster seat in the back seat of the car since he is now ≥1 year of age

96. A 4-week-old male infant born at term presents with emesis, dehydration, and poor weight gain. The pediatrician evaluating the child palpates an olive-sized mass in the child's

epigastrium. She believes the infant may have pyloric stenosis. Which of the following clinical presentations is most consistent with pyloric stenosis?

a. projectile nonbilious emesis
b. bilious emesis
c. bloody diarrhea
d. violent episodes of intermittent colicky pain and emesis
e. right lower quadrant abdominal pain

97. A 5-year-old boy presents to the emergency department with complaints of dizziness and confusion. Three days before presentation he developed a low-grade fever and vomited twice. Since then, the fever and vomiting have resolved, but the patient has passed 8 to 10 loose, foul-smelling stools per day. The boy's mother has been afraid to give him anything but water or diluted juice due to his history of vomiting. Deep tendon reflexes are diminished throughout. This patient's ataxia and confusion are most likely due to which of the following electrolyte imbalances?

a. hypomagnesemia
b. hyperkalemia
c. metabolic alkalosis
d. hypochloremia
e. hyponatremia

98. A 13-year-old male presents to the office with short stature. Growth data demonstrates that he has been growing between the 3rd and 5th percentile at a steady rate since age 4 years. His father started shaving at age 17 and completed his growth at age 19 years. What examination and workup would support the diagnosis of constitutional delay of growth and puberty?

a. acne and axillary hair, Tanner III pubic hair, testicular volume 12 cc, bone age 14 years, TSH 1.5 (0.5 to 4.8), IGF-I 340 (152 to 540)
b. no axillary hair, Tanner I pubic hair, testicular volume 4 cc, bone age 11 years, TSH 12 (0.5 to 4.8), IGF-I 200 (152 to 540)
c. scant axillary hair, Tanner II pubic hair, testicular volume 5 cc, bone age 11 years, TSH 2.1 (0.5 to 4.8), IGF-I 420 (152 to 540)
d. no axillary hair, Tanner I pubic hair, testicular volume 4 cc, bone age 11 years, TSH 3.1 (0.5 to 4.8), IGF-I 62 (152 to 540)

99. A 24-month-old male in your office for his regular health maintenance visit has the following results on screening tests: hemoglobin 9.6 g/dL; capillary blood lead level 16 mcg/dL. He lives in Section 8 housing in poor repair built before 1960. Which of the following is the most appropriate next course of action?

a. Counsel the family regarding lead removal and recheck the level in 6 months.
b. Refer the family to the local governmental lead management agency.
c. Obtain a venous lead level for confirmation.
d. Start the patient on oral succimer on an outpatient basis.
e. Obtain neurodevelopmental testing for the patient.

100. A 10-year-old girl presents with a linear streaks of thickened and indurated skin on the right arm and trunk. The linear streak on the right arm has a longitudinal orientation and extends from the upper arm to the dorsal aspect of the hand, whereas the linear streak on the trunk is transversely oriented. The lesions are surrounded by a halo of erythema with a violaceous appearance. The central portion is hyperpigmented and thickened. Which of the following complications is this child most likely to develop?

a. esophageal dysfunction
b. pulmonary fibrosis
c. contracture of the right elbow
d. raynaud phenomenon
e. digital necrosis

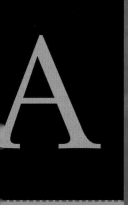

Answers

1. b (Chapter 1)

Epinephrine is used for asystole, bradycardia, and/or pulseless VT or ventricular fibrillation. Epinephrine increases systemic vascular resistance, chronotropy, and inotropy, thereby increasing cardiac output and systolic and diastolic blood pressure. By increasing systolic blood pressure, cerebral blood flow is increased; by increasing diastolic blood pressure, coronary perfusion is increased. Epinephrine may change fine ventricular fibrillation to coarse ventricular fibrillation and promote successful defibrillation.

2. a (Chapter 6)

Turner syndrome is relatively common, with an incidence of 1 in 2,500. Female patients present with short stature and delayed puberty caused by primary ovarian failure. Other stigmata, including webbed neck, a low hairline, and increased carrying angle, may not be present. Patients with Cushing syndrome present with other physical characteristics, including moon facies, buffalo hump, and abdominal striae. In isolated growth hormone deficiency and familial short stature, patients do not have delayed puberty. Patients with Addison disease present with fatigue, weakness, nausea, and vomiting. In the acute setting, they may present with cardiovascular shock.

3. d (Chapter 9)

The child has a 25% chance of acquiring the autosomal recessive disorder. Because each parent is a carrier for the disorder, each parent has one normal allele and one mutant allele. The probability of the child receiving an affected allele is 0.5 from each parent. Therefore, the child has a 25% risk (0.5 × 0.5).

4. d (Chapter 10)

Hydroxyurea maintenance therapy has been shown to reduce the number and severity of vaso-occlusive crises in individuals with sickle cell disease. Children with sickle cell disease, like all children, require all routine childhood vaccinations. Despite penicillin prophylaxis, children with sickle cell disease are still at high risk of sepsis caused by *Streptococcus pneumoniae*. These children require both the pneumococcal conjugate vaccine (7-valent) during infancy and the pneumococcal polysaccharide vaccine (23-valent) at 4 to 6 years of age. Gallstones typically develop during adolescence as a result of chronic hemolysis. Dactylitis, or hand-foot syndrome, is the earliest manifestation of vaso-occlusive disease. It is caused by avascular necrosis of the metacarpal and metatarsal bones and requires analgesics, not antibiotics. Acute chest syndrome requires both supportive care (supplemental oxygen, red blood cell transfusions) and antibiotics.

5. a (Chapter 16)

Children with vegan diets are at risk for vitamin B_{12} deficiency, iron deficiency, and, if exposed to inadequate sunlight, vitamin D deficiency as well. A child who lives in New Mexico and spends a lot of time outdoors can be assumed to have adequate vitamin D levels. Calcium is unlikely to be a concern if the child is indeed eating many dark green, leafy vegetables. Finally, the boy is fed iron-fortified grains regularly, so unless a screening hematocrit is low, iron stores are likely sufficient. Vitamins B_{12} and B_6, niacin, and riboflavin are all B vitamins. Of these, vitamin B_{12} is found only in foods of animal origin, so vegans in particular are at risk for deficiency of this substance.

6. b (Chapter 3)

Functional or "innocent" murmurs are heard in up to 80% of children at some point, and represent normal blood flow through a structurally normal heart. They are accentuated by increased cardiac output (i.e., during exercise, with fever, or with anemia). A Still's murmur is the most common innocent murmur. It has a low-pitched, vibratory quality and is heard best in the supine position. A bicuspid aortic valve is associated with an S2 click. If stenosis or regurgitation is present, an associated murmur will be heard. The murmur of a ventricular septal defect is higher frequency and occurs throughout systole. Small VSDs may have pronounced murmurs and a thrill and not uncommonly undergo spontaneous closure during the first 2 years of life. An atrial septal defect is characterized by fixed and wide splitting of S2, due to delayed closure of the pulmonary valve. A soft systolic ejection murmur may be present, due to increased flow across the pulmonary valve. The hallmark findings in coarctation of the aorta are discrepant pulses and blood pressures in the upper and lower extremities. A systolic ejection murmur may be present at the left upper sternal border. Continuous murmurs may also be present across the chest or back, if collateral arteries are present.

7. a (Chapter 20)

Upper airway obstruction in the neonate can result from all the conditions listed. However, the child does not turn blue when crying (mouth breathing). The inability to pass the NG tube in this clinical setting is virtually diagnostic of bilateral choanal atresia or significant stenosis. There is no communication between the nose and pharynx, and thus no air flow. Bilateral choanal atresia is an emergency. This patient will likely require endotracheal intubation and surgery to correct the defect. Vocal cord paralysis may result from recurrent laryngeal nerve damage during delivery. If this were the case, the infant should have a soft, hoarse cry, and stridor might be noted. Subglottic stenosis and laryngeal web would also result in stridor. In all three of these conditions, passage of the NG tube would not be impeded.

8. c (Chapter 6)

The child with diabetic ketoacidosis (DKA) usually exhibits some combination of polyuria, polydipsia, fatigue, headache, nausea, emesis, and abdominal pain. When DKA occurs, ketones are formed in the blood and cleared in the urine. Hyperglycemia, and not hypoglycemia, is typical. Primary metabolic acidosis with secondary respiratory alkalosis is noted (decreased venous blood pH and hypocarbia). Dehydration results in an elevated BUN level. When DKA is present, the patient's total body potassium is depleted from significant potassium loss in the osmotic diuresis. However, serum potassium measurements at presentation may appear high, low, or normal.

9. a (Chapter 14)

Although >99% of males have bilateral descended testes by 12 months of age, testes that do not descend on their own by 3 to 6 months of age are unlikely to do so. Testes that remain outside the scrotum develop ultrastructural changes and impaired sperm production resulting in possible infertility. There is also an increased risk of malignancy, even after the testis is surgically relocated (and even in the contralateral testis).

Ninety percent of patients with cryptorchidism also have inguinal hernias. Cryptorchidism may occur as an isolated defect or be part of a genetic syndrome; however, there is no known increase in the risk of microphallus in these patients.

10. a (Chapter 19)

Legg-Calve-Perthes (LCP) disease. Although LCP can have associated hip or knee pain, it is commonly known as "the painless limp." The peak age of onset is 3 to 8 years. Slipped capital femoral epiphysis (SCFE) is incorrect because the peak age range of this disorder is peripubertal, approximately ages 8 to 14 years. SCFE typically has pain associated. A "toddler's fracture" is a nondisplaced fracture of the tibia in children aged 2 to 4 years which is often not appreciated on plain films at presentation. Most are healed within 4 weeks, and any associated limp would disappear by 2 months. Septic arthritis is usually acute in presentation and has associated pain, fever, inability to walk, and elevations of C-reactive protein and erythrocyte sedimentation rate. Juvenile idiopathic arthritis (JIA) rarely presents in the hip; the most common location is the knees. Morning stiffness is a common complaint with JIA.

11. c (Chapter 10)

Pulmonary embolism (PE) is a potentially fatal complication of deep vein thrombosis (DVT). The classic signs and symptoms of PE include sudden chest pain, dyspnea, anxiety, and cyanosis. Hemoptysis is uncommon. A helical CT (spiral CT) or a ventilation/perfusion (V/Q) scan is the recommended diagnostic study. While small emboli can be managed by anticoagulation therapy and close monitoring, massive PE may require thrombolytic therapy with recombinant tissue plasminogen activator (r-tPA) or thrombectomy. Venous insufficiency is also a common complication noted after DVT but is not a significant issue in the acute setting. Limb overgrowth, edema and gangrene from a venous ulcer are all potential complications of DVT.

12. d (Chapter 15)

Women who are taking carbamazepine or valproic acid are at an increased risk of producing a child with a neural tube defect if they are treated with this drug during their pregnancies. The mechanism for this is unclear. The other anticonvulsants listed do not increase the risk for neural tube defects specifically, although they may be associated with a higher risk for other birth defects. Other drugs which do increase the risk of neural tube defects include aminopterin, pyrimethamine, trimethoprim, sulfasalazine, methotrexate, phenothiazines, and cyclophosphamide.

13. b (Chapter 1)

With probable supraventricular tachycardia, the best course of action listed is to administer IV adenosine by rapid bolus to temporarily block the AV node and interrupt the likely reentrant circuit causing the SVT. In a hemodynamically unstable patient, synchronized cardioversion 0.5 to 1.0 J/kg is recommended with an increase to 2 J/kg if initial cardioversion is unsuccessful. The use of epinephrine is indicated in cases of asystole, bradycardia, pulseless VT or VF. The use of atropine is indicated in cases of bradycardia and atrioventricular block. Calcium may be used for hypocalcemia, hyperkalemia, hypermagnesemia, and calcium channel blocker overdose. Sodium bicarbonate may be used if the infant is acidotic secondary to decreased perfusion and oxygen delivery to the tissues.

14. b (Chapter 15)

Infantile spasms typically present between 2 and 7 months of age and may be idiopathic or associated with other neurologic or developmental diseases. Hypsarrhythmia, characterized by widespread random, high-voltage slow waves and spikes that spread to all cortical areas, is the characteristic EEG finding in infantile seizures. All children with infantile seizures should receive a Wood lamp exam to determine whether ash-leaf spots, the lesions described here, are present. Ash-leaf spots are the earliest manifestation of tuberous sclerosis, a neurocutaneous disease which may present with infantile spasms. Von Recklinghausen disease and bilateral acoustic neurofibromatosis are forms of neurofibromatosis. Café-au-lait spots, which are hyperpigmented, are seen in these diseases. Von Hippel-Lindau disease presents in adolescence. Infants with Sturge-Weber may have seizures, but the port wine stain is present at birth and is the primary skin lesion.

15. b (Chapter 12)

She needs a fourth dose of DTaP, a fourth dose of Hib, and a fourth dose of pneumococcal conjugate vaccine. She needs the MMR and varicella vaccines unless there is a reliable history that she has had chickenpox. She has already completed the required vaccination courses for hepatitis A and hepatitis B. Three doses of IPV are appropriate for her age.

16. e (Chapter 4)

Speech delay is the most common developmental concern raised by parents. As many as 15% of children have some sort of speech/language delay at one time or another during the preschool years. Any child with suspected language delay should receive a full audiologic assessment, followed by referral to a speech pathologist for further workup and treatment (if indicated). The most common cause of mild to moderate hearing loss is young children in otitis media with effusion, but this child has clear, mobile tympanic membranes, so a tympanogram is unnecessary. Evaluation of the boy's ability to understand and produce language, as well as speak fluently, is part of a comprehensive speech assessment following the hearing test.

17. c (Chapter 8)

Functional abdominal pain is best treated with a biopsychosocial model. Medical treatment might include acid reduction therapy for pain associated with dyspepsia, antispasmodic agents, smooth muscle relaxants, or low doses of tricyclic psychotropic agents for pain or nonstimulating laxatives or antidiarrheals for pain associated with altered bowel pattern. A CT scan and endoscopy are unlikely to identify abnormalities based on the history and physical examination. A diet history and elimination diet are unlikely to provide additional insight since the pain is not related to meals. Psychiatric referral is premature and sends the message that there is only an emotional component to these symptoms.

18. a (Chapter 9)

The clinical description is that of a patient with trisomy 21, or Down syndrome. Common dysmorphic facial features include flat facial profile, upslanted palpebral fissures, a flat nasal bridge with epicanthal folds, a small mouth with a protruding tongue, micrognathia, and short ears with downfolding earlobes. Other dysmorphic features are excess skin on the back of the neck, microcephaly, a flat occiput (brachycephaly), short stature, a short sternum, small genitalia, and a gap between the first and second toes ("sandal gap toe"). Anomalies of the hand include single palmar creases (simian creases) and short, broad hands (brachydactyly) with fingers marked by an incurved fifth finger and a hypoplastic middle phalanx (clinodactyly). Features of trisomy 18 include hypertonia, microcephaly, corneal opacities, micrognathia, and rocker bottom feet. Features of trisomy 13 include microcephaly, occipital scalp defects, iris coloboma, microphthalmia, cleft lip and palate, and clenched hands. Boys with Klinefelter syndrome do not have physical features identifiable at birth that could lead to suspicion of the disorder. Girls with Turner syndrome have a webbed neck, low posterior hairline, wide-spaced nipples, cubitus valgus (wide carrying angle), and edema of the hands and feet.

19. a (Chapter 2)

Asymptomatic patients with blood lead levels >45 μg/dL require chelation within 48 hours. EDTA (edetate calciumdisodium) is an appropriate treatment for asymptomatic patients with blood lead levels between 45 and 69 μg/dL. It is administered in the hospital. Outpatient oral succimer is also an option in this patient. BAL (intramuscular dimercaprol) is added to EDTA when a patient's blood lead level reaches 70 μg/dL or greater. The family should be removed from the home while decontamination is taking place. Siblings of any patient with elevated lead levels should be tested, and nutritional therapy is certainly not contraindicated; however, patients with levels exceeding 45 μg/dL require chelation treatment per American Academy of Pediatrics and Centers for Disease Control recommendations.

20. b (Chapter 16)

Breastfed infants should receive oral vitamin D supplementation beginning in the weeks after birth to prevent rickets, a condition in which developing bone fails to mineralize due to inadequate 1,25-dihydroxycholecalciferol. Rickets is rare in breastfed infants but does occur. Dark-skinned infants and those exposed to limited sunlight in northern latitudes are particularly at risk. Rickets in breastfed infants becomes clinically and chemically evident in late infancy; rickets due solely to vitamin D deficiency begins to respond to supplementation within weeks. The American Academy of Pediatrics recommends exclusive breastfeeding during the first 6 months of life and continuation of breastfeeding during the second 6 months for optimal infant nutrition. Studies have shown that breastfed infants have a lower incidence of infections, including otitis media, pneumonia, sepsis, and meningitis. Breastfed infants are less likely to experience feeding difficulties associated with allergy (eczema) or intolerance (colic).

21. c (Chapter 17)

Although all of the choices are possible presentations of Hodgkin disease, choice C is the most common presentation, occurring in approximately 80% of patients. Approximately two-thirds of patients will have mediastinal lymphadenopathy, and 20% to 30% will experience "B" symptoms. Pruritus, fatigue, and anorexia are also common presenting symptoms. The pruritus is often extremely difficult to control prior to diagnosis, but resolves very rapidly once chemotherapy begins. Patients will often have more than one of the presenting signs or symptoms listed here.

22. d (Chapter 20)

The preferred therapy regimen for a patient ≥12 years with persistent asthma (symptoms [before treatment] >2 days per week or waking with symptoms >2 nights per month, or use of an inhaled β agonist >2 times per week) that is not well-controlled on step 2 (low-dose inhaled steroids) is daily low-dose inhaled corticosteroid and a long-acting inhaled β2-agonist. Answer a is most appropriate for patients with intermittent asthma, who can control their sporadic symptoms with an inhaled β2-agonist as needed. Answer b is the preferred therapy for a patient with mild persistent asthma. Answer c is an acceptable step 4 treatment. Nedocromil is an older drug and presumed mast cell membrane stabilizer that may be an alternative to low-dose inhaled corticosteroids in patients with mild persistent asthma.

23. a (Chapter 5)

Measles is caused by a paramyxovirus and characterized by malaise, high fever, cough, coryza, conjunctivitis, Koplik spots, and an erythematous maculopapular rash. Koplik spots are small, irregular red spots with central gray or bluish-white specks that appear on the buccal mucosa. Rubella is caused by rubella virus and is characterized by mild fever and erythematous maculopapular rash, with generalized lymphadenopathy, especially of the posterior auricular, cervical, and suboccipital nodes. Roseola infantum is caused by herpesvirus 6 and is characterized by high fever followed by a maculopapular rash that starts on the trunk and spreads to the periphery. The fever typically resolves as the rash appears. Erythema infectiosum is caused by parvovirus B19 and is characterized by marked erythema of the cheeks ("slapped cheek" appearance) and an erythematous, pruritic, maculopapular rash starting on the arms and spreading to the trunk and legs. Hand-foot-and-mouth disease is caused by coxsackie A virus and is characterized by ulcers on the tongue and oral mucosa and a maculopapular vesicular rash on the hands and feet. Chickenpox is caused by varicella-zoster virus and is characterized by fever and a pruritic papular, vesicular, pustular rash starting on the trunk and spreading to the extremities. The infected child is infectious until the last lesion is crusted over. Zoster, or shingles, is caused by reactivation of varicella-zoster virus from the dorsal root ganglion and is characterized by fever and painful pruritic crops of vesicles along a dermatomal distribution in an individual with previous varicella-zoster infection.

24. b (Chapter 12)

High-dose amoxicillin is the recommended first-line antibiotic treatment for acute otitis media. Children who have been treated with antibiotics within the past month are eligible for second-line therapy with amoxicillin-clavulanate, an oral second- or third-generation cephalosporin, or IM ceftriaxone. The most common bacteria that cause acute otitis media are *Streptococcus pneumoniae*, *Haemophilus influenzae*, and *Moraxella catarrhalis*. Azithromycin, erythromycin, and trimethoprim-sulfamethoxazole are minimally effective against beta-lactamase-producing strains of *H. influenzae* or *M. catarrhalis*. Dicloxacillin is not active against gram-negative organisms such as *H. influenzae* and *M. catarrhalis*.

25. b (Chapter 13)

Infants with neonatal sepsis or pneumonia typically have normal surfactant production and do not benefit from surfactant replacement therapy. Preeclampsia is associated with acceleration of lung maturation and surfactant production. Full-term infants with neural tube defects have normal lung maturation. Newborns with trisomy 21 are at risk for pulmonary hypertension due to delayed development of the pulmonary vasculature, but typically have appropriate surfactant production. Infants of diabetic mothers, especially those with poor control, have delayed maturation of surfactant production and are at increased risk for neonatal respiratory distress syndrome at any gestational age.

26. d (Chapter 14)

A child with a suspected UTI and positive leukocyte esterase on dipstick urinalysis should be treated for presumptive UTI until culture results become available. Children older than 5 years of age with a recurrent UTI warrant further workup to rule out anatomic abnormalities (renal ultrasound) and vesicoureteral reflux (VCUG). A nontoxic-appearing child of this age does not need to be admitted to the hospital for treatment. On the other hand, empiric treatment should never be withheld in a febrile child with a suspected UTI and a dipstick urinalysis which is positive for leukocyte esterase.

27. a (Chapter 3)

The central feature of tetralogy of Fallot is a malaligned ventricular septal defect. The malalignment in the septum is characterized by an anteriorly displaced infundibulum (the septal muscle in the outlet area). This leads to subpulmonary narrowing and an aorta that appears to over-ride the inferior portion of the septum. The amount of pulmonary stenosis (right ventricular outflow obstruction) varies in patients with TOF. Right ventricular outflow obstruction leads to right ventricular hypertrophy in these patients. Atrial septal defect, aortic stenosis, coarctation of the aorta, mitral valve prolapse, and left ventricular hypertrophy are not associated with tetralogy of Fallot. Left ventricular hypertrophy may be found in patients with coarctation of the aorta or aortic stenosis.

28. c (Chapter 10)

Fresh frozen plasma (FFP) is indicated for replacement of missing coagulation factors when the specific factor concentrate is unavailable. FFP is prepared by either separating the liquid portion of whole blood or by collecting the liquid portion of the blood by apheresis technology and freezing it within 8 hours of collection. FFP contains all of the normal coagulation factors and naturally occurring inhibitors of coagulation. Cryoprecipitate is a rich source of fibrinogen and clotting factors VIII and XIII. Granulocyte infusions are usually used in the neonate or infant with prolonged neutropenia and life-threatening sepsis. Platelet transfusions are effective in cases of thrombocytopenia or functional platelet defects. DDAVP is used in von Willebrand disease or mild hemophilia A patients.

29. c (Chapter 21)

The typical sequence of pubertal events in the male begins with testicular enlargement from the prepubertal size of about 2.5 mm in length. This is followed in rapid succession by pubic hair growth, penile enlargement, and maximal height growth velocity (approaching 9 cm/year).

30. e (Chapter 20)

A patient with an acute asthmatic episode who has already taken multiple dosages of albuterol at home should still receive a trial of another dose in the emergency department. Failure to respond to initial treatment and the presence of hypoxemia signal a moderate to severe acute asthma episode that will require more aggressive treatment. The addition of the anticholinergic agent ipratropium results in significant improvement in a large percentage of patients. The lack of response to initial treatment also is an indication to begin treatment with systemic corticosteroids to help relieve airway inflammation. Supplemental oxygen will help relieve the hypoxemia caused by ventilation perfusion mismatch and can also produce mild bronchodilation.

31. d (Chapter 14)

This patient displays the characteristic findings of acute renal failure due to the use of ibuprofen in a subject with decreased renal perfusion. He would be expected to have decreased renal perfusion based on symptoms and signs of mild to moderate dehydration (tachycardia, decreased urine output). In the presence of decreased renal perfusion, the intrarenal vasodilatory prostaglandins comprise a powerful mechanism for maintenance of glomerular filtration rate. Interference with this compensatory mechanism, by the use of nonsteroidal anti-inflammatory drugs as in this case, is a common mechanism that can precipitate intrinsic acute renal failure. This patient does not have hemolytic uremic syndrome since his complete blood count is normal (no hemolysis, thrombocytopenia, or schistocytes). He does not have any evidence for pyelonephritis (no costovertebral angle tenderness, no white blood cells in the urine, no bacteria in the urine). He does not display any clinical features characteristic of interstitial nephritis (no skin rashes, no white blood cells in the urine) or urinary tract obstruction (normal kidney ultrasound).

32. a (Chapter 11)

This child most likely has classical systemic lupus erythematosus given that she fulfills 6 out of 11 criteria for the classification for the condition: malar rash, photosensitivity, oral ulcers, arthritis, cytopenias, and active urine sediment. A positive ANA is present in essentially all patients with SLE; therefore, the correct answer is a. Anti-double-stranded DNA antibodies are present in up to 70% of patients with active SLE, anti-Smith antibodies in up to 50%, anti-Ro antibodies in up to 60%, and rheumatoid factor is rare in SLE. Anti-double-stranded DNA and anti-Smith antibodies are highly specific for SLE; therefore its presence is highly suggestive of SLE.

33. a (Chapter 1)

The primary assessment is the initial evaluation of the critically ill or injured child when life-threatening problems are identified and prioritized. The proper order of the primary

ANSWERS

survey or initial assessment is airway, breathing, circulation, disability, and exposure. After the primary survey is complete, resuscitation should occur if the condition is life-threatening. Once the life-threatening issues are addressed, the secondary survey should be performed.

34. d (Chapter 10)

The most likely diagnosis is immune thrombocytopenic purpura. Isoimmune thrombocytopenia is noted in newborns, not in children. Isoimmune IgG antibodies are produced against the fetal platelet when the fetal platelet crosses the placenta and has antigens that are not found on the maternal platelet. The maternal antibodies cross the placenta and attack the fetal platelets. Leukemia, sepsis, and hypersplenism may all cause thrombocytopenia in the child's age group, but are unlikely in this case. The white blood cell count is normal, and no immature white cells are seen on the peripheral smear. Sepsis is unlikely given that the child appears well and is hemodynamically stable. Hypersplenism is unlikely when the spleen is normal on palpation.

35. b (Chapter 9)

Microdeletion of 22q11.2 has been found in 90% of children with DiGeorge syndrome, in 70% of children with velocardiofacial syndrome, and in 15% of children with isolated conotruncal cardiac defects. Although the above-mentioned names are still in use, the more general term *22q11.2 deletion syndrome* more appropriately encompasses the spectrum of abnormalities found in these children. Its prevalence in the general population is 1 per 4,000 live births. The deletion can be inherited (8% to 28% of cases), but more typically occurs as a de novo event. However, if a parent has the deletion, the risk to each child is 50%. The microdeletion can be detected using fluorescent in situ hybridization (FISH) probes. Classic cardiac features of this spectrum of disorders include conotruncal defects such as tetralogy of Fallot, interrupted aortic arch, and vascular rings. Other common findings are absent thymus, hypocalcemic hypoparathyroidism, T-cell-mediated immune deficiency, and palate abnormalities. These children usually have feeding difficulties, cognitive disabilities, and behavioral and speech disorders.

36. e (Chapter 12)

Palivizumab is an RSV monoclonal antibody approved for monthly injection during the winter months in infants at high risk for severe RSV disease. These include children younger than 24 months who are former premature infants or have chronic pulmonary disease (bronchopulmonary dysplasia) requiring oxygen therapy within the last 6 months. RespiGam is an intravenous polyclonal immunoglobulin with high RSV antibody concentration which is also appropriate for administration in children at high risk for complicated RSV infections;

however, palivizumab is preferred because it is easier to administer and is not a blood product. Neither the nasal nor the injectable influenza vaccine is approved for infants younger than 6 months of age. Ribavirin is not appropriate for prophylactic use.

37. c (Chapter 16)

Formula-fed infants do not require supplementation with vitamins, minerals, additional caloric sources, or free water during the first 6 months of life, regardless of local climate. Dilution of the formula is potentially harmful to an infant under 6 months of age due to the inability of the immature kidney to fully dilute urine. If this infant is feeding well, growing appropriately, and tolerates the formula, there is no reason to switch to a soy protein-based formula at this time.

38. c (Chapter 18)

The absence of a red reflex on funduscopic examination (also called leukocoria, for "white" pupil) calls for immediate consultation with a pediatric ophthalmologist. The most common cause is a congenital cataract, which may occur spontaneously, secondary to a genetic predisposition, or as a result of metabolic disease or intrauterine infection. Retinoblastoma, congenital glaucoma, and toxocariasis may also cause leukocoria but are much less common than congenital cataracts.

39. d (Chapter 15)

The child in the vignette is initially diagnosed with adrenal insufficiency, which can be associated with adrenoleukodystrophy. Treatment of the insufficiency does not help with the personality changes and declining cognitive faculties. His difficulty with walking is likely due to increasing spasticity. The first three disorders listed are all gray matter degenerative diseases which present earlier in life with hypotonia, mental retardation, and seizures. Rett syndrome is a disease of general cerebral atrophy which presents almost exclusively in girls early in the second year of life.

40. d (Chapter 15)

Absence seizures begin between ages 4 and 9 years and consist of brief episodes of staring associated with altered consciousness. The typical duration is 5 to 10 seconds. Often, the staring is accompanied by subtle clonic activity in the face or arms or simple automatisms (such as eye blinking, chewing, or perseverative motor activity). Absence seizures start and stop abruptly and have no postictal phase. Although brief, absence seizures can occur in clusters many times a day and interfere with learning and socialization. In a typical absence seizure, the EEG shows abrupt onset and offset of 3-per-second generalized symmetric spike-and-slow-wave complexes. In a child with untreated absence epilepsy, 3 to 5 minutes of hyperventilation will often precipitate a typical absence seizure. Valproic acid and ethosuximide have equal efficacy for treatment of childhood absence epilepsy; lamotrigine is more effective than placebo but has not been compared head-to-head with the other medications. For children with partial-onset epilepsy, oxcarbazepine should be considered for initial monotherapy based on current efficacy evidence. Considering all factors, including cost, carbamazepine, valproic acid, topiramate, and phenytoin are other reasonable choices to treat partial-onset seizures. Methylphenidate is a stimulant medication which is often beneficial in the treatment of attention-deficit/hyperactivity disorder.

41. e (Chapter 9)

Turner syndrome occurs in 1 per 5,000 live births. Approximately 98% of fetuses with Turner syndrome expire in utero; only 2% are born. Therefore, the recurrence risk for parents who have a child with Turner syndrome is no higher than that of the general population. Dysmorphic features include lymphedema of the hands and feet, a shield-shaped chest, widely spaced hypoplastic nipples, a webbed neck, low hairline, cubitus valgus (increased carrying angle), short stature, and multiple pigmented nevi. Additional abnormalities include gonadal dysgenesis, gonadoblastoma, renal anomalies, congenital heart disease, autoimmune thyroiditis, and learning disabilities. Gonadal dysgenesis, present in 100% of patients, is associated with primary amenorrhea and lack of pubertal development due to loss of ovarian hormones. The gonads are appropriately infantile at birth but regress during childhood and develop into "streak" ovaries by puberty. In mosaics with a Y chromosome in one of their cell lines, gonadoblastoma is common. Therefore, prophylactic gonadectomy is necessary in these patients. Renal anomalies, usually duplicated collecting system or horseshoe kidney, occur in 40% of those with Turner syndrome. Congenital heart disease occurs in 20% of patients; common defects include coarctation of the aorta, aortic stenosis, and bicuspid aortic valve. As a consequence of having only one functional X chromosome, females with Turner syndrome display the same frequency of sex-linked disorders as males. The diagnosis is made by karyotype and fluorescent in situ hybridization. Because of their mosaicism, some girls suspected of having Turner syndrome have a 46,XX karyotype in the peripheral blood, and a skin biopsy may be necessary to make the diagnosis.

Short stature has been successfully treated using human growth hormone. Secondary sexual characteristics develop after estrogen and progesterone administration. As mentioned earlier, gonadectomy is indicated in patients with dysgenetic gonads and the presence of a Y chromosome. With the rare exception of a few mosaics, women with Turner syndrome cannot become pregnant.

42. d (Chapter 2)

Oral N-acetyl cysteine is the antidote for acetaminophen ingestion. It is most effective if administered within 8 to 10 hours of ingestion. Multiple doses are required. If the patient refuses, a nasogastric tube may be placed. The administration of N-acetyl cysteine should not be delayed until after the 4-hour acetaminophen level is drawn if the patient presents prior to this time. Activated charcoal may be beneficial if used within 4 hours of ingestion and is often followed by whole bowel irrigation, but neither of these is considered an antidote specific to acetaminophen poisoning. Neither hemodialysis nor atropine sulfate, which is used in cases of organophosphate poisoning, affects blood levels of acetaminophen.

43. e (Chapter 2)

Fractures which are highly specific for abuse include bilateral fractures, bucket handle fractures, metaphyseal chip fractures, and fractures of the (especially posterior) ribs, scapula, sternum, or spinous processes. Fractures that occur before ambulation are usually inflicted. Bruises on the chest, head, neck, or abdomen and bruises on a nonambulatory child are extremely suspicious for abuse. Vigorous shaking may lead to shaken baby syndrome (SBS), which results from acceleration/deceleration forces to the head. Virtually pathognomonic injuries include intracranial (subdural) hemorrhage, diffuse axonal injury, and widespread retinal hemorrhages, which may result in permanent vision loss. SBS has the highest mortality rate of any reported form of child abuse. Falls from beds, changing tables, cribs, counters, or toilet seats do not cause the injuries seen in SBS. Injuries in different stages of healing occur in chronic or repeated abuse.

44. c (Chapter 8)

Painless rectal bleeding sufficient to lower hemoglobin in a 2-year-old is a common presentation of Meckel diverticulum. A colonoscopy would not reveal this since the bleeding point is sufficiently proximal to the ileocecal valve. Transfusion is not needed at this time. However, close monitoring and the availability of packed red blood cells as proper management. Gastric lavage would likely not identify a source of bleeding since the most likely cause is distal to the ligament of Treitz. Bacterial colitis is usually associated with bloody diarrhea, not painless rectal bleeding.

45. c (Chapter 6)

This infant presents with classic clinical and biochemical evidence of adrenal crisis from congenital adrenal hyperplasia (21-hydroxylase deficiency). This classic presentation consists of hypotension, hypoglycemia, hyponatremia, hyperkalemia in a 2- to 6-week infant, typically male (females are usually identified in the newborn period with ambiguous genitalia). All emergency personnel should think of adrenal insufficiency when a child presents in this fashion. These infants need fluid, salt, dextrose and stress dosing of hydrocortisone for survival. Answer A (azithromycin) is not a wide-spectrum antibiotic or one that is considered a drug of choice for sepsis in the infant. The infant's

HCO$_3$ level is not low enough to warrant the consideration of IV bicarbonate. Albumin could help improve intravascular volume but would not add any additional therapeutic benefit beyond the fluid resuscitation that was already provided. Hypocalcemia is not generally present in patients with adrenal insufficiency. If the patient has cardiovascular issues related to hyperkalemia, calcium is a useful adjunct to stabilize the myocardium as the extracellular potassium level is lowered.

46. c (Chapter 5)

The patient described in the question has psoriasis. The scaly red plaques concentrated on her trunk demonstrate the Auspitz sign which is pinpoint bleeding when the scale is removed. Nail pitting is a common finding in patients with psoriasis. Psoriasis is a chronic disease but is often exacerbated by infection in many patients, particularly group A β-hemolytic *Streptococcus* (GAS) in genetically susceptible patients. In addition, GAS may be the precipitating factor in a subtype of psoriasis known as guttate psoriasis. Recognizing and treating streptococcal pharyngitis in guttate psoriasis may improve the patient's outcome. Patients with psoriasis are also directed to try and avoid exacerbating factors such as streptococcal infections.

Because this patient has psoriasis, a bacterial (a) or fungal (b) culture of the plaques would not be necessary and could be misleading if a skin contaminant was found. Tzanck smears (d) are used to look for multinucleated giant cells consistent with herpes viruses such as HSV-1 and -2 or varicella, neither of which is associated with psoriasis. A complete blood count (e) would not be necessary in patients with psoriasis and, if checked, should be normal.

47. a (Chapter 4)

The goal of pharmacologic therapy for ADHD is sustained symptom reduction throughout the day with a tolerable minimum of adverse effects. Atomoxetine is a highly specific norepinephrine reuptake inhibitor; its nonstimulant status sets it apart from the stimulants commonly used to treat ADHD (methylphenidate, dextroamphetamine, and mixed amphetamine salts). Unlike the psychostimulants, atomoxetine has a generally low incidence of side effects and low abuse potential. In the United States, atomoxetine carries a "black box" warning mandated by the FDA alerting physicians and patients to the risk of suicidal ideation. Individuals with ADHD should continue to take their medications over the weekends and during holidays for good control of symptoms in academic and nonacademic settings. Pharmacologic intervention should be administered along with behavioral management and support for the patient and family in order to achieve the best possible outcome.

48. c (Chapter 12)

Roseola is a febrile illness caused by human herpesvirus 6. Children have elevated temperatures for 3 to 5 days, followed by a rash that develops after an abrupt defervescence. The rash consists of erythematous, maculopapular lesions that begin on the trunk and subsequently spread to the neck, face, and extremities.

The characteristic rash of erythema infectiosum (fifth disease; human parvovirus B19) is facial erythema giving a "slapped cheek" appearance, followed by spread to the extremities in a reticular pattern. Measles is a confluent, erythematous, maculopapular rash that starts on the head and progresses caudally. Children with measles have high fever and associated cough, coryza, and conjunctivitis. The rash of chickenpox begins as pruritic, erythematous macules that evolve to vesicles and later crust. As initial lesions resolve, new crops form so lesions in different stages are observed simultaneously. The rash of scarlet fever, caused by group A beta-hemolytic streptococci, is an erythematous, "sandpaper-like" rash which first appears on the neck or trunk, spreads to the extremities, and may desquamate 10 to 14 days later. Fever and pharyngitis accompany the rash.

49. c (Chapter 15)

Febrile seizures are typically brief, generalized seizures with fever which occur in up to 5% of otherwise healthy children ages 6 months to 6 years. Febrile seizures, even when recurrent, are not considered epilepsy. However, children with febrile seizures have an increased risk of developing epilepsy. Between 2% and 7% of all children with febrile seizures develop epilepsy if followed to age 25 years. Overall, the morbidity and mortality associated with febrile seizures is extremely low. Only about a third of patients with an initial febrile seizure will experience recurrent febrile seizures. Anticonvulsant medication is not indicated in the vast majority of patients with initial or even recurrent febrile seizures. By definition, the diagnosis of febrile seizure excludes children with intracranial infection or prior history of nonfebrile seizure.

50. d (Chapter 10)

The most likely diagnosis is hemophilia A. Hemophilia A is an X-linked disorder that is caused by deficiency of factor VIII. Hemophilia B is also an X-linked disorder and is caused by factor IX deficiency. Hemophilias A and B are characterized by spontaneous or traumatic hemorrhages, which can be subcutaneous, intramuscular, or within joints (hemarthroses). Life-threatening internal hemorrhages may follow trauma or surgery. The PTT is prolonged, the PT is normal, and in hemophilia A the factor VIII coagulant activity (VIII:c) is decreased. Other than their factor replacement regimens, there is no distinguishable difference between hemophilias A and B. Idiopathic thrombocytopenic purpura is unlikely in this patient, since the platelet count is normal at 150,000. With no history of epistaxis, gingival bleeding, or cutaneous bruising, von Willebrand disease is unlikely. Hemarthroses are not typical for von Willebrand disease. Vitamin K deficiency occurs in the neonate who is exclusively breastfed and has not received prophylactic vitamin K injection after birth or in the child with significant fat malabsorption. In vitamin K deficiency and in liver disease, there is a prolonged PT and normal factor VIII coagulant activity. The most appropriate therapy for complications of hemophilia A is to infuse factor VIII concentrate.

51. a (Chapter 7)

This patient has a metabolic acidosis (pH ≤7.4) with an increased anion gap ([134 + 4.5] − [106 + 10] = 22.5, outside the normal range of 12 ± 4). Metabolic acidosis with an increased anion gap usually results from increased acid production (such as in diabetic ketoacidosis), decreased acid excretion (renal failure), or inborn errors of metabolism. Chronic diarrhea usually causes either normal anion gap acidosis or, less commonly, metabolic alkalosis. Pyloric stenosis also results in metabolic alkalosis (HCl loss via vomiting). Children with cystic fibrosis may exhibit alkalosis. Renal tubular acidosis results in a metabolic acidosis with a normal anion gap.

52. c (Chapter 11)

This child has a chronic arthritis as evidenced by the presence of joint swelling, limitation of movement, limping, and morning stiffness of more than 6 weeks' duration. Of note, pain is commonly absent in chronic arthritis (in contrast to acute arthritis or mechanical derangements). The most common cause of chronic arthritis in childhood is juvenile idiopathic arthritis (JIA). The involvement of less than five joints indicates oligoarticular JIA. About 70% of children with oligoarticular JIA have a positive antinuclear antibody test. A common complication is chronic, nongranulomatous anterior uveitis in up to 30% of individuals (C). This form of uveitis is asymptomatic but can lead to severe sequelae including blindness. For this reason, frequent surveillance slit-lamp examinations are indicated. These children are not at risk for the development of SLE and its complications (for example, glomerulonephritis or hemolytic anemia). Acute anterior uveitis with conjunctival injection, severe pain, and photophobia occurs most commonly in patients with HLA-B27-associated disease but not in the context of oligoarticular JIA. Rheumatic heart disease is a consequence of acute rheumatic fever, but not of JIA.

53. a (Chapter 12)

Cases of suspected bacterial pneumonia that are complicated by large (compromising) pleural effusions (or pleural abscesses) are most likely caused by *Staphylococcus aureus*.

Streptococcus pneumoniae is the most common cause of bacterial pneumonia after infancy and can result in an effusion; however, the effusions seen with *S. pneumoniae* (and the other pathogens listed) are usually small.

Bilateral diffuse interstitial infiltrates are common in pneumonia due to *M. pneumoniae*. Focal abnormalities such as lobar consolidation and small effusions may occur. The effusions seen in pneumonia due to nontypeable *H. influenzae* are usually small. Diffuse interstitial infiltrates may be present in pneumonia due to *C. pneumoniae*. Pleuritis and small pleural effusions may occur. *Klebsiella pneumoniae* is an uncommon cause of lobar pneumonia in children. It may cause pneumonia in adults with underlying problems such as alcoholism, diabetes mellitus, and chronic obstructive pulmonary disease.

54. d (Chapter 14)

This patient most likely has primary essential hypertension. Given her obesity and family history, the hypertension is most likely to benefit from weight loss and exercise.

This patient has sustained hypertension. Reassurance or further observation is inappropriate, since the high blood pressure has already been verified with the appropriate technique. The kidney function is normal, and an underlying renal etiology is unlikely. The cardiac examination is normal and four extremity blood pressures are equally elevated, so an urgent cardiology evaluation is not needed. If the blood pressure is not controlled by exercise and weight loss, then this patient may benefit from diuretic therapy.

55. d (Chapter 16)

Feeding intolerance may lead to food aversion and failure to thrive; the most significant cause is cow milk protein intolerance or allergy. Allergy may be accompanied by eczema or wheezing. A severe local allergic reaction within the bowel results in colitis, indicated by anemia and/or obvious blood in the stools. Other possible nonspecific symptoms include vomiting, irritability, and abdominal distention. If there is no evidence of any underlying disease in formula-fed infants with characteristic symptoms, substitution of a protein hydrolysate formula is recommended. Soy formula is not an appropriate initial substitution because as many as 25% of children with cow milk protein allergy are also intolerant of soy protein. Whole cow milk should not be given to infants younger than 1 year of age, and would contain the same offending protein. Parenteral alimentation is not indicated for protein intolerance but may be necessary following surgery for another gastrointestinal condition (intussusception, volvulus).

56. b (Chapter 21)

A portion of the adolescent health maintenance visit is dedicated to interviewing the parent and child together to evaluate family dynamics, explore past medical and family history, and gather nonsensitive health-related information. Additional time should be set aside to interview and evaluate the adolescent alone, which permits open discussion of more sensitive issues. Laws regarding confidentiality and consent vary from state to state, but in all cases, behaviors that represent a serious threat to the adolescent's health must be disclosed. These include being subjected to physical or sexual abuse and plans to harm oneself or others. That said, the physician can ask the patient's permission to disclose information to the parents when he or she deems it in the best interest of the child. For instance, patients may be willing to discuss issues related to their sexual behavior, drinking, or drug use with their parents in the presence of a supportive physician that they would never bring up at home. Depending on the state, adolescents under the age of 18 years can provide consent for their own healthcare regarding (1) contraception, prenatal care, and sexually transmitted diseases, and (2) issues related to mental health and/or substance abuse evaluation and treatment. In addition, various states grant "mature" or "emancipated" minors (those who have children, are married, are enlisted in the service, or are living apart from their parents) the right to consent to or decline healthcare.

57. c (Chapter 20)

Polysomnography is not always necessary to diagnose obstructive sleep apnea, but it is the gold standard. This test usually is performed in the hospital overnight and includes monitoring of the respiratory effort, airflow, oxygenation, sleep state, and heart rate. Bronchoscopy would show enlarged adenoids but does not measure airflow. Overnight EEG monitoring may be done in children who have central sleep apnea or are suspected of having certain types of seizures (nocturnal seizures). Pulse oximetry monitoring is performed as part of polysomnography. Fluoroscopy has no role in the diagnosis of obstructive sleep apnea.

58. b (Chapter 18)

Gonococcal ophthalmia neonatorum has an onset of symptoms at 2 to 4 days of age. Characteristic features include bilateral involvement, purulent discharge, marked eyelid edema, and chemosis. Diagnosis is suggested by Gram stain and confirmed on conjunctival culture plated on chocolate or Thayer-Martin agar. The infant must be treated with parenteral antibiotics to prevent blindness and other complications. The great majority of gonococcal eye infections are prevented by the instillation of silver nitrate or erythromycin in the neonatal nursery. Chlamydial infections of the eye may usually present at 4 to 10 days of life with unilateral or bilateral mucopurulent discharge and conjunctival injection. Group B *Streptococcus* does not typically cause of ophthalmia neonatorum, although it can cause sepsis and other complications in the neonatal period. Congenital toxoplasmosis can cause chorioretinitis that persists long term. Congenital syphilis does not have any characteristic findings on eye examination.

59. c (Chapter 2)

Based on presentation and physical examination, this patient most likely has overdosed (accidentally or intentionally) on a narcotic. Opiates cause bradycardia, hypotension, respiratory depression, somnolence, and pinpoint pupils. Naloxone is the antidote for opiate poisoning. Atropine and pralidoxime chloride are indicated for organophosphate poisoning. Physostigmine is used to counteract the effects of anticholinergic agents. Deferoxamine (desferrioxamine) chelation is beneficial in patients with iron ingestions.

60. b (Chapter 2)

Aspiration is the accidental inspiration of foreign material into the respiratory tract. Foreign body aspiration is most common in children 6 to 30 months old. Food, coins, and small toys constitute the most commonly aspirated objects. Aspiration into the lower airways is much more common than tracheal obstruction. While the angle of the right mainstem bronchus in adults favors right-sided aspiration, no such propensity exists in children given the symmetric bronchial angles in this age group. Patients who do not acutely obstruct their airways may present up to a week after the initial event with no witnessed episode of choking. Wheezing and respiratory distress may be mistaken for asthma; pneumonia is a consideration when breath sounds are decreased. Of note, findings on auscultation in cases of foreign body aspiration are localized to one side of the chest only. In cases of complete obstruction, the chest radiograph demonstrates significant one-sided atelectasis, and the heart is drawn toward the affected lung throughout the entire respiratory cycle. However, a partial obstruction allows air to enter during inspiration, where it becomes trapped (ball-valve obstruction). In these cases, the inspiratory film may appear normal, but the expiration radiograph will show a hyperinflated obstructed lung with mediastinal shift away from the blockage.

61. c (Chapter 4)

This patient exhibits behaviors that are consistent with the diagnosis of an autism spectrum disorder. He has impaired social interaction, does not communicate with others, and engages in repetitive, stereotypic behavior (rocking). Patients with Down syndrome have developmental delay but socialize with others and attempt to communicate at this age; their development is not described as deviant, as this patient's could be. A child with an isolated hearing impairment would communicate nonverbally but clearly and, depending on the severity, may be unable to repeat works spoken to him, as this child does. Although rocking and other self-stimulatory behaviors are found in developmentally normal children as well as those with autism and other disorders, its presence in this setting lends support for the diagnosis of autism spectrum disorder.

62. b (Chapter 7)

Normal serum potassium levels range from 3.5 to 5.5 mEq/L. This patient has symptomatic hypokalemia. The two studies which are most helpful in categorizing hypokalemia are patient blood pressure and urine potassium value. Both blood pressure and urine potassium levels are elevated in patients with Cushing syndrome and renovascular disease. Normotensive patients with decreased potassium levels may be anorexic or losing potassium from the skin or gastrointestinal track (e.g., laxative abuse). Renal tubular acidosis is the only condition listed for which you would expect the patient to have a normal blood pressure and elevated urine potassium measurement.

✗ 63. b (Chapter 9)

Functional and structural abnormalities in children with trisomy 21 include generalized hypotonia (obstructive sleep apnea), cardiac defects (endocardial cushion defects and septal defects are seen in 50% of cases), gastrointestinal anomalies (duodenal atresia and Hirschsprung disease), atlantoaxial instability, developmental delay, moderate mental retardation, and hypothyroidism. There is a higher frequency of leukemia in children with trisomy 21 than in the general population.

64. e (Chapter 13)

Congenital malformations causing fetal bowel obstruction frequently lead to polyhydramnios. Most tracheoesophageal fistulas are accompanied by esophageal atresia. Congenital or genetic defects that impair fetal swallowing also promote polyhydramnios. Therefore, hydrocephalus with myelomeningocele is also correct. Fetal urine production is a major contributor to amniotic fluid volume. Renal agenesis causes profound oligohydramnios or absence of amniotic fluid.

65. c (Chapter 8)

The history, physical examination, and abdominal radiograph are classic for a diagnosis of intussusception, the "telescoping" of a proximal segment of bowel into a more distal segment. In cases of intussusception, air or double-contrast enema demonstrates a coiled spring appearance to the bowel in the right lower quadrant. The contrast or air enema results in hydrostatic reduction of the intussusception in 75% of cases.

66. a (Chapter 8)

The most common cause of rectal bleeding in toddlers is an anal fissure. If there were significant upper GI tract bleeding from peptic ulcer disease or a Mallory-Weiss tear, the child would likely have melena instead of blood-streaked stool. Inflammatory bowel disease and necrotizing enterocolitis could both cause lower GI tract bleeding (hematochezia or blood-streaked stool) but are unlikely in an 18-month-old.

67. d (Chapter 17)

This is a classic presentation of Wilms tumor. Patients with Wilms tumor may come to medical attention after abdominal trauma. The trauma causes hemorrhage into the tumor, resulting in pain, abdominal distention, and hematuria. The patient may also have an associated anemia, depending on the degree of hemorrhage. Hypertension is frequently found in patients with Wilms tumor and resolves with treatment.

68. e (Chapter 19)

This clinical picture is most consistent with idiopathic talipes equinovarus. Dorsiflexion at the ankle is not possible in patients with this disorder. Metatarsus adductus, or in-toeing of the forefoot, is a less severe condition that often responds to regular passive stretching. Talipes equinovarus will result in a severe limp and foot ulcerations if correction is not achieved by the time the child begins to ambulate. Many but not all cases do require surgical repair; serial bracing or casting has enjoyed a revival of sorts in recent years. One in 7 patients with talipes equinovarus will have an associated congenital malformation.

69. b (Chapter 8)

Evaluation for other conditions (e.g., bacterial colitis, *C. difficile* infection) is important before starting therapy directed against IBD. Similarly, complications of IBD may require antibiotics or surgery rather than anti-inflammatory drugs (e.g., prednisone). Cancer risk is somewhat increased in long-standing Crohn disease. Therapy with mercaptopurine and azathioprine will not provide symptom relief for weeks. Therapy with anti-TNF alpha antibody may be helpful but other options may be preferable and excluding an abscess is the first order of business. A capsule endoscopy is helpful for occult small intestinal disease but less likely to be the test of choice in an acute setting.

70. c (Chapter 7)

Food allergy is an IgE-mediated clinical response triggered by antigen-specific IgE bound to mast cells and basophils, resulting in cellular degranulation and the resultant immediate clinical response. While skin prick tests measure the wheal-and-flare response of food-specific IgE bound to skin mast cells, this response is frequently false positive. As such, a positive test has to be followed by the development of clinical symptoms in response to oral challenges to the implicated food (but not the placebo) via a double-blind placebo-controlled food challenge, a procedure that must be performed in a hospital/office setting equipped to respond to acute life-threatening anaphylaxis. Food-specific IgE levels can often be falsely positive and should not be used alone to diagnose food allergy. Open-label food challenges are often helpful but not used for definitive diagnosis. Finally, an endoscopy is useful to examine the presence of gastrointestinal anatomy and pathology but does not diagnose food allergy.

71. a (Chapter 19)

Scoliosis in a premenarchal female is likely to progress and should be treated aggressively. Curvature of 25 to 45 degrees requires bracing to halt progression of the curve. If external bracing is not successful and the curve progresses to greater

ANSWERS

than 40 to 50 degrees, surgery is required. Stretching exercises are not effective in the treatment of scoliosis.

72. c (Chapter 19)

A fracture through the growth plate that extends into the epiphysis and into the joint space is consistent with a Salter-Harris Type III fracture. If the fracture extended into the metaphysis only, this would constitute a Type II fracture. Fractures through both the metaphysis and epiphysis into the joint space are Type IV. Type I fractures occur along the growth plate only, whereas Type V fractures result from compression of the growth plate. Type III fractures such as the one described in the vignette may require open reduction and fixation but have a relatively good prognosis.

73. b (Chapter 10)

Based on the information provided, this patient most likely has hereditary spherocytosis (HS) which gives a positive result on the osmotic fragility test. Patients with HS have a history of neonatal jaundice, occurring usually in the first 24 hours of life. HS is caused by a defect in the red blood cell membrane proteins (spectrin, ankyrin, or band 3 protein). Inheritance is usually autosomal dominant, but 25% of cases are caused by new mutation or autosomal recessive forms. None of the other listed diagnoses would give positive results on the osmotic fragility test.

74. d (Chapter 21)

The examination described is most consistent with Tanner stage IV development (see Table 21-2). Stage III is characterized by enlargement and elevation of the breast and areola without separation of their contours, and pubic hair spread sparsely over the pubis which is less dark and curly than adult pubic hair. In stage V, the areola regresses to the general contour of the breast, and pubic hair is adult in texture and amount and has spread to the medial thighs.

75. b (Chapter 17)

The chemotherapy used in AML is more intense than that used in ALL, and the myelosuppression is severe. Patients require hospitalization for aggressive supportive care until they begin to show signs of count recovery. Hyperleukocytosis is more likely to by symptomatic in AML (and thus more likely to require treatment) than in ALL because AML blasts are larger and stickier than ALL blasts. Patients with Down syndrome and AML have an excellent overall survival rate, while secondary AML is extremely difficult to treat and outcomes are poor. Not all patients with AML will go on to bone marrow transplantation. Low-risk AML is treated with chemotherapy alone.

76. c (Chapter 8)

Crohn disease typically is associated with transmural inflammatory disease resulting in fistulae or stricture formation.

Lesions may be found from the mouth to the anus but most commonly appear in the ileum and/or colon involvement with skip lesions, rectal sparing, segmental narrowing of the ileum (string sign), granuloma, perianal disease, and growth failure. Ulcerative colitis typically is characterized by rectal involvement, rectal bleeding, and diffuse superficial mucosal ulceration. Ulcerative colitis is associated with an increased the risk of colon cancer.

77. d (Chapter 2)

Carbon monoxide poisoning presents with lethargy, irritability, confusion, dizziness, headache, and nausea. Signs include irregular breathing, cyanosis, and mental status changes. Unconscious patients are severely affected and have a high risk for death. Oxygen is considered an antidote for carbon monoxide poisoning; immediate administration of oxygen is indicated for affected patients. While all the other options listed should also be performed in this patient, the most immediate need is oxygen.

78. a (Chapter 12)

Epiglottitis consists of inflammation and edema of the epiglottis and aryepiglottic folds. Most cases occur during the winter months in children 3 to 5 years of age. Fever, sore throat, hoarseness, and progressive stridor develop over 1 to 2 days. On examination, the child appears toxic, drools, and leans forward to maximize airway patency. Epiglottitis is considered a life-threatening emergency because of the propensity of the swollen tissues to result in sudden and irreversible airway occlusion.

Children with croup typically experience the sudden onset of a hoarse voice, barky cough, and inspiratory stridor, which may progress to respiratory distress. Patients may have a prodrome consisting of low-grade fever, and rhinorrhea 12 to 24 hours prior to the onset of stridor. Children with bacterial pneumonia may present with nonspecific constitutional complaints, including fever, irritability, vomiting, abdominal pain, and lethargy. Abrupt onset of fever, chills, dyspnea, and chest pain is typical. Drooling and other symptoms related to the upper airway are rarely present. The onset of diphtheria may be abrupt, with a low-grade fever, sore throat, mild pharyngeal injection, and development of a membrane on the tonsils. The membrane may extend to involve the nasopharynx and laryngotracheal areas. Due to the use of the diphtheria-tetanus-acellular pertussis vaccine, diphtheria is a rare disease in most areas of the world. Anaphylaxis is a life-threatening immunoglobulin E-mediated allergic reaction that may occur with foods, medicines, and other triggers. Children often present with respiratory distress, wheezing, pruritis, and hives.

79. d (Chapter 21)

Although guns are often bought with the intention of making a home safer, they actually increase the risk of gun death in family members living in the home. Adolescents who live in a home with a gun are three times more likely to die of homicide and 10 times more likely to commit suicide with a gun than their peers who live in homes without guns.

80. b (Chapter 4)

A 36-month-old child with typical development should be able to pedal a tricycle, broad jump, copy a circle, use five- to eight-word sentences, and know his or her own age and gender. Two-year-old children can jump with 2 feet off the floor and copy straight lines but cannot broad jump or copy circles. In contrast, 4-year-old children can generally balance on one foot, copy a cross, dress themselves, and wash and dry hands. At age 5 years, a child can skip with alternating feet, draw a person with six or more body parts, and name four colors. Six-year-olds can ride bikes and write their own names.

81. c (Chapter 7)

This child, judged to be 10% dehydrated, is 3,000 mL behind on fluids (3 kg). 540 mL is subtracted from the deficit, leaving 2,460 mL to be given over the next 24 hours. Half of this is provided over the first 8 hours (1,230 mL at 153 mL/hr) along with maintenance fluids (67 mL/hr). The most appropriate fluid choice for a child this age is D_5 0.2 normal saline (with 20 mEq/L KCl to be added after the patient has urinated). If the child had hypernatremic dehydration, the deficit would need to be replaced over a longer period.

82. a (Chapter 8)

Both celiac disease and Crohn disease are possible. Anemia may be present with both. The tissue transglutaminase assay (IgA) should be elevated in celiac disease. Inflammatory markers such as elevated CRP and platelet count are often elevated in Crohn disease. Physical examination does not justify a CT scan next. A urinary tract infection, hydronephrosis or cystic fibrosis may be the etiology of the complaint but a laparotomy is not yet indicated. Colonoscopy and upper endoscopy are not yet indicated but either or both may be in the next round of testing. Without a history of diarrhea, the symptoms and signs are unlikely due to bacterial or parasitic infection.

83. a (Chapter 17)

The leukemias account for the greatest percentage of childhood malignancies. Acute leukemias constitute 97% of all childhood leukemias and are divided into acute lymphocytic leukemia (ALL) and acute myelogenous leukemia (AML). ALL accounts for 75% of all childhood acute leukemias. A history of fever, pallor, anorexia, bone pain, lymphadenopathy, petechiae, and hepatosplenomegaly is consistent with ALL. Leukemic cell dissemination results in bone marrow failure, reticuloendothelial system infiltration, and penetration of sanctuary sites (CNS and testicles). Marrow infiltration results in crowding out of normal marrow blood cell precursors, which then results in anemia (pallor) and thrombocytopenia (petechiae). Infiltration of the reticuloendothelial system results in lymphadenopathy and hepatosplenomegaly. Bone pain is caused by expansion of the marrow cavity, destruction of cortical bone by leukemic cells, or metastatic tumor. Although fever and petechiae are consistent with aplastic anemia, bone pain, lymphadenopathy, and hepatosplenomegaly are not.

84. e (Chapter 19)

Observation is the best answer because this girl is skeletally mature and her curve is unlikely to progress significantly in the future. If no progression is seen in 1 year on radiograph, then minimal further follow-up would be indicated, and she should have an essentially normal spine in the future. Posterior spinal fusion is only indicated for scoliosis over 40 to 50 degrees in skeletally mature patients. Intensive physical therapy has not been shown to alter the natural history of scoliosis. Bracing is only indicated for curves over 25 to 30 degrees in patients who are still growing. Spinal manipulation has not been shown to effect scoliosis curve progression.

85. d (Chapter 12)

The boy's history and clinical picture are most consistent with Rocky Mountain spotted fever or ehrlichiosis. He is significantly ill (and vomiting) and should be admitted to the hospital. Both Rocky Mountain spotted fever and ehrlichiosis are rapidly progressive; treatment should be initiated immediately when these diseases are suspected. Delay in treatment can be fatal. Because this boy has no history of a tick bite and is sufficiently ill, empiric antibiotic treatment should include coverage for Rocky Mountain spotted fever and ehrlichiosis (doxycycline) and meningococcemia (cefotaxime or ceftriaxone).

86. d (Chapter 11)

Henoch-Schönlein purpura (HSP) is the most common vasculitis in childhood and the classic tetrad of findings consists of skin (purpura), joint (acute arthritis), gastrointestinal (abdominal pain, GI bleeding), and kidney disease. Approximately 20% of patients will have renal involvement early in the disease course, most often microscopic hematuria. Severe renal involvement with azotemia is rare (less than 5% of cases). Autoantibodies are negative. Even though HSP is an IgA-mediated immune complex disease, C3 and C4 levels are usually normal.

87. a (Chapter 10)

The adjusted reticulocyte count (ARC) = [(measured hematocrit)/(normal hematocrit for age)] × reticulocyte count. An ARC less than 2.0 suggests ineffective erythropoiesis, whereas an ARC greater than 2.0 signifies effective erythropoiesis. Anemia caused by a lack of production of red blood cells will therefore have an ARC less than 2.0, whereas anemias resulting from hemolysis or chronic blood loss will have an ARC greater than 2.0. The mean corpuscular volume (MCV) is used to describe the anemia as microcytic, macrocytic, or normocytic. All of the anemias noted in the question result from decreased red cell production and have an inadequate reticulocytosis (ARC <2.0). Decreased red cell production is due to either deficiency of hematopoietic precursors or bone marrow failure. The microcytic anemia described in the question is most likely due to iron deficiency, which is not only the most common microcytic anemia, but also the most common cause of anemia during childhood. It is most often seen between 6 and 24 months of age. Thalassemia syndromes are also microcytic anemias but are less common than iron-deficiency anemia. Anemia of chronic disease may be microcytic or normocytic. Transient erythrocytopenia of childhood is a normocytic anemia that is an acquired red cell aplasia. Parvovirus B19 aplastic crisis is a normocytic anemia that results from parvovirus B19 marrow suppression of erythropoietic precursors.

88. a (Chapter 17)

The clinical description is most consistent with Ewing sarcoma. Unlike osteosarcoma, Ewing sarcoma tends to involve systemic symptoms, such as fever, weight loss, and fatigue. Ewing sarcoma usually involves the diaphyseal portion of the long bones. The most common sites for Ewing sarcoma are the midproximal femur and the bones of the pelvis. The most common sites of osteosarcoma are the distal femur, proximal tibia, and proximal humerus. Benign bone tumors and eosinophilic granuloma are generally not painful. Chronic osteomyelitis may present with fever, pain, and localized swelling, but weight loss is unlikely.

89. a (Chapter 18)

A positive cover test is consistent with strabismus or misalignment of the eyes. This child is at risk for amblyopia (reduced vision in the affected eye) and loss of depth perception. She should be referred to a pediatric ophthalmologist for evaluation and treatment, which may include surgical realignment. Leukocoria describes a white pupil (that is, absence of the red reflex). Retinoblastoma is a potential cause of leukocoria. Nasolacrimal duct obstruction occurs in infancy and presents with tearing.

90. b (Chapter 15)

In older patients with acute courses, the signs of hydrocephalus with increased intracranial pressure are relatively clear and include morning headache that improves after upright positioning or vomiting; irritability and/or lethargy; and papilledema and diplopia (CN VI palsy). Spasticity, clonus, and hyperreflexia most prominent in the legs are additional neurologic signs of hydrocephalus. The Cushing triad, consisting of hypertension, bradycardia, and slow irregular respirations, is a late and ominous sign of increased intracranial pressure implying imminent risk of brain herniation. Hypotension and tachycardia would

not be expected. The anterior fontanelle typically closes prior to age 2 years. Erythema migrans is a rash associated with Lyme disease (Chapter 12); although Lyme disease can be associated with abducens nerve palsy, the presence of additional signs and symptoms of increased intracranial pressure on examination make this etiology more likely.

91. a (Chapter 14)

This patient displays the characteristic findings of prerenal acute renal failure due to decreased renal perfusion from dehydration. She has tachycardia, decreased urine output, and a low fractional excretion of sodium. Recognition and prompt treatment of prerenal failure is essential to prevent progression to intrinsic renal failure. The treatment of choice is restoration of renal perfusion by correcting the intravascular volume deficit with an intravenous bolus of normal saline. This will usually result in restoration of kidney function and urine output as well as correction of the acidosis and hyperkalemia.

The metabolic acidosis does not require urgent specific correction with bicarbonate. The patient does not display signs of significant fluid overload and therefore does not require furosemide (which may cause more harm than good in this situation). The gastroenteritis is most likely viral in etiology, and does not require immediate antibiotic therapy. Dialysis would be indicated only if the patient has persistent fluid overload, hyperkalemia, or acidosis that is unresponsive to other medical therapies.

92. e (Chapter 16)

Colic is a syndrome of recurrent irritability that occurs most commonly in infants 3 weeks to 3 months of age. The episodes occur daily and persist for several hours, usually in the late afternoon or evening. During the attacks, the child draws the knees to the abdomen and cries inconsolably. The crying resolves as suddenly and spontaneously as it begins. Colic is often mistaken for cow milk protein allergy, although the latter typically occurs in slightly older infants and may involve bloody stools, an eczematous rash, poor growth, abdominal distention, and vomiting. Intussusception is rare in a child this young and is not temporally cyclical. Hirschsprung disease is unlikely as the child is stooling normally.

93. e (Chapter 19)

Breech presentation or family history of developmental dysplasia of the hip (DDH), either of which warrants a hip ultrasound. The remaining options are all minor risk factors for DDH.

94. a (Chapter 21)

As many as 40% of patients with anorexia nervosa develop mitral valve prolapse, evidenced by a midsystolic click and/or murmur. Other cardiac abnormalities (arrhythmias) can occur as a complication of anorexia but are less common. Anorexic patients will often present with bradycardia; however, bradycardia alone does not result in a click or murmur. A prolonged QTc interval may develop in patients who purge by vomiting (which is more common in bulimia) due to hypokalemia.

95. a (Chapter 2)

The routine use of seat belts and child car seats has been shown to be highly effective in reducing the incidence of severe injury and death in the pediatric population. All states require car seat restraint of passengers under 40 pounds. Children who are both ≥20 pounds and 1 year of age or older may ride facing forward, whereas lighter/younger infants must face the rear. When a child passenger has reached the height/weight limit for his or her car seat (usually up to 40 lbs.), a booster seat should be employed. The child should be restrained in a booster seat until the standard lap belt fits correctly (across the chest and thighs) and the child is tall enough for the legs to bend at the knees with the feet hanging down. This usually does not occur until the child is 8 to 12 years old or approximately 57 inches in height. Because air bags are designed primarily for adults, children should always ride belted in the back seat.

96. a (Chapter 8)

Projectile nonbilious vomiting is the cardinal feature seen in virtually all patients with pyloric stenosis. Physical findings vary with the severity of the obstruction. The classic finding of an olive-sized, muscular, mobile, nontender mass in the epigastric area occurs in most cases. Dehydration and poor weight gain are common when the diagnosis is delayed. Hypokalemic, hypochloremic metabolic alkalosis with dehydration is seen secondary to persistent emesis in the most severe cases.

97. e (Chapter 7)

Children who lose electrolytes in their stool and are supplemented with free water of very dilute juices are prone to the development of hyponatremia. Symptoms of hyponatremia include anorexia, nausea, confusion, and lethargy. The ataxia may be due to weakness or may be due to lethargy. Hypomagnesemia is uncommon unless the patient has been receiving medication or parenteral nutrition. Hyperkalemia presents with symptoms of paresthesias and weakness but is less likely given the history of present illness. Patients with protracted vomiting and those who are being treated with loop or thiazide diuretics may develop metabolic alkalosis, but acidosis would be expected in this patient. This patient may indeed have hypochloremia, but it is unlikely to be the primary cause of his symptoms.

98. c (Chapter 6)

Scant axillary hair/Tanner II pubic hair, testicular volume 5 cc, and bone age of 11 years with normal screening labs describe a boy with prepubertal physical exam findings, a delayed bone age, and likely euthyroid with normal growth hormone screening parameters. Answer a is a more pubertal advanced boy with an advanced bone age. Answer b describes a boy with pubertal delay but with biochemical evidence of hypothyroidism. Answer d describes answer a delayed but with biochemical concerns that may suggest growth hormone deficiency.

99. c (Chapter 2)

Lead poisoning is an ideal condition for which to screen given its lack of early symptoms, its harmful effect on cognitive development at preclinical levels, and its amenability to treatment. Children ages 9 months to 6 years should be assessed for an increased risk of lead exposure with a questionnaire developed by the Centers for Disease Control (2001). Current recommendations vary depending on practice location, with most areas under universal screening coverage, which involves testing all children at the ages of 12 and 24 months. Research is under way to determine how to better define and target high-risk groups and decrease the number of tests performed on the general population. Many offices screen for elevated blood lead levels by performing a capillary micro-lead measurement. Any capillary blood level >10 µg/dL must be confirmed by a venous blood lead test due to a relatively high false positive rate. All elevated screening (capillary) blood tests should be confirmed with a venous sample before treatment is initiated unless the child is acutely symptomatic.

100. c (Chapter 11)

This child has linear scleroderma, a condition characterized by linear streaks of indurated and thickened skin and underlying soft tissues. Major sequelae include growth restriction and limitation of the affected areas. In this case, there is a high risk for the development of a right elbow contracture as the linear scleroderma extends over the elbow joint. The child is at very low risk for the development of systemic sclerosis, a condition in which internal organ disease, such as esophageal dysfunction, cardiopulmonary disease, severe Raynaud phenomenon, and peripheral arterial disease is commonly seen.

ANSWERS

Index

Page numbers followed by *t* refer to tables; page numbers followed by *f* refer to figures.